Basic Open Rhinoplasty

Fabio Meneghini

Basic Open Rhinoplasty

Principles and Practical Steps for Surgeons in Training

Springer

Fabio Meneghini
Villa Torri Hospital
BOLOGNA
Bologna
Italy

ISBN 978-3-030-61826-1 ISBN 978-3-030-61827-8 (eBook)
https://doi.org/10.1007/978-3-030-61827-8

This Springer imprint is published by the registered company Springer Nature Switzerland AG
The registered company address is: Gewerbestrasse 11, 6330 Cham, Switzerland

Acknowledgments

I wish to thank the following friends, colleagues, and mentors for their help, support, and guidance.

The medical and all patient care staff at Maria Cecilia Hospital, Humanitas Castelli, and Villa Donatello. In particular, Andrea and Iulian for the countless photographs taken in the operating room.

My close collaborators, doctors Elisabetta Sarti and Carlo Ghilardi. Working with them is always pleasant and instructive.

The many surgeons who joined me in the operating room and adding their expertise for better patient treatment. In particular, Paolo Bonan, Alessandro Colli, Vittorio Dallera, Daniele Fasano, Marketa Koka, Gianfranco Niedda, Giuseppe Rampino, Leone Rigo, Giuseppe Spinelli, Alexandra Tommasi, and Diletta Vitali.

Doctors Jose Carlos Neves from Lisbon and Süreyya Seneldir from Istanbul for having recently accepted me in their operating rooms and for sharing so many useful details and ideas on rhinoplasty with me.

My colleague, friend, and wonderful mentor Paolo Gottarelli. His help and guidance have accompanied me in most of my 30-year professional journey.

Dr. Itala Brancaleone for the revision of the English text.

My lucky experience with Springer started in 2004 in Vienna where I met informally Dr. Gabriele Schröder who would become the editor of my first scientific book titled *Clinical Facial Analysis: Elements Principle Techniques*. Today the collaboration continues, and I want to warmly thank my current editor Dr. Juliette R. Kleemann and Mrs. Depika Devan of Springer Nature for their help in this new project.

Contents

1 Introduction: Why this Book?

Rhinoplasty is not learned on books but in the operating room.

Generally speaking, I agree, or at least I understand the profound meaning of this sentence: a frequent attendance in the operating room is mandatory to prepare to be a rhinoplasty surgeon. But there is still another phrase that comes first, a phrase that once in our life we have said to ourselves or perhaps we are about to say: "*Someday I will be a nose surgeon.*"

For those who have not yet entered or are just taking their first steps in the world of rhinoplasty, I thought of writing this book. Reading a text and, on the same day, watching what happens in the surgical field is fundamental. Or better yet, studying what you see in the operating room in a book and asking the experienced surgeon anything that is not clear is fundamental. To start, the key is to have a mentor and have a book!

For more than 30 years I have had the fortune to devote myself to surgery of the face and of the nose in particular. I have had the fortune to attend the operating room of more experienced colleagues and to talk with them about every aspect of the profession. I have had the fortune to study books and articles on the subject, to participate in cultural meetings and to seek personal solutions to the problems I encountered.

Together with many colleagues I shared the feeling of difficulty and uncertainty of dealing with rhinoplasty with the aim of giving our patients a high level of performance in human, medical, and surgical terms.

In the journey, as often happens in other professional fields, the greatest difficulty is starting, taking the first steps and believing in oneself. So the first goal of this book is to help young surgeons, provide them with a blueprint or, I hope, a basic method and some selected techniques to follow so they can them grow professionally and make nasal surgery the passion of their working life.

Another objective is to recognize the standardizable aspects of a practice that has a high variability. Juxtaposing the terms "standard" and "variability" may seem strident and sound like an oxymoron but a basic discipline with rules applicable to the majority of clinical cases is an indispensable point from which to start. If many aspects of the clinical pathway are standardized (note "standardized" and not "simplified," as there is no room for simplification in rhinoplasty), the surgeon will have more freedom when he needs to customize the treatment details. The discipline of Basic Open Rhinoplasty (BOR) therefore intends to offer a set of fixed points that have solid foundations in logic and clinical experience while allowing both the surgeon and the patient to explore the individual characteristics of the personalized surgical project.

To become a good rhinoplasty surgeon, it is undoubtedly necessary to have great enthusiasm,

F. Meneghini, *Basic Open Rhinoplasty*, https://doi.org/10.1007/978-3-030-61827-8_1

which should not be kept to ourselves but shared with our closest collaborators, mentors, and the patients we will meet.

1.1 Recognizing One of Our Enemies

In rhinoplasty, **certainty** is one of the enemies of professional growth. **Certainty** ultimately blinds you, sets fixed limits and creates "automatic habits." The surgeon guided by his **certainties** is closed off to learning and far removed from innovation and progress in the discipline. One goal of this book is to help young surgeons to put aside their need for **certainty** and replace it with curiosity, daily commitment, critical spirit, and continuous study of their clinical results. All this, with authentic self-confidence.

In rhinoplasty there is also a positive **certainty**: each nose that we will meet in everyday professional practice is different from any other. It is unique. And the time we dedicate to rhinoplasty will be all the more interesting if we consider it from the perspective of an ever-changing and challenging practice.

1.2 Is There Still Room for Improvements in Rhinoplasty?

Working in the operating room, I discovered that in the world of rhinoplasty there is wide space for improvements. Here is a simple example: for years, as I had always seen my colleagues do so, I collected the cartilage fragments harvested at the beginning of the operation in a stainless steel surgical cup containing sterile saline solution. The shape of the surgical cup is unstable due to its narrow base and there is a real risk of inadvertently knocking it over onto the floor during surgery. For this reason, for a few years now, I have no longer used the smallest bowl to collect the cartilage. I no longer accept the risk of it sooner or later falling onto the floor together with its precious contents. I have therefore replaced it with a low, flat Teflon container with a round base and, again for safety reasons, I have also made a perfectly fitting cap, also in Teflon (Fig. 1.1). The choice of construction material was easy: for years I had a small Teflon cartilage-cutting block among my instruments. Some surgical hammers and surgical instruments also have Teflon parts. It is an autoclavable, heavy, robust, and safe material that is stable over time. Before mass production of the final object, I made some wooden prototypes (Fig. 1.2). A square-based version was discarded as the final product would have been more expensive without offering any advantage in return.

My current standard requires that every cartilage fragment harvested during rhinoplasty is

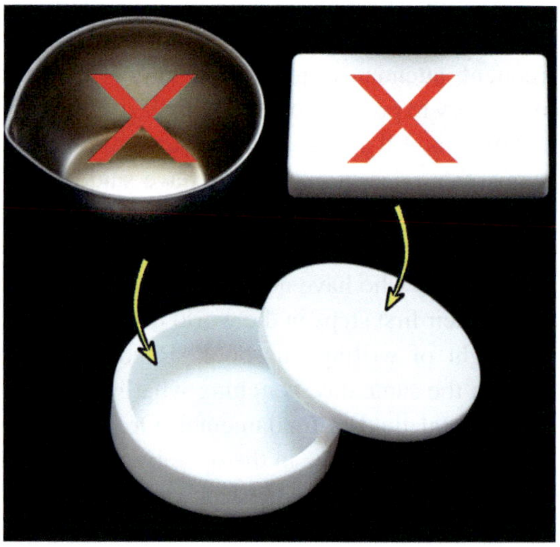

Fig. 1.1 Low, round-based Teflon cartilage container with its cover

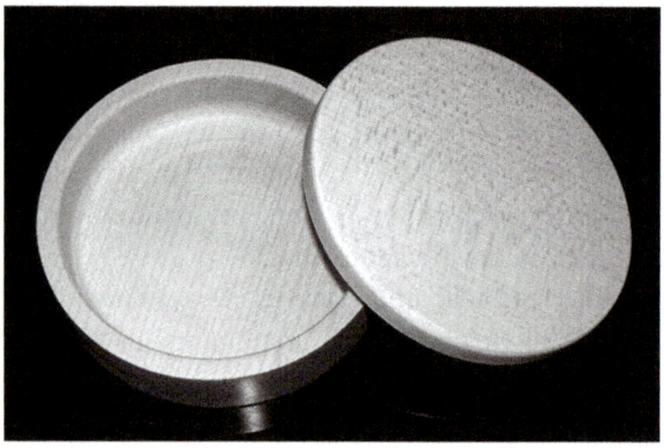

Fig. 1.2 Round cartilage container (wooden prototype)

gently cleaned by the nurse with a wet gauze and immersed in sterile saline solution inside the Teflon container closed with its cover, where it will remain until use (Fig. 1.3). The same round cover has also replaced the old cutting block used for cutting and carving the cartilage to be utilized as a graft (Figs. 1.4 and 1.5).

This useful little work tool is part of a more general principle that I have been following for a long time: strive to create something useful for your work every year. Sometimes it is a simple useful object, other times an innovative surgical instrument. But also the publication of an article or a scientific book, a presentation at a conference, an anatomical dissection course for a small group of students, a lecture on rhinoplasty for postgraduate students at your university, an educational poster for your colleagues on how to take standard pictures of patients' faces, a small information book to give your next patients, new contents on your website, and many other things will do fine.

If every year you realize one project related to your work, in 20 years' time you will have realized 20 projects!

Of course this book is my project for 2020.

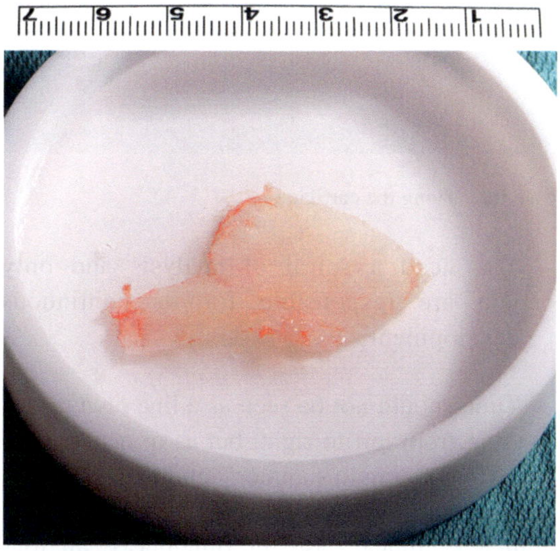

Fig. 1.3 Septal cartilage cleansed and immersed in sterile saline solution

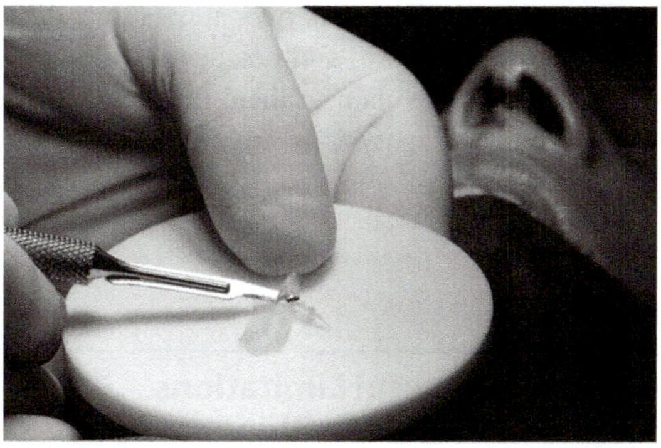

Fig. 1.4 The cover of the cartilage container is utilized as a base for carving the cartilage graft before its insertion in place

1.3 The Spiral of Clinical Analysis

A large part of this book has been reserved for the clinical and photographic study of the patient's nose. In rhinoplasty, the results come from good documentation and accurate analysis. Learning from personal clinical experience is an essential, unavoidable, and central aspect for the entire professional life of a nose surgeon. I think of it as a rising spiral (Fig. 1.6).

The never-ending process of clinical analysis in rhinoplasty can be divided into four consecutive steps: the preoperative, the intraoperative, the early postoperative, and the late postoperative analysis. The final step, known as the follow-up, which concludes the process for a given patient or group of patients, is functional to the next preoperative step with a new patient, creating the positive spiral of analysis. This is probably the best self-teaching exercise we do. To create a positive spiral of analysis, one must respect the following rules:

- Document with clinical photographs and written notes every new patient as best you can, whether or not he or she will be treated later.
- Continue to document during the intraoperative, early, and late postoperative phases utilizing, as a template, the initial materials to ensure the best comparative value to the clinical case.
- Continue to schedule your old patients about once a year to perform the late follow-up. By seeing the patient again, you are obliged to

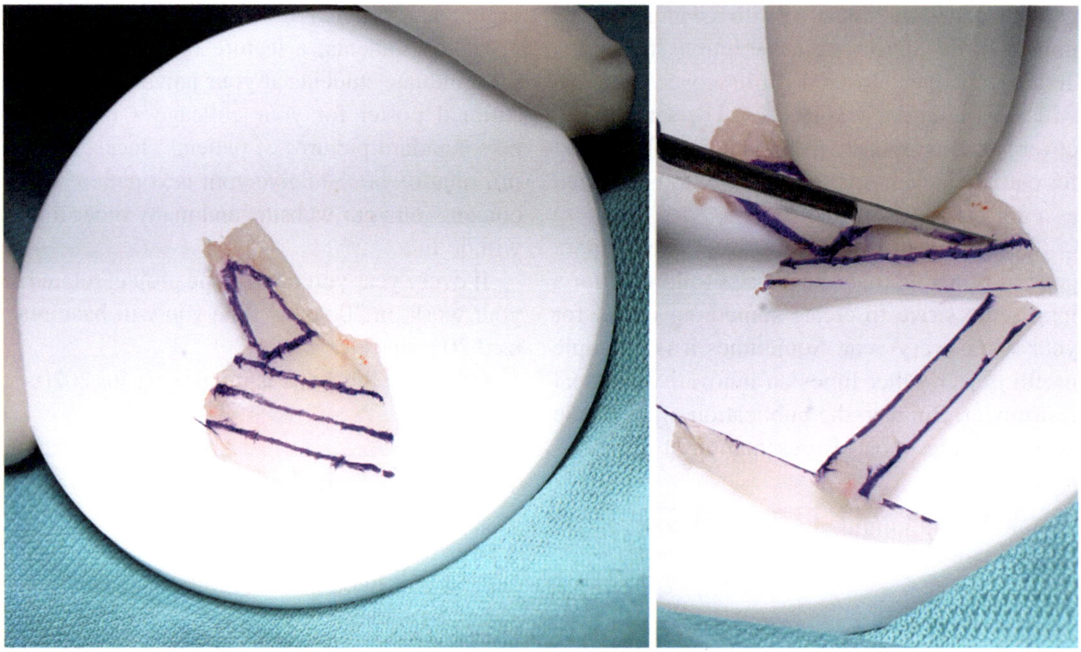

Fig. 1.5 The cover of the cartilage container is utilized as a base for carving the cartilage

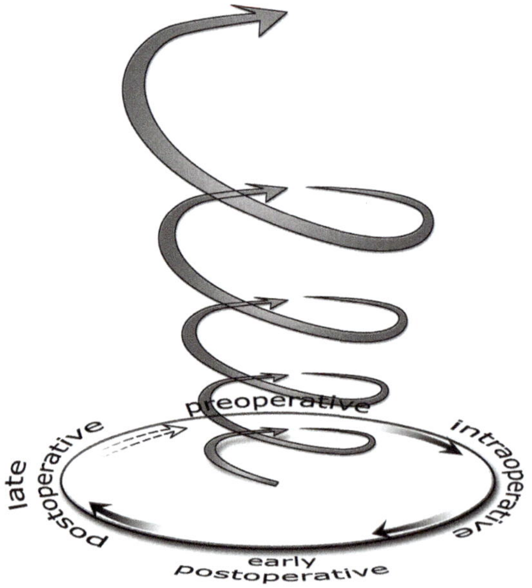

Fig. 1.6 The spiral of clinical analysis

review the case immediately before and during the consultation. Nothing is so effective for your memory than reviewing the case with the patient himself.
- Collect and store the materials in the best way you can, remembering that you need these data as a working instrument.
- You need a spiral of analysis and only you are responsible for its continuous development.

Time should not be seen as a line on a graph, running from left to right, but as in nature, running from spring to summer, autumn, and winter. To complete a cycle, 1 year for nature and a complete clinical case for rhinoplasty, all four "seasons" must be started and finished. Our experience is of more value if we can personally follow the entire cycle.

Sometimes, when I ask my patients for authorization to use the pre- and postoperative images of their faces, I explain to them the significance of the spiral of analysis as a component of the general process of a surgeon's continuing medical education.

1.4 The Useful Limitations of a Book on Rhinoplasty

Dr. Rodolphe Meyer, a great master of rhinoplasty, wrote on the back cover of the second edition of his "Secondary Rhinoplasty":

With its 36 chapters, this book is the most complete work about nose surgery in the world.

It is a monumental text with 1800 figures and about 2000 bibliographical references. Also his previous work from 1967, recently reprinted, recalls the encyclopedia format. No doubt, nasal surgery is a wide field of knowledge with a long history despite the small size of the anatomical nose.

In writing this book, instead, my goal was to address a young audience of professionals. For this reason, the choice of topics, principles, and surgical techniques has been reduced to a minimum and optimized predicting that, if the reader decides to further devote himself to rhinoplasty, he will have a basic knowledge from which to set out on his journey.

Further Reading

Books

For those interested in the historical evolution of rhinoplasty surgical techniques: Deneke HJ, Meyer R. Plastic surgery of head and neck. Berlin: Springer; 1967; Meyer R. Secondary rhinoplasty. 2 edn. Berlin: Springer; 2002.

Articles

Three editorial articles written by Rod Rohrich on how to be an expert in surgery: Rohrich RJ. So you want to be an expert. Plast Reconstr Surg. 2009;124(5):1719–21; Ramanadham SR, Rohrich RJ. Mentorship: a pathway to succeed in plastic surgery. Plast Reconstr Surg. 2019;143(1):353–5; Rohrich RJ. I want my trophy: setting expectations for life. Plast Reconstr Surg. 2007;119(4):1363–4.

2 Approaching the Patient for Nasal Surgery

This chapter discusses how to approach a new patient for rhinoplasty. It is necessary, in a relatively restricted period of time, to gain a clear understanding of his needs and provide basic information in an accurate and simple manner. Where to meet the patient and the organization of the office are also aspects addressed in this chapter.

The ideal room—with three separate areas dedicated for the interview, the clinical examination, and clinical photography—is described in detail.

The first consultation is divided into various steps: entrance, interview, direct clinical examination, photographic documentation, and final communication. The subsequent preoperative consultations are also considered.

2.1 The Single Room Concept

Communication between the patient and the doctor, the direct clinical examination, and the taking of clinical photographs require three dedicated areas of the office. After a variety of experiences, I strongly favor concentrating all three areas in the same room. Figure 2.1a–c shows the floorplan of my current office.

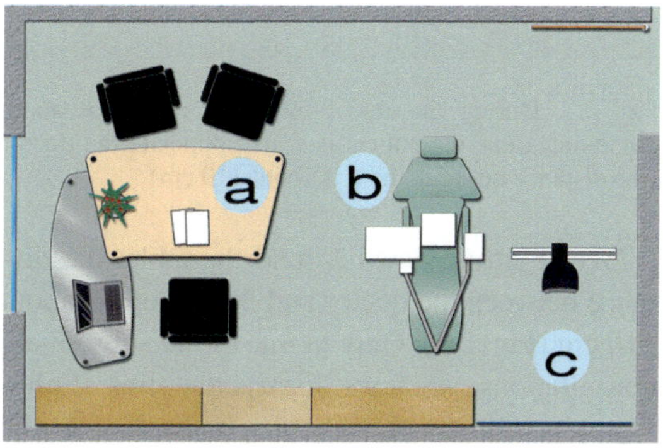

Fig. 2.1 Floorplan of the room in my current office with the three areas dedicated to the interview (**a**), the clinical examination (**b**), and the clinical photographs (**c**)

2.2 The Interview Area

For the initial and subsequent consultations, most of the time is spent in the interview area. A large table, with a lateral extension for the computer, the printer, a plant, and the telephone, are centered under a diffuse, but not too intense, light; care is taken to avoid any visual obstruction preventing eye contact. Adequate extra space around the table is needed when other colleagues and accompanying persons are attending the interview.

F. Meneghini, *Basic Open Rhinoplasty*, https://doi.org/10.1007/978-3-030-61827-8_2

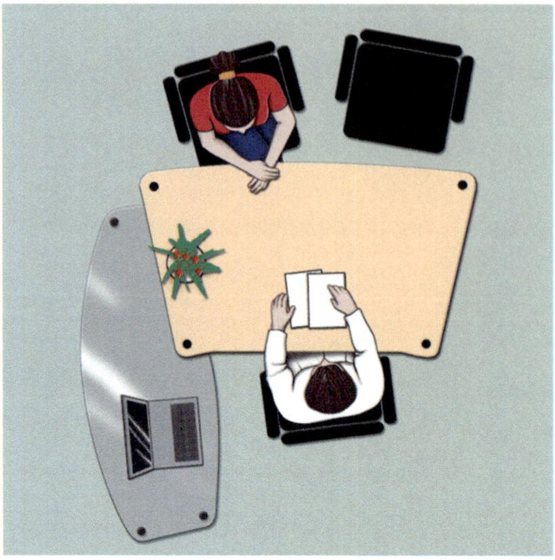

Fig. 2.2 During the initial interview and subsequent communication, the patient is seated opposite the doctor (the distance between them is about 110 cm)

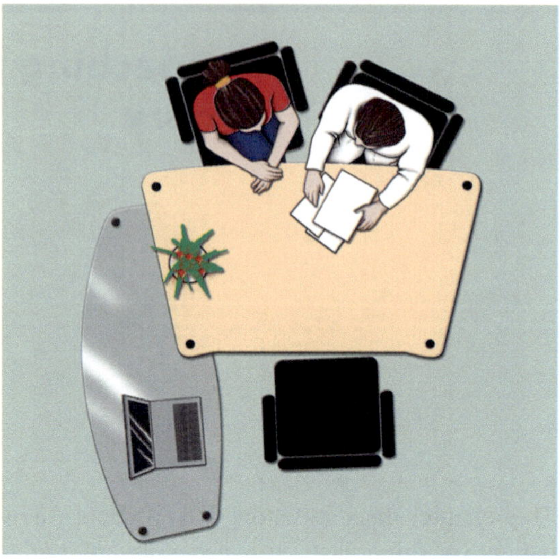

Fig. 2.3 Only when discussing the clinical photographs and the treatment plan in detail is the doctor seated beside the patient, reducing the distance to about 60 cm

When sitting down around the table, the distance between the doctor and the patient is about 110 cm (Fig. 2.2). Only in one of the subsequent consultations, when we discuss the clinical photographs and the treatment plan in detail, does the doctor sit beside the patient, reducing the distance to about 60 cm (Fig. 2.3).

2.3 The Clinical Examination Area

A modified dental chair and two different lighting systems occupy the room's central area, which is dedicated to the clinical examination.

The main characteristics of the chair are:

- It is adjustable in height and inclination. As I remain in a standing position during the direct clinical examination, I can elevate the chair in order to have my eyes at the same height as the patient's eyes, so that I may help him to maintain the natural head position (Fig. 2.4).
- Instead of the original dental instruments, there is a small work tray useful for holding a nasal speculum, a facial mirror, a camera, a ruler, or other useful small objects.
- It is equipped with a vacuum tube.
- It is easily adjusted to the Trendelenburg position.

One large, ceiling-mounted lighting system produces a diffuse and intense white light. This is preferred for the external examination due to the complete absence of dark shadows. The other lighting system is adjustable and produces an intense light beam that is very helpful for the anterior nasal and intraoral examination. There is enough space around the chair to see the patient's face from any viewpoint and at any distance.

When the patient is seated in the examining chair, the mean distance between the doctor and the patient is about 60 cm (Fig. 2.4).

2.4 The Clinical Photography Area

The space for clinical photography is rather limited and occupies a corner of the room. The lighting equipment and technique for capturing the images are described in Chap. 3, whereas Chap. 4 illustrates how to acquire a complete set of clinical facial photographs.

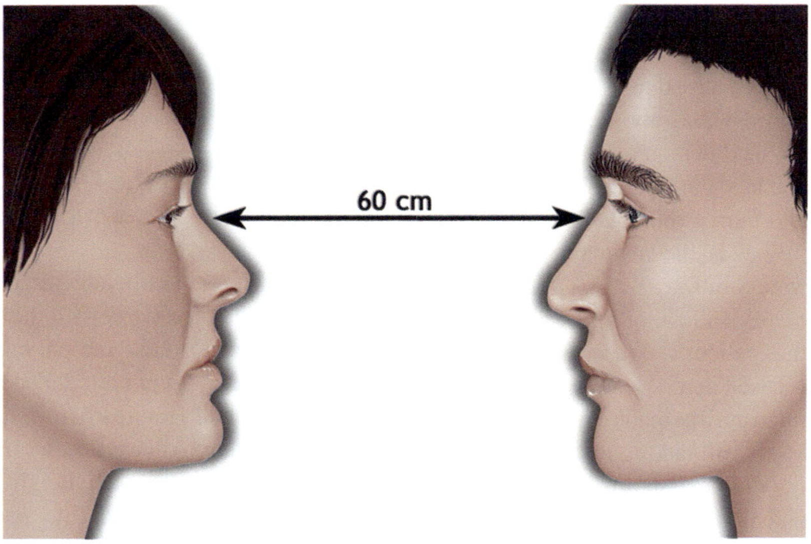

Fig. 2.4 During the clinical facial examination, the doctor's eyes should be at the same height as the patient's eyes and the distance between them is about 60 cm

2.5 Approach to the First Consultation

The first 10 min spent with a new patient are the most decisive in establishing the best line of communication. In that brief period of time, personal impressions about each other are created and are later changed only with great difficulty. So, exceed patient expectations on their initial consultation.

When I meet a new patient, I need to know in advance a few important facts. She has had two contacts with my staff before: the first, a telephone call or an email for the booking a few days earlier, and the second, at the entrance to the office, a few minutes before. These are two perfect opportunities to ask her:

- Her name, email address, and telephone number.
- The most suitable day and time for her consultation.
- The reason for the consultation.
- Which of my patients, friends, or colleagues referred her to my practice (I must reward this person soon!).

Each topic addressed during the call or written in the contact email must be recorded in the new patient's personal folder and is available to the surgeon. This simple knowledge will allow me to direct the approach and the information towards her needs.

Also, the patient needs to know in advance something about the competence, care, and specializations of my practice, and the first telephone contact should be an important opportunity to offer this, as well as other, information. To provide adequate preliminary information about nasal surgery, we send by email my guide book entitled "Your Rhinoplasty" or we instruct the patient on how to download it for free from the author's professional website.[1]

When one of my nurses introduces the patient and the accompanying persons into my room, I am in another workroom and I come in after a few seconds. I prefer this more dynamic type of introduction rather than the other, where the doctor is waiting, sitting in a relaxed position on his chair. In this manner, I greet the patient with a handshake, smile and introduce myself before sitting in front of her.

[1]Fabio Meneghini: La Tua Rinoplastica, Tutto quello che vorresti sapere sulla chirurgia del naso. First italian edition 2014. Tempo al Libro – Faenza, Italy. English edition on fourth Italian edition: YOUR RHINOPLASTY—All you need to know about nasal surgery. 2019. Tempo al Libro – Faenza, Italy (English translation by Fabio Leopardi).

2.6 The Interview

I have learned to ask questions to establish a rapport. Even if my secretary has informed me that the next person requested a consultation because she has a nose that she considers to be too large and I am a rhinoplasty surgeon, I start by asking "What is the main reason you are here today, Mrs. Smith?"

My following open questions concentrate on the patient's concerns and I want to remain focused on that aspect, resisting the temptation to interrupt the patient often in this early phase if she is still talking.

The next step is to help the patient organize and dictate her personal patient's priority list, her way of communicating problems, needs, wishes, and expectations. I write this down personally in an itemized way to make the order of importance given by the patient clear at every point. Avoid "translating" into strict medical language everything she says and be sure not to suggest undetected problems at this time.

Beginning with this fixed scheme, I avoid any improvisation in the first 10 min, which means loss of control and insecurity in the patient's eyes. As Tardy and Thomas pointed out, "... *two relative strangers proceed to make judgments about each other: the patient about whether she can have unqualified confidence in the surgeon consulted, and the surgeon about whether a favorable outcome is likely to be achieved that will result in a satisfied and happy patient*".[2]

The interview continues in order to obtain information about general health status, taking of aspirin and other drugs, allergies, previous medical and surgical treatments and to offer detailed information about the subsequent direct clinical examination and clinical photographic documentation. I provide the patient with a brief and clear explanation of why I have to ask many questions, touch her nose and take photographs of her face. During the interview, I always say that an important objective for me is to produce an in-depth clinical analysis from both the functional and esthetic points of view, which serves as a basis for an individually tailored treatment plan.

[2]Tardy ME, Regan Thomas J. Facial aesthetic surgery. St Louis: Mosby Year Book; 1995. p. 148.

2.7 The Direct Clinical Examination

The "unofficial" direct clinical examination of the face starts with the interview, even if I prefer not to make the patient aware of my interest in her nose or chin. I also avoid commenting on any facial features before the patient is sitting in the chair. After elevating the chair to put her eyes at almost the same height as mine, I instruct her on how to obtain the natural head position and, reviewing her priority list, I examine the facial features. Sometimes I give her a facial mirror, which helps in communicating ideas and points to each other.

The direct examination continues with some maneuvers, which I carry out utilizing a pair of examining gloves; these are specific to the clinical case (e.g., palpation of the nasal dorsum and tip in rhinoplasty patients to explore the length of the nasal bone and the resilience of the cartilaginous skeleton). Intranasal and intraoral examinations are mandatory in almost every case; to reassure and obtain the consent of the patient, I never forget to inform her about what I am doing.

Again, also in this more "practical" step of the consultation, I must resist the temptation to interrupt the patient when she is telling me something she thinks is important.

2.8 The Clinical Photographic Documentation

The taking of clinical photographs must be performed after the interview and the direct examination in order to decide which series of specific views should be added to the basic one. Chapters 3 and 4 illustrate, respectively, how to position and illuminate the patient's head and which views should be taken to obtain a complete photographic documentation.

2.9 Final Communications and Remarks

The final phase of the first consultation is conducted around the table, as for the interview. In the previous stages my listening activity was dominant, now is the time to answer all the questions the patient wishes to ask and inform her about the next preoperative steps, the treatment plan, the indications and limits of the procedure proposed, and many other general points.

Basically, I must decide if I want this patient in my practice, and if this is the case, if I can finalize my preoperative analysis into a complete and individually tailored treatment plan now or schedule a second consultation with the patient.

When dealing with facial esthetics, I am cautious about putting a right profile view into the monitor of my personal computer to show, in a spectacular way, how I could cut the nasal hump and project the chin. Moving quickly on to a definitive treatment plan requires two conditions: a doctor with long experience and a well-motivated "ideal" patient.

Almost always, I favor giving written information about the treatment proposed and schedule a second consultation with the patient.

Specifically for nasal surgery, in May 2014, I published "La Tua Rinoplastica" (English edition title: "Your Rhinoplasty") a book dedicated to anyone seeking clear and simple information about nasal surgery from an esthetic, functional, and reconstructive perspective. The book is composed of these main sections:

- Your nose and how it works
- Rhinoplasty surgery
- Preparing for your operation
- What to do after your operation

I give all my rhinoplasty patients a copy of "La Tua Rinoplastica" during the first consultation, reserving the discussion on the optimal treatment plan for the next visit.

A good last phrase before the final greeting is "Please read the book and write down any questions for the next consultation."

2.10 The Time Spent in Organizing the Next Consultation

Ideally, the patient is scheduled for her second consultation 1 or 2 weeks later in order to give her time to complete the preoperative instrumental examinations requested (e.g., CT scan). I prefer not to exceed 1 month because, even if I have several methods to review in my mind, waiting for longer is counterproductive, both because the patient forgets what has been previously discussed and because the wait prolongs her psychological stress.

In any case, this time is necessary for me to organize the clinical images and data collected, and to debate the feasible treatment options. The main steps are:

- For each photographic view, select the best image, optimize its contrast and brightness, and print it on A4 format paper, as described in detail in Chap. 10.
- Confirm or partially modify and enrich the findings obtained with the direct clinical examination and also perform the analysis on photographs.
- Create one or more nasal profile simulations and print them on A4 format paper.

The doctor's priority list is an itemized list of the findings (not only problems!) obtained, in order of importance. In this way, positive aspects like a beautiful and proportioned nasal tip or a well-balanced chin/neck profile are also detected and noted as things that need to be conserved.

2.11 Approach to the Second (and Subsequent) Consultations

The following preoperative consultations are quite different to the first for two reasons. First, I do not need a standard and sometimes rigorous approach because, knowing the person, her problems and needs, it is time to personalize the approach. Second, my previous role of "listener" should move into a new and more active role of the surgeon, who produces the best treatment plan for the patient.

Immediately before meeting the patient, I comment on the CT scan images with simple words, review the patient priority list, the doctor (my) priority list, the provisional treatment plan, and all the documents collected or developed and the instrumental exams delivered by the patient. To show and explain my findings and treatment purposes, I sit alongside the patient and utilize extensively her clinical photographs and CT scan images.

The principles and method suggested for preparation of the final treatment plan will be described in Chaps. 9 and 10.

2.12 How to Enhance Patient/Physician Communication

Good communication is vital for a constructive patient/physician relationship as well as for the clinical facial analysis. How well you explain your ideas and understand the needs of the patient directly influences all your subsequent work. The cornerstones of communication are:

- Greet your patient with a handshake, and sit down in front of her during the consultation.
- Listen, really listen to your patient. Listen to understand. Listening requires us not only to hear what the other person is saying, but to comprehend it as well. Improve your ability to listen by videotaping yourself and noting how many times you mistakenly stop the patient when she is talking to you.
- Maintain eye contact. Be sure to look directly at the patient and to any accompanying person.
- Smile and offer reassuring comments such as "I understand," "Okay, right," "Yes." Echo what she has said to show you are paying attention.
- Utilize some visual aids or simple little drawings to explain the relevant aspects of the treatment. A high percentage of what we remember, we recall because we associate it with images.
- Use general and simple examples to reinforce your ideas.
- Avoid excessive pessimism and unrestrained optimism in delivering any information.
- Review the main points before the end of the consultation. Repetition is the doctor's way of emphasizing crucial points and it is not necessarily redundancy.
- Work cooperatively with your staff to further enhance communication.
- Do not forget to communicate the positive aspects of your work as well as your commitment in doing it.

To further improve communication with my patients I wrote a small book focused on rhinoplasty for them. It is a special gift full of information and advice written in simple words. In my personal experience, this is the best way to start talking about the journey to arrive at an informed and aware decision whether or not to perform such a complex surgery as rhinoplasty.

2.13 The Single Operator Concept

All patients want a coordinator and a leader to approach their problems. They feel negatively towards different people conducting the assessment and the planned surgery, in particular rhinoplasty.

The single operator concept emphasizes the importance of your patient being followed by you in all the main clinical steps with the ideal coordination of information and activity with the medical team and office personnel.

If you need to consult a more experienced colleague or a different specialist, you must directly organize, present, and actively coordinate the meeting, to underline the importance and the support you continue to give the case.

Further Reading

In the following chapters, the principles and techniques of patient-centered communication will be repeated several times. For further information, a basic book is: Moreno NJ. Patient-centered communication: the seven keys to connecting with patients. New York: Thieme; 2020. ISBN-13: 978-1684201839.

3 Techniques for Clinical Facial Photography

The realization of a standardized and good-quality photographic documentation of the face, both preoperative and postoperative, is a mandatory objective for the surgeon who is dedicated to rhinoplasty. This activity cannot be delegated to the office staff or external professionals since the time spent in direct contact with the patient is essential to establish and maintain a relationship of mutual knowledge and trust. Even the few minutes dedicated to taking preoperative clinical facial photographs are important to signify the surgeon's willingness to follow and help personally the patient.

Several times I have observed my colleagues getting annoyed because of a less than perfect result obtained with the latest high-ended camera. What are the weak points in clinical facial photography? The principal variables are the technical features of the camera, the quality of the lighting, the lens, and the background panel. Patient positioning and camera positioning (framing) during the photographic shoot are also a difficult task and must be considered peculiar abilities of the nasal surgeon.

After years of direct experience and commitment, I am convinced that the most demanding aspects of clinical photography are patient lighting—the main topic of this chapter—and patient positioning and framing, which are discussed in Chap. 4.

A portable and inexpensive alternative to performing facial clinical photographic documentation will be presented at the end of this chapter.

3.1 Professional Lighting Techniques for Clinical Facial Photography[1]

The taking of clinical photographs, to record and to utilize during surgery, is an essential part of the activities of every professional practice or facial surgery department. The narrowness of the office, the cost of the equipment, and a vague lack of time do not constitute excuses for less precise patient documentation.

To obtain the best quality and consistency of results, many suggest the use of a professional lighting system composed of two or more flash units. Thus an entire room or a large part of it should be permanently reserved for this use.

In the past 20 years, I have utilized a system of lighting based on a unique source of light (monolight flash), which is ceiling-mounted in a corner of a room also dedicated for other activities, with good results. The next sections present a description of the key technical

[1] Adapted from Meneghini F. Clinical facial photography in a small office: lighting equipment and technique. Aesthetic Plast Surg. 2001;25:299–306.

F. Meneghini, *Basic Open Rhinoplasty*, https://doi.org/10.1007/978-3-030-61827-8_3

points and the rationale for using single-light equipment.

3.2 Equipment and Technique

The studio lighting equipment consists of a single professional flash (System 300 professional compact flash by System Imaging Ltd., UK), which is ceiling-mounted on a straight rail parallel to the background panel. The total length of the rail is 0.95 m. The distance of the flash unit from the background is fixed at 1.6 m. A pantograph (Friction Pantograph 3250 by I.F.F., Calenzano–Firenze) holds the monolight and allows unrestricted vertical adjustment. A rectangular 0.75 × 0.35 m soft box (75 Light Bank by System Imaging Ltd., UK) fits onto the flash unit, softening and diffusing the light. An alternative smaller and more practical soft box, 0.4 × 0.3 m (Chimera Lightbanks, Boulder, Colorado, USA), has also been utilized during the past few years.

The distance from the monolight to the subject is fixed (about 1.1–1.2 m), so each photograph is taken at the same F-stop of 16 to enhance the depth of field of the portrait subject. The lighting is directed towards the subject in all views, maintaining the flash unit at a high level. The rectangular soft box is held in a horizontal position. In order to eliminate the problem of shadows on the submental region and under the nasal base, the patient holds, with her hands, a small rectangular reflecting panel of 0.35 × 0.7 m (Fig. 3.1). This panel is positioned horizontally against the chest, just under the collarbone.

The ceiling-mounted rail allows the adjustment of the monolight to a side or central position. It easily follows the rotation of the subject from the frontal to oblique and lateral views. Figure 3.2a–c shows the basic positions of the flash unit used in the different views to achieve the best results. An important rule is to maintain the subject's position close to the background panel itself in order to avoid the need for an additional flash unit to light the background panel.

For a routine set of photographs consisting of full-face portraits and close-up views, I use the 105 mm Micro Nikkor lens mounted on a full-frame digital camera.

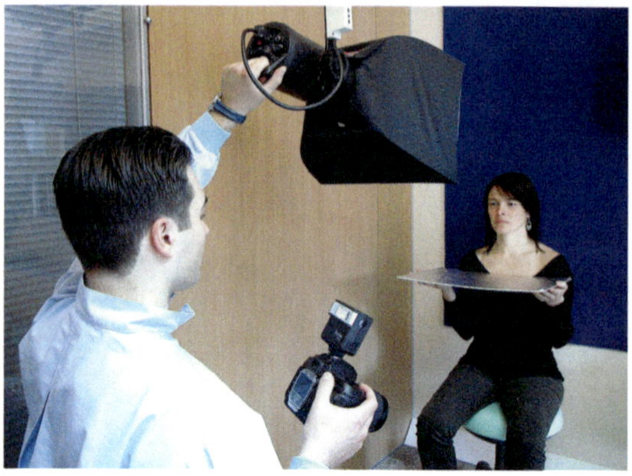

Fig. 3.1 Photographic set. The patient holds, with her hands, a small rectangular reflecting panel positioned horizontally against the chest, just under the collarbone. The operator easily adjusts the monolight vertically and horizontally

I personally do not use a camera tripod for stability because of the very short time of light emission by the flash unit. Focusing is done by moving the camera back and forth. A camera tripod also interferes with the positioning of the monolight and the patient's head. In almost every case, I directly help the patient during positioning, touching her chin with my hand (Fig. 3.3). On the other hand, a viewfinder grid screen is highly recommended to help the surgeon orient the camera precisely.

To avoid using a direct wire connection to the monolight, a small on-camera electronic flash, oriented in a reverse direction, gives the input to the built-in slave unit of the main flash. The space reserved for clinical photography in the room is rather narrow, as illustrated in the previous chapter. Due to the combination of movements permitted by the pantograph and the ceiling-mounted rail, the flash unit can be easily positioned high up, near the ceiling, and on the left wall of the room when not in use, to leave space for other activities. The blue background panel, 0.95 m wide and 1.10 m high, is made from a sheet of plastic material for outdoor use. An advantage of this panel is that it is washable without running the risk of losing or changing the color. The

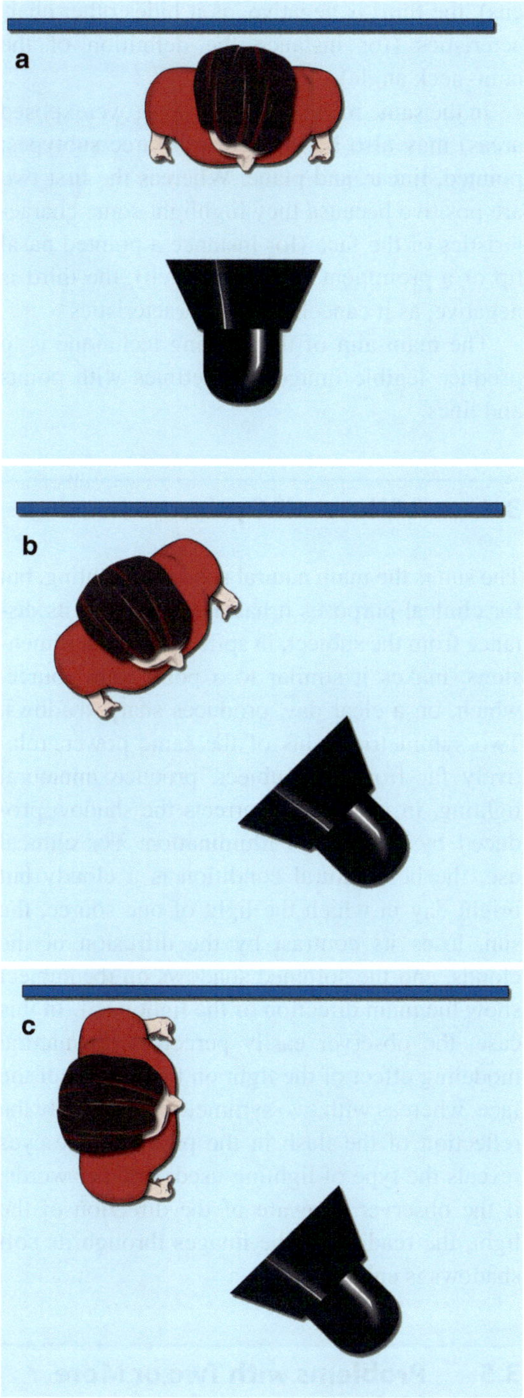

Fig. 3.2 (**a–c**) The three main patient/monolight positions utilized to capture the various facial views. (**a**) Setting utilized for frontal, basal, and face-down views. (**b**) Setting utilized for oblique right view. (**c**) Setting utilized for profile right view

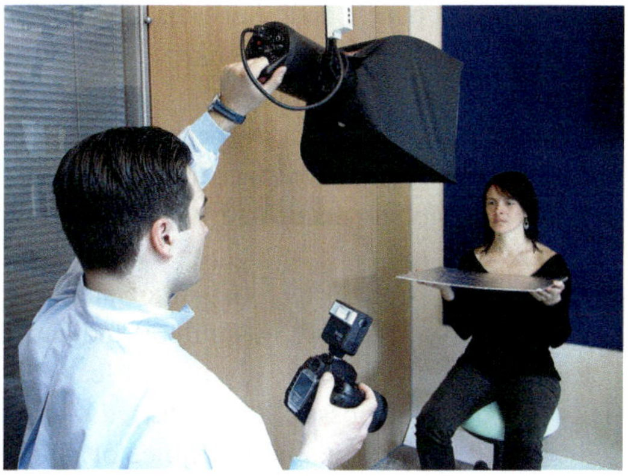

Fig. 3.3 Direct and unrestricted positioning of the patient's head

patient and I sit on rotating stools with rollers. The chairs are easily adjusted in the vertical position in order to maintain the subject and the camera at the same height during the capture of the images.

I usually take my clinical photographs personally, without the aid of an assistant, and the entire procedure requires no more than 5 min. For better efficiency and to save time, I follow a specific sequence:

- I ask the patient to meet me in the photo area, turn on the monolight, instruct her on how to use the reflecting panel correctly, and adjust her height on the stool, close to the blue background panel.
- I pick up my camera, turn on the small on-camera electronic flash and set the standard shutter speed/aperture combination of 1/125 s–F16 with the monolight adjusted to full-power light emission.
- I shoot the frontal view first, with the patient and the flash unit oriented as in Fig. 3.2a.
- I position the patient's head for the extended and basal views and take the photographs. The position of the monolight remains unchanged.
- I position the patient for the right oblique views, taking care to maintain her close to the blue background panel. The monolight is oriented as in Fig. 3.2b, and the photos are taken.
- I position the patient for the right profile view, taking care to maintain her close to the blue

background panel, and shoot the photo. The position of the flash unit remains unchanged, as depicted in Fig. 3.2c.
– I repeat the two latter steps for the left oblique and profile views, orienting the patient's head and the monolight accordingly.

During the procedure, I help the patient to assume a relaxed face and no smile, if indicated. For each view, I systematically take at least two shots to reduce the possibility of blurred photos, and generally to ensure a better choice of photos later.

Some authors have investigated lighting techniques for facial photographs in rhinoplasty patients and, in particular, the effects of different positioning of two main frontal lights on the nasal tip. Both articles point out that any changes in lighting produce a different type of reflection. Simply by moving the lights further laterally, increasing the angle of incidence, the nasal tip appears more pointed, whereas an asymmetric positioning produces an asymmetric reflection on the tip, which could be mistaken for a real anatomical asymmetry. Even in a dedicated room for patient photography, with fixed light sources and a camera mounted on a fixed tripod, the variable of the patient position remains. Not surprisingly, Jack Sheen stated that: "There is no doubt that photographs can be manipulated. And lighting is probably the easiest, most effective way to manipulate an image."[2]

3.3 Point, Line, and Plane

Generally speaking, a photograph may be illegible due to underexposure (too much black) or overexposure (too much white). In clinical facial photography, the shadows (underexposed areas) may be divided into three subtypes: pointed, linear, and plane. Whereas the first two are positive because they underline some characteristics of the face (for instance a depressed scar or a sulcus), the third is negative, as it hides other characteristics (for instance the definition of the chin–neck angle).

In the same manner, the reflexes (overexposed areas) may also be divided into three subtypes: pointed, linear, and plane. Whereas the first two are positive because they highlight some characteristics of the face (for instance a pointed nasal tip or a prominent zygomatic arch), the third is negative, as it cancels other characteristics.

The main aim of the lighting technique is to produce legible images, sometimes with points and lines.

3.4 A "Natural" Option

The sun is the main natural source of lighting, but for clinical purposes it has a weak point: its distance from the subject, in spite of its great dimensions, makes it similar to a point light source, which, on a clear day, produces sharp shadows. Two symmetric lights of the same power, relatively far from the subject, produce unnatural lighting, in which one corrects the shadow produced by the other's illumination. For clinical use, the best natural condition is a cloudy but bright day in which the light of one source, the sun, loses its contrast by the diffusion of the clouds, and the softened shadows on the subject show the main direction of the light itself. In this case, the observer easily perceives the natural modeling effect of the light on the surface of the face, whereas with two symmetric lights, only the reflection of the flash in the pupils of the eyes reveals the type of lighting used. In other words, if the observer is aware of the direction of the light, the reading of the images through its soft shadows is enhanced.

3.5 Problems with Two or More Lights

In my personal experience, the use of two or more flash units is counterproductive and unnecessary. The negative aspects of a multiple light system are:

[2]Cited by: Daniel RK, Hodgson J, Lambros VS. Rhinoplasty: the light reflexes. Plast Reconstr Surg. 1990;85:859.

- Increased cost (almost double).
- It occupies more space.
- More complex technique (increases the parameters that potentially require adjustments).
- The effects of any single light source are difficult to assess due to the presence of other lights.

In a single flash system, the orientation of the light is easily adjusted from one view to another because the operator directly controls the shadows and the reflection on the face with the aid of the floodlighting. The reflecting panel, held by the patient, does not require any adjustment during the change from one view to another (keep the variables to a minimum!).

3.6 Avoid False Facial Asymmetry

The main views used to confirm or exclude the presence of facial asymmetry are frontal, extended, and basal. For that reason, any differences in side-to-side lighting during the shooting of these particular images may produce an erroneous conclusion. In any system using two main lights, the power output of the two units, the type of soft boxes utilized, the orientation, the distance from the subject, the angles of incidence, and the height of the tripods must be identical. In other words, six different parameters set on the right unit must be reproduced exactly on the left. Any deviation from a perfect equilibrium produces a false asymmetric patient, or changes the appreciation of a true asymmetry.

With the author's approach to lighting, symmetry is easily achievable in frontal, extended, and basal views, positioning the monolight directly in front of the subject at a higher level and asking the patient to hold the reflecting panel horizontally against her chest, just under the collarbone. In each case, the camera must be positioned perfectly frontal to the subject.

3.7 The Importance of Soft Box Size

The selection of the size of the soft box has repercussions on the quality and the ease of use. In particular, the large light-banks (0.75 × 0.35 m) produce softer light and, because of their wide and homogeneous lighting, permit easy subject positioning. The small light-banks (0.30 × 0.40 m), on the contrary, produce harder light and enhance the texture of the skin, and it is difficult to obtain the ideal position because the area covered with homogeneous light is smaller and there is an increased likelihood of undesired shadows.

With the same emission power and distance from flash to subject, the smaller light-bank also provides higher intensity and hence greater depth of field (the range within which objects are in focus).

3.8 Advantages of Ceiling-Mounted Equipment

The advantages of ceiling-mounted equipment are sound. The floor is completely free of cables, tripod, stands, or other objects. The pantograph and rail system permit unrestricted horizontal and vertical movement of the monolight, while maintaining a relatively fixed distance from the subject and the background. Access to the area is easier for the patient and, at the end of the procedure, the equipment can be set aside to gain space for other activities within seconds.

3.9 The Six Rules of Multiple Shots

1. Document every new patient with multiple shots whether or not she will be treated later.
2. Multiple shots of the same view ensure that you have plenty of perfectly focused images to choose from.
3. After a rigorous capture of the standard view set, if you wish, perform multiple shots to

document, in a personalized manner and without restrictions, the features of the face.
4. Use the skin marker to point out any particular deformity or lesion and perform multiple shots from different points of view to avoid shadows and reflections.
5. During capture of the full-face oblique view and full-face basal view, perform multiple shots in conjunction with small differences in head position.
6. Today, with digital cameras, the extra cost of multiple shots is small (one or ten shots cost roughly the same).

The methodology for better documentation must be cultivated daily, applying the six rules of multiple shots, which also help to develop greater photographic skills. Clinical facial photography is largely a rigorous procedure, which requires rules to assure clarity and consistency but, unfortunately, it is also, to a small extent, an art.

3.10 A Portable and Inexpensive Alternative

Preoperative and postoperative clinical facial photography is mandatory in nasal surgery. The equipment described in the previous paragraphs requires a dedicated area of the office and has a relatively high initial cost. For young surgeons as well as for those who do not have in their office an area dedicated to clinical photography, a complete documentation can be realized with a small digital camera equipped with a built-in flash and a zoom lens, such as the one shown in Fig. 3.4. All the figures of Chap. 10 are realized with this small and relatively inexpensive digital camera.

The main rules to be respected during shooting are:

- Choose among the walls of the room a uniform and opaque background to avoid distracting elements and unwanted reflections.
- All views are captured at a distance of 1 m or more utilizing the built-in flash as the main light source.
- The zoom is always adjusted to telephoto.

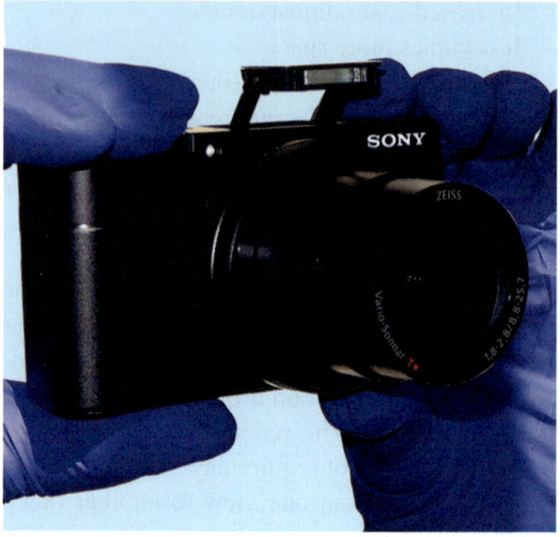

Fig. 3.4 Compact digital camera with built-in flash and zoom lens adjustable to telephoto

- The automatism is set on aperture priority. To obtain adequate depth of field, the diaphragm aperture is set to 8 or 11.
- The camera must be maintained at the same level of the subject's face as well as oriented perpendicularly. This is probably the most demanding task for the photographer.
- For the frontal, basal, and face-down views, the camera is maintained in a perfect horizontal position.
- For the right oblique and profile views, the camera is rotated clockwise vertically for a better lightening of the subject by the built-in flash.
- For the left oblique and profile views, the camera is rotated counterclockwise vertically for a better lightening of the subject by the built-in flash.

Patient positioning, another demanding task, will be presented in the next chapter.

Further Reading

Beker DG, Tardy ME. Standardized photography in facial plastic surgery: pearls and pitfalls. Facial Plast Surg. 1999;15(2):93–9.

Meneghini F. Clinical facial photography in a small office: lighting equipment and technique. Aesthet Plast Surg. 2001;25:299–306.

4 Views of Clinical Facial Photography for Nasal Surgery

The photographic documentation of our patients must have the following important features: completeness, standardization, and quality. All physicians dealing with facial esthetics need these documents for analysis, patient communication, planning, as an intraoperative tool, for early and late follow-up, for self-teaching and teaching objectives as well as for medico-legal purposes.

The previous chapter described a personal technique used to obtain standardization and quality in lighting of the face. This chapter illustrates how to position the patient's head and which views should be taken to obtain a complete photographic documentation for nasal surgery.

4.1 Natural Head Position

The natural head position (NHP) is a standardized and reproducible orientation of the head achieved when one is looking at a distant point in front of oneself, at eye level. The great majority of clinical photographs and direct clinical examination steps require the NHP; in addition, patient positioning for cephalometric analysis should be the NHP. The simplest way to obtain the NHP is to instruct the patient to look straight ahead at a point at eye level on the wall in front of him.

Sometimes the orientation obtained seems unnatural to the examiner but, on asking the patient to tilt the head upwards and downwards and then return to looking straight ahead at the point at eye level, we have noted that the final spatial orientation is very similar to the initial one.

The NHP is of paramount importance in facial analysis due to its reproducibility and, most importantly, because it is extremely simple to obtain. In contrast, the Frankfort horizontal and the other constructed planes utilized to orient the head and based on internal skeletal landmarks, are "unnatural" and difficult to obtain clinically.

4.2 How To Obtain Life-Size Photographs

Sometimes the preoperative case study needs a soft tissue cephalometric analysis on life-size photographs. I place an opaque white ruler close to the subject while shooting the images, taking care that both are perfectly focused to ensure the accuracy of the enlargement. With the digital camera, a quick and simple method is:

The pictures in this chapter are taken from the scientific poster "Views of Clinical Facial Photography," conceived and realized by F. Meneghini in May 2003, whereas the text is modified from Chapter 3 of the book: Meneghini F. Clinical Facial Analysis. Berlin Heidelberg: Springer-Verlag; 2005.

F. Meneghini, *Basic Open Rhinoplasty*, https://doi.org/10.1007/978-3-030-61827-8_4

- Transfer the image to the personal computer.
- With Adobe Photoshop software, adjust contrast and brightness.
- Save in JPEG format for storage.
- Import the image into a Microsoft Word document and enlarge or reduce it to obtain a life-size dimension.
- Insert the date, the name of the patient and any useful clinical notes.
- Print on A4 paper (210 × 297 mm) format to obtain space around the life-size image for all future hand-written notes.

4.3 The Poster "Views of Clinical Facial Photography"

The experience acquired documenting thousands of patients and teaching at the maxillofacial surgery postgraduate course at the University of Padua convinced me to realize and print in multiple copies a poster to inform my patients and instruct my young colleagues about clinical facial photography (Fig. 4.1). Its dimensions are 0.70 m wide and 0.50 m high. A free printable full-size electronic copy, in JPEG format, can be requested from the author by email.[1]

The background consists of a drawing of a large open left hand. On the palm, the 11 basic views taken for all patients during the initial examination and subsequent postoperative follow-up assessments are illustrated, independently of the type of treatment planned. On the thumb, we see the five views added to the previous basic series in the case of documenting the nasal features; on the index finger, the five views used for documenting dentofacial deformities and/or orthodontic problems are added; on the middle finger, the seven views used for documenting orbital and lid features; and on the ring finger, the three views needed for documenting ear features. Thus, there are a total of 31 standard facial pictures illustrated in the poster and only four of these are not in the NHP.

The small piece of 35 mm film, on the little finger, is a reminder of the necessity to take any other useful photographs required by a particular clinical case.

I recommend hanging the poster up in the examining room, near the blue background panel utilized for facial photography. The goals obtained by using this visual tool are to:

- Strengthening the doctor's skills, as a communicator, during the first consultation.
- Helping the patient to understand the need for complete facial documentation, and to cooperate actively during the shooting.
- Assisting the doctor in following a rigorous method and sequence in patient documentation so that no views are forgotten and no technical errors made.

4.4 Shooting a Complete Set of Clinical Facial Photographs for Rhinoplasty

The ideal time for a complete set of clinical photographs during the first consultation with a new patient is described in Chap. 2. Before asking the patient to sit on the rotating stool with rollers, I illustrate the basic and specific views utilizing the poster, underlining the fact that I will take two or three shots for each view to avoid the problem of blinking. When we are both sitting face to face, I instruct him on how to obtain the NHP and then start the set, taking the 11 basic views.

This series of pictures is fundamental and should be taken for all patients. All the basic views presented in this chapter are taken at a fixed subject–camera distance of 1.5 m with a digital camera mounted with the 105 mm Micro Nikkor lens. Care should be taken to maintain the camera at the same height as the subject.

The first two or three shots are the full-face frontal view (Fig. 4.2). The patient is instructed to look at the lens of the camera, which is held perfectly frontal to the subject. I do not always continue with the next view but I prefer to review these in the monitor of the digital camera to check the exposure, the shadows, the patient positioning, and the occurrence of blinking. Setting a good full-face frontal view is essential

[1] info@fabiomeneghini.it

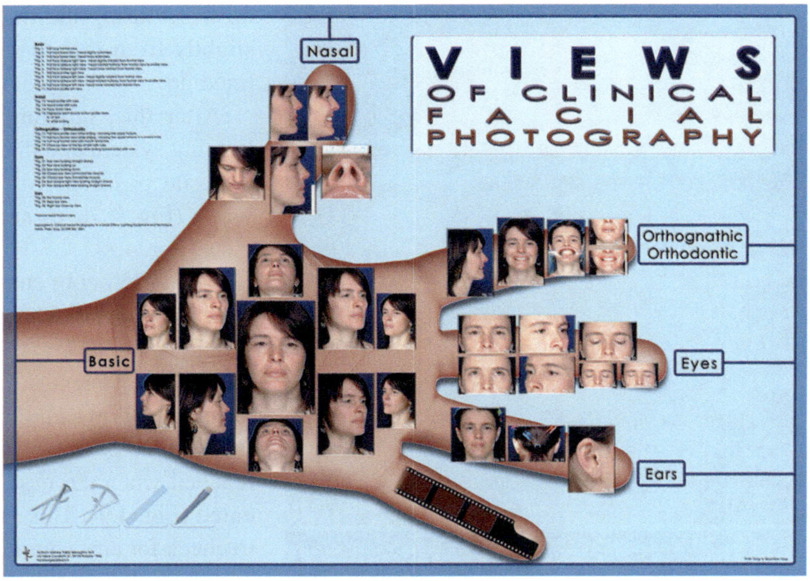

Fig. 4.1 The author's poster "Views of Clinical Facial Photography"

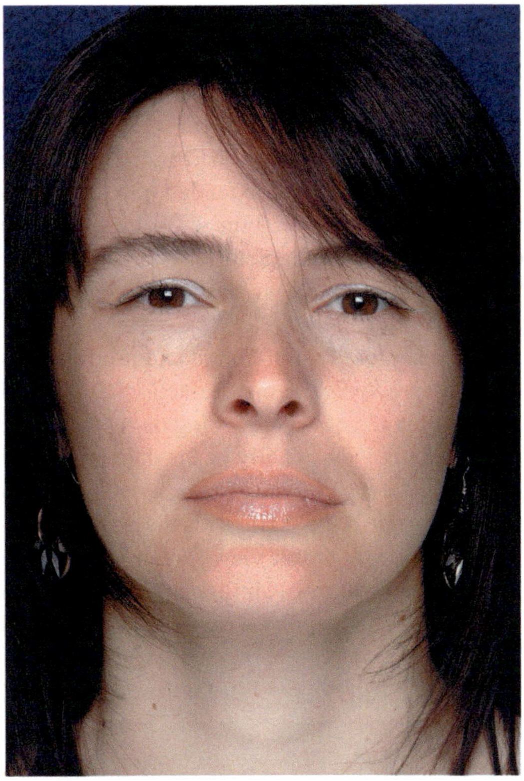

Fig. 4.2 Full-face frontal view

because many of the parameters do not change during the next steps of the procedure.

The next view is the full-face basal view (Fig. 4.3a, b). These photographs are taken with two or three small differences in the degree of head extension due to the difficulty in reproducing the same non-NHP orientation at the time of follow-up. The more extended position (Fig. 4.3b) is ideal for the analysis of the nasal base and the shape and symmetry of the zygomatic arches and the inferior border of the mandible, but note that the dorsal profile of the nose is hidden completely by the nasal base compared with the less extended position (Fig. 4.3a).

For the next step, I ask the patient to return to the NHP and rotate the stool for the three full-face oblique right views (Fig. 4.4a–c). For a more precise head orientation, I find an object on the wall in front of the patient or a small part of it, at the same level as the patient's eyes, and I suggest that he looks at this point during shooting. Once the flash unit is oriented, I take these pictures, moving my camera from side to side to obtain three views with more or less rotation from the frontal view (to obtain these I prefer to change the camera position instead of moving the patient's head).

These three oblique right views are taken to obtain more material for an in-depth analysis as well as to allow for the difficulty in reproducing the same head orientation in the future. Furthermore, each small difference in head rotation for the oblique views hides some facial details and highlights others; for example, the

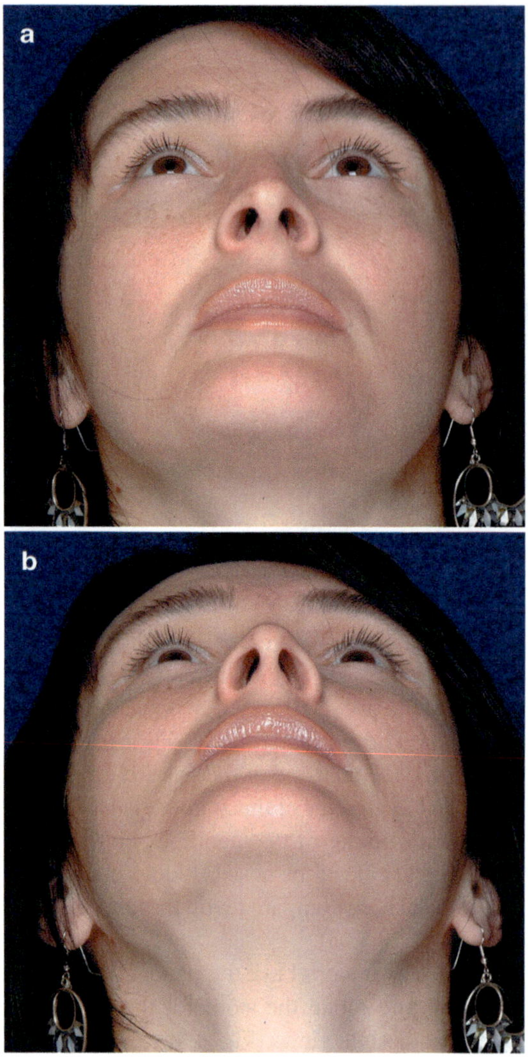

Fig. 4.3 Less extended (**a**) and more extended (**b**) full-face basal views

best oblique view to study the nasal outline is quite different from the best one to study the malar eminence, as depicted in Fig. 4.5a, b.

The full-face profile right view (Fig. 4.6) is taken next, taking care to orient the camera exactly perpendicular to the subject. In order to do that, during the framing, I move the camera slightly from side to side until the eyebrows are lined up.

After this, utilizing the same technique, the lighting system and the patient are oriented in the opposite positions for the full-face oblique left views (Fig. 4.7a–c) and the full-face profile left view (Fig. 4.8).

For an in-depth study of nasal features, as in the case of a rhinoplasty patient, five nasal views should be added.

With the patient sitting facing me, I ask him to tilt his face down and look at the reflecting panel; the perfect position for the face-down view is reached when the nasal dorsum is vertically oriented (Fig. 4.9). This view is important clinically to check for any asymmetry or external deformity of the nasal dorsum.

The next two nasal views are all close-up with a subject–camera distance less than 1.5 m and the presence inside the frame of a ruler, to permit printing at a 1:1 scale for subsequent analysis and precise surgical planning. The nasal base with ruler view (Fig. 4.10) is taken with the head in a more extended position, similar to that utilized for Fig. 4.3b, in which the dorsum is hidden completely by the nasal base. The right nasal profile with ruler view (Fig. 4.11) is taken in the NHP.

The last pictures, the frontal and profile views of the depressor septi muscle action, are useful for studying the effect of smiling on the tip of the nose caused by the activity of the depressor septi muscle. The two pictures are shot in rapid sequence and in the NHP with the patient positioned for a right profile view (Fig. 4.12a, b). The frontal view during smiling is depicted in Fig. 4.13. The depressor septi muscle action views are also important for studying the range of movement of the upper lip (smile analysis) and the nostrils.

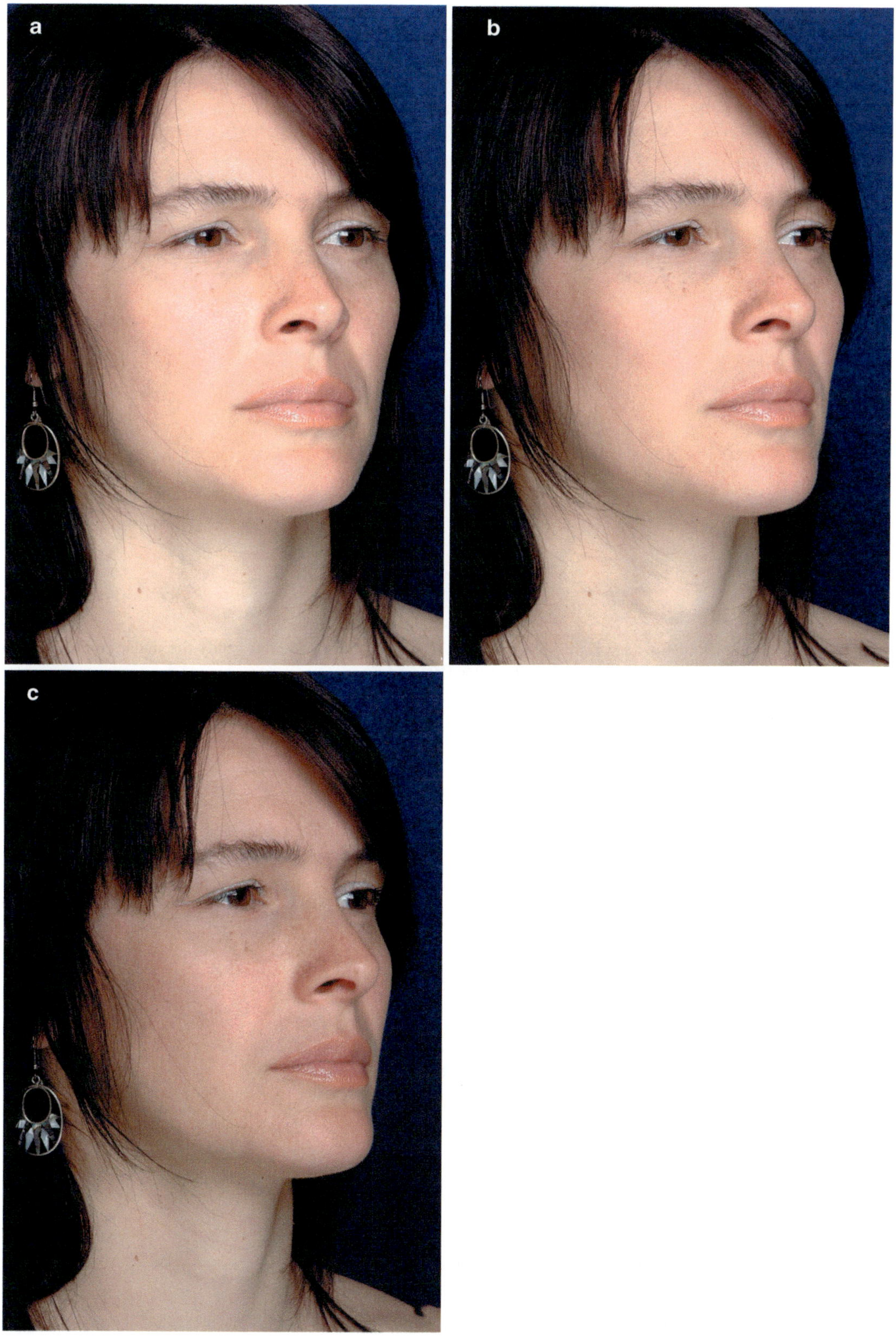

Fig. 4.4 (**a–c**) Full-face right oblique views. By rotating the subject's head it is possible to highlight or hide some facial features

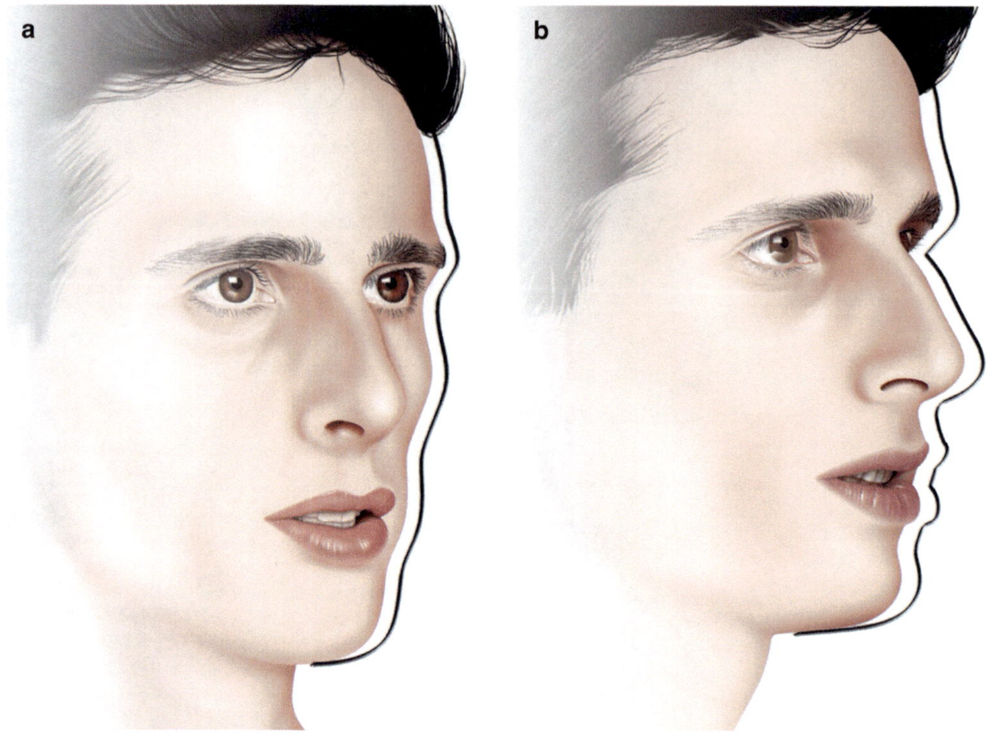

Fig. 4.5 (**a**, **b**) Examples of full-face right oblique views. The best oblique view to study the malar eminence (**a**) is quite different from the best one to study the nasal outline (**b**)

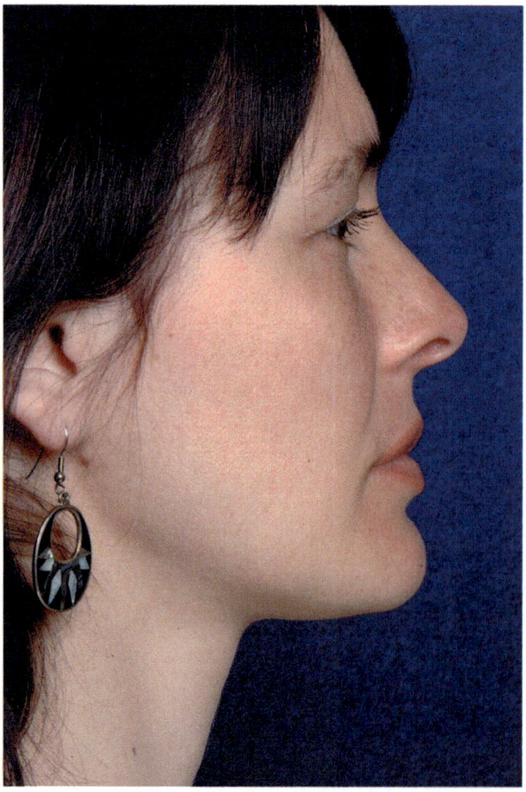

Fig. 4.6 Full-face right profile view

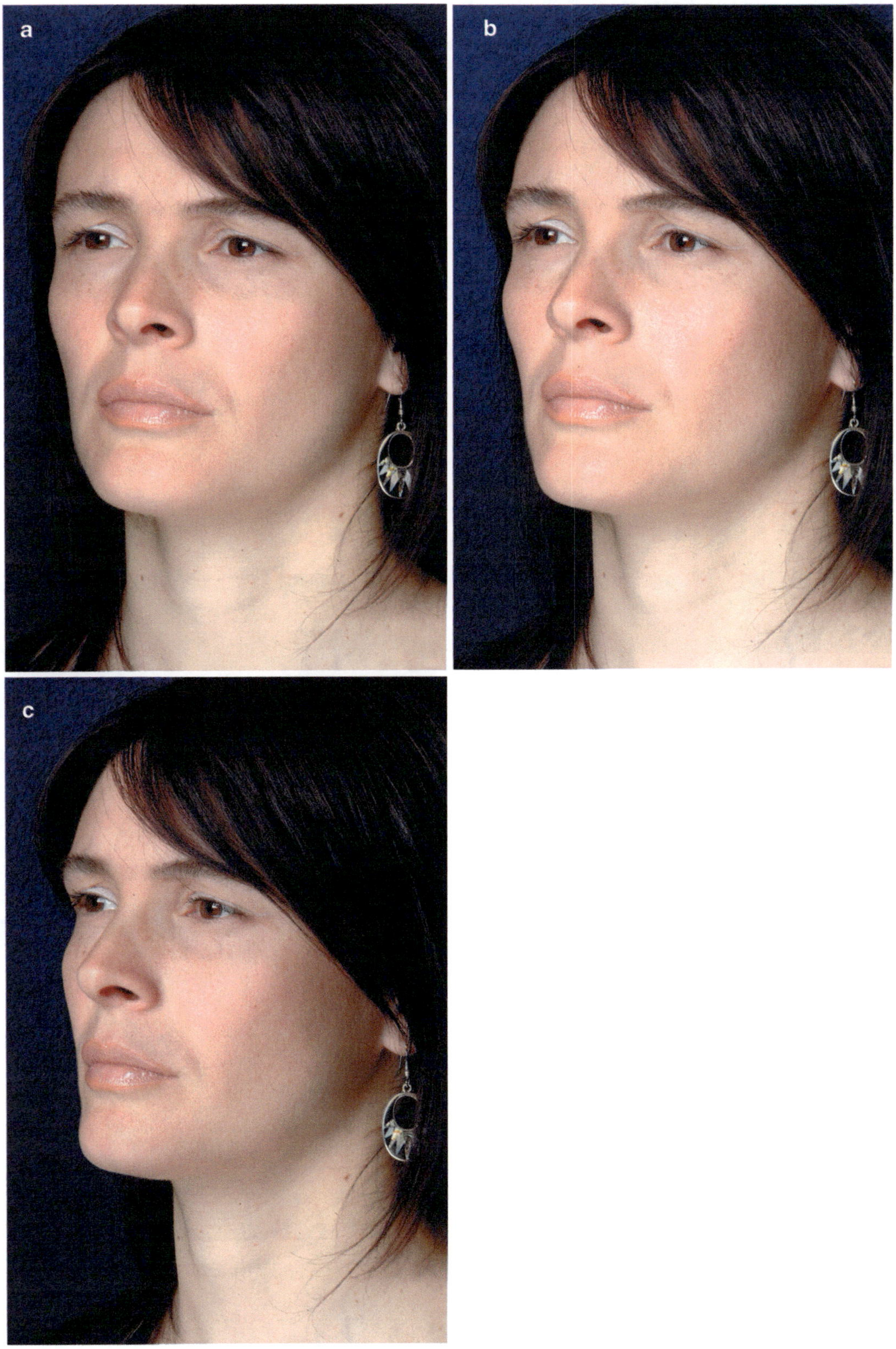

Fig. 4.7 (**a–c**) Full-face left oblique views

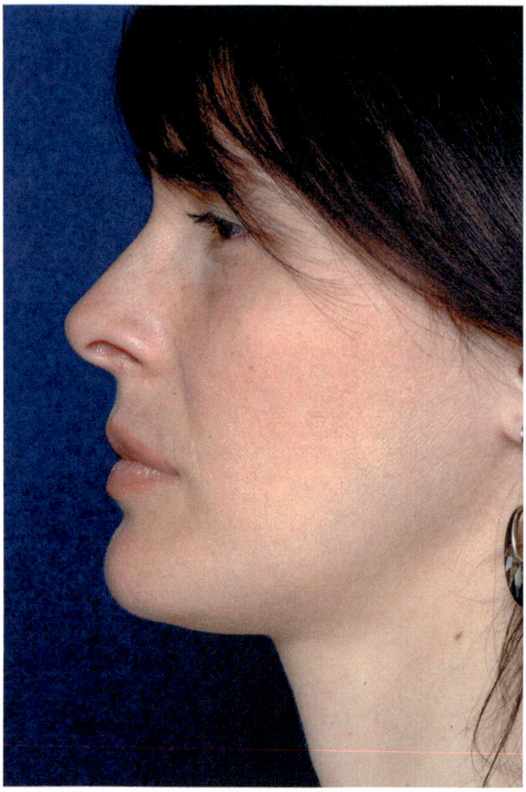

Fig. 4.8 Full-face left profile view

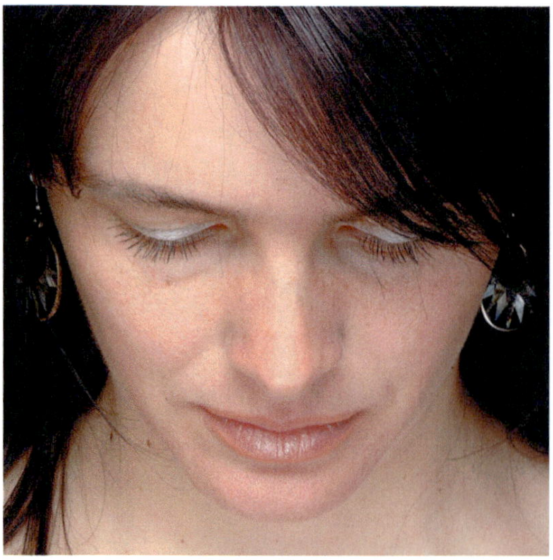

Fig. 4.9 Face-down view (also named helicopter view)

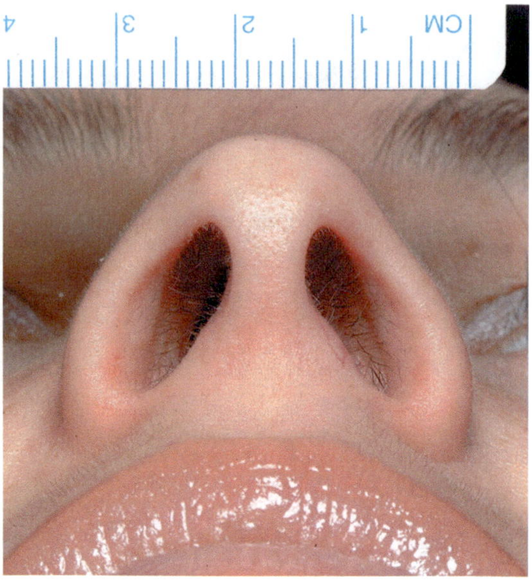

Fig. 4.10 Nasal base view (with ruler)

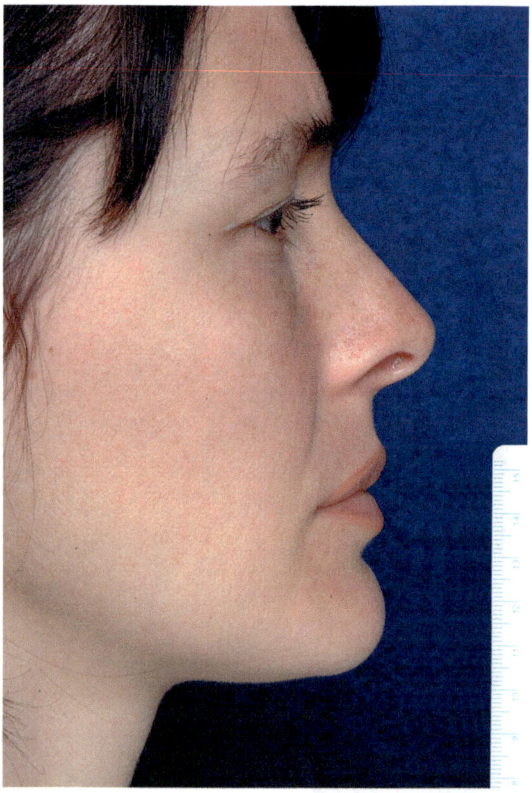

Fig. 4.11 Right profile view (with ruler)

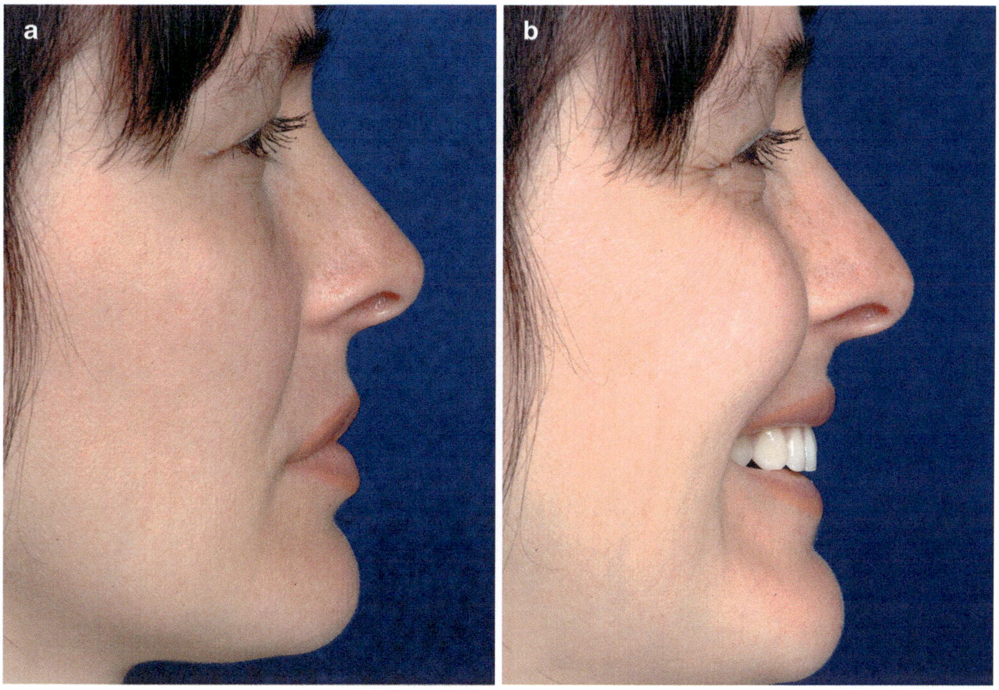

Fig. 4.12 Right profile views at rest (**a**) and during smiling (**b**)

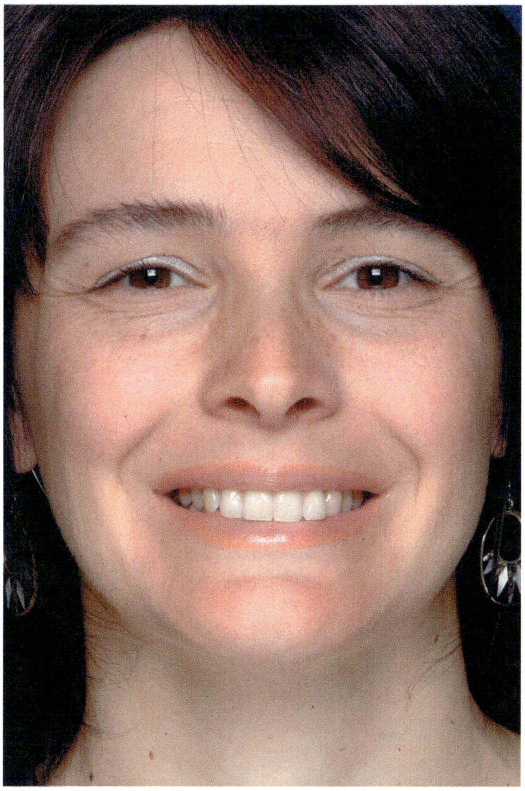

Fig. 4.13 Full-face frontal view during smiling (depressor septi muscle action)

Further Reading

To deepen the study of the standard frames used for other areas of the face, such as the auricles, the orbital region and the lower third of the face, it is possible to consult another book by the same author: Meneghini F. Clinical facial analysis. Berlin: Springer; 2005.

5 Facial and Nasal Clinical Analysis

5.1 Regions of the Face and Neck

The surface of the face and neck can be divided into basic regions or frames as follows:

1. Forehead region
2. Temporal region
3. Zygomatic arch
4. Malar region
5. Orbital region
6. Infraorbital region
7. Nasal region
8. External ear
9. Parotid-masseteric region
10. Buccal region
11. Oral region
12. Chin region
13. Mandibular border region
14. Mandibular angle region
15. Suprahyoid region
16. Submandibular triangle
17. Carotid triangle
18. Retromandibular fossa
19. Median cervical region
20. Sternocleidomastoid region

The landmarks of these anatomical regions are not always obvious, as depicted in Fig. 5.1.

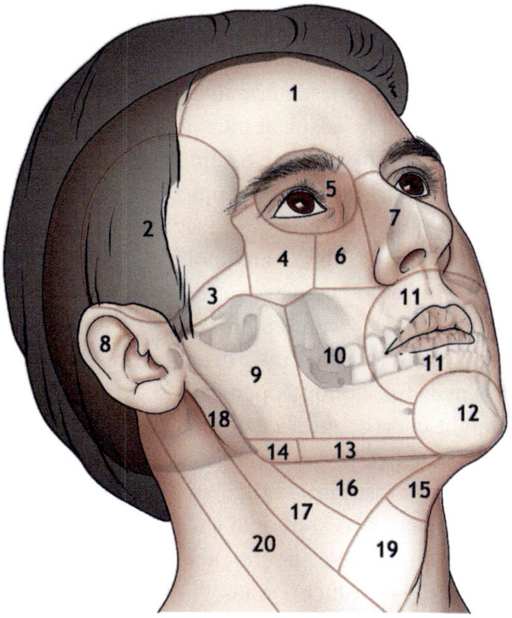

Fig. 5.1 Regions of the face and neck: *1* forehead region, *2* temporal region, *3* zygomatic arch, *4* malar region, *5* orbital region, *6* infraorbital region, *7* nasal region, *8* external ear, *9* parotid-masseteric region, *10* buccal region, *11* oral region, *12* chin region, *13* mandibular border region, *14* mandibular angle region, *15* suprahyoid region, *16* submandibular triangle, *17* carotid triangle, *18* retromandibular fossa, *19* median cervical region, *20* sternocleidomastoid region

F. Meneghini, *Basic Open Rhinoplasty*, https://doi.org/10.1007/978-3-030-61827-8_5

5.2 Basic Qualitative Facial Analysis (Without Measurements)

The preliminary analysis—the most important—of a clinical case first requires exploring some basic facial features without taking any metric or angular measurements. These quantitative measurements are frequently at variance with each other: the same nasal tip can be 2 mm under-projected utilizing the norms proposed by Doctor JX, 1 mm under-projected utilizing the parameters of Doctor JJ, or normal utilizing the data of Doctor JK! Furthermore, are the subject's sex, age, height, weight, race, hormonal balance, head positioning, and many other variables all taken into account in these normative data? I think not. So, a general assessment must be created without comparing it to normative values or a given template but using only simple adjectives and referring them to the whole face and to the main facial subunits, lines, and points. Some of the most utilized adjectives are: normal, symmetric-asymmetric, present-absent, long-short, large-small, wide-narrow, deep-shallow, convex-concave, full-hollow, open-closed, acute-obtuse, straight-curved, projected-depressed, balanced-unbalanced, deviated-centered. A particular effort is made to recognize which areas are in an ideal position and have a normal shape and volume, as they will be used as a reference in evaluating and comparing the other regions.

5.3 Frontal View Analysis

Frontal analysis starts by assessing the transverse and vertical facial dimensions and general symmetry. The relationship between the bitemporal, bizygomatic, bigonial, and mental widths, also in comparison with facial heights, determines the facial form, which varies from wide to narrow, from long to short, and from square to triangular (Fig. 5.2a, b). The grade of angularity and skeletonization of the facial form should also be noted.

Symmetry is always checked. Many patients are unaware of minor facial asymmetries and if they discover these in the postoperative period, it will lead to patient dissatisfaction and misunderstanding. My preferred way to document and show all the facial asymmetries to the patient requires the marking of the midline skin points, using a fine-tip surgical skin marker and taking the frontal, basal, and face-down views again (Fig. 5.3a–c). If the facial asymmetry is located in a lateral structure and not in the midline, as in the case of unilateral upper lid ptosis, a simple picture taken in frontal view is the best way to communicate this to the patient.

My attention is almost always focused on the central oval of the face. This extended facial region is also of interest in every basic facial analysis. The central oval of the face comprises the eyes, the eyebrows, the zygoma, the nose, the mouth, and the chin, as depicted in Fig. 5.4.

5.4 Basal View Analysis

The basal views offer an additional check in the evaluation of general facial symmetry. The shape of the nasal base, the projection of the nasal tip and eye globes, and the shape of the zygomatic arches and chin are all evaluated and judged utilizing the basal view (Fig. 5.5).

5.5 Oblique View Analysis

There are multiple oblique views because, from the pure frontal to the pure profile views, we can find 89 different head positions to the right and 89 different head positions to the left by making small intermediate rotations of one degree.

As recommended in Chap. 4, in every clinical case, I prefer to take at least three different right and left oblique views, changing the camera position and maintaining the position of the subject, with the lighting system fixed.

Ideally, an oblique view should be considered as being composed of two distinct components, which need to be analyzed separately. The first one (Fig. 5.6) is the half of the face that is facing the camera (or the eyes of the observer) and is a great aid in the evaluation of the lateral components of the face such as the temporal, zygomatic,

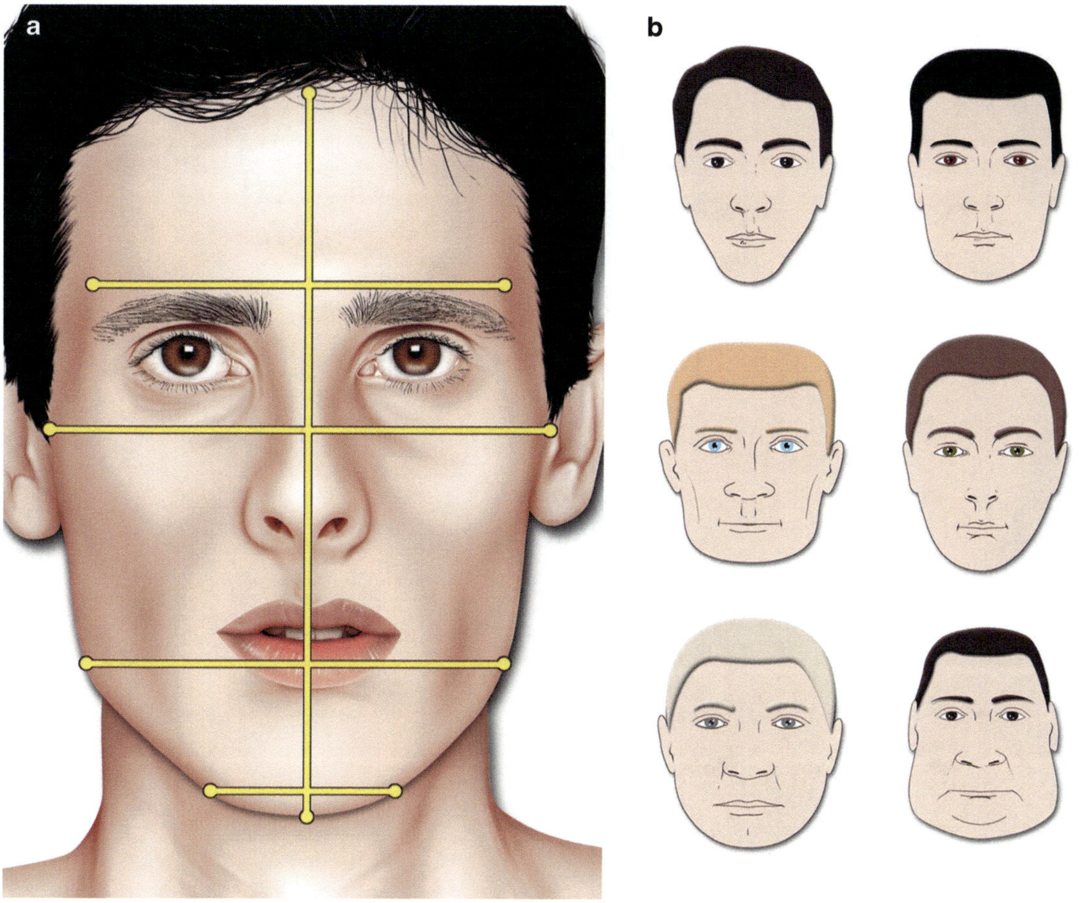

Fig. 5.2 (**a**, **b**) The bitemporal, bizygomatic, bigonial, and mental widths, and the total facial height (**a**). Examples of differences in facial form obtained by varying the width of the face at different levels (**b**)

orbital, cheek, paranasal, preauricular, and mandibular angle. This component is usually familiar to the patient, as is the frontal view, so it is utilized extensively during communication with her. The second component (Fig. 5.7) is the profile of the opposite side of the face that emerges on the background panel. In a youthful subject, it is composed of a series of gentle curves, which resembles the outline of an ogee. Here is how J. William Little describes these curves: "*The youthful facial ogee typically arises from a high, subtle lid–cheek interface and rises gradually and gracefully to a broad, uniform convexity that peaks near or above the nasal tip. It then continues as a descending convex curve to the level of the upper lip, where it rapidly reverses itself through the occlusal plane, entering a limited concavity that rises slightly at the mandibular border before curving acutely around that structure into the neck.*"

5.6 Profile View Analysis

The profile view is the most utilized by the doctor and the least known by the patient herself. Without a couple of mirrors specifically oriented or a photographic camera, nobody can observe their own profile. How many pictures, captured in profile view, do you have in your personal album? And how many times have you looked at your profile, using two mirrors, in the last year? For that reason, even if the profile view analysis is fundamental for planning and visualizing the treatment goals, it must not be overemphasized to

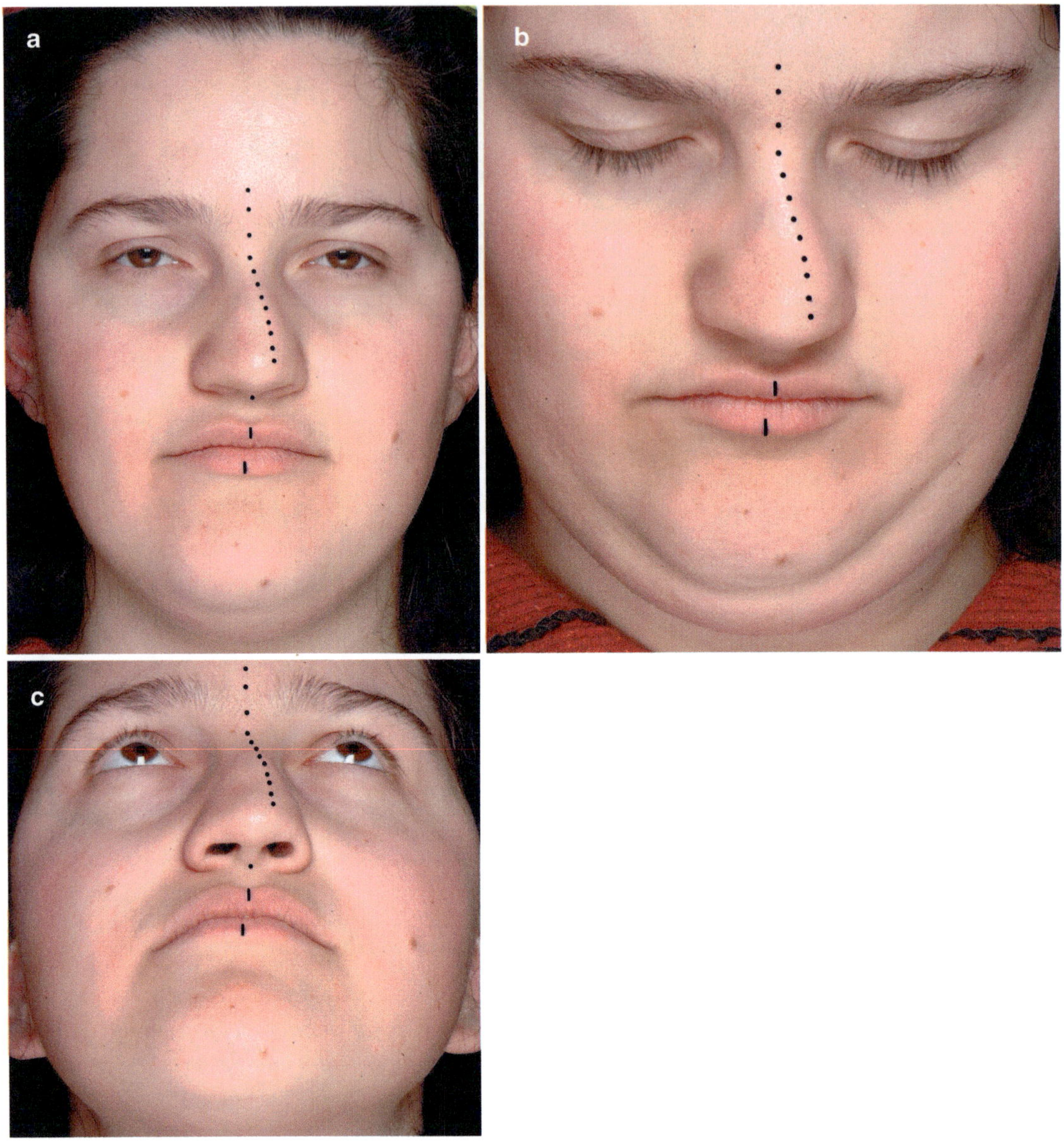

Fig. 5.3 (**a–c**) Frontal (**a**), face-down (**b**), and basal (**c**) views with midline facial points, marked with blue ink, in a clinical case of posttraumatic nasal asymmetry

the patient, stating that it is only in the eyes of the beholder. In all cases, the profile view is essential to judge some basic facial parameters, such as:

- The total face height; the heights of the upper, middle, and lower facial thirds separately; as well as the heights of the basic regions of the face (forehead, orbit, nose, upper lip, lower lip, and chin).
- The sagittal (posteroanterior) projection of the orbital ridges, zygoma, nasal radix and tip, lips, and chin.
- The slope of forehead, nasal, infraorbital, columellar, upper and lower lip, submental, mandibular border, and neck outlines.
- The
- general shape of the facial profile itself in terms of concavity/convexity.

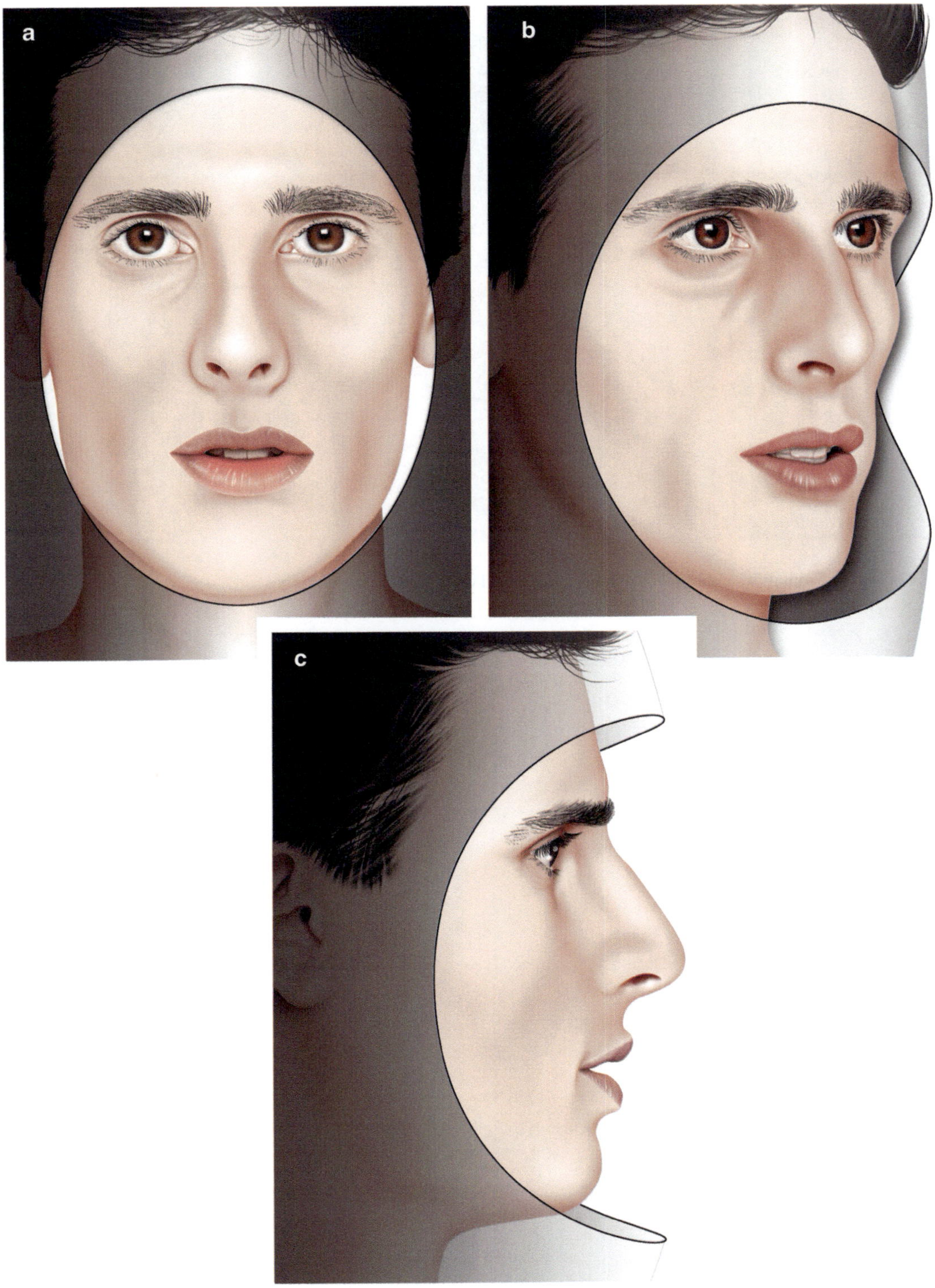

Fig. 5.4 (**a–c**) The central oval of the face in frontal (**a**), oblique (**b**), and profile views (**c**)

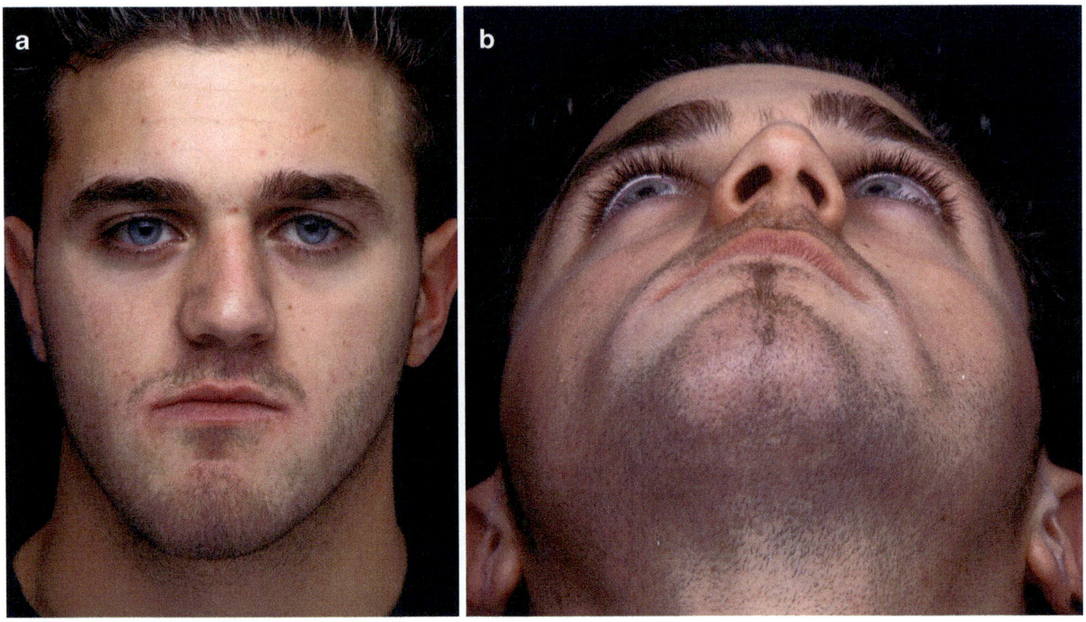

Fig. 5.5 (**a**, **b**) Frontal (**a**) and basal (**b**) views in a clinical case of facial asymmetry

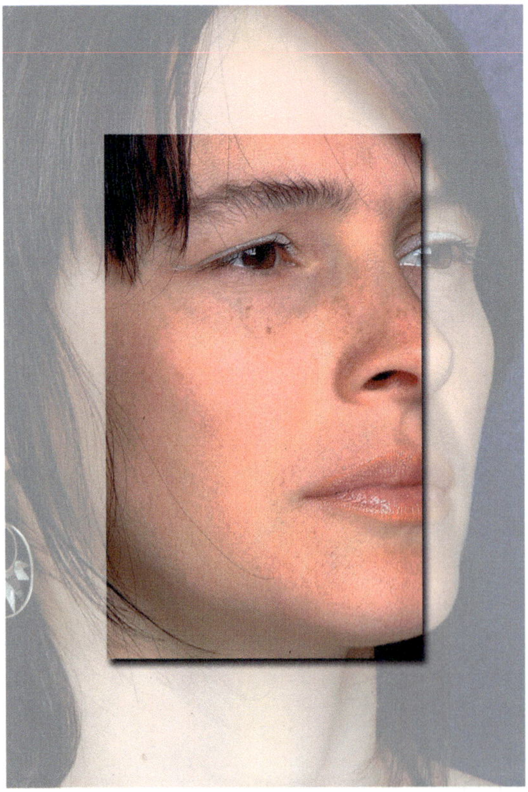

Fig. 5.6 The first component of the oblique views is facing the camera or the observer's eyes. It is a great aid in the evaluation of the lateral regions of the face such as the temporal, zygomatic, orbital, cheek, preauricular, and mandibular angle

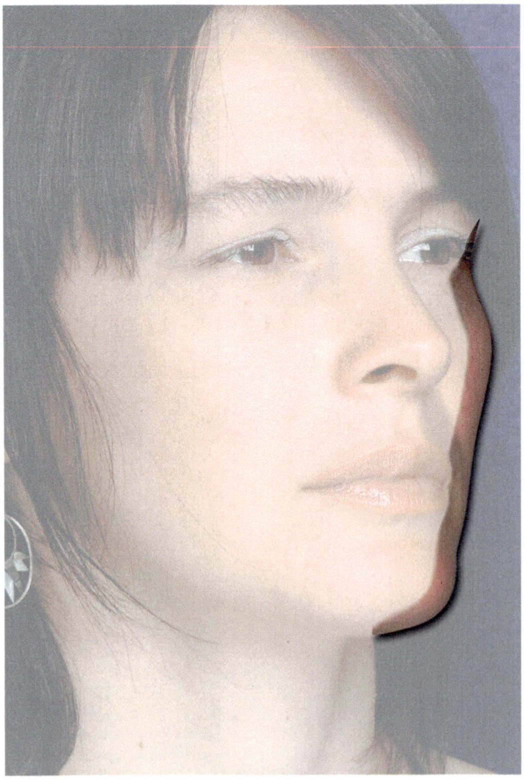

Fig. 5.7 The second component of the oblique views is the opposite profile of the face that emerges on the background panel. In a youthful subject, it is composed of a series of gentle curves, which resembles the outline of an ogee

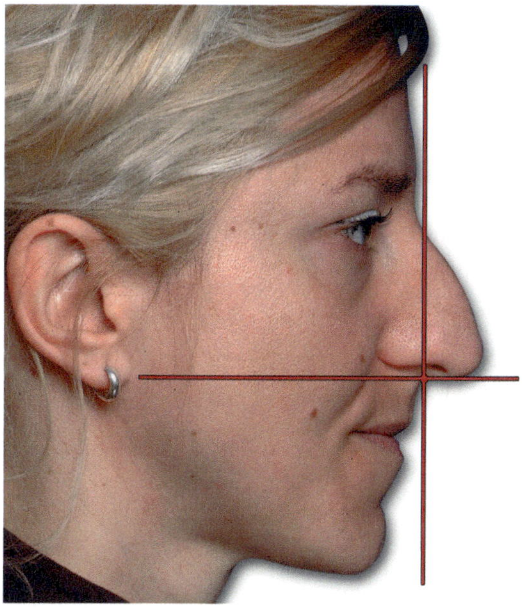

Fig. 5.8 In this photograph, taken in profile view with the subject in the natural head position, horizontal and vertical reference lines, both passing through the subnasale point, aid evaluation of the facial features

For a better evaluation of the profile view, I suggest adding two reference lines, one horizontal and one vertical, both passing through the subnasale point, as depicted in Fig. 5.8. With this approach, the vertical and sagittal position of many points, as well as the incline of some facial outlines can be studied and recorded.

5.7 The Facial Angles

The construction and assessment of facial angles is a fundamental part of basic analysis. Again, the comparison of a clinical case with an average template or normative data is seldom necessary. The most utilized photographic and radiographic view is the profile view, but all of the clinical views are suitable for an analysis by angles (Figs. 5.9a, b and 5.10a–c).

For the angles constructed utilizing views taken in the natural head position, I favor break-

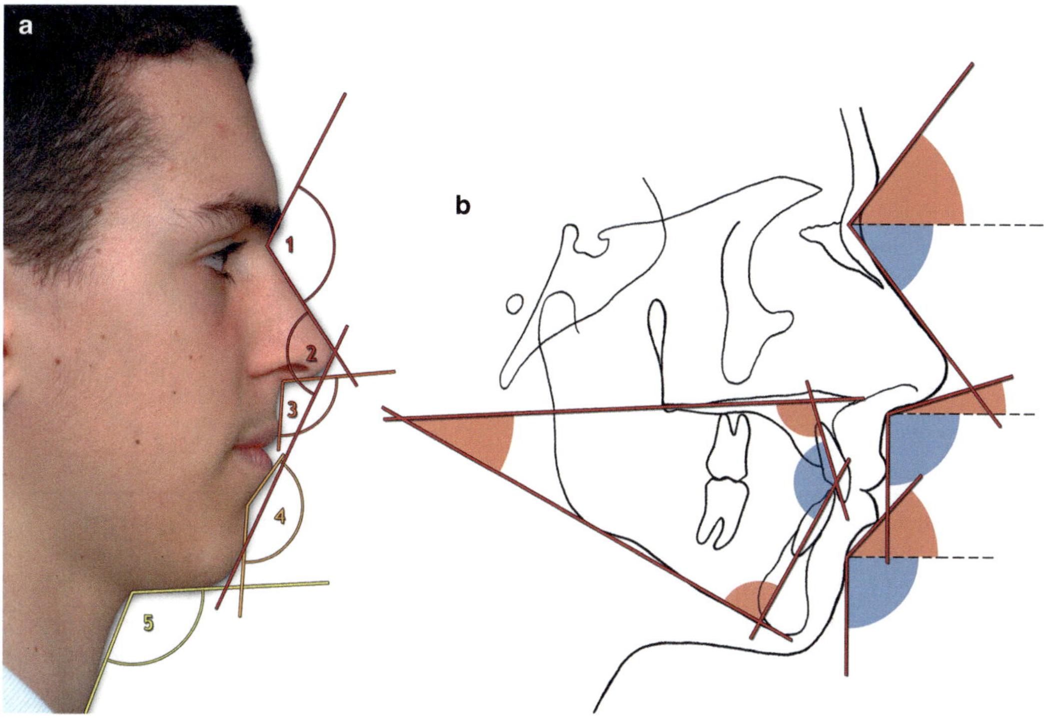

Fig. 5.9 (a, b) Angles constructed over a photographic (a) and cephalometric tracing (b) profile view of the same patient

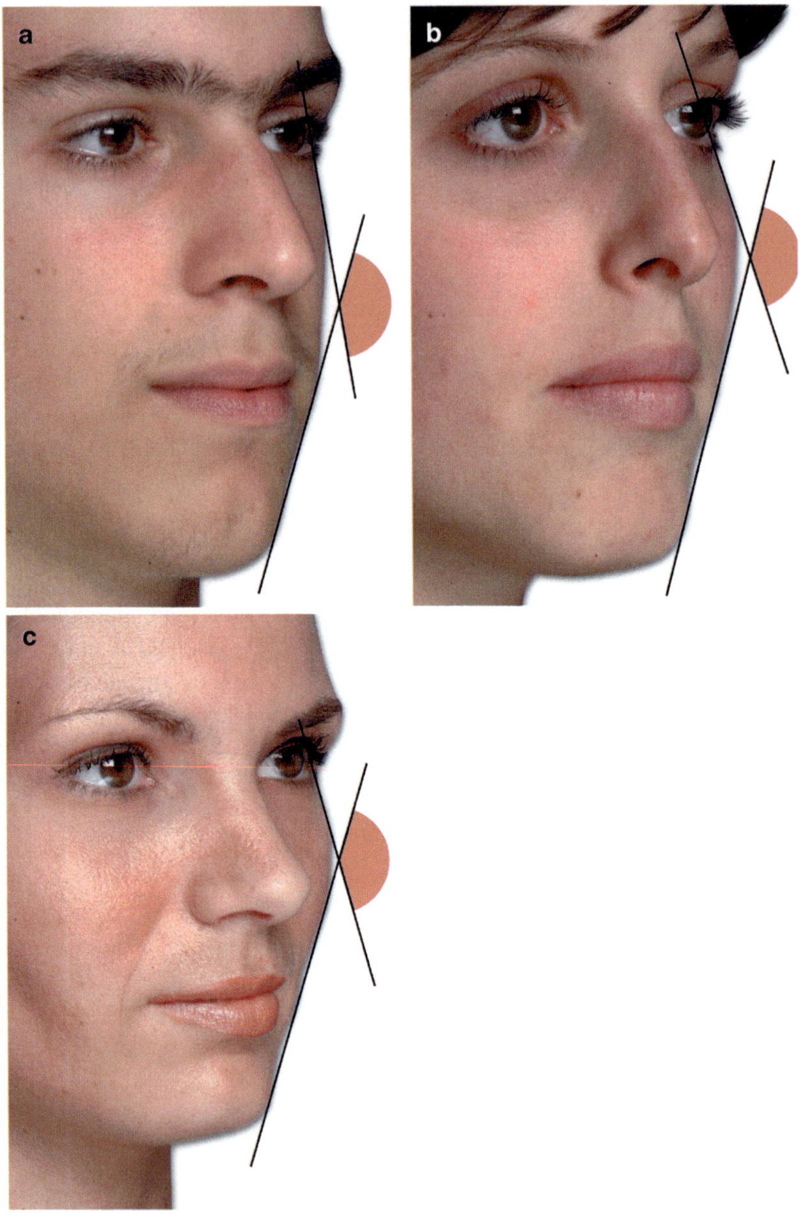

Fig. 5.10 (**a–c**) The same angle constructed over the ogee curve of three different young subjects in which the projection of the malar eminence increases from (**a**) to (**c**). There are three parameters to consider: the degree of the angle, the background area between the angle and skin profile, and the vertical level of the face at which the angle is positioned. In these three cases, from left to right, the degree of the angle decreases, the background area also decreases, and the vertical position of the angle is higher

ing up the angle into its two elementary components by dividing it with a horizontal or vertical line, as depicted in Fig. 5.11a, b. In this manner, each incline can be assessed independently from the other.

5.8 The Supporting Skeleton Assessment

Figure 5.12a–c illustrates the three main supporting structures of the facial soft tissue envelope:

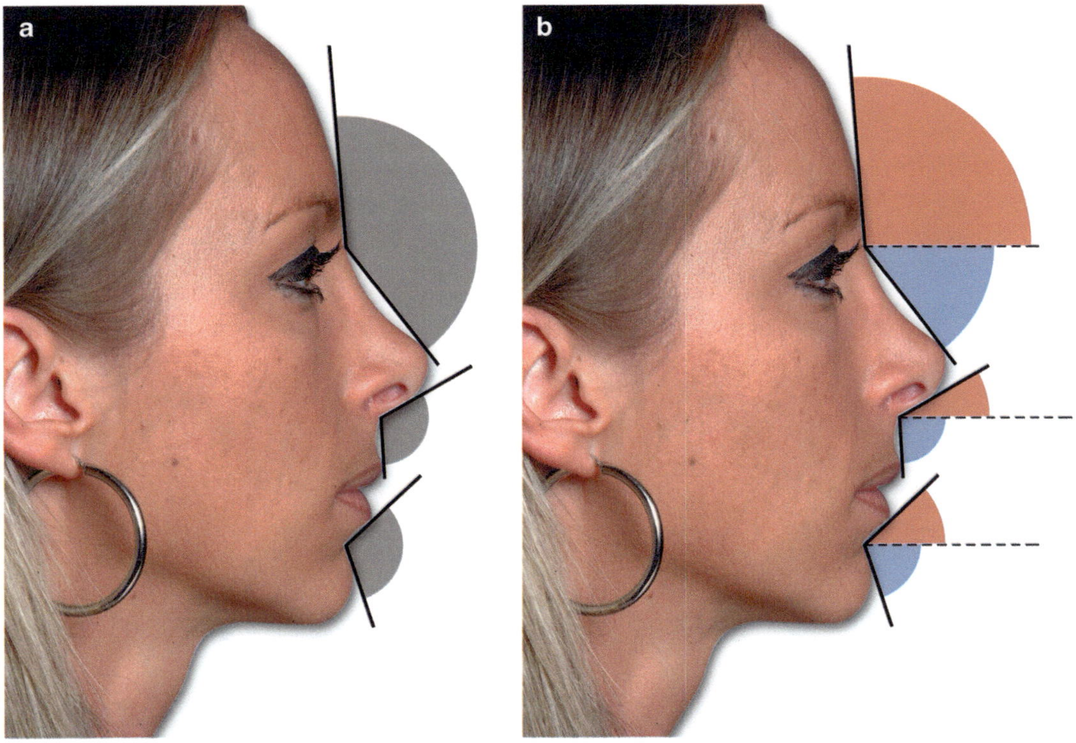

Fig. 5.11 (**a**, **b**) The absolute value of some facial angles (**a**) can be broken up into their two elementary components by a horizontal or vertical line (**b**). For example, the excessively wide subnasale angle of this clinical case is due more to an upward rotated columella and less to a clockwise rotated upper lip

the bony, the cartilaginous, and the dental structures. It can be noted that the major determinant of facial support and shape is a relatively small portion of these three components (Fig. 5.12b, c). The eye globe, with its fixed spatial position, may be assumed to be a skeletal supporting structure for the lids.

5.9 From Specific to General: A Reversed Approach to Basic Analysis

Basic facial analysis is mainly conducted observing the entire face. But often we need the input offered by a small particular to discover or confirm a general feature of the whole face. In other words, we should combine two key clinical approaches: "from general to specific" and its reverse, "from specific to general."

An example of the latter is given by the presence of the inferior scleral show. This is the presence of a small portion of white sclera between the iris and the lower lid margin in a subject examined with the natural head position and straight gaze. Tilting the head down or orienting the gaze upwards can produce a false scleral show (Fig. 5.13a–c). A true scleral show can be a sign of regional problems, such as a retracted lower lid or exophthalmia, but also of a whole facial problem such as a hypoplasia of the middle third of the face (Fig. 5.14a, b).

5.10 Points, Lines, and Subunits of the External Nose

As for the whole face, the surface of the nasal pyramid offers some points, lines, and areas for consideration (Fig. 5.15a–d):

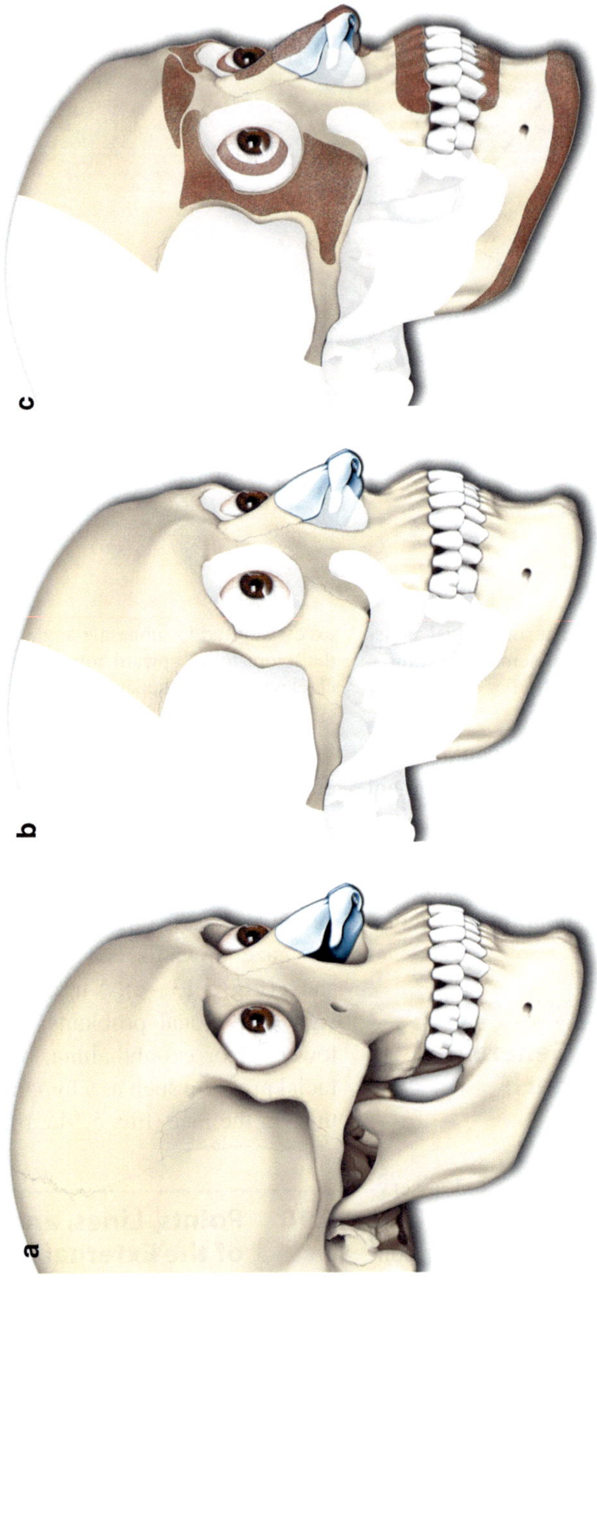

Fig. 5.12 (**a–c**) The portions of the bony skeleton (pale yellow), the teeth (white) and the nasal cartilage (pale blue) as well as the eye globe responsible for the "esthetic" support of the facial soft tissue envelope are illustrated (**a**). In (**b**) and (**c**), the main support structures are highlighted

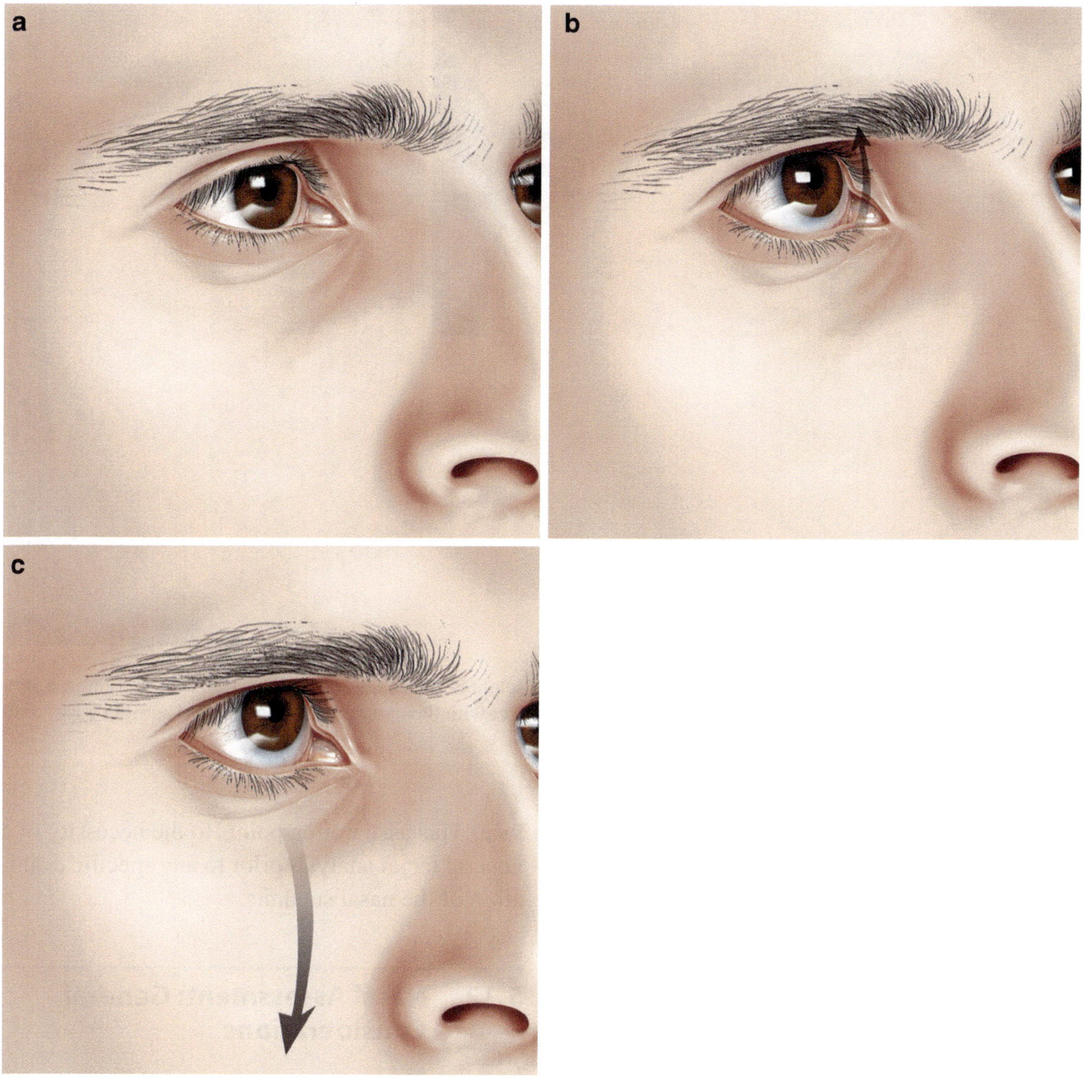

Fig. 5.13 (**a–c**) Errors in detecting the inferior scleral show. Oblique close-up view taken in the natural head position and straight gaze with no evidence of scleral show (**a**). The same subject in upward oriented gaze (**b**) and in head tilted down position (**c**) with the appearance of a false scleral show

1. Alar base width
2. Alar crease junction
3. Alar groove
4. Alar rim
5. Columella
6. Columellar base
7. Columella outline
8. Footplates of the medial crura
9. Glabella
10. Nasal base line
11. Nasal dorsum outline
12. Nasal lobule
13. Nasal lobule outline
14. Nasal radix outline
15. Nasal "unbroken" line
16. Nasion
17. Nostril sill
18. Rhinion (clinically this is evaluated with direct palpation of the dorsum)
19. Soft triangle or facet

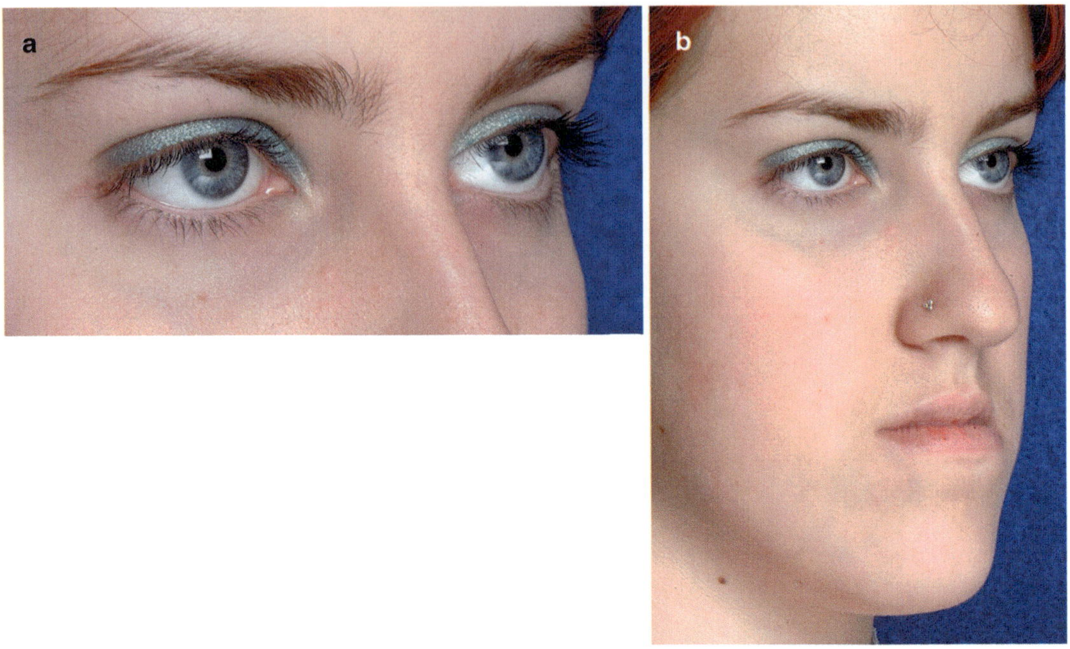

Fig. 5.14 (**a**, **b**) A clinical case in which the scleral show (**a**) is a sign of marked maxillary hypoplasia (**b**). The scleral show is the presence of a small portion of the white sclera between the iris and the lower lid margin in a subject with the natural head position and straight gaze

20. Subnasale
21. Supratip area or supratip break-point in clinical cases where a clear step over the nasal tip is present
22. Nasal tip
23. Tip defining points

5.11 Direct and Photographic Clinical Analysis for Nasal Deformities

A note reporting the major findings regarding nasal esthetics, determined by visual inspection and palpation only, is made during the first consultation. The subsequent revision and enhancement of the definitive form is written when the photographic documentation, either in a printed form or on a wide monitor, is also available.

Defining a nose as short or long, narrow or wide should also be related to the sex, height, physique, and primarily to the whole face of the subject. A "balanced" nose exists only for a given face! This assumption points to the necessity of a general facial analysis prior to any specific evaluation of the nasal subunits.

5.12 Nasal Assessment: General Considerations

The first step is the assessment of the general symmetry of the face and nose utilizing one reliable horizontal reference line. The most commonly utilized horizontal references are the lines connecting the medial canthus, the upper palpebral folds, or the apex of the eyebrow, which are easy to detect and draw; the next step is the creation of a unique vertical midline that should bisect the glabella, the nasal bridge, the nasal tip, and the Cupid's bow (Fig. 5.16a–d). In a complex case, instead of a unique vertical midline, it is necessary to trace several small midline segments for every facial subunit to evaluate better the role of nasal asymmetry in the context of an asymmetric face (Fig. 5.17a–d).

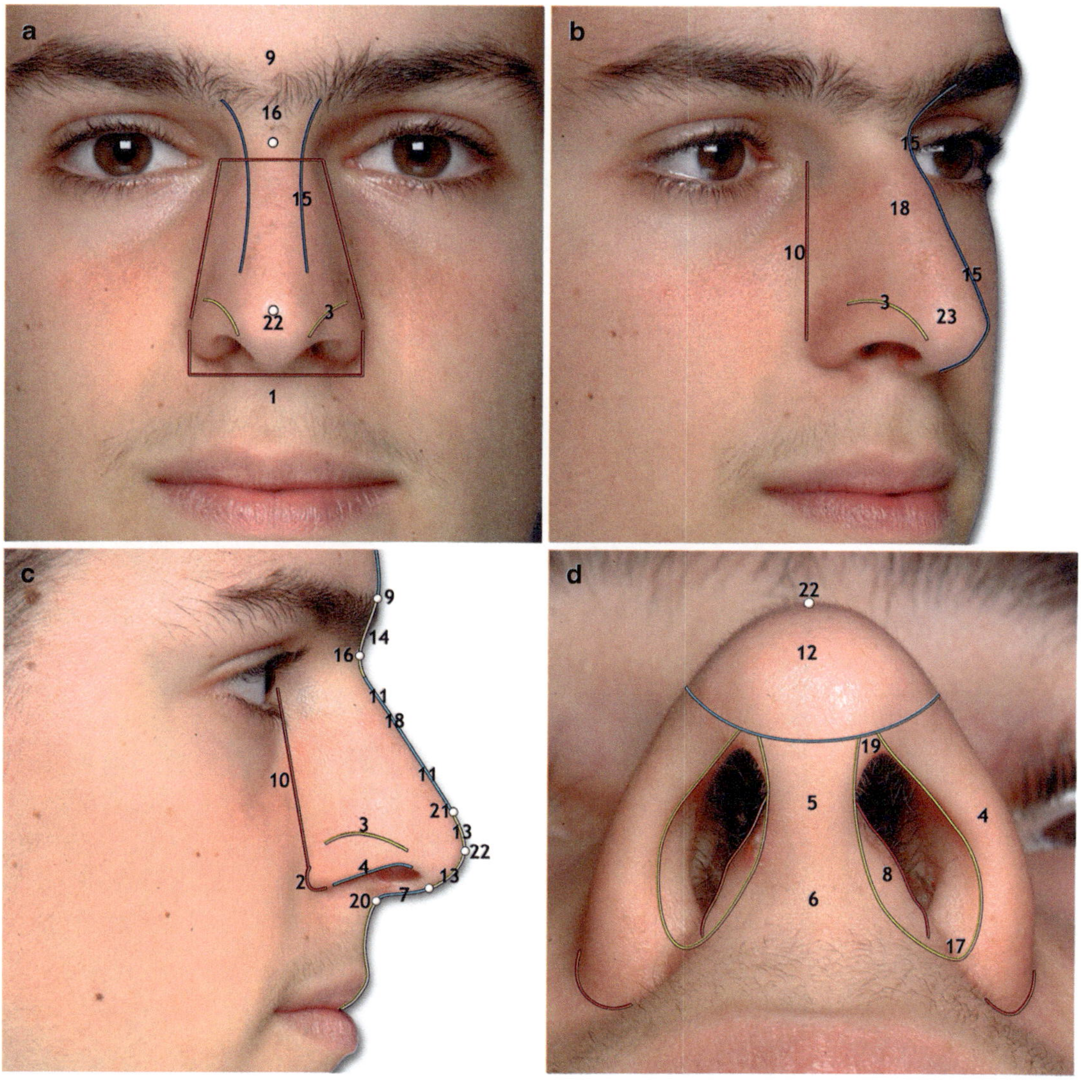

Fig. 5.15 (**a–d**) Points, lines, and subunits of the nasal surface in frontal (**a**), oblique (**b**), profile (**c**), and basal view (**d**). The numbers refer to the list reported in the text

The skeletal boundaries of the nose must be evaluated in order to recognize the surrounding structures from which the nasal pyramid emerges. Figure 5.18a–c shows these boundaries in a subject with an adequate supporting base, whereas Fig. 5.19a–d depicts three cases of depressed paranasal region due to maxillary hypoplasia and a case of an excessively protruding anterior nasal spine that greatly influences how the observer sees the shape and the projection of the nose.

Utilizing the oblique views, the entire nasal outline must be evaluated, searching for the presence of a bilateral symmetric "unbroken" line. In the attractive nose, this line descends gracefully from the supraorbital ridge onto the nasal dorsum and the nasal tip (Fig. 5.20). In the case of a deviated nose, dorsal irregularities, a dorsal hump or a dorsal saddle, this line is "broken," creating one or two steps or a strong curve, as depicted in Fig. 5.21a–c. Utilizing the nasal outline obtained

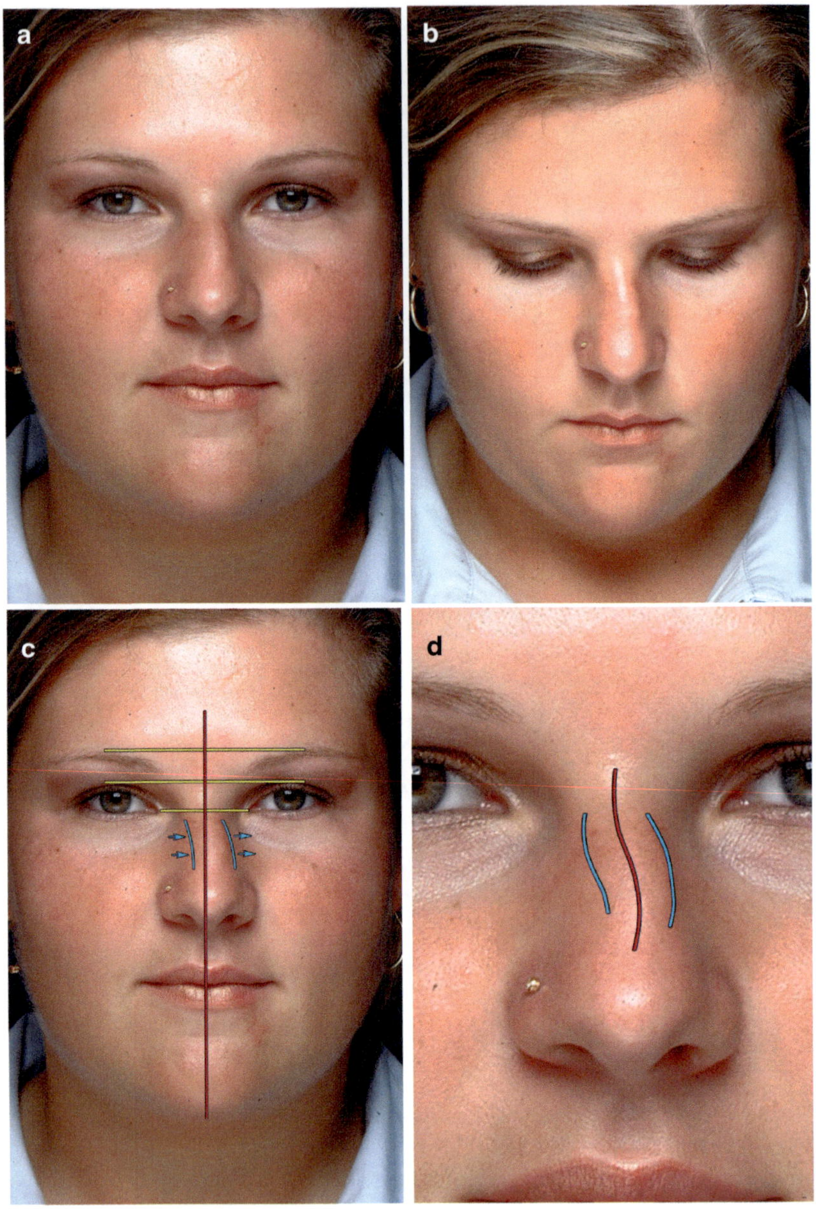

Fig. 5.16 (**a–d**) An example of a symmetric face with an asymmetric nose secondary to a previous trauma (**a–d**); in this case, the horizontal reference lines are reliable in constructing the vertical midline

from the oblique view helps in the assessment of the type, grade, and location of the deformity.

The nasal profile slope should be assessed clinically and utilizing the full-face profile view for a better comparison with the whole facial profile. In many cases, identifying and drawing the dorsal line is an easy task and the difficulties that can remain lie only in the construction of a correct facial plane (Fig. 5.22).

In some nasal and dentofacial deformities, the assessment of nasal slope can be difficult. In a posttraumatic nose with dorsal irregularities, as in a combination of bone hump and cartilage saddle, more than one dorsal line can be considered (Fig. 5.23a, b). Furthermore, none of these lines can be utilized as guidance for the visualization of the treatment goals as they reflect the actual situation measured at different levels (bony nasal

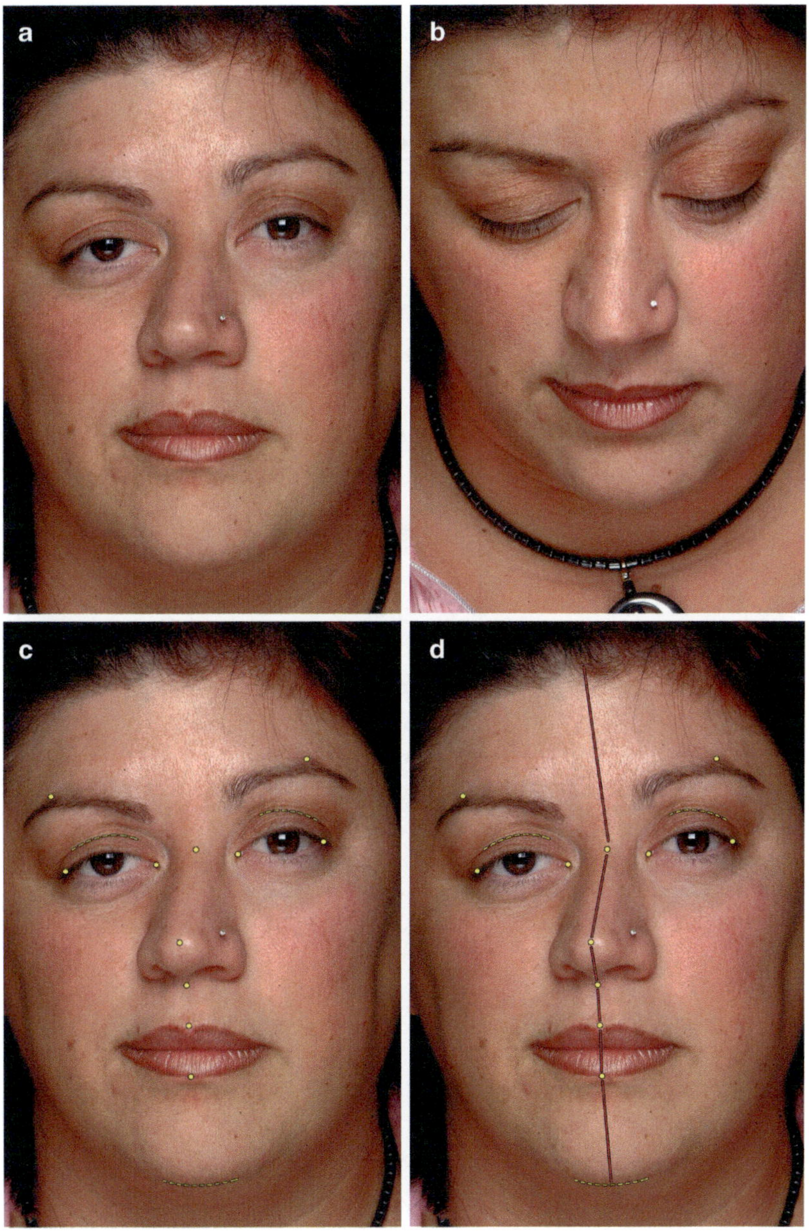

Fig. 5.17 (**a–d**) In a complex asymmetric case, instead of a unique central vertical line, it is necessary to trace several small midline segments for every facial subunit (**a–d**) in order to evaluate better the role of the nose in the whole asymmetry

dorsum, cartilaginous nasal dorsum, and nasal lobule outline) and not the ideal slope for this subject.

The difficulty in assessing the nasal slope increases in the case of obvious nasal deformity combined with an equally obvious dentofacial deformity. Tracing some reference points and lines helps the observer to distinguish and grade the severity of each deformity (Fig. 5.24). In the sections dedicated to specific nasal regions, such as radix and lobule, more of the factors affecting the real and perceived nasal slope are explored.

The next step consists of the appreciation of nasal widths. It should be done considering eight different basic parameters:

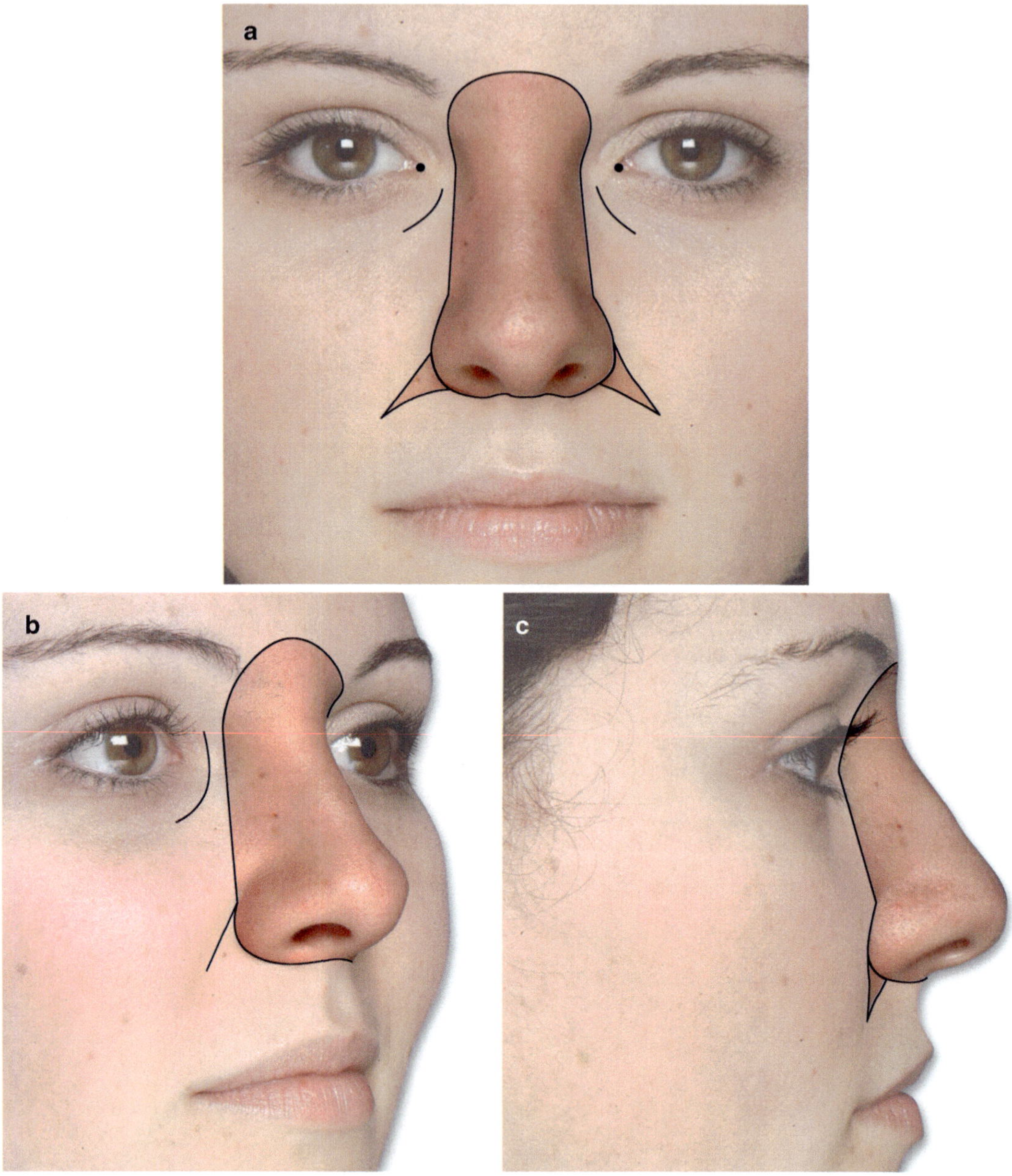

Fig. 5.18 (**a–c**) The skeletal boundaries of the nasal pyramid in frontal (**a**), oblique (**b**), and profile view (**c**)

- Whole nasal width.
- Radix width at the level of the base.
- Radix width at the level of the profile.
- Dorsal width at the level of the base.
- Dorsal width at the level of the profile.
- Alar base width.
- Nasal tip width.
- Columellar base width.

Figure 5.25a, b shows a case of a large nose in which all eight widths are depicted.

The general nose assessment is not finished without examining the overlaying skin and without the information obtainable by palpation. The skin assessment is a very important step; from radix to tip, along the midline, the thickness of the soft tissue envelope is thick

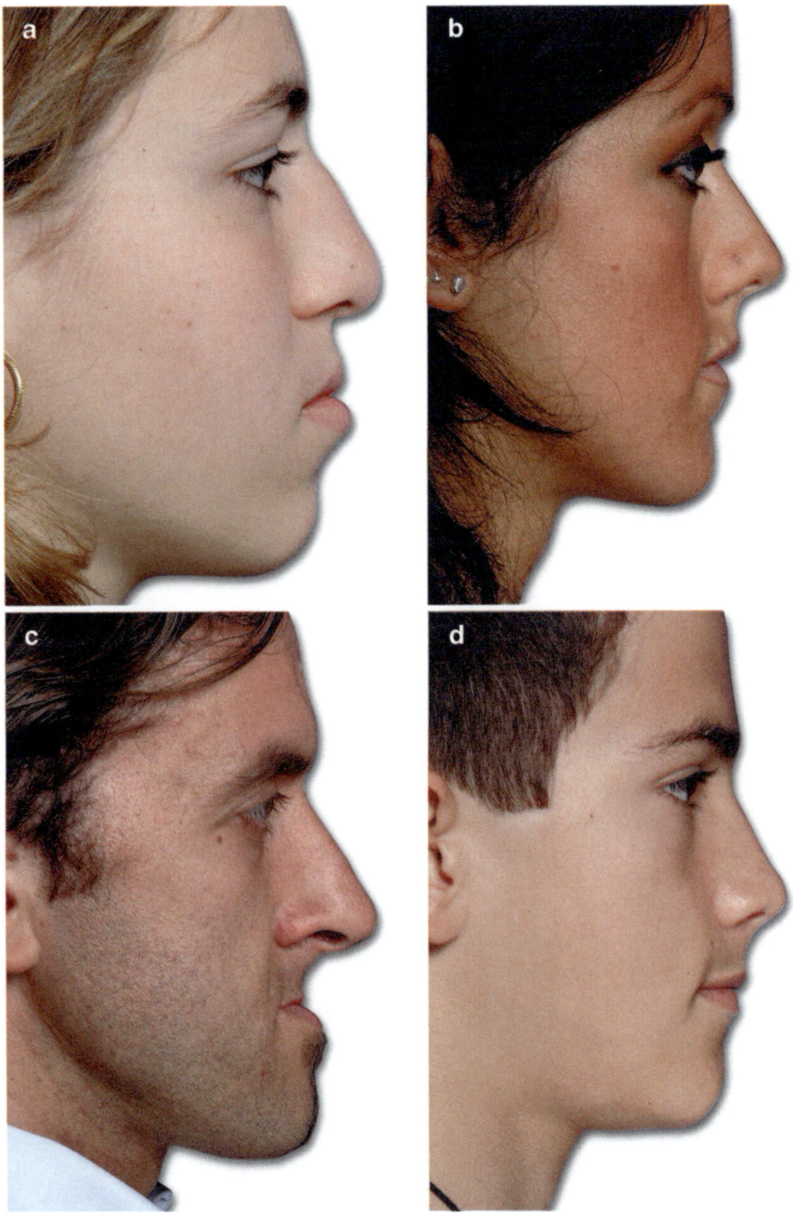

Fig. 5.19 (**a–d**) Three cases of depressed paranasal region due to maxillary hypoplasia (**a–c**) and a case of an excessively protruding anterior nasal spine (**d**) that greatly influences how the observer sees the shape and projection of the nose

over the glabella and radix break-point, thinner over the rhinion, and thick again at the supratip area (Fig. 5.26a). Moving from the midline to the nasal base line, at the level of the radix and osteocartilaginous dorsum, the skin thickness increases (Fig. 5.26b). The skin thickness at the level of the lobule and the base of columella is highly variable and must be assessed precisely in each case (Fig. 5.27a–d).

Utilizing the thumb and the index finger of the dominant hand (Fig. 5.28a–f), the nose is palpated in order to establish:

- The length of the nasal bones (Fig. 5.28a).
- The presence of any bony or cartilaginous irregularities (Fig. 5.28b–c).
- The level of the most anterior-inferior aspect of the septal cartilage profile with respect to

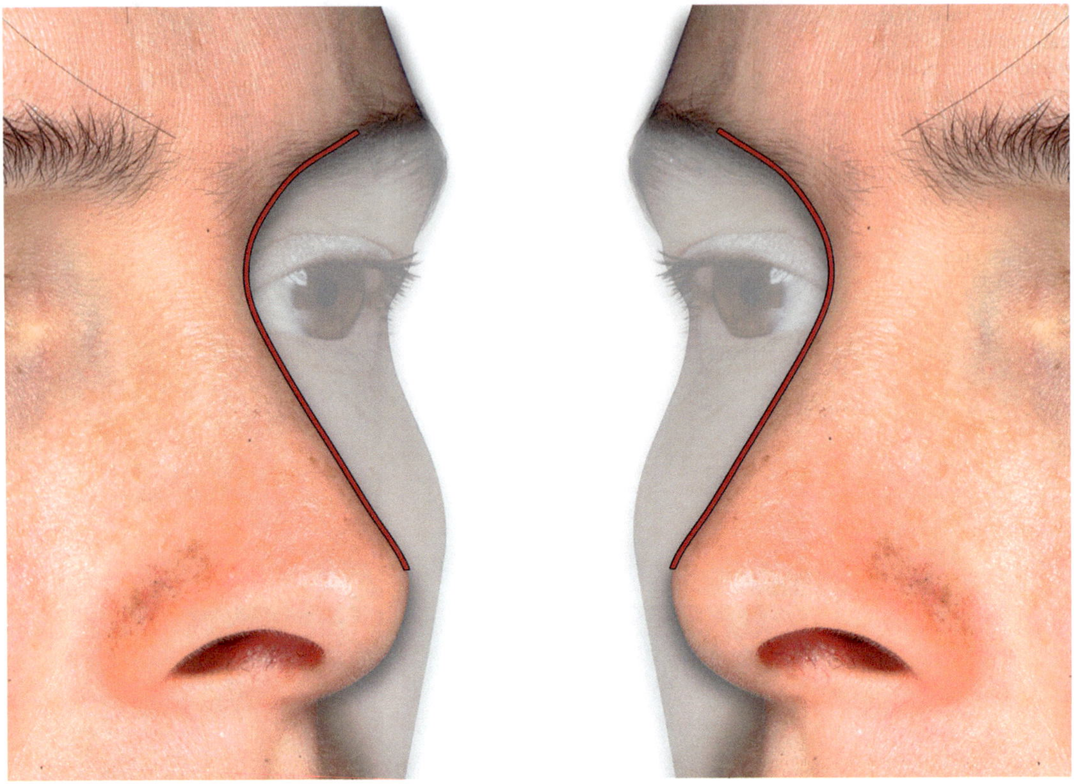

Fig. 5.20 The nasal unbroken line is the outline of the nasal pyramid in oblique view. In the attractive nose, this line descends gracefully and symmetrically from the supraorbital ridge onto the nasal dorsum and the nasal tip

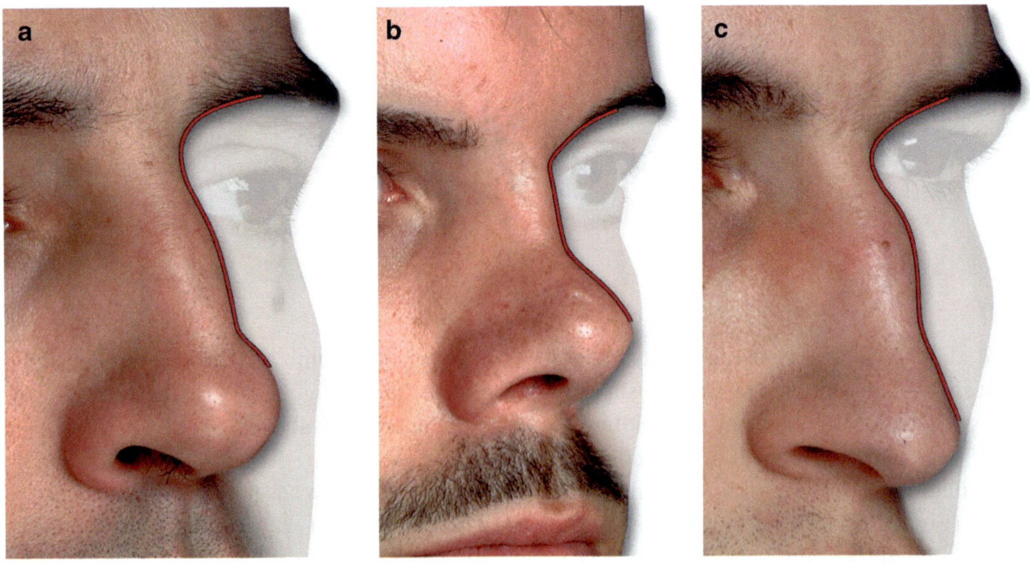

Fig. 5.21 (**a–c**) The nasal outline in oblique view of a dorsal hump (**a**), a dorsal saddle (**b**), and a crooked nose (**c**)

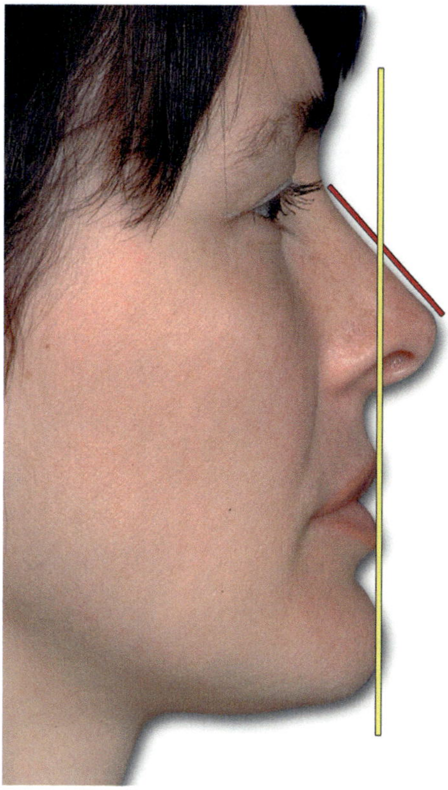

Fig. 5.22 Identifying and tracing the dorsal line can be relatively easy to do in the case of a straight dorsal outline. In this patient, the main difficulty is recognizing the projection of the chin that alters the facial plane. A vertical reference line passing through the subnasale point helps in the visualization of the excess chin projection

the most projecting point of the lobule (Fig. 5.28d).

- The resistance offered by the cartilaginous dorsum and nasal tip to posterior displacement by pressure as well as the speed with which the tip returns to its normal configuration upon release (Fig. 5.28e, f).
- The grade of passive mobility of the skin over the skeletal framework.

Other points to consider regarding the nasal soft tissue envelope are the presence of scars, the grade of elasticity and atrophy, as well as the presence of telangiectasia.

5.13 Nasal Upper Third Assessment

Identifying the spatial location of the radix break-point and the definition of the nasofrontal angle is a fundamental part of nasal analysis.

The radix break-point is the most posterior point of the outline between the nasal dorsum and the frontal bone. Any change in the radix break-point influences how the observer judges the length as well as the slope of the entire nose. It is best assessed utilizing the corneal plane, the glabella, and the superior palpebral fold as references, even if each of these references should critically be checked for its reliability (Fig. 5.29a–f).

The nasofrontal angle is not necessarily measured and can be assessed simply by drawing (or imaging) two lines on the profile. The upper line is based on the mean inclination of the outline from glabella to the radix break-point, whereas the lower one is based on the mean inclination of the outline from the radix break-point to the supratip area. Figure 5.30a–c shows the nasofrontal angle of the three clinical cases presented in Fig. 5.29a–f.

The profile of the bony portion is usually one-third of the entire nasal dorsum and should be palpated to identify the real length of the nasal bones. Any convexity/concavity, symmetry/asymmetry, unilateral/bilateral lateral hump must be assessed visually.

5.14 Nasal Middle Third Assessment

The clinical analysis of the central portion of the nasal pyramid considers the symmetry, outline, slope, volume, and shape of the cartilaginous dorsum. A particular mental exercise, that correlates the external aspect of the nasal dorsum at every level with the corresponding structural bony or cartilaginous architecture, can be very helpful (Fig. 5.31a–f).

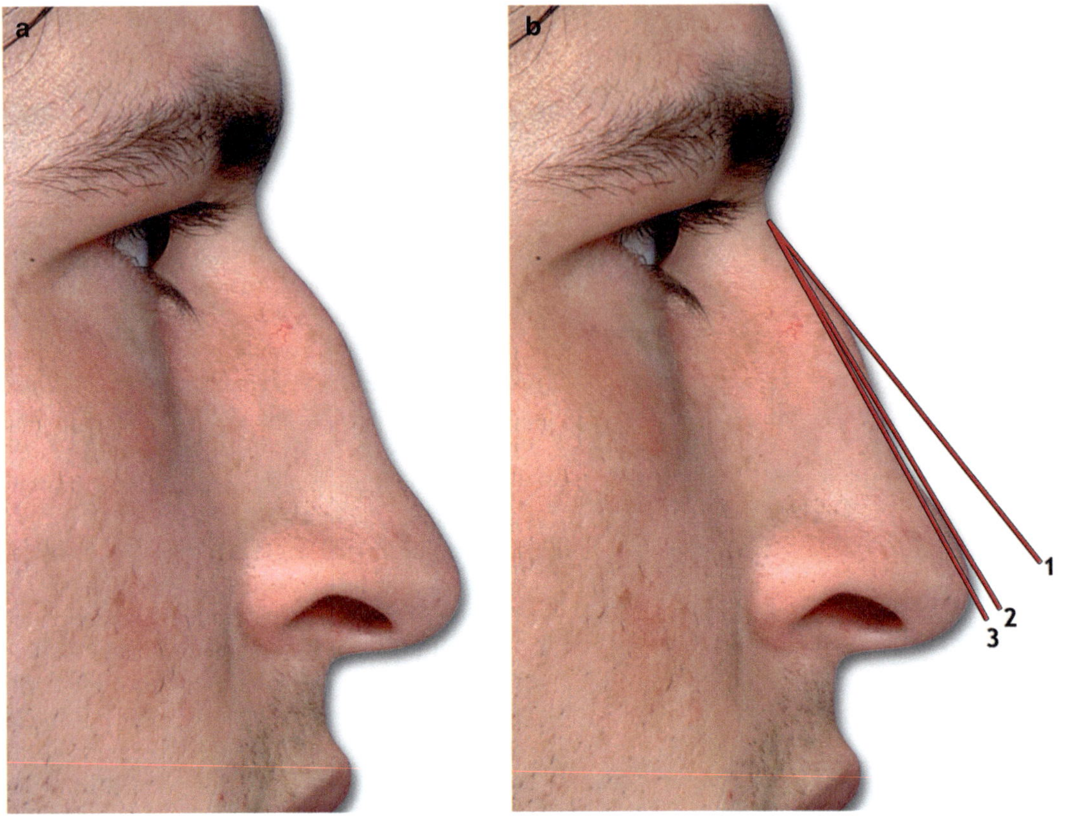

Fig. 5.23 (**a**, **b**) A case in which the outcome of nasal trauma results in a bone hump and a cartilaginous saddle (**a**). The construction of the dorsal profile line can be done in different ways (**b**): line 1 is superimposed on the nasal bone outline, line 2 is superimposed on the lobule outline, and line 3 is superimposed on the cartilaginous dorsum outline. None of these lines can be utilized as guidance for the visualization of the treatment goals as they reflect the actual situation measured at different levels (bony nasal dorsum, cartilaginous nasal dorsum, and nasal lobule outline) and not the ideal slope for this subject

The separation between bony and cartilaginous dorsum has its value in that the surgeon needs to treat these two "materials" differently at the time of surgery; however, from the point of view of any other observer, such as the patient, the dorsum is best considered as a unique, highly visible structure connecting the radix to the tip.

The great difficulty in assessing the dorsum often lies in the visual influence of the radix and the tip, which are rarely ideal. So, after the general assessment, it is preferable to reconsider the analysis of the dorsum, when the "construction" of the correct radix and tip is done.

5.15 Nasal Lower Third Assessment

The clinical assessment of the nasal tip must consider these parameters:

- Projection
- Rotation
- Position
- Volume
- Definition
- Width
- Shape

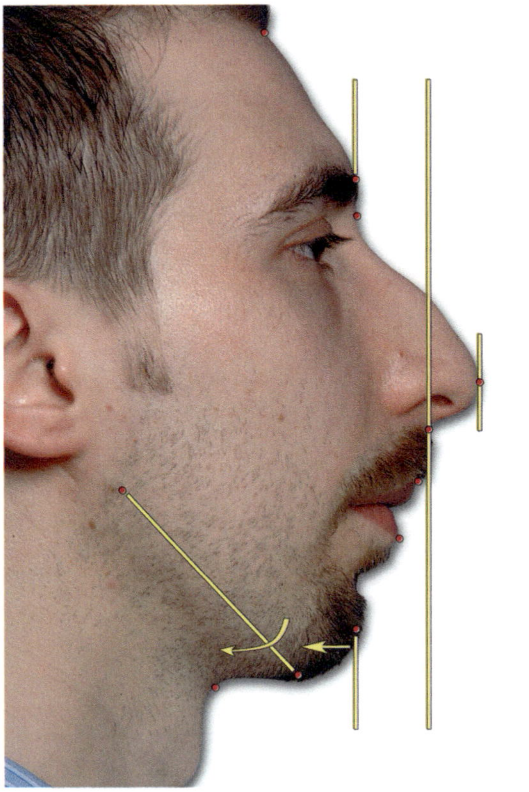

Fig. 5.24 A clinical case combining a clear nasal and dentofacial deformity. Tracing of some reference points and lines helps to distinguish and grade the severity of each deformity. On understanding the degree of the microgenia and mandibular clockwise rotation, the extent of the counterclockwise rotation of the nasal slope is not as great as may appear on initial examination

The tip projection is measured from the alar crease junction (ACJ) to the most anterior point of the nasal tip (T) and can be divided into intrinsic and extrinsic projection. The intrinsic projection is related to the lobule portion of the tip, whereas the extrinsic projection is related to the length of the ala and the columella (Fig. 5.32a–e).

The angle of tip rotation is measured between the ACJ–T line and the vertical reference; its normative mean value is 105° for females and 100° for males (Fig. 5.33a–d). The data obtained by this analysis must be added to those emerging from the evaluation of columella incline, the alar profile incline, as well as the incline and the length of the upper lip (see also the next section) (Fig. 5.34).

The tip position refers to the location of the tip along the dorsal line (Fig. 5.35). This assessment helps in judging the actual length of the nose, as well as any planned surgical modification of the dorsal profile (shortening or lengthening) varying the tip.

The tip volume, definition, width, and shape are considered intrinsic characteristics of the nasal lobule. The tip volume refers to the size of the lobule and is primarily related to the shape, dimension, and orientation of the lateral crura of the lower lateral cartilage (Fig. 5.36a).

The tip definition is related to the transition between the most anterior projecting section of the lower lateral crura, the domal segment, and the nearest portion of the lateral crura. In particular, at surgery, the convexity of the dome should turn into a slight concavity on the lateral crura to create a well-defined tip (Fig. 5.36b).

The tip width refers to the distance between the paired domes (Fig. 5.36c).

The classification of the nasal tip based on its external form has produced many shape-related terms such as boxy tip, bulbous tip, and pinched nose. In the basal view, the shape considered to be ideal resembles a triangle (Fig. 5.36d).

Figure 5.37a–h shows a case of a "boxy" tip deformity that is apparent only in frontal and basal views, whereas Fig. 5.38a–d illustrates a secondary deformity concerning the whole nose, with a tip defined in the literature as "pinched."

The columellar show is the area of visible columella under the alar rim (Fig. 5.39a). It is best evaluated in profile view and its normal range is between 2 and 4 mm; as well as the measurement, however, the ala and columellar profile should be analyzed in depth, considering the different combinations of the relationship between ala and columella categorized by Gunter et al. A reduced columellar show can be produced by a hanging ala (Fig. 5.39b), a retracted columella (Fig. 5.39c), or the combination of these two conditions, whereas an increased columellar show can be produced by a retracted ala (Fig. 5.39d), a hanging

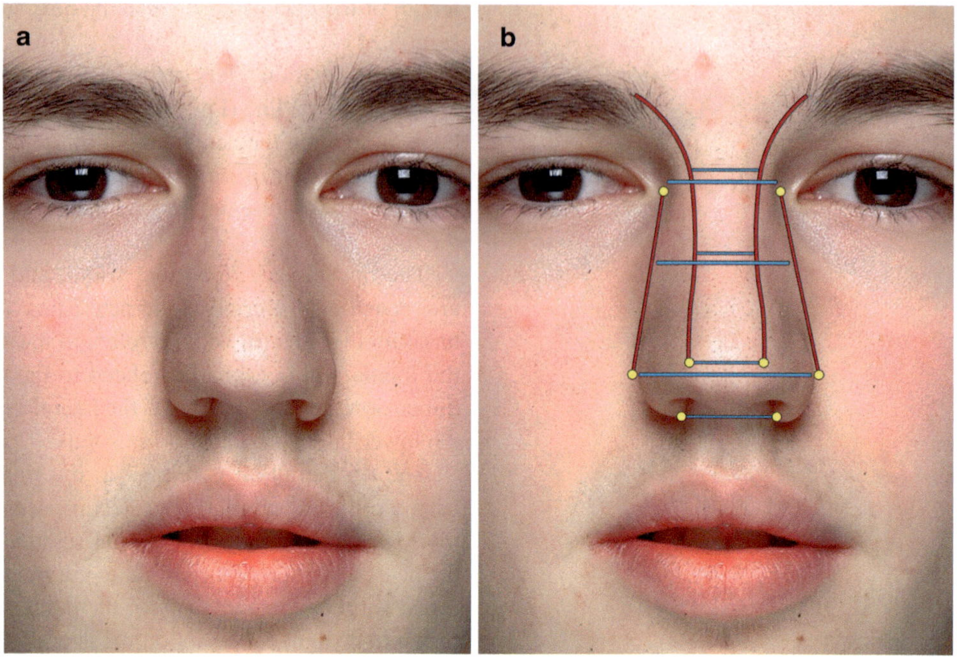

Fig. 5.25 (**a**, **b**) Frontal view of a "large nose" in a teenager (**a**). The analysis of nasal width should consider eight different basic parameters (**b**): whole nasal width, radix width at the level of the base, radix width at the level of the profile, dorsal width at the level of the base, dorsal width at the level of the profile, alar base width, nasal tip width, columellar base width

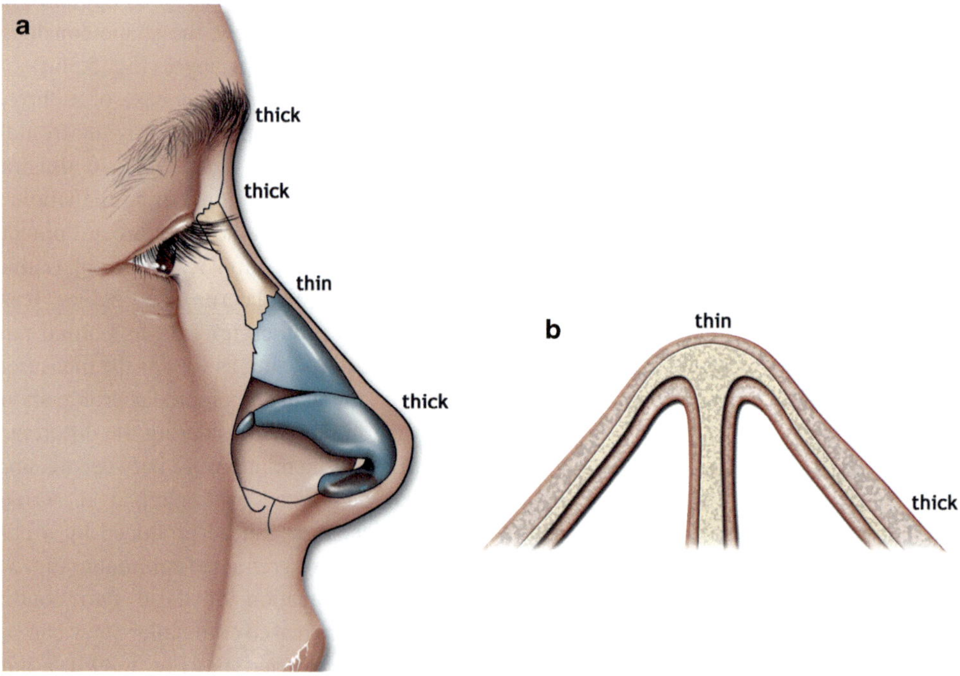

Fig. 5.26 (**a**, **b**) From radix to tip, along the midline, the thickness of the soft tissue envelope is thick over the glabella and radix break-point, thinner over the rhinion and thick again at the supratip area (**a**). Moving from the midline to the nasal base line, at the level of the radix and osteocartilaginous dorsum, the skin thickness progressively increases (**b**)

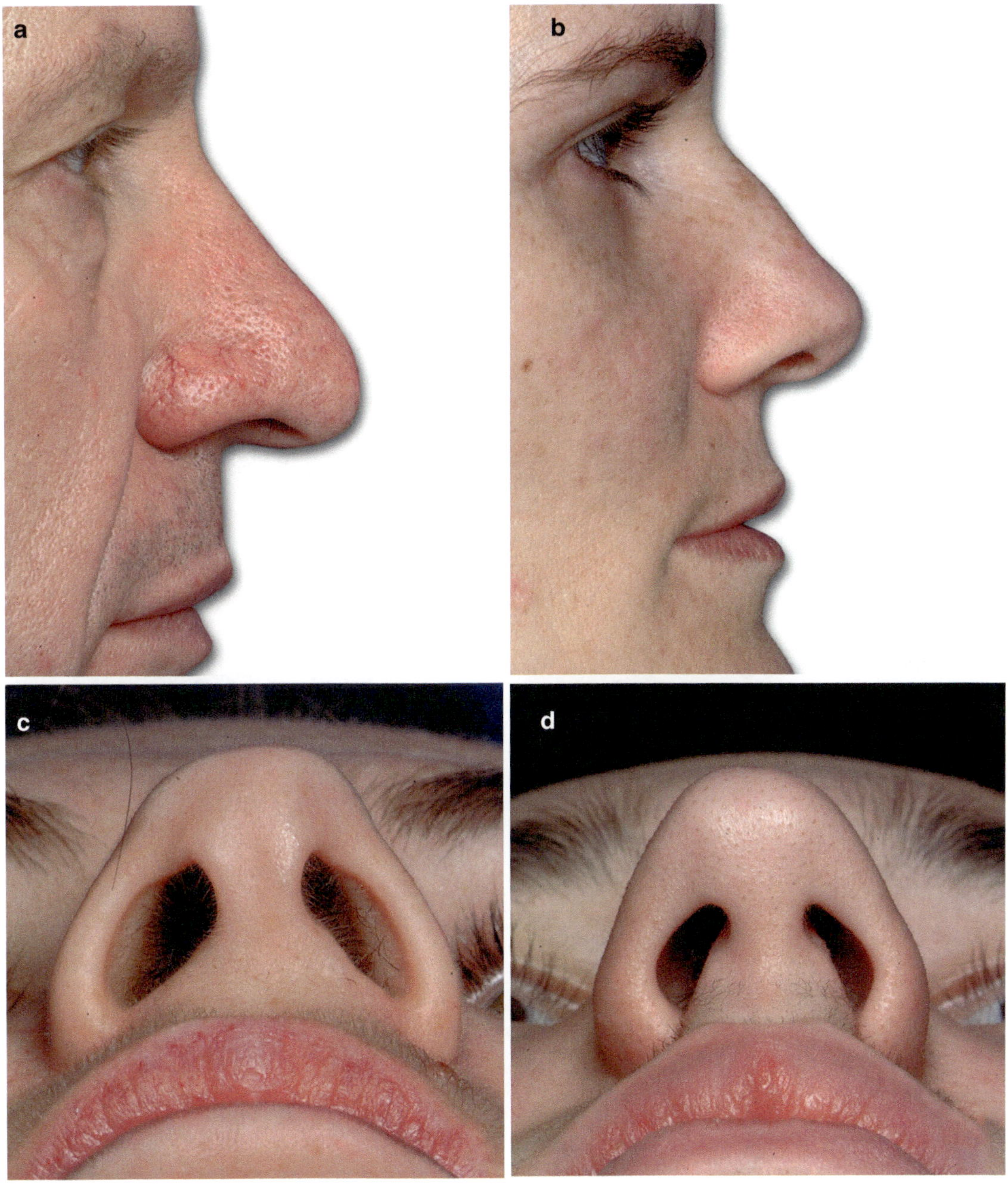

Fig. 5.27 (**a–d**) A case of thick sebaceous skin that hides the underlying cartilaginous skeleton of the nasal tip (**a**) and the opposite condition in which the shape and volume of the lower lateral cartilage are easily assessed through the skin (**b**, **c**). A clinical case presenting a large columellar base due to increased soft tissue envelope thickness (**d**)

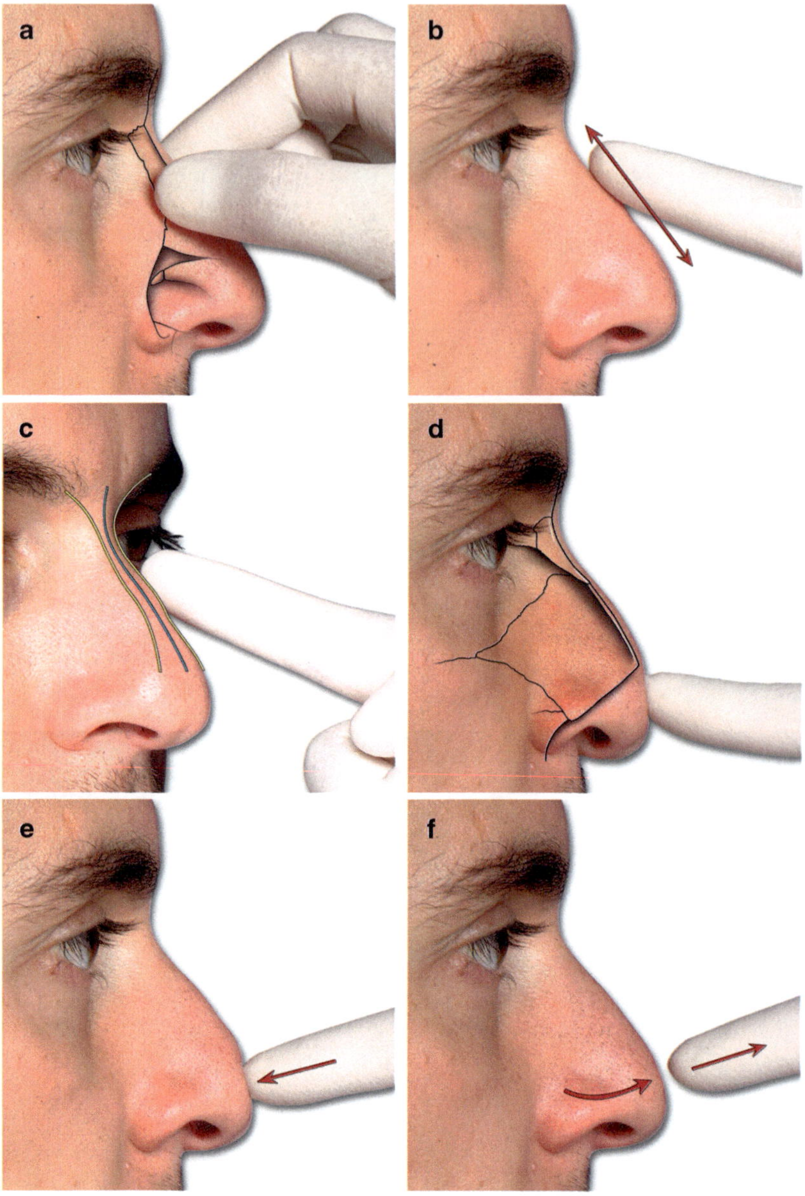

Fig. 5.28 (**a–f**) Utilizing the thumb and the index finger of the dominant hand, the examiner can feel the distal end of the paired nasal bones (**a**), detect any bony or cartilaginous irregularities on the midline or the lateral aspects of the dorsum otherwise not evident (**b**, **c**), evaluate the distal portion of the septal cartilage outline normally hidden between the two domes (**d**), feel the amount of resistance offered by the cartilaginous dorsum and nasal tip to posterior displacement, and observe the speed with which the tip returns to its normal configuration upon release (**e**, **f**)

columella (Fig. 5.39e), or the combination of these two conditions. The ideal outline of the paired nasal alar rims and the columella, in frontal view, should resemble the figure of a gull in flight (Fig. 5.39f). A different condition, similar to the retracted ala, is the notched alar rim, in which the gentle curvature of the alar outline is lost with the formation of an evident angle (Fig. 5.40).

5.16 The Close Relationship Between the Nose and the Upper Lip

Simply changing the observer's point of view in front of the subject changes the relationship between the columella and the upper lip, the nostril show and also the light reflex over the tip.

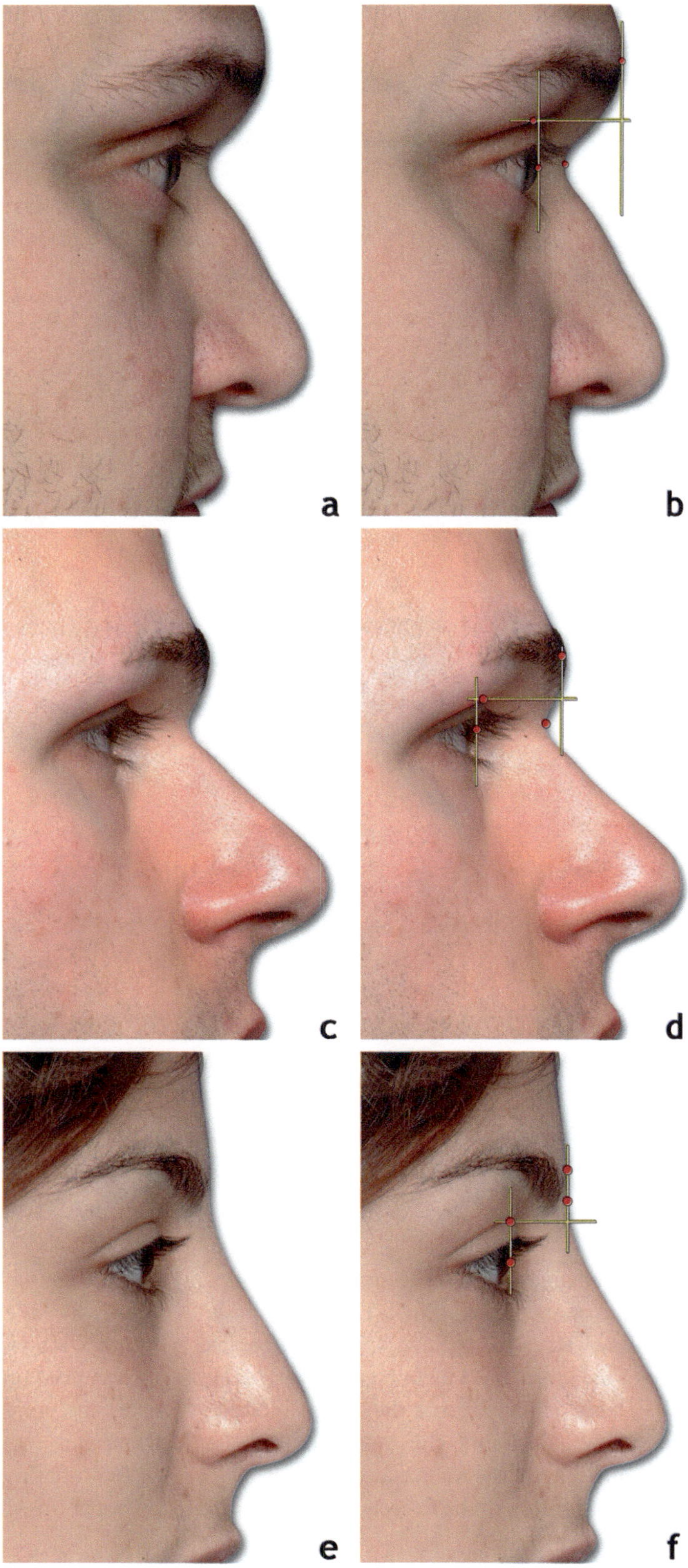

Fig. 5.29 (**a–f**) Profile views of three different clinical examples of nasal radix. A excessively posterior and inferior nasal radix near the corneal plane and well below the superior palpebral fold; the anteriorly positioned glabella is in part secondary to the pneumatization of the frontal sinus (**a**, **b**). An inferior positioned radix break-point, clearly below the superior palpebral fold, which can be mistakenly judged as being too posterior; in this case the distance between the corneal plane and the nasal outline is not reduced (**c**, **d**). A shallow nasal upper third outline with an excessively anterior and superior radix break-point, which makes the nose appear too long (**e**, **f**)

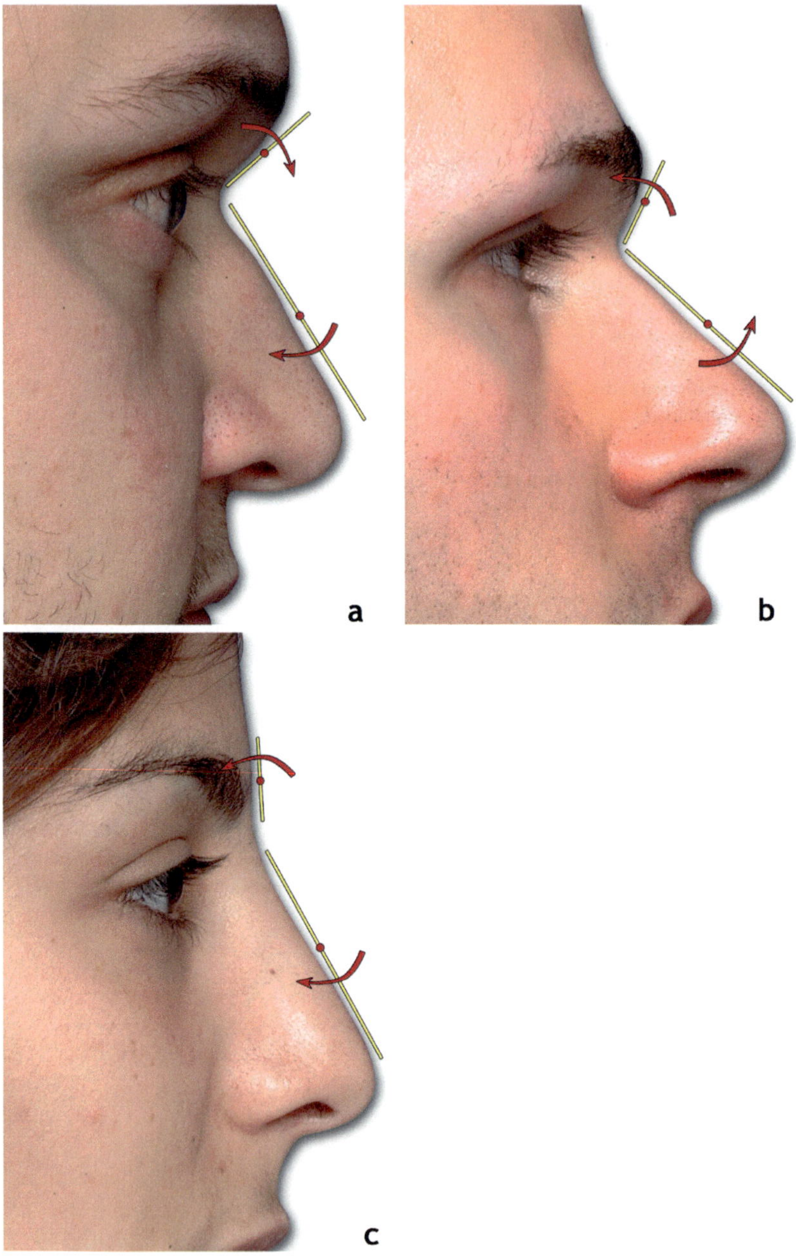

Fig. 5.30 (**a–c**) The construction of nasofrontal angle can be simply done by drawing (or imaging) two lines. The upper line is based on the mean inclination of the outline from glabella to the radix break-point, whereas the lower one is based on the mean inclination of the outline from the radix break-point to the supratip area. Nasofrontal angles of similar degrees can be rotated clockwise (**a**) or counterclockwise (**b**) resulting in very different nasal patterns. In the case of a wide nasofrontal angle, the transition from the forehead to the nose is not so evident (**c**)

Every change in the volume, length, slope, and shape of the lower third of the nose influences how we see the volume, length, slope, and shape of the upper lip. The opposite is also true.

The basic knowledge of the visual interplay between the nasal tip, the columellar–lobular profile and length, the subnasale point or curve, the alar rim profile, the upper lip profile and length, and the labrale superior point can be simplified by altering one parameter at a time. Figure 5.41a–d shows the visual effects of changing the nasal tip rotation, the upper lip length, the upper lip projection, and the profile contour at subnasale.

The mobility of the lower third of the nose and the upper lip when smiling is always assessed and

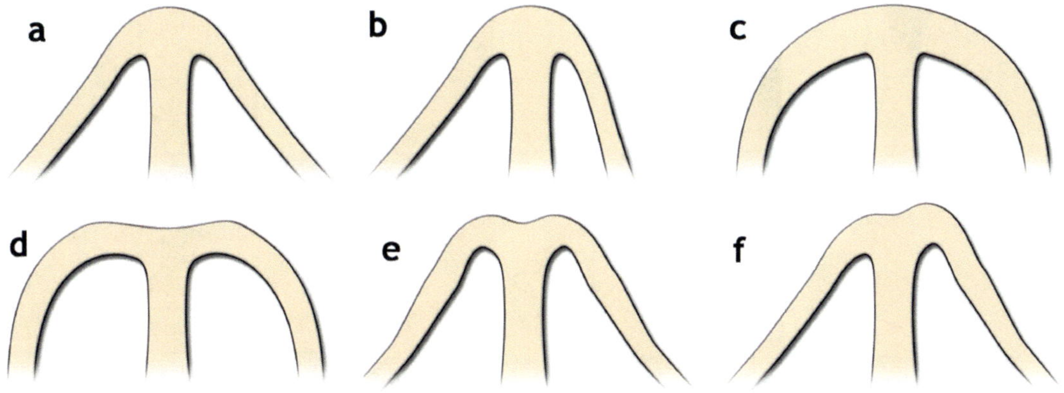

Fig. 5.31 (a–f) Various types of structural bony and cartilaginous architecture of the nasal dorsum

documented with at least two profile photographs. With a range of movement that differs between cases, the tip of the nose is displaced down and posterior, revealing the inferior dorsal profile of the cartilaginous septum, whereas the ala, at the alar crease junction, rises (Fig. 5.42a, b).

5.17 External Deformities and Nasal Airway Obstruction

The external esthetic analysis must be associated with a complete medical "nasal" history, anterior rhinoscopy, and CT scan to detect problems related to the nasal airway. It is interesting that many of the external details found during the esthetic analysis, such as crooked or saddle dorsum, midline deviation of the nasal framework, narrowing of the base of the nasal pyramid, nostril asymmetry, pinching of the alae, caudal septum deviation, broad columellar base, loss of tip support, excessive down rotation of the nasal tip, nasal skin scars, maxillary hypoplasia, long face, etc. can be a sign of an underlying airway obstruction. Even if a patient wanting rhinoplasty assures the surgeon that her breathing through the nose is good, every effort must be made to reveal and treat any structural cause of obstruction.

5.18 Basic Facial Analysis: Preferred Terms

In this paragraph, the reader will find an alphabetically ordered glossary that gives the essential terminology relative to facial features used in the text.

- **Bigonial width**. The width of the face, measured between the skin outline at the level of the mandibular angles, in frontal view.
- **Bimental width**. The width of the face, measured between the skin outline at the level of the chin, in frontal view.
- **Bitemporal width**. The width of the face, measured between the skin outline at the level of the temporal region, in frontal view.
- **Bizygomatic width**. The width of the face, measured between the two zygomatic arches at their maximal distance, in frontal view.
- **Central oval of the face**. The extended central region of the face. It is comprised of the eyes, the eyebrows, the zygoma, the nose, the mouth, and the chin.
- **Concave/convex profile**. The anterior–posterior relationship of the whole facial profile. It varies from concave, due to a relative posteriorly positioned middle third, to convex, due to a relative anteriorly positioned middle third.

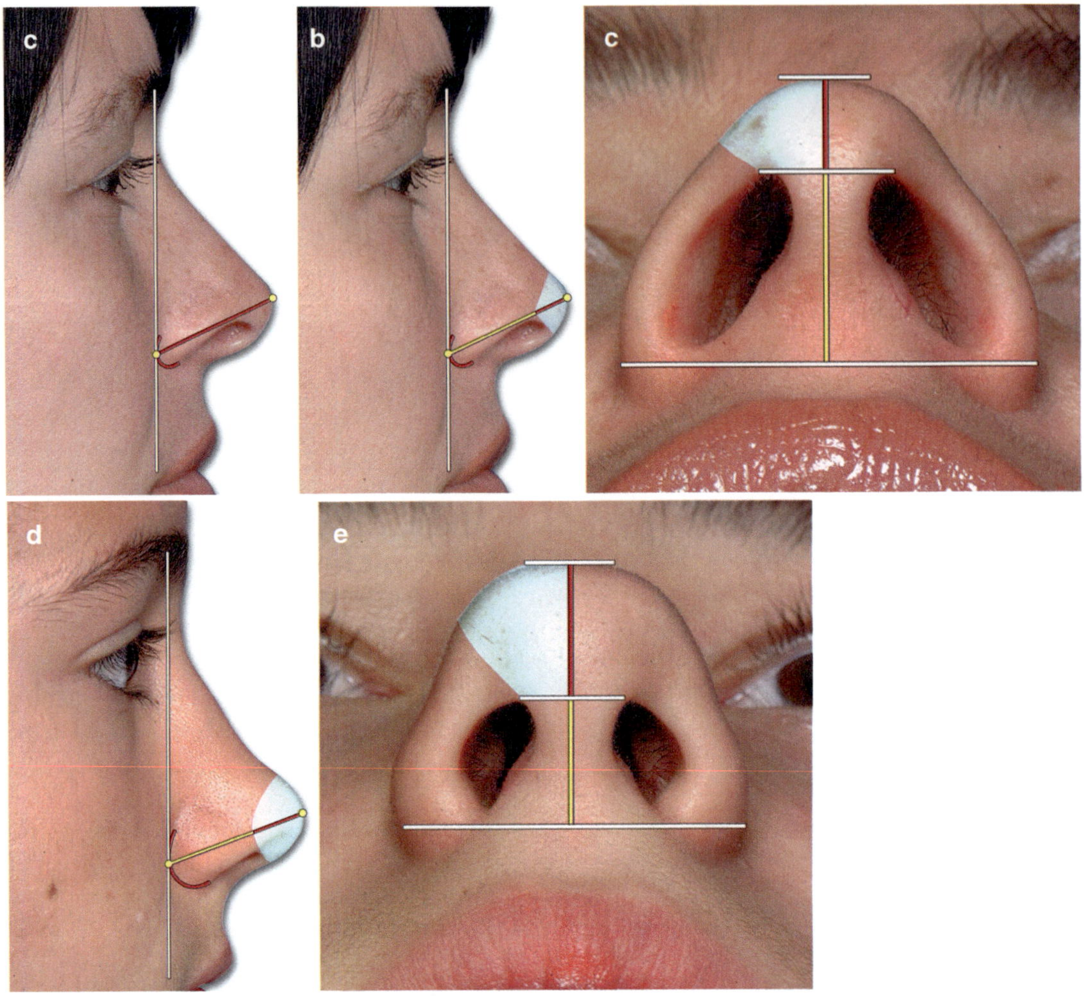

Fig. 5.32 (**a–e**) The tip projection is the distance between the alar crease junction (ACJ) and the most anterior point of the nasal tip (T) and can be divided into intrinsic and extrinsic projections. The intrinsic projection is related to the lobule portion of the tip, whereas the extrinsic projection is related to the length of the ala and the columella (**a–c**). A clinical case in which the total tip projection is mainly sustained by the lobule portion (**d**, **e**)

This classification does not define which third of the face is responsible for the deformity.

- **Facial height** (total facial height). The distance between the trichion and soft tissue menton.
- **Hairline**. The edge of hair round the face.
- **Wide/narrow face**. The predominance and the reduction, respectively, of the four widths of the face over the total facial height.
- **Long/short face**. The predominance and the reduction, respectively, of the total facial height over the four widths of the face.
- **Menton** (soft tissue menton). Lowest point on the contour of the soft tissue chin. In cephalometric analysis it is found by dropping a perpendicular from the horizontal plane through the skeletal menton.
- **Subnasal**. The point at which the columella merges with the upper lip in the midsagittal plane. It varies widely in relation to the caudal septum prominence and nasal spine morphology.
- **Malar eminence**. The point of maximal outer projection of the malar region.
- **Mandibular border outline**. The skin contour line that separates the mandibular body from the submental and submandibular ones.

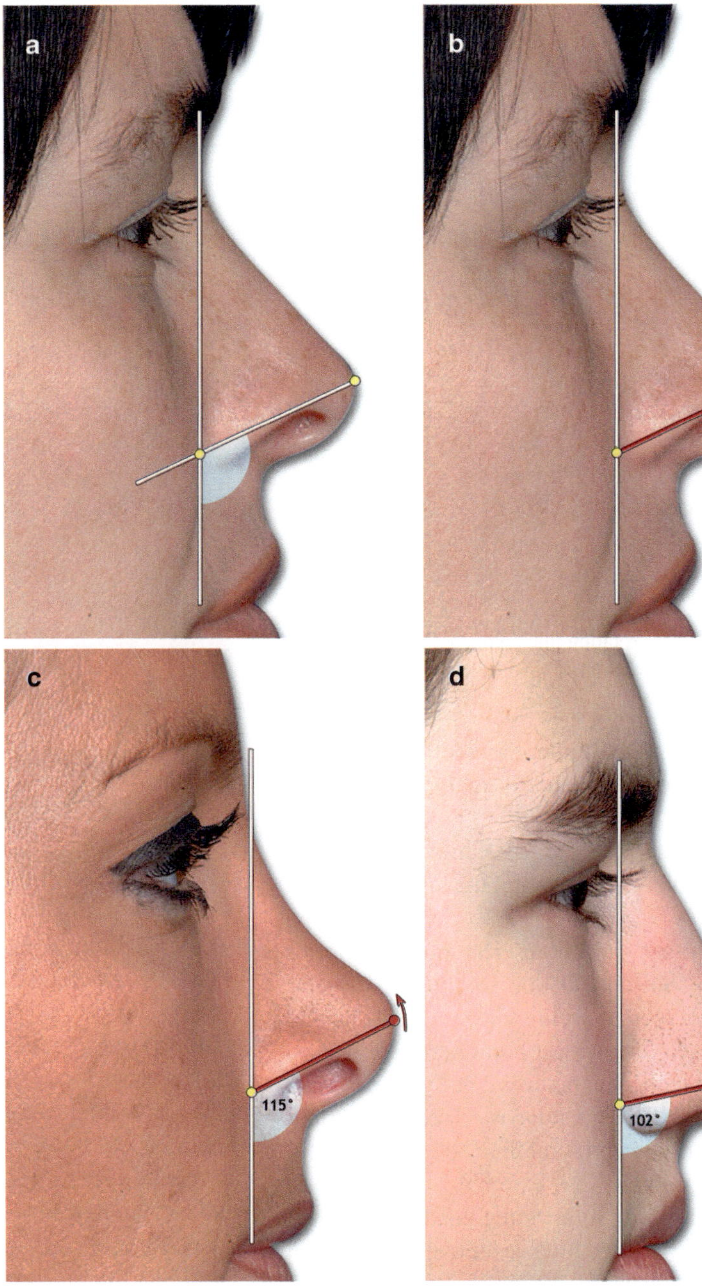

Fig. 5.33 (**a–d**) The angle of tip rotation is measured between the ACJ–T line and the vertical reference (**a**, **b**); its normative mean value is 105° for females and 100° for males. A clinical case of an excessive upward rotation in a secondary nasal deformity (**c**) and a normally rotated tip in a male teenager (**d**)

5.19 Nasal Analysis: Preferred Terms

In this section, the reader will find an alphabetically ordered glossary that gives the essential terminology relative to nasal features used in the text.

- **Accessory cartilages**. Small cartilages of nasal alae found in the space between the lateral ends of the lateral crura and the pyriform aperture edge.
- **Ala** (Alae). Ala literally means "wing." It is the lateral wall of the nostril that extends from the tip to join the upper lip and cheek.

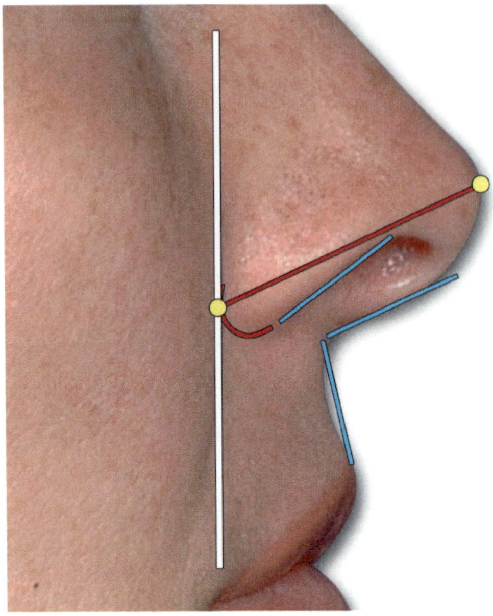

Fig. 5.34 The tip rotation line compared with the profile lines of the columella, nasal ala, and upper lip

- **Alar base width** (Interalar width). The width of the nose measured at the alar–cheek junction.
- **Alar crease**. The curved skin crease formed by the ala when joining the upper lip and cheek.
- **Alar crease junction**. The most posterior point of the curved line formed by the alar crease as seen in profile view.
- **Alar flare**. The widest point between the two ala. It usually occurs several millimeters above the alar crease. Interalar width is usually less than alar flare and sometime coincides with it.
- **Alar groove**. The external, oblique skin depression that follows the caudal margin of the lateral crus as it leaves the alar rim to run in a more cephalic direction. It separates the tip from the thickened portion of the ala that joins the face at the superior cheek–lip junction.
- **Anatomic dome**. The junction of the medial and lateral crus. It is the more anterior projected portion of the lower lateral crura.
- **Anterior nasal spine**. The median bony process of the lower rim of the pyriform aperture.

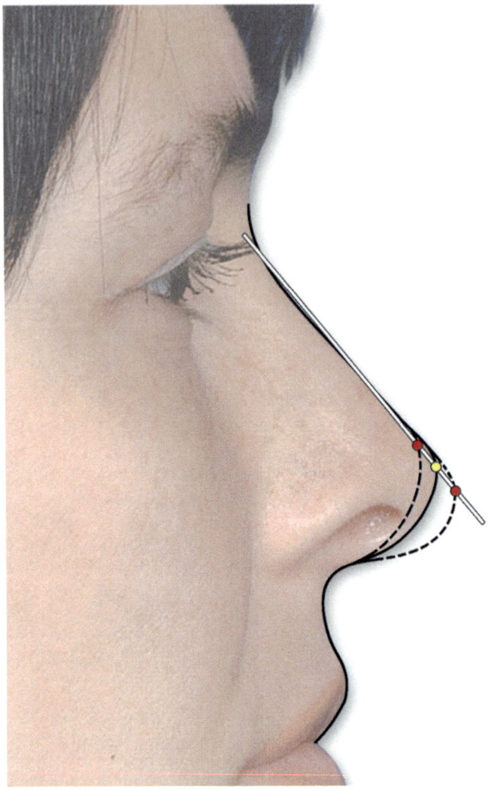

Fig. 5.35 The tip position assessment refers to the location of the nasal tip along the dorsal line

- **Anterior septal angle**. The junction of the anterior and caudal margins of the cartilaginous septum.
- **Bifid Tip.** Visible separation of the paired lower lateral cartilages at the level of the domes. A more common condition in thin skin patient.
- **Boxy Tip**. It is characterized by strong, convexly curved lower lateral cartilages. The strong convex curve of the lower laterals gives width in frontal and basal views and is responsible for the flat, box-like tip appearance.
- **Caudal septum**. The free inferior border of the quadrangular cartilage.
- **Caudal**. Means the same as inferior when referring to the nose.
- **Cephalic**. Means the same as superior when referring to the nose.
- **Clinical dome**. The most anterior projecting portion of the lower cartilage. The exter-

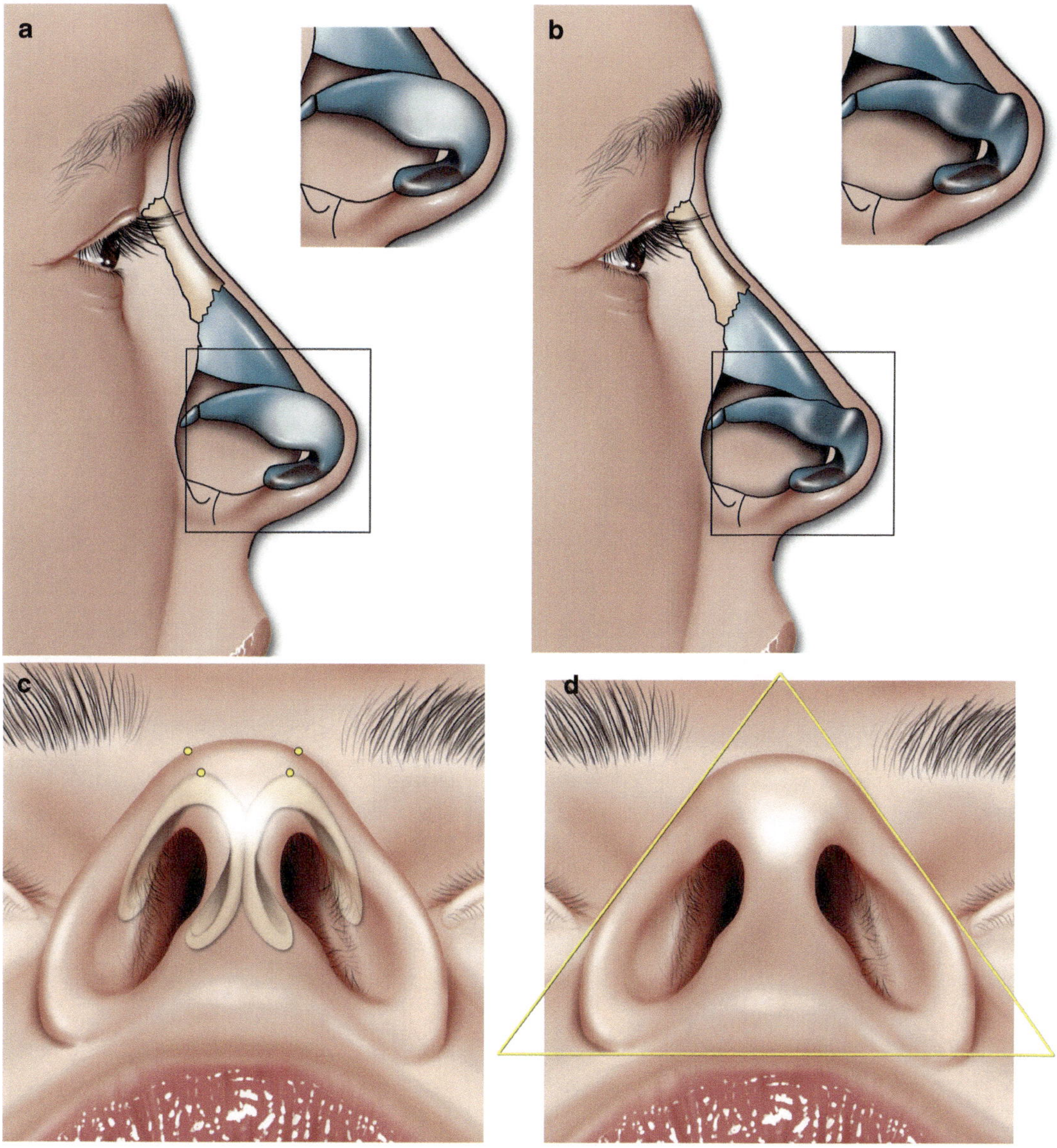

Fig. 5.36 (**a–d**) The tip volume refers to the size of the lobule and is primarily related to the shape, dimension, and orientation of the lateral crura of the lower lateral cartilage (**a**). The tip definition is related to the transition between the most anterior projecting section of the lower lateral crura, the domal segment, and the nearest portion of the lateral crura; in a well-defined tip the convexity of the dome should turn in a concavity on the lateral crura (**b**). The width of the tip refers to the distance between the paired domes (**c**). In the basal view, the nasal shape considered ideal resembles a triangle (**d**)

nal projection of the dome is the tip defining point.

- **Columella**. The column at the base of the nose separating the nostrils. Its posterior portion, the columella base, is usually wider.
- **Columellar–labial angle**. Curved junction of the columella with the lip. See also subnasale and nasolabial angle.
- **Columellar–lobular angle**. The angle between the infratip lobule and the columella.

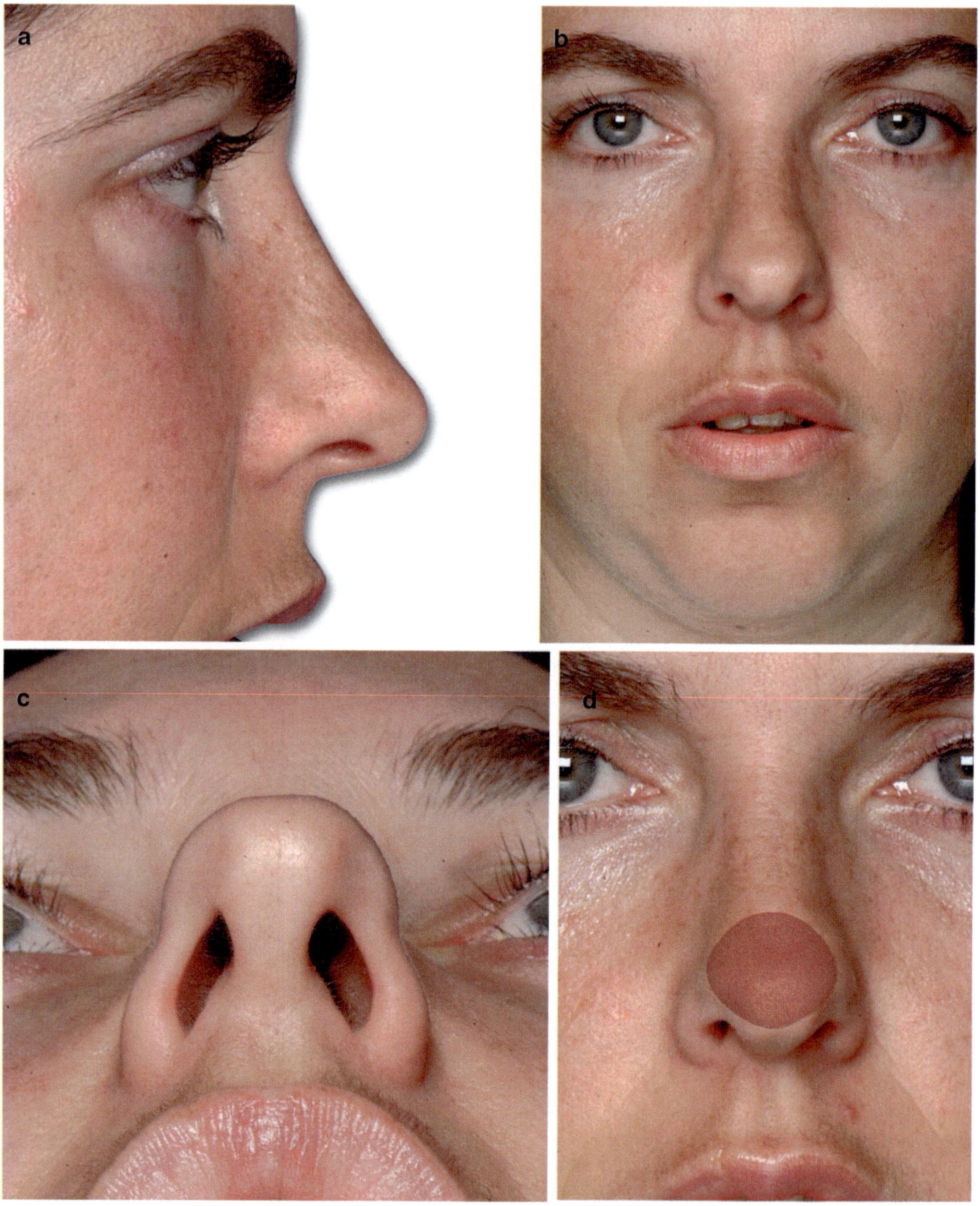

Fig. 5.37 (**a–h**) A clinical case of intrinsic tip deformity. In close-up profile view, the nasal outline appears to be quite good (**a**) but the frontal and basal views (**b**, **c**) show a large nasal tip. The increased volume of the lobule (**d**), the lack of definition and angularity (**e**), the increased interdomal distance (**f**) and a shape, recognized as "boxy" (**g**), characterize this nasal lobule. The full-face profile view permits the surgeon to understand the whole facial imbalance due to the severe class II dentofacial deformity (**h**)

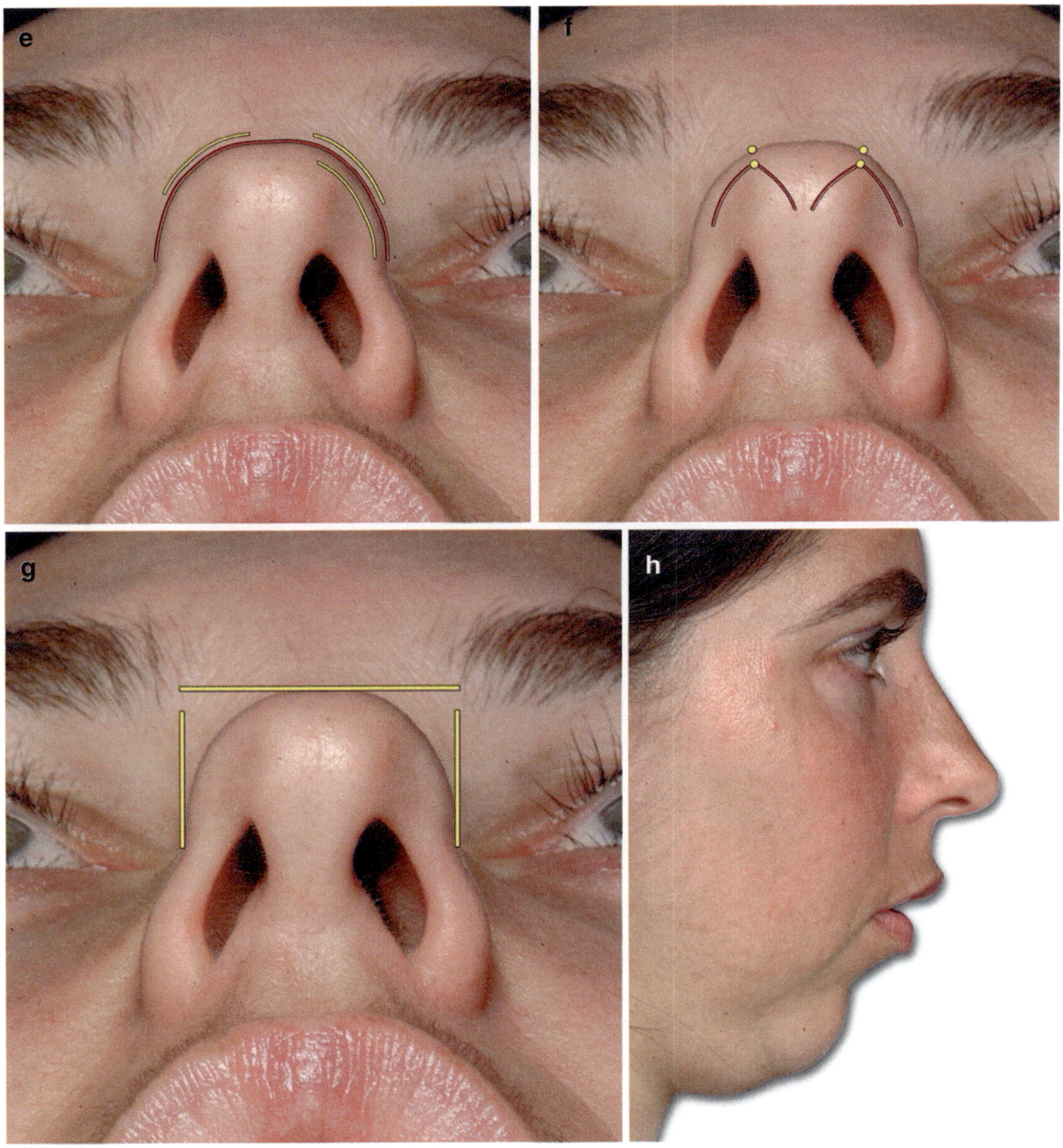

Fig. 5.37 (continued)

- **Corneal plane**. A coronal plane tangential to the surface of the cornea.
- **Crooked nose**. A nose in which any break or deviation of dorsal nasal contour lines may give a crooked or irregular appearance.
- **Deviated nose**. A nose that varies from the straight vertical orientation of the face.
- **Dorsal hump**. A pronounced convexity of the dorsal profile of the nose. Cartilaginous framework, bony framework, or more frequently both can sustain it.
- **Dorsum of the nose**. Where the lateral surfaces of the upper two-thirds of the nose join the midline. It is comprised between the tip and the radix.
- **External nasal valve.** The volume of the first tract of the nasal airway comprised from the nostril aperture and the internal nasal valve.

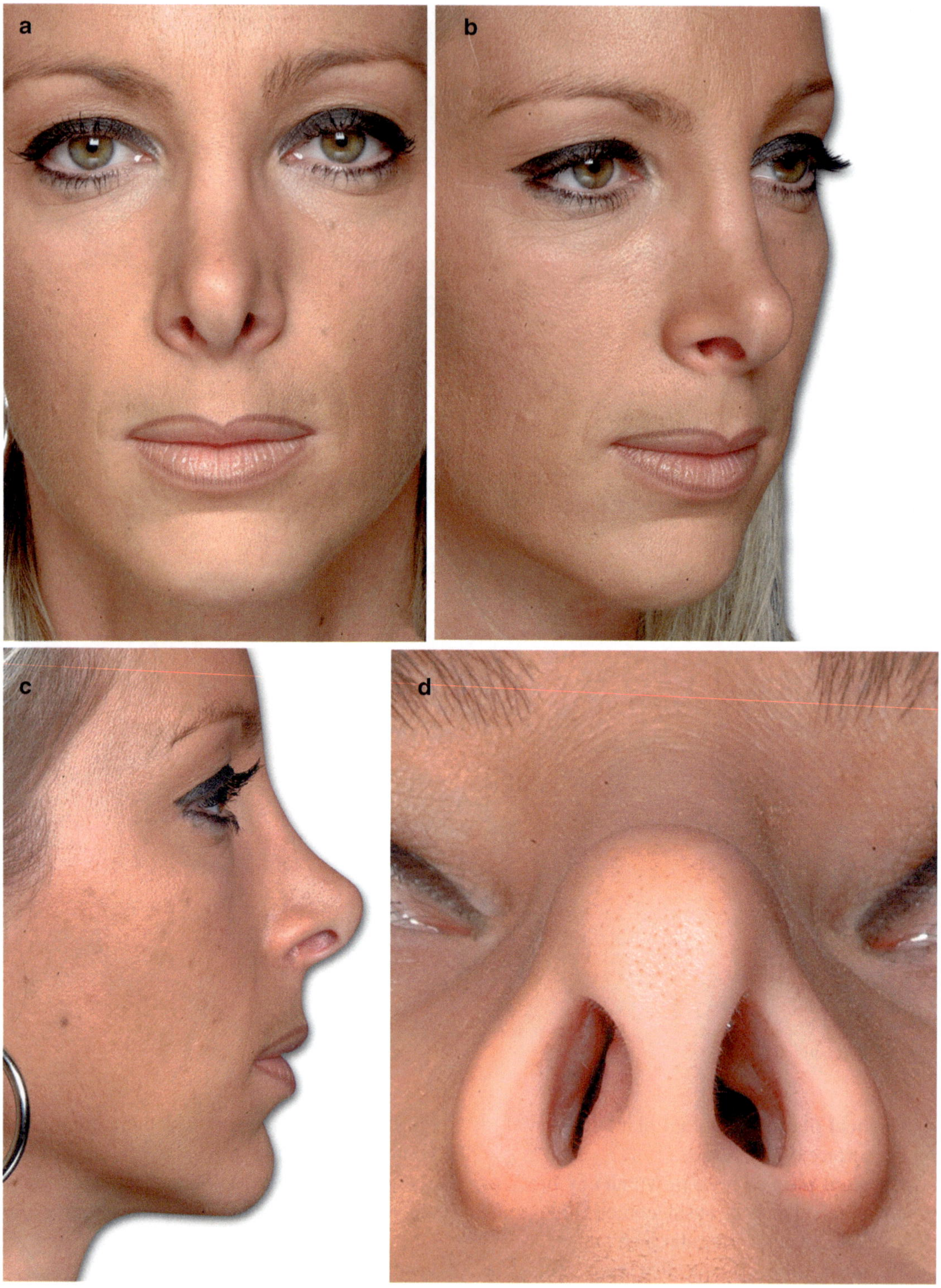

Fig. 5.38 (**a–d**) A secondary deformity following aggressive nasal surgery. In the frontal view, the bilateral dorsal lines are interrupted at the level of the cartilaginous dorsum, the nostril show is increased on each side, and the lobule appears bilaterally pinched (**a**). The oblique right view confirms the distortion of the left "unbroken" line due to the dorsal saddle (**b**). In the profile view, the absence of a radix break-point, the excessive concave dorsal outline, the over-rotated and over-projected intrinsic tip, the retracted right ala, and the long upper lip are evident (**c**). The basal view confirms the pinched aspect of the lobule and reveals the reduction of the right nostril aperture (**d**)

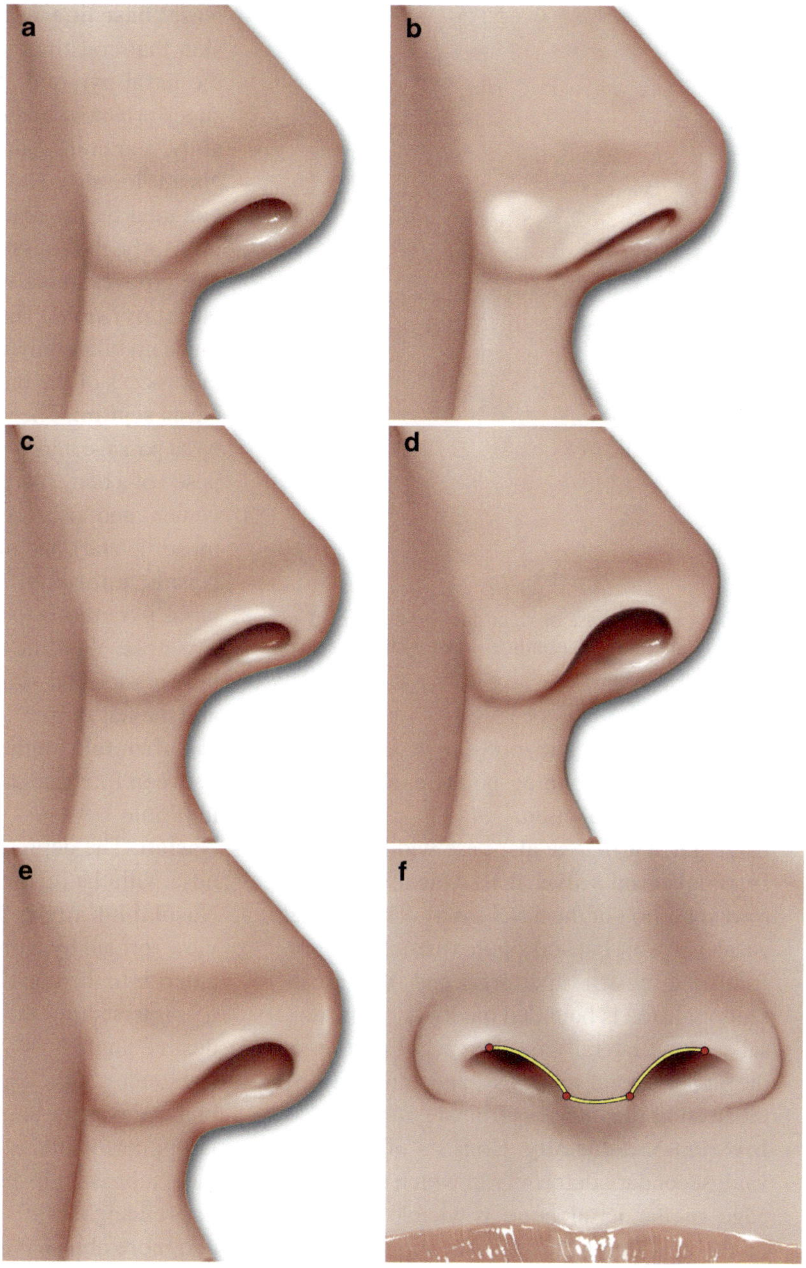

Fig. 5.39 (**a–f**) The columellar show is the area of visible columella under the alar rim (**a**). A reduced columellar show can be produced by a hanging ala (**b**), a retracted columella (**c**), or the combination of these two conditions, whereas an increased columellar show can be produced by a retracted ala (**d**), a hanging columella (**e**), or the combination of these two conditions. The ideal outline of the paired nasal alar rims and the columella, in frontal view, should resemble the figure of a gull in flight (**f**)

The borders of this volume are the nostril aperture caudally, the septum and medial crura medially, the alar cartilage and fibrofatty tissue anterolaterally, and the internal nasal valve opening posteriorly.

- **Facet**. See soft triangle.
- **Glabella** (soft tissue glabella). The most prominent anterior point in the midsagittal plane of the forehead. It is influenced by pneumonization of the frontal sinus and varies widely in the posteroanterior position.
- **"Greek nose."** A particular nasal profile in which the forehead and nasal dorsum are almost in line and the nasofrontal angle is almost 180°. The radix break-point is excessively projected and difficult to identify.

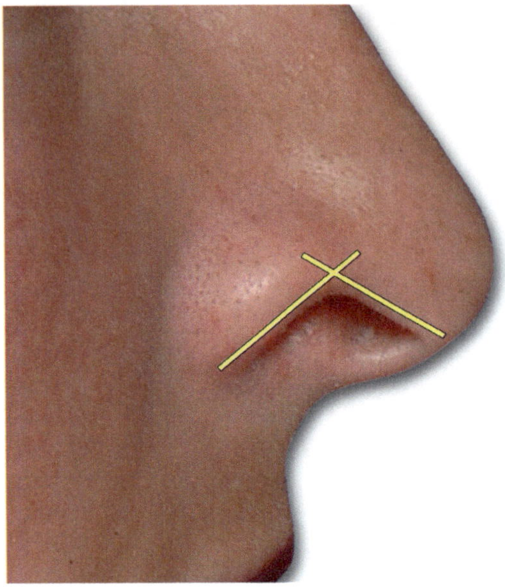

Fig. 5.40 A clinical case of right notched alar rim. The gentle curvature of the alar outline is lost with the formation of an evident angle

- **Infratip lobule**. The portion of the lobule between the tip defining points and the columellar–lobular junction.
- **Interalar width**. See alar base width.
- **Internal nasal valve.** It is typically the narrowest portion of the nasal cavity. The internal nasal valve is located approximately 1.3 cm from the nostril apertures and the cross-sectional area is bounded medially by the dorsal septum, laterally by the caudal portion of the upper lateral cartilage, and inferiorly by the head of the inferior turbinate.
- **Inverted-V deformity**. Consists of a middle vault secondary deformity in which the caudal edge of the nasal bone is visible in broad relief. It is due to inadequate support of the upper lateral cartilages and/or inadequate osteotomy of the nasal bones.
- **Keystone area**. The junction of the perpendicular plate of the ethmoid with the septal cartilage at the dorsum of the nose.
- **Limen vestibuli**. The lower free edge of upper lateral cartilage seen intranasally.
- **Lower lateral cartilage**. The paired inferior nasal cartilages consisting of the medial, middle, and lateral crura.
- **Nasal base line**. A slightly oblique line on the skin that constitutes the lateral boundaries of the nasal pyramid. The nasal base line starts superiorly near to the medial canthus and ends at the alar crease junction.
- **Nasal lobule**. The lower part of the nose bounded by the anterior nostril edge postero-inferiorly, the supratip area superiorly, and the alar grooves laterally.
- **Nasal pyramid**. The bony portion of the nose made up bilaterally of the nasal bone and frontal process of the maxilla.
- **Nasal septum**. The vertical wall that divides the nasal passage into two distinct tunnels. It is composed of a bony (perpendicular plate of ethmoid, vomer, and premaxillary crest), cartilaginous (quadrilateral), and membranous portion.
- **Nasal "unbroken" line**. The outline of the nasal pyramid in oblique view. In the attractive nose, this line descends gracefully from the supraorbital ridge onto the nasal dorsum and the nasal tip.
- **Nasofrontal angle**. Angle of demarcation between forehead and nasal dorsum, best seen in profile.
- **Nasion**. The depression at the junction of the nose with the forehead.
- **Nasolabial angle**. The angle seen on lateral view formed by a line drawn through the most anterior to the most posterior point of the nostril, intersecting the vertical facial plane. The desired angle is 90–95° in males and 95–100° in females. Other authors identify the nasolabial angle as the angle defined by the columellar point-to-subnasale line intersecting with the subnasale-to-labral superior line; the desired angle is 90–120°, more acute in males and more obtuse in females.
- **Nostril aperture**. The paired apertures of the nose; their area is outlined by the nostril sill, the columella, and the margin of nasal alae and represent the anterior portion of external nasal valve.
- **Nostril sill**. The skin area forming the base of the nostril. It is comprised between the columellar base and the alar base.
- **Pinched nose** (pinched nasal tip). A nasal tip deformity secondary to collapse of the alar

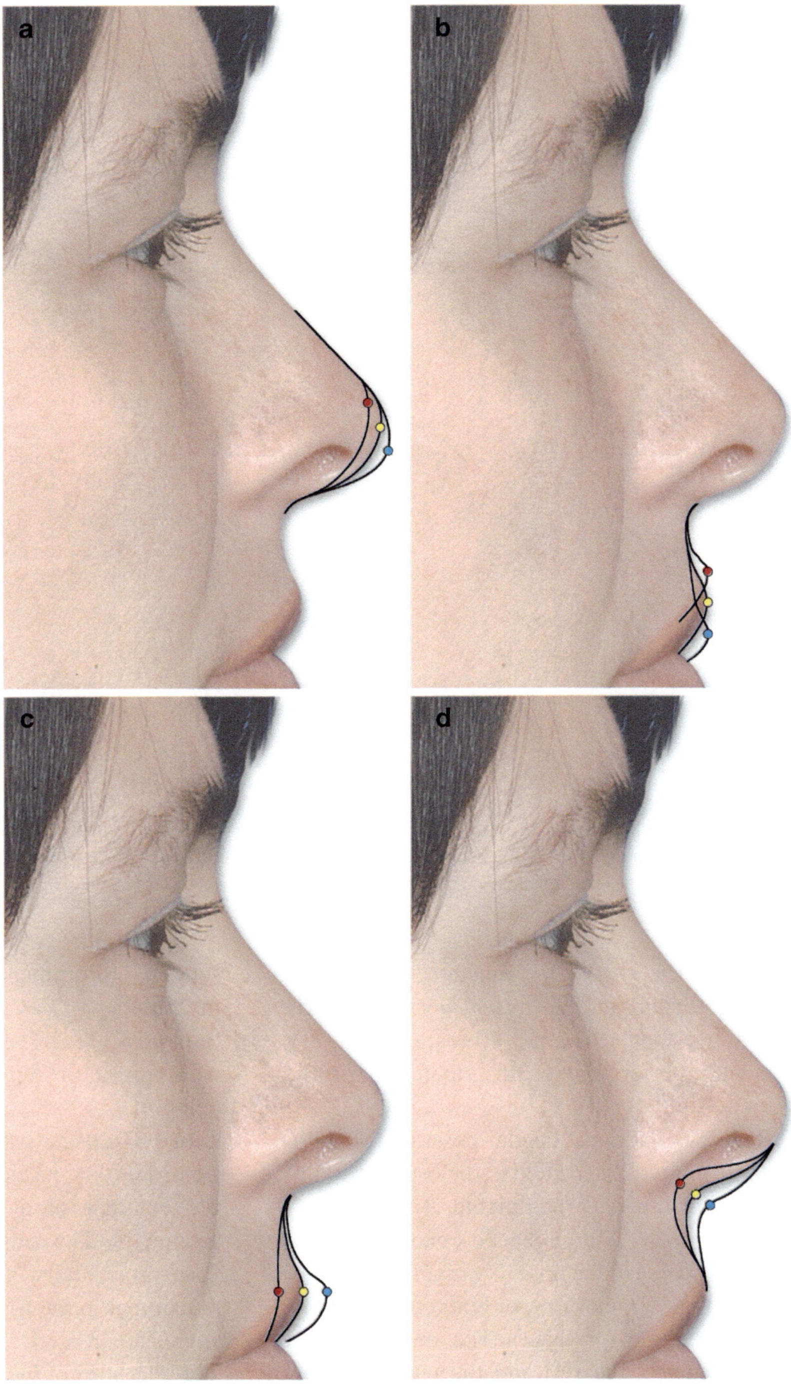

Fig. 5.41 (**a–d**) The visual effects of changing the nasal tip rotation (**a**), the upper lip length (**b**), the upper lip projection (**c**), and the profile contour at subnasale (**d**)

rims subsequent to loss of lateral crural support from either congenital or acquired causes.

- **Pyriform aperture**. The pear-shaped external bony opening of the nasal cavity.
- **Pollybeak nasal deformity**. Secondary deformity refers to postoperative fullness of the supratip region, with an abnormal tip–supratip relationship.

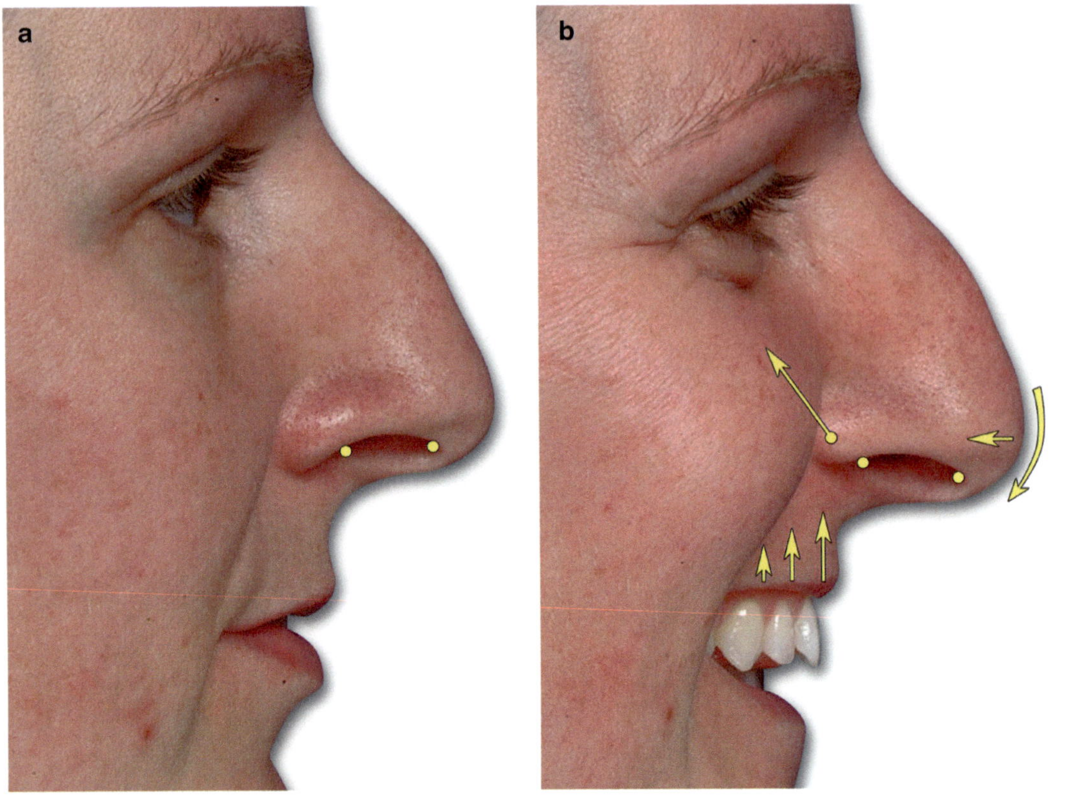

Fig. 5.42 (**a**, **b**) The act of smiling produces a specific pattern of movements on the face and nose. From the relaxed position (**a**) to the smiling one (**b**) the characteristic downward displacement of the lobule is associated with the rising up of the ala at the alar crease junction

- **Radix**. The area of the junction between the nasal dorsum and the frontal bone, inferiorly to the glabella. The radix break-point is the most posterior point of this junction in profile view.
- **Rhinion**. The most caudal point of the intranasal suture. It is located at the osseocartilaginous junction over the dorsum of the nose.
- **Saddle nose**. A pronounced concavity of the dorsal profile of the nose. Cartilaginous framework, bony framework, or both can sustain it.
- **Soft triangle** (or facet). The thin skin fold between the alar rim and the curved caudal border of the junction of the medial and lateral crura. When this is well defined, it is referred to as a facet.
- **Subnasale**. The point at which the columella merges with the upper lip in the midsagittal plane. It varies widely in relation to caudal septum prominence and nasal spine morphology.
- **Supratip area**. The area just superior to the nasal tip at the inferior aspect of the nasal dorsum.
- **Tension nose** (prominent-narrow pyramid syndrome). A particular deformity in which the external nasal pyramid is abnormally prominent. The length and the height of the nose are usually greater than normal. The radix break-point is shallow and the nasolabial angle is increased.
- **Tip**. The apex of the lobule, but it is frequently used when referring to the lobule.
- **Tip defining points**. The most projecting area on each side of the tip, which produces an external light reflex.
- **Tip projection**. The horizontal component of the distance from the most anterior point of

the nasal tip and the most posterior point of the nasal–cheek junction (Alar crease junction).

- **Tip rotation**. Determined by the tip angle as measured from a vertical line at the alar crease to the tip, with the norms being 105° for females and 100° for males. Tip rotation can also be referred to the movement of the tip cephalad or caudal pivoted at the alar base on the profile view.
- **Upper lateral cartilage** (or triangular cartilage). The paired superior nasal cartilages, triangular in shape extending laterally from the dorsal septum making up the lateral walls of the middle third of the nose.
- **Weak triangle** (or Converse triangle). The area immediately cephalad to paired domes. As other nasal areas, it lacks a cartilaginous or bony framework support.

Further Reading

Little JW. Volumetric perceptions in midfacial aging with altered priorities for rejuvenation. Plast Reconstr Surg. 2000;105:252–66.

Gunter JP, Rohrich RJ, Hackney FL. Correction of the pinched nasal tip with alar spreader grafts. In: Gunter JP, Rohrich RJ, Adams WP, editors. Dallas rhinoplasty. Nasal surgery by the masters. St. Louis: Quality Medical; 2002.

What are the more interesting reference points and lines of the external—visible—part of the face? How can some of these elements, spontaneously perceived by our patients as well, be used for a better communication? The experience gained with the classical studies on eye movements and visual perception can help the rhinoplasty surgeon in identifying and prioritizing the points and the lines most interesting for our patient and concentrate the clinical analysis on these aspects. The author has devoted a chapter of his previous book to the application of these theoretical studies to everyday clinical practice: Meneghini F. The facial point of interest. In: Meneghini F, editor. Clinical facial analysis. Berlin: Springer; 2005. p. 35–40.

Open access article on preoperative nasal analysis: Brito ÍM, Avashia Y, Rohrich RJ. Evidence-based nasal analysis for rhinoplasty: the 10-7-5 method. Plast Reconstr Surg Glob Open. 2020;8:e2632. https://doi.org/10.1097/GOX.0000000000002632. Published online 26 Feb 2020.

Book chapter on preoperative nasal analysis: Rohrich RJ, Ahmad J, Gunter JP. Nasofacial proportions and systematic nasal analysis. In: Rohrich RJ, Adams WP Jr, Ahmad J, Gunter JP, editors. Dallas rhinoplasty: nasal surgery by the masters. 3rd edn. St. Louis. Quality Medical; 2014. p. 85–110.

6 Dentofacial Analysis for Rhinoplasty Patients

Facial harmony and proportion are greatly influenced by the spatial relationships between maxilla and mandible together with their degree of development as well as by the shape and size of the nose.

Many patients seeking a nose correction have a more or less evident dentofacial deformity, but also the contrary is true: many patients in treatment for dentofacial deformities present a nasal deformity. So, even if the surgeon who dedicates himself to nasal surgery does not necessarily have to be a surgeon who treats dentofacial deformities, it is essential that he must be able to diagnose them and work in a team with at least two other "facial" specialists: the maxillofacial surgeon and the orthodontist. Without these extended diagnostic skills and a team approach the risk of poor clinical treatment of many clinical cases is high.

6.1 Basic Assessment of Dental Occlusion

The basic elements of dental occlusion need to be known because of the important role played by the dental structures in supporting and shaping the lower third of the face. The sagittal, vertical, and transversal relationship of the two arches during occlusion, as well as any crowding, loss, or abnormal shape of the teeth should be noted as a matter of routine during the direct facial lower third examination. Figure 6.1a, b shows the dental cast of a subject with optimal dental occlusion.

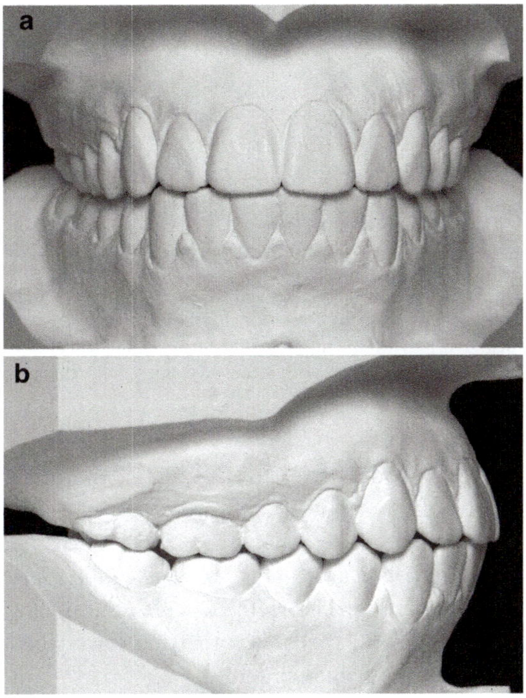

Fig. 6.1 (**a**, **b**) Frontal (**a**) and profile right (**b**) views of the dental cast of a subject with optimal dental occlusion. Note that the upper arch is wider than the lower one, there is no space between adjacent teeth (diastema), there is no space between the two arches (normal overbite and absence of open bite), the upper incisors are in front of the lower incisors (normal overjet), the upper and lower dental midlines coincide, and there is no teeth rotation or abnormal teeth inclination

Figure 6.2a–c shows the three basic sagittal relationships between the incisors (overjet). In

F. Meneghini, *Basic Open Rhinoplasty*, https://doi.org/10.1007/978-3-030-61827-8_6

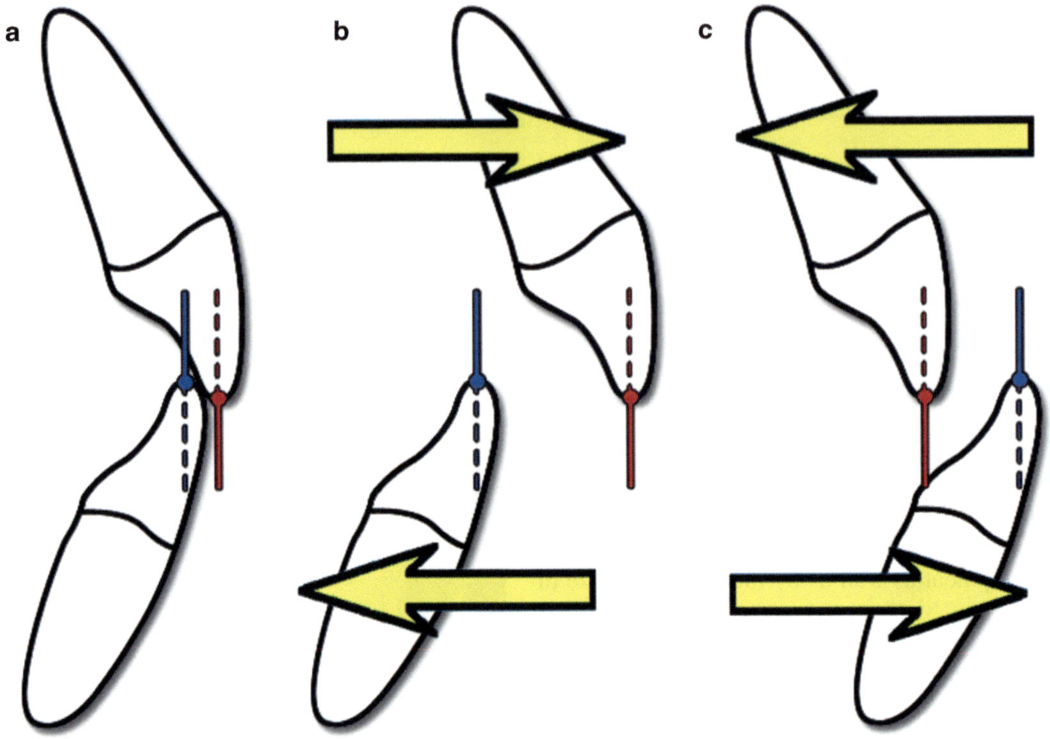

Fig. 6.2 (**a–c**) Sagittal relationship between the incisors: ideal overjet with the upper teeth in front of the lower ones (**a**), increased overjet with excessive horizontal distance between the teeth (**b**), reverse overjet with the lower teeth in front of the upper ones (**c**)

the case of ideal overjet (Fig. 6.2a), the upper incisors are in front of the lower ones with little or no space between them. The increased overjet (Fig. 6.2b) consists of an excessive horizontal distance between the teeth, whereas the reverse overjet (Fig. 6.2c) requires that the lower teeth are in front of the upper ones.

The sagittal relationships between the dental arches can be divided into three main classes. Class I presents the ideal posteroanterior relationship between the two dental arches (Fig. 6.3a). Class II is a too anterior upper dental arch and/or a too posterior lower dental arch (Fig. 6.3b). Class III is a too posterior upper dental arch and/or a too anterior lower dental arch (Fig. 6.3c).

Figure 6.4a–c shows the three basic vertical relationships between the upper and lower incisors (overbite). In the case of ideal overbite, the upper incisors are in front of the lower ones with a limited overlap between them of 1–2 mm (Fig. 6.4a). The deep bite consists of an excessive overlap between the teeth (Fig. 6.4b), whereas the open bite (Fig. 6.4c) requires the presence of a vertical separation between the teeth.

Assessment of the occlusal transversal relationships considers the presence of a midline deviation between the dental arches, a cross-bite between opposite teeth, and/or a cant of the occlusal plane (Fig. 6.5a–c).

One important task of the examiner is to correlate the intraoral findings with the external facial appearance of the subject in order to establish the role of dental occlusion on the facial esthetics. The long-term support effect of particular teeth on the lips and cheeks is also considered. With aging, the esthetics of the soft tissue envelope is progressively more dependent on the skeletal support offered by well-aligned and correctly inclined frontal teeth and the surrounding alveolar bone (Fig. 6.6).

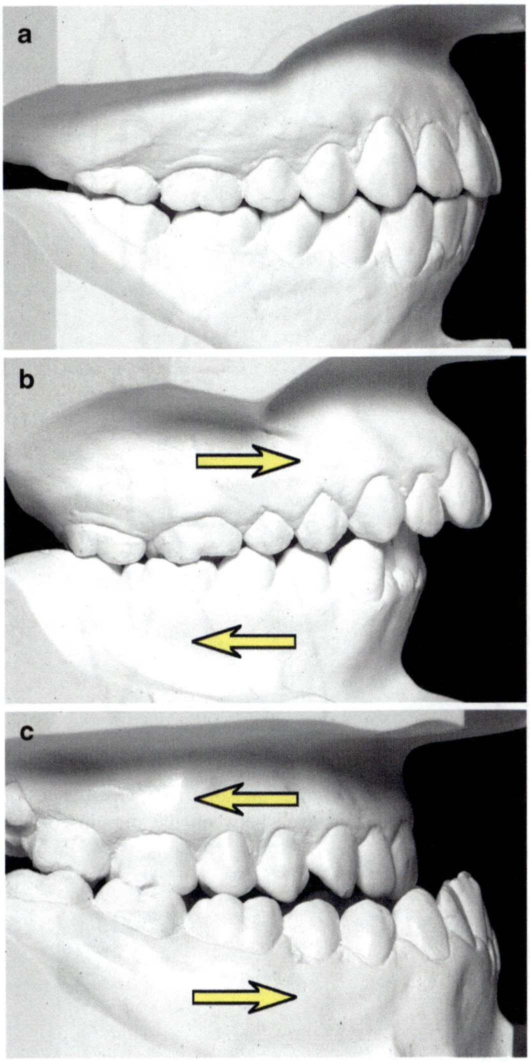

Fig. 6.3 (**a–c**) Sagittal classification of dental occlusion. Class I: ideal posteroanterior relationship between the two dental arches (**a**). Class II: too anterior upper dental arch and/or too posterior lower dental arch (**b**). Class III: too posterior upper dental arch and/or too anterior lower dental arch (**c**)

6.2 Upper Frontal Teeth Assessment

The upper frontal teeth need special attention in all patients, even if they are not mentioned in the patient priority list. Their role in overall facial esthetics is so important that a qualitative and sometimes quantitative analysis can add many details that help in planning treatment. The upper frontal teeth consist of the four incisors, the two canines, and the four premolars; these teeth should occupy the larger part of the smile. The teeth's shape, color, alignment, and symmetry must be evaluated, as well as the architecture and color of their gingival margin. Figure 6.7a–d shows the detail of well-proportioned and aligned upper frontal teeth.

One of the most difficult and at the same time most important aspects to assess is the anteroposterior projection of the upper teeth relative to the facial profile. The orthodontic literature has called this topic "anterior limit of dentition." Clinically and using photographs, the full facial profile view at rest must be compared with the same during a posed smile. Figure 6.8a–c shows the assessment of the anterior projection of the upper incisors in three different clinical cases.

Two particular esthetic problems of the upper incisors are the midline diastema and the black triangle. The midline diastema is represented by a space between the two upper incisors (Fig. 6.9b), whereas the so-called black triangle is a base-up triangular space bounded by an excessive mesial inclination of the two upper first incisors (Fig. 6.9c). In both cases, the observer and the patient usually perceive the dark shadow between the teeth as an esthetic problem.

6.3 Lip Assessment

The first problem in the assessment of the lips is to obtain a truly relaxed position from the patient. When reviewing a complete set of photographs of a clinical case, it is not unusual to discover that the lip position is not constant but changes from a complete seal, most frequently at the start of the photographic session, to a more relaxed (habitual!) one with the presence of a more or less wide space between the two lips (Fig. 6.10a, b). A partial nasal obstruction should be suspected when the subject has the habit of maintaining a space between the lips and breathing through the mouth.

Figure 6.11a, b shows a case of lip incompetence with absence of lip seal at rest due to an increased overjet with mandibular hypoplasia. In

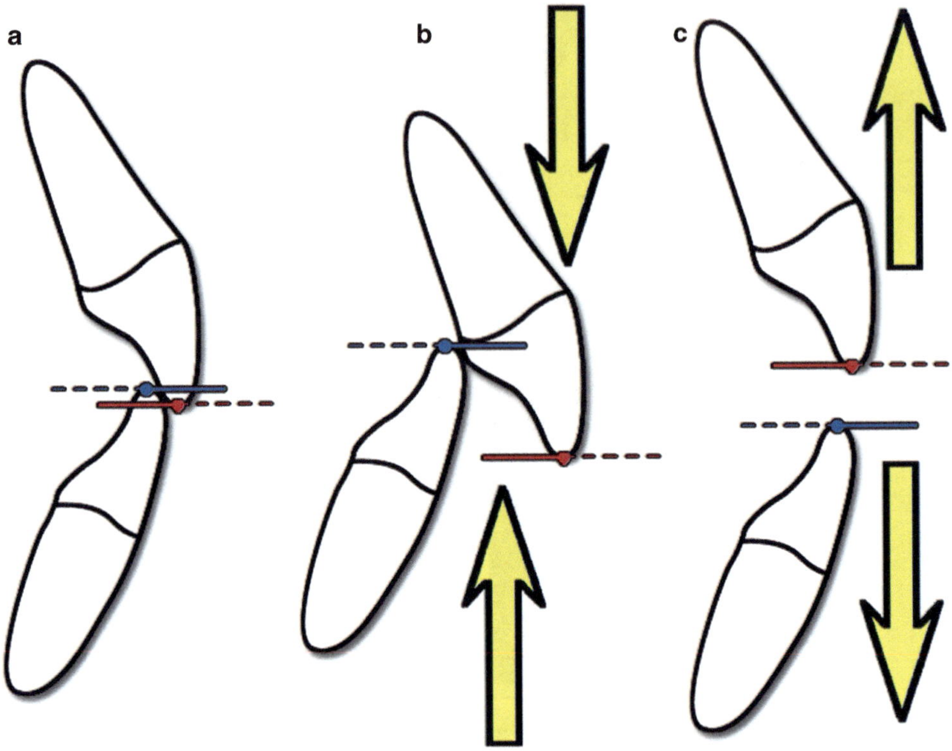

Fig. 6.4 (**a–c**) Vertical relationships between the upper and lower incisors. Ideal overbite with a limited overlap of 1–2 mm between the incisors (**a**). Deep bite or excessive overlapping between the incisors (**b**). Open bite or excessive vertical distance between the margins of the incisors (**c**)

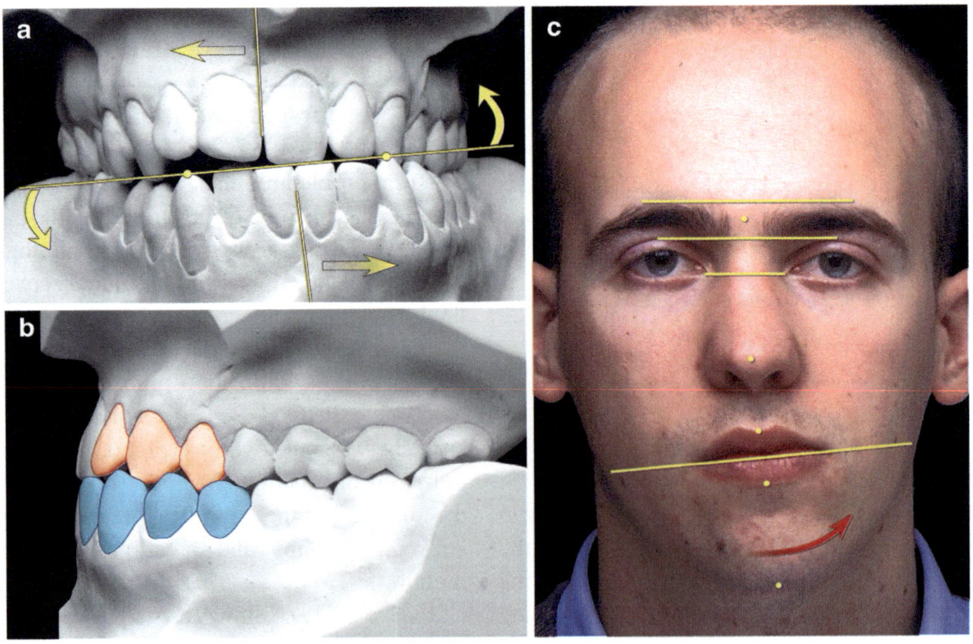

Fig. 6.5 (**a–c**) Dental malocclusion with mandibular deviation on the left, cant of the occlusal plane (**a**), dental cross-bite of some teeth (**b**) associated with facial asymmetry and cant of the lip commissures (**c**)

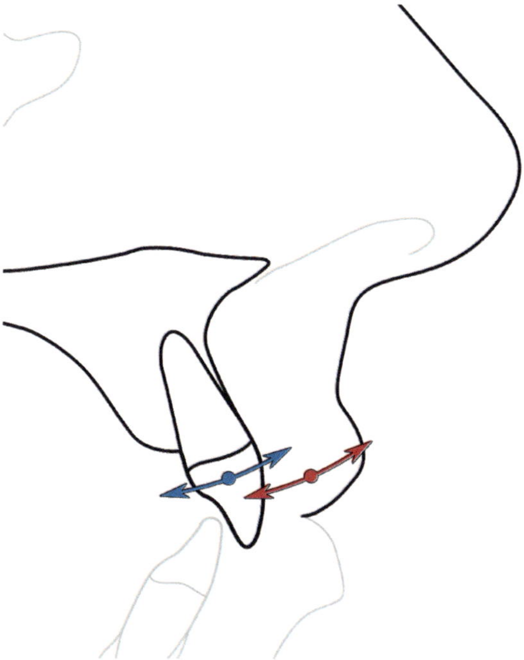

Fig. 6.6 The tracings show the intimate relationship between the inclination of the upper incisors and the upper lip position

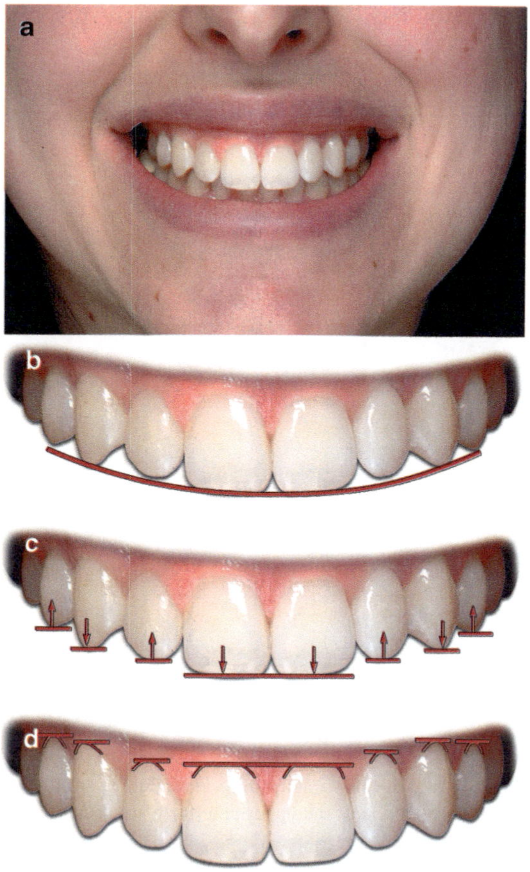

Fig. 6.7 (**a–d**) Smiling view of a well-proportioned and aligned upper frontal teeth group (**a**). It can be noted that: the outline created by the occlusal margin forms a gentle curve (**b**), adjacent teeth have different marginal vertical positions (**c**), and the gingival margins also have a different shape and position (**d**)

these cases, maintaining perfect lip closure requires a voluntary contraction that results in the flattening of the lip profile curves.

Knowing a prototype of younger, "healthy" and attractive female lips helps us to understand the roles and effects of intrinsic lip problems and any possible correlation with a dentofacial deformity, the aging process, or an acute lip trauma; it also helps to define the younger, "healthy" attractive male lips.

Figs. 6.12a, b and 6.13 show this prototype in frontal and profile views, as well as the preferred anatomical terms of the perioral region. The characteristics of attractive female lips can be summarized as follows:

- Mouth width or distance between the two lips.
- The nasolabial sulcus is almost undetectable when the patient is in the rest position.
- The skin linear reliefs of the philtrum columns, the Cupid's bow, and the upper and lower lip rolls are all present and well defined.
- The vermillion area and volume of the lower lip exceed those of the upper lip.
- The most anterior lower lip points in the profile view (labrale inferior) lie slightly anterior to the upper ones (labrale superior).
- The upper lip profile from subnasale to labrale superior is never vertically or posteriorly oriented but forms a gentle, anteriorly projected, concave curve.
- From the nasal tip to the soft tissue menton, there is a series of gentle curves, without

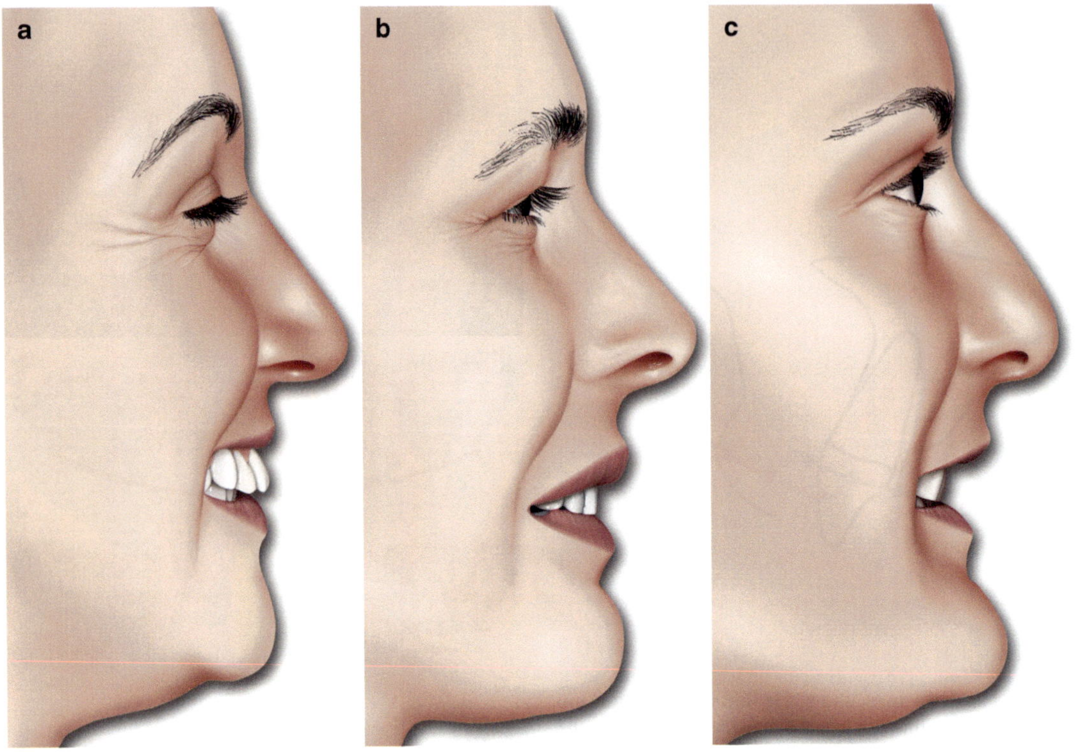

Fig. 6.8 (**a–c**) Full facial profile view during smiling. Clinical examples of excessive (**a**), ideal (**b**), and reduced (**c**) sagittal projection of the upper anterior teeth relative to the facial profile

straight traits, and a unique well-defined angle at the stomion (Fig. 6.13).

- The Ricketts E-line, the reference line connecting the tip of the nose with the soft tissue pogonion (Fig. 6.13), passes about 4 mm in front of the upper lip and 2 mm in front of the lower lip.

For comparison, the main differences in the attractive male lips are:

- The upper lip is higher and less anteriorly inclined. The height of the vermillion portion is reduced compared with that of the skin portion.
- The profile from the nasal tip to the soft tissue menton may show the presence of angles instead of gentle curves, in particular a more defined passage from lower lip to chin (labiomental fold).
- The distances between the lips and the Ricketts E-line are greater with a flatter profile.

6.4 Smile Analysis

The smile may be either posed or spontaneous. The differences between the two are important because the posed smile is voluntary, not elicited by an emotion, static, unstrained, and fairly reproducible. The unposed (spontaneous) smile is involuntary, induced by joy or mirth, and is not sustained (it is dynamic). It is often characterized by more lip elevation than the posed smile. When a subject is forced to mimic an unposed smile, this cannot be sustained and will appear strained and unnatural. So, we mainly conduct the analysis utilizing the posed smile because of the need for reproducible features.

The upper and lower lips frame the display zone that contains the teeth and the gingival scaffold. The soft tissue determinants of the display zone are lip thickness and marginal profile, intercommissure width (mouth width during smiling), smile index (width/height), and gingi-

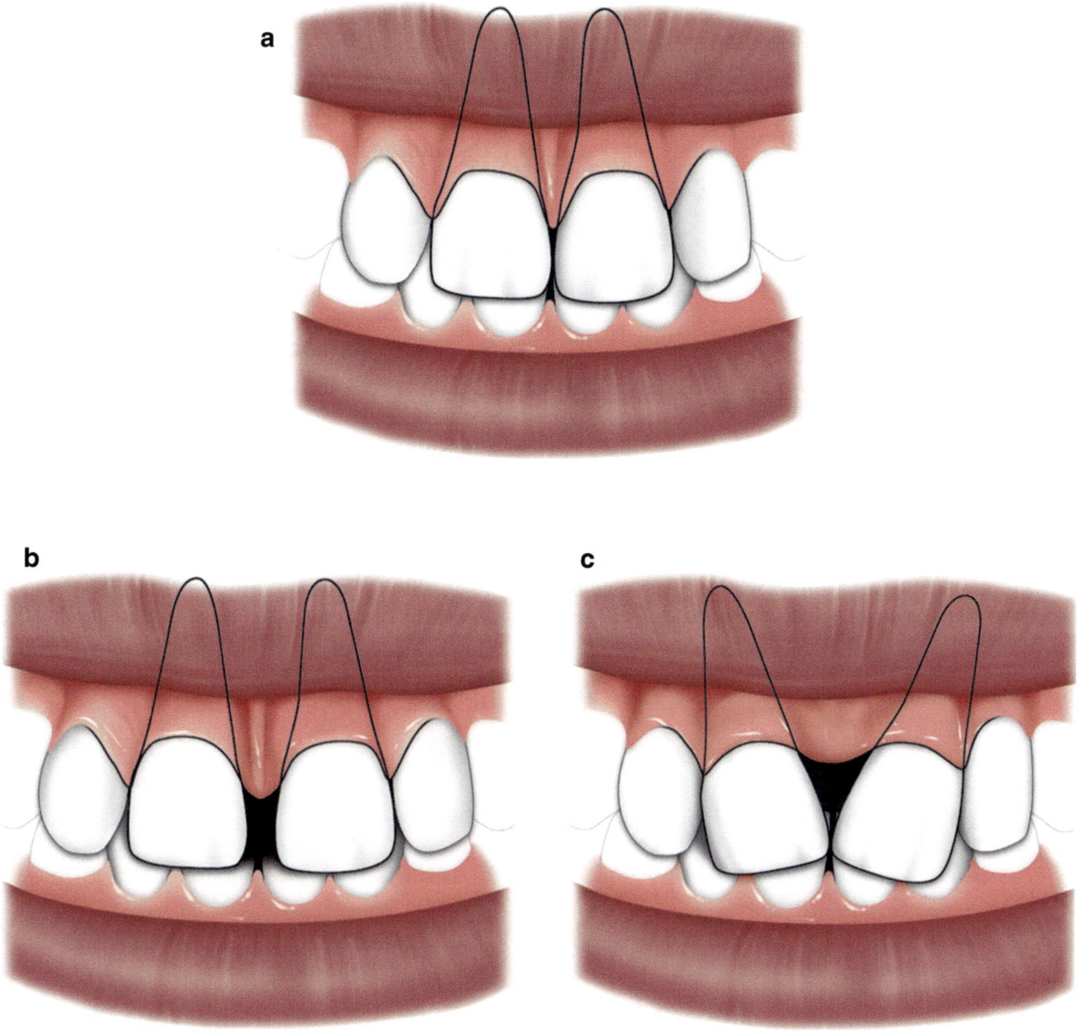

Fig. 6.9 (**a–c**) The most favorable esthetic relationship between the upper incisors, as well as other teeth, requires considerable contact between the two parallel structures (**a**). The presence of a midline dark shadow between upper central incisors may be a diastema (**b**), or a "black triangle" (**c**)

val architecture (Fig. 6.14a). Figure 6.14b–f shows the variability in the shape and total area of the display zone, utilizing five clinical examples.

An important characteristic of the smile is the presence of the buccal corridors, the so-called negative space described in the orthodontic literature (Fig. 6.14a), which are the bilateral dark shadows situated between the buccal (vestibular) surface of the posterior teeth and the inner commissure of the lips. The perceived dimensions and depth of the shadows in this space depend on several factors, such as the width of the dental arches, the sagittal position of the dental arches, the range of horizontal movements produced at the lip commissure, and the type of lighting utilized during the assessment and photographic session. Both the absence and the enlargement of the buccal corridors negatively affect the esthetics of the face. The smile with a lack of buccal corridors is called a "denture smile."

The assessment of a smile is not complete without evaluation of the smile arc. This is the relationship between the curvature of the incisal

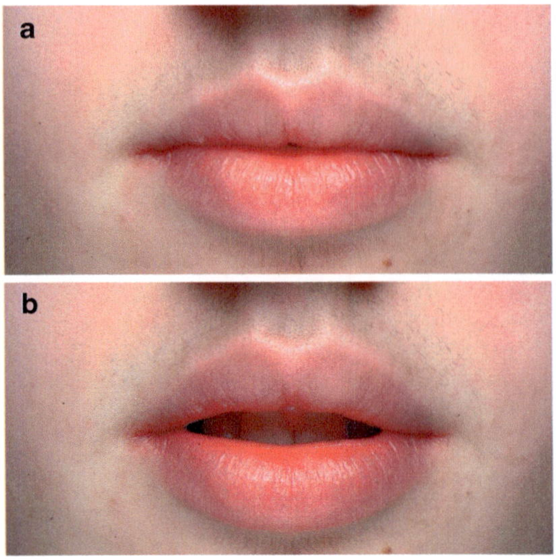

Fig. 6.10 (**a**, **b**) These photographs were taken in sequence during the same sitting without requesting the patient to take a particular lip position. After a few seconds in which the patient maintained a lip seal sustained with some muscular contraction (**a**), he returned to his habitual relaxed position with loss of contact between the lips (**b**)

edges of the maxillary incisors and canines to the curvature of the lower lip in the posed smile. It is defined as "consonant" when the maxillary incisal curve is parallel to the curvature of the lower lip on smiling, as in Fig. 6.14a, and "nonconsonant," or flat, when the incisal curvature is flatter than the curvature of the lower lip on smiling, as in Fig. 6.14b.

6.5 The Attractive Female Smile

The characteristics of the attractive female smile can be summarized as follows:

- Generous display of the upper anterior teeth.
- Noticeable lip movement from the relaxed position of the lips to the smiling one.
- Prevalence of the transverse dimension of the display zone of the smile over the vertical one.
- Absent or limited display of inferior teeth.

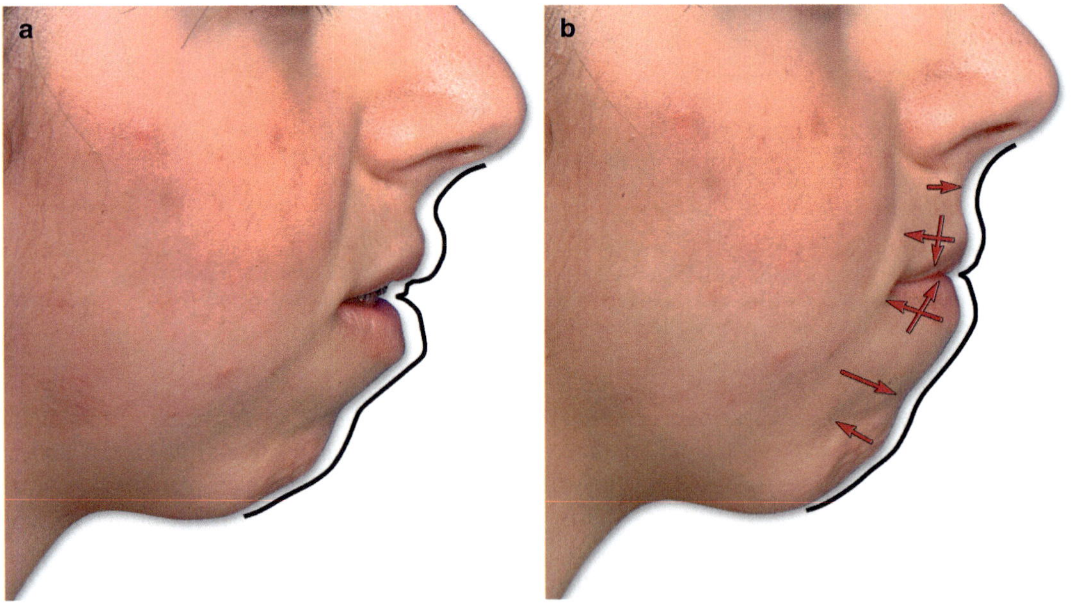

Fig. 6.11 (**a**, **b**) A case of lip incompetence with absence of lip seal at rest due to an increased overjet with mandibular hypoplasia (**a**). In these cases, maintaining perfect lip closure requires a voluntary contraction that results in the flattening of the lip profile curves (**b**)

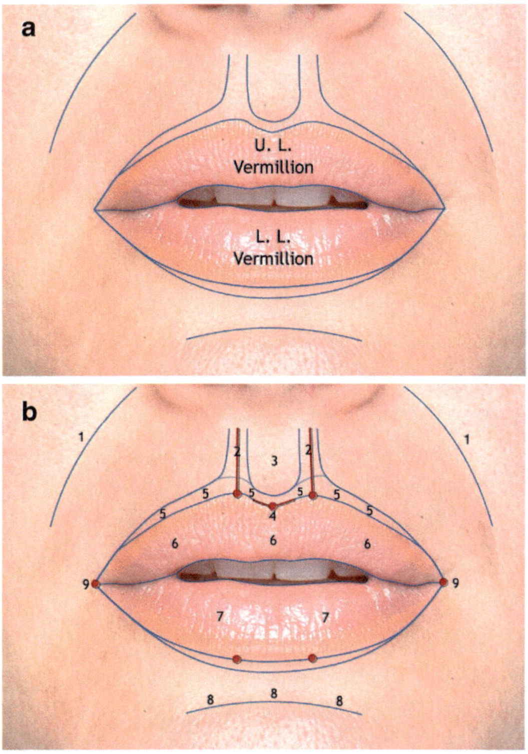

Fig. 6.12 (**a**, **b**) Frontal views of younger, "healthy," attractive female lips (**a**, **b**). Perioral soft tissue determinants (**b**): *1* nasolabial sulcus, *2* philtrum columns, *3* philtrum, *4* Cupid's bow, *5* lip white roll, *6* upper lip vermillion (its central and more projecting portion is also called the upper lip tubercle), *7* lower lip vermillion, *8* labiomental sulcus, *9* lip commissures (the distance between the two commissures is defined as mouth width)

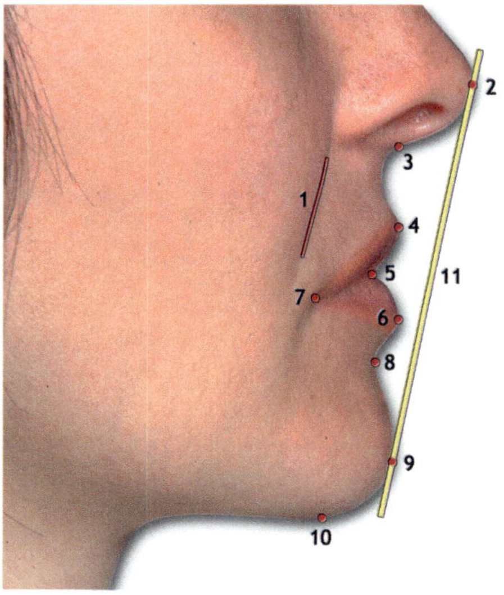

Fig. 6.13 Profile view of younger, "healthy," attractive female lips. Reference points and Ricketts lips projection reference E-line: *1* nasolabial sulcus, *2* nasal tip, *3* subnasale, *4* labrale superior, *5* stomion, *6* labrale inferior, *7* lip commissure, *8* labiomental sulcus, *9* soft tissue pogonion, *10* soft tissue menton, *11* Ricketts E-line. The series of gentle curves from nasal tip to soft tissue menton characterize the lips profile

- Presence of a variable amount of upper gingival display (this is also correlated with the age of the subject).
- Presence of a moderate amount of buccal corridors.
- Presence of a consonant smile arc. Figure 6.15a, b shows two clinical cases of attractive female smiles with less and more gingival display.

6.6 The "No-Smile Patient"

An uncommon but serious facial deformity is the inability to produce a smile. An example of this is shown in Fig. 6.14f, where the outline of the upper anterior teeth is barely visible even though the subject is trying to elevate the upper lip as high as possible. The factors involved in this dynamic deformity, which is evident to observers only during smiling, are multiple and can be classified as follows:

- Vertically long upper lip at rest, due to an increment of the skin area only (the vermillion area is frequently reduced).
- Poor upper lip elevation during smiling.
- Small size of upper anterior teeth or loss of anterior teeth.
- Posterior positioned upper incisors.
- Posterior inclined upper incisors.
- Posterior positioned maxilla (maxillary deficiency).
- Vertically short maxilla (short middle third of the face).

It is clear that the "no-smile patient" facial deformity is a mix of soft tissue, dental, and skeletal problems, which needs a team approach to diagnose and treat completely (Fig. 6.16a–f).

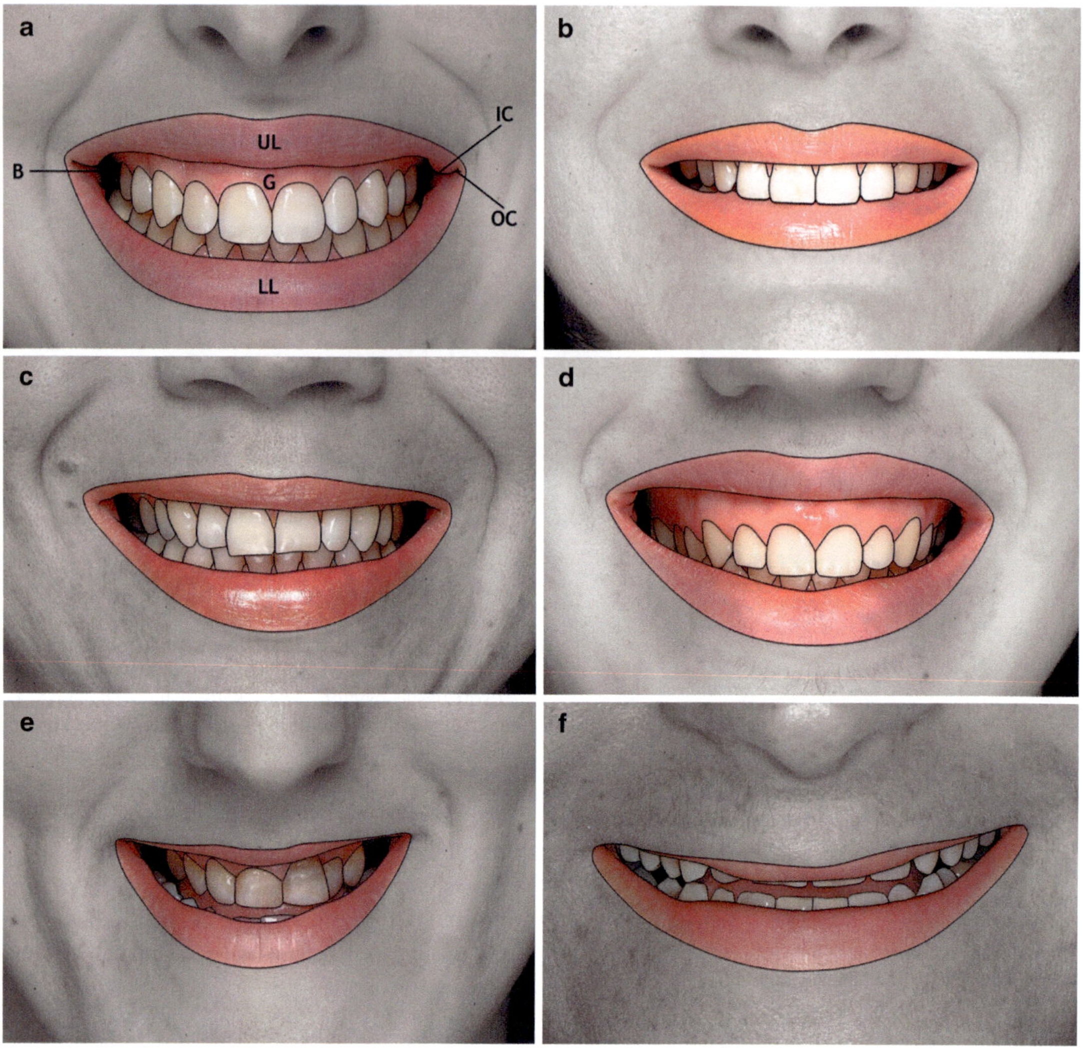

Fig. 6.14 (**a–f**) The smile components and the display zone: *B* buccal corridors, *OC* outer commissure, *IC* inner commissure, *G* gingival, *UL* upper lip vermillion, *LL* lower lip vermillion (**a**). Display zones of five different subjects (**b–f**)

6.7 Chin Assessment

An in-depth direct and photographic study of the chin should be done with the lips in a relaxed position (in many clinical cases this means without contact between the lips), lips in an unforced contact position (lip seal), and during smiling.

The first step considers the balance of the chin with the other facial subunits, mainly the nose, the lips, the submental, and the neck; it is essential to distinguish between an isolated chin deformity and one that is combined with dentofacial or nasal deformities. The chin shape must also be related to the sex, the general proportion of the face, and the height of the subject.

Discerning between the underlying skeletal bony contour and the thickness of the soft tissue envelope must be done by palpation. The soft tis-

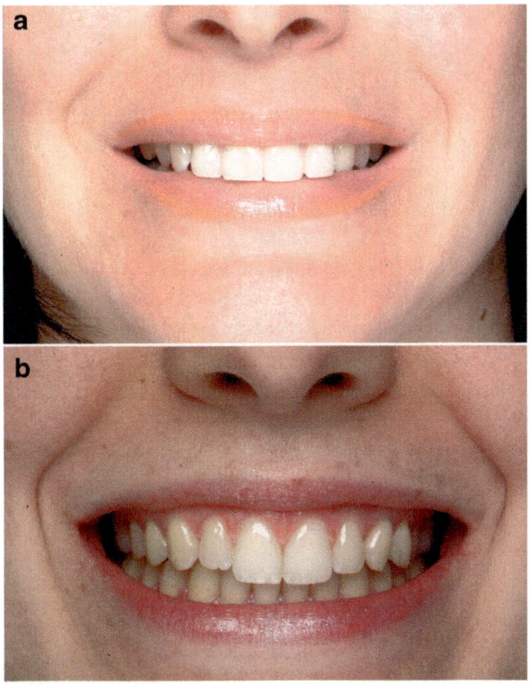

Fig. 6.15 (**a**, **b**) Frontal view of attractive female smile (**a**). An increased display of gingival tissue (**b**) gives a more youthful appearance

sue thickness must also be palpated off the midline because the chin soft tissue is thinnest at the center; the normal thickness of the chin pad soft tissue is 8–10 mm. The labiomental fold divides the lower facial height into two distinct segments, the chin pad and the lower lip. A high or low positioned labiomental fold changes the lengths and the relationships between the two segments (Fig. 6.17).

The cephalometric analysis of the lateral view can be helpful in distinguishing between skeletal and chin pad deformity. Figure 6.17 shows the basic measurements obtainable from a cephalometric tracing in the lower teeth—mandibular symphysis region, whereas Fig. 6.18a–f shows different patterns of chin morphology with the relative soft tissue outline.

An asymmetric deformity can also be related to the shape of the bony structure, the thickness of the soft tissue, or an asymmetric muscular contraction (dynamic chin asymmetry).

6.8 The Basic Components of Dentofacial Deformities

The study of dentofacial deformities is based on three different analyses:

- Direct and photographic clinical facial analyses, which dictate the need for surgery to change the facial appearance.
- Intraoral and dental cast analysis, which is necessary to assess the malocclusion in its two components: intra-arch and inter-arch relationships. The basic elements of dental analysis are described in Sect. 6.1. In particular, the dental cast is the most utilized and easiest solid reproduction of a portion of the human body to obtain; it is also familiar to the patient himself and, for these reasons, we utilize it extensively as a visual tool during the patient communication process.
- Cephalometric analysis, which can add new data, measure some parameters, and permit, by enabling visualization of treatment objectives, an in-depth study of the effects of jaw surgery on skeletal, dental, and soft tissue spatial position.

Understanding a clinical case of dentofacial deformity can be made easier by the identification of its basic components:

- Anterior vertical excess or deficiency.
- Class III or II sagittal discrepancy.
- Transverse discrepancies and asymmetry.

6.9 Anterior Vertical Excess

The anterior vertical excess has been given many other names, such as vertical maxillary excess, hyperdivergent skeletal pattern, high angle case, long face, and skeletal open bite.

Figure 6.19a–e shows a clinical case in which many of the external morphological and skeletal characteristics of the anterior vertical excess are present. Analyzing the frontal view (Fig. 6.19a),

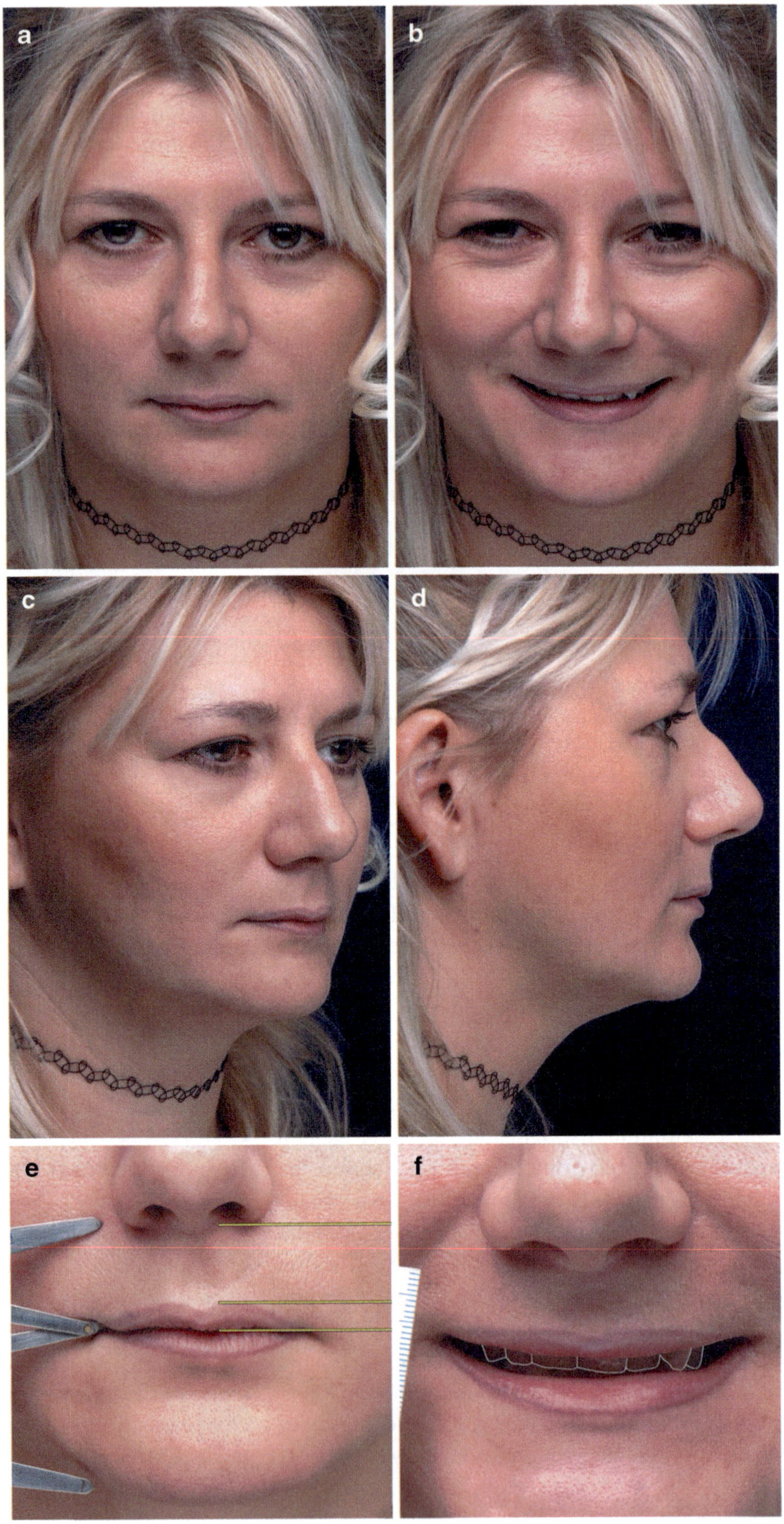

Fig. 6.16 (**a–f**) A clinical case of a "no-smile patient." The frontal (**a**), frontal during smiling (**b**), oblique right (**c**), and profile right views (**d**) show the vertically long upper lip at rest, the poor upper lip elevation during smiling, the clockwise rotation and the flattening of the upper lip profile. The frontal lips close-up view at rest (**e**) highlights that the skin area of the upper lip greatly exceeds the small vermillion area, whereas the close-up frontal smile (**f**) demonstrates that the upper incisors are hidden under the upper lip

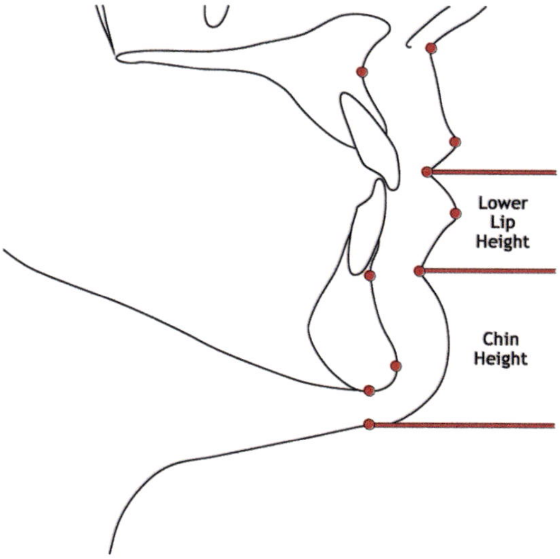

Fig. 6.17 The bony and soft tissue parameters to consider in chin cephalometric tracing are the vertical position of the labiomental fold, which determines the height of the lower lip and chin pad segments, the thickness of the tissue around the bony chin, and the shape of the chin profile

we note a clear elongation of the vertical axis of the face with a reduction in the facial widths. The mandibular outline is asymmetric at the angles and a general impression of flatness of the malar, infraorbital, paranasal, cheek, and chin regions is perceived.

The oblique view (Fig. 6.19b) confirms the flattening of the malar, infraorbital, cheek, paranasal, and chin regions. In particular, the ogee curve outline, in all its components, is constituted of long and nearly straight tracts joined together with open angles.

The profile view (Fig. 6.19c) adds the following important diagnostic elements:

- The total anterior facial height is augmented.
- All the anterior facial thirds appear to be augmented.
- The flatness of the malar, infraorbital, paranasal, cheek, and chin regions is confirmed.
- The nose appears to be long.
- The upper lip outline is clockwise rotated with a lack of anterior projection.
- The labiomental fold is flat.
- The mandibular border outline is partially hidden and clockwise rotated.
- The total chin–throat–neck outline length is reduced with an open cervicomental angle.

The intraoral view (Fig. 6.19d), despite the external facial morphology, shows a molar class I, an anterior dental malocclusion with no anterior open bite.

The cephalometric tracing (Fig. 6.19e), obtained from the cephalograms in the lateral view, permits the correlation of the facial profile with the shape and spatial position of some of the dental and skeletal supporting structure.

6.10 Anterior Vertical Deficiency

The anterior vertical deficiency is characterized by the opposite features of the vertical excess and is also called vertical maxillary deficiency, hypodivergent skeletal pattern, low angle case, short face, and skeletal deep bite.

Figure 6.20a–e shows a clinical case in which many of the external morphological, skeletal, and dental characteristics of the anterior vertical deficiency are present. Analyzing the frontal view (Fig. 6.20a), we note a short vertical axis of the face with a large reduction of the lower facial third height and the relative increase of all facial widths.

The oblique view (Fig. 6.20b) confirms the large reduction of the lower face height, also drawing attention to the long and over-projected nose.

The profile view (Fig. 6.20c) confirms and adds some important diagnostic elements such as:

- Reduction of the lower anterior face height; conversely, the central and upper anterior facial third may appear augmented.
- The nose appears to be long.
- The upper lip outline is counterclockwise rotated and excessively concave.
- The labiomental fold is extremely deep and unnatural.

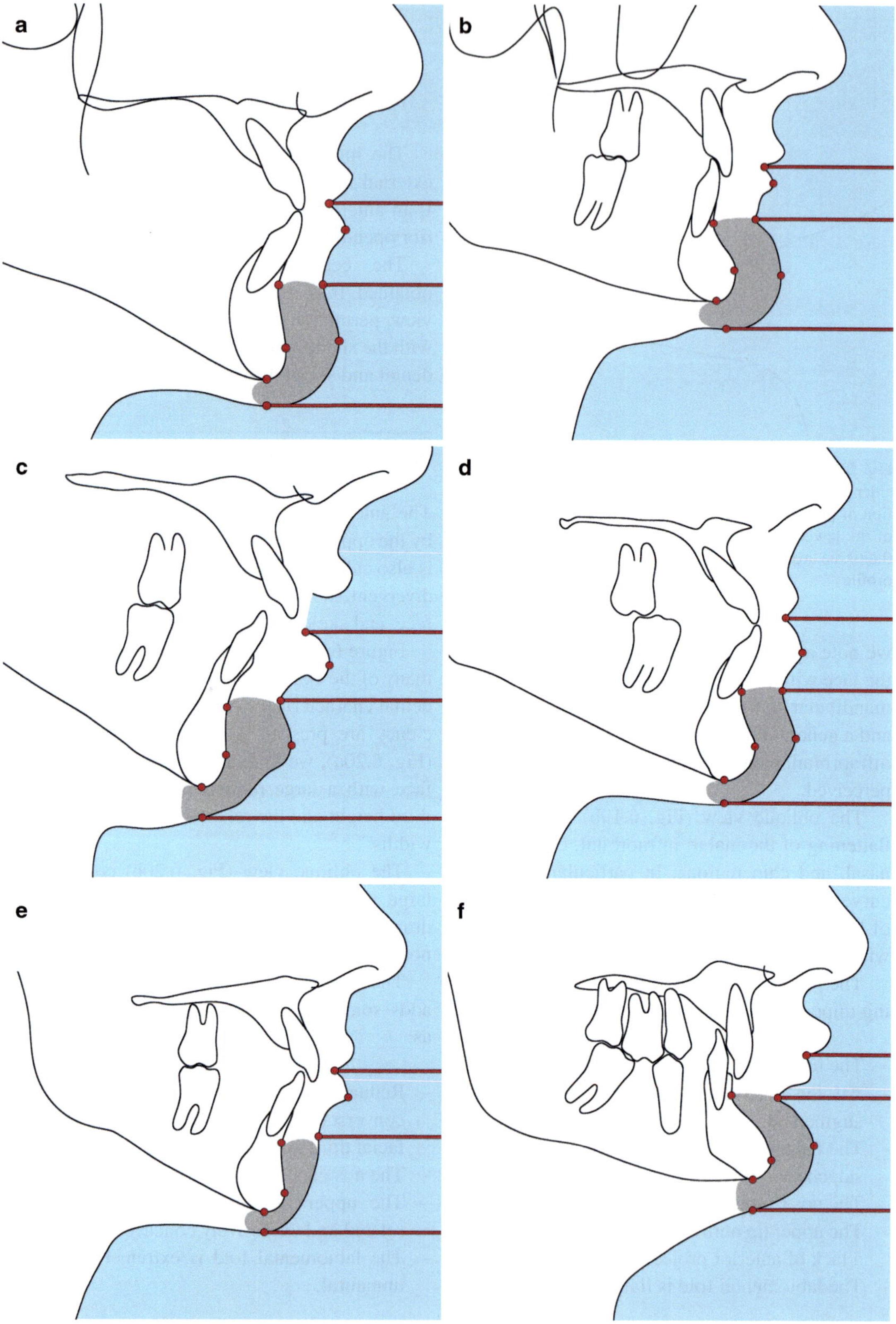

Fig. 6.18 The morphology of the bony chin as well as the overlying soft tissue varies greatly (**a–f**)

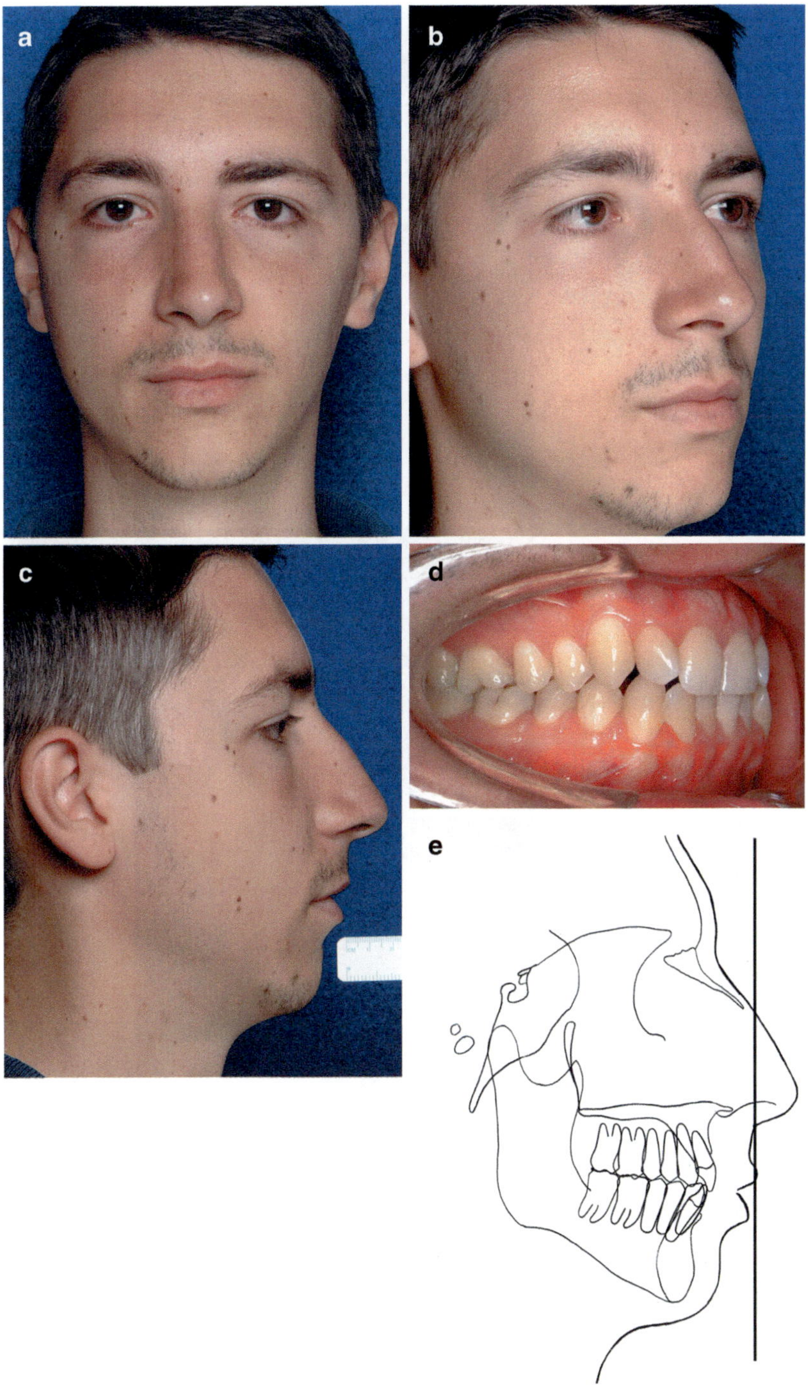

Fig. 6.19 (**a**–**e**) A clinical case of anterior vertical excess. Frontal (**a**), oblique right (**b**), profile (**c**), intraoral right views (**d**), and cephalometric tracing (**e**)

- The mandibular border outline is counterclockwise rotated in a nearly horizontal position. This affects the chin projection, which seems to be increased; nevertheless this is not sufficient to obtain a pleasant cervicomental angle.
- The throat length is extremely short.

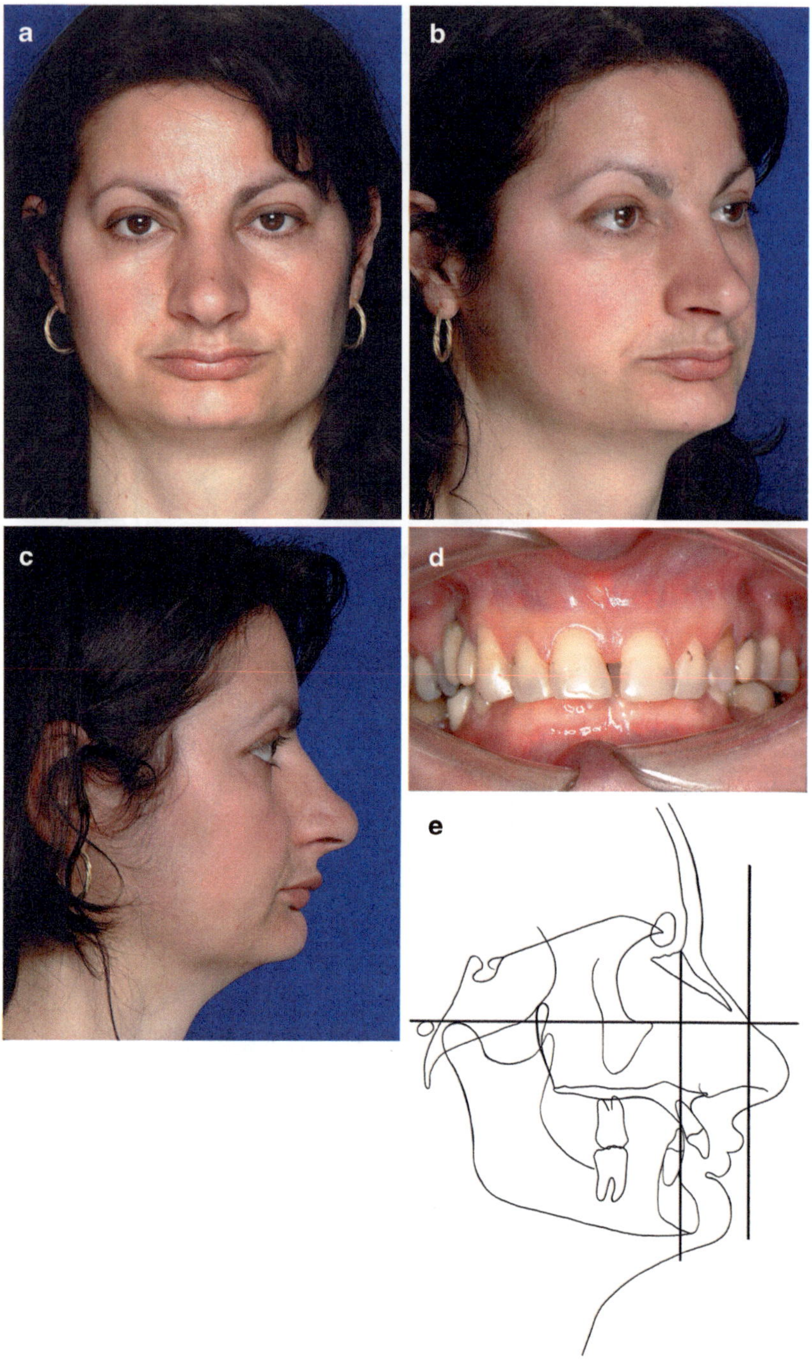

Fig. 6.20 (**a–e**) A clinical case of anterior vertical deficiency. Frontal (**a**), oblique right (**b**), profile (**c**), intraoral anterior views (**d**), and cephalometric tracing (**e**)

The frontal intraoral view (Fig. 6.20d), according to the external facial morphology, shows the anterior dental deep bite (the lower teeth are totally hidden by the upper incisors and cuspids). The cephalometric tracing (Fig. 6.20e), obtained from the cephalograms in the lateral view, permits the correlation of the facial profile with the shape and spatial position of some of the dental and skeletal supporting structure.

6.11 Class III Sagittal Discrepancy

The class III sagittal discrepancy brings together many deformities common to an anteriorly positioned lower third of the face and/or a posterior positioned middle third.

Figure 6.21a–e shows a clinical case in which many of the external morphological, skeletal, and dental characteristics of the class III sagittal discrepancy are present. Analyzing the frontal view (Fig. 6.21a), we note the depressed infraorbital and paranasal regions with a tendency towards an inferior scleral show. The total facial height and the facial widths seem proportioned, whereas a general impression of flatness of infraorbital, paranasal, and cheek regions is perceived.

The oblique view (Fig. 6.21b) confirms the flattening of the infraorbital, cheek, and paranasal regions; in particular, the ogee curve outline shows the tendency towards a concave face due to midface retrusion.

The profile view (Fig. 6.21c) confirms and adds some important diagnostic elements such as:

- The total anterior facial height appears to be increased.
- The flatness of malar, infraorbital, cheek, and paranasal regions is confirmed.
- The lower third of the nose appears to be normal in spite of the lack of skeletal support.
- The upper lip outline is clockwise rotated.
- The chin is slightly over-projected.
- The labiomental fold is normally shaped.
- The mandibular border outline is well defined and clockwise rotated.
- The total chin–throat–neck outline length, as well as the cervicomental angle definition and degree, are pleasing.

The oblique right intraoral view (Fig. 6.21d) shows a dental malocclusion with molar and canine class III, partial anterior reverse overjet, and anterior dental crowding of the lower anterior teeth.

The cephalometric tracing (Fig. 6.21e), obtained from the cephalograms in the lateral view, permits the correlation of the facial profile with the shape and spatial position of some of the dental and skeletal supporting structure.

6.12 Class II Sagittal Discrepancy

The class II sagittal discrepancy brings together many deformities common to a posteriorly positioned lower third of the face (more frequent) and/or an anteriorly positioned middle third (less frequent).

Figure 6.22a–d shows a clinical case in which many of the external morphological, skeletal, and dental characteristics of the class II sagittal discrepancy are present. Analyzing the frontal view (Fig. 6.22a), we note an evident facial asymmetry, a large and deviated nose, and a reduced chin width.

The right oblique view (Fig. 6.22b) reveals the flat malar, infraorbital, cheek, paranasal, and chin regions. The ogee curve outline, in this particular case, helps the observer to recognize the extreme grade of the chin under-projection.

The profile view (Fig. 6.22c) adds the following important diagnostic elements:

- The facial profile is convex, which is primarily due to the clockwise over-rotated mandible.
- The flatness of the malar, infraorbital, cheek, paranasal, and chin regions are confirmed.
- The upper lip outline is slightly clockwise rotated.
- The labiomental fold is flat.
- The chin is severely under-projected.
- The mandibular border outline is clockwise rotated.
- The total chin–throat–neck outline length is reduced with an open cervicomental angle.
- The throat length is extremely short.

The cephalometric tracing (Fig. 6.22d), obtained from the cephalograms in lateral view, shows the presence of overjet between the upper and lower incisors, as well as the molar class II relationship, and confirms the clockwise rotation of the mandible and the chin under-projection.

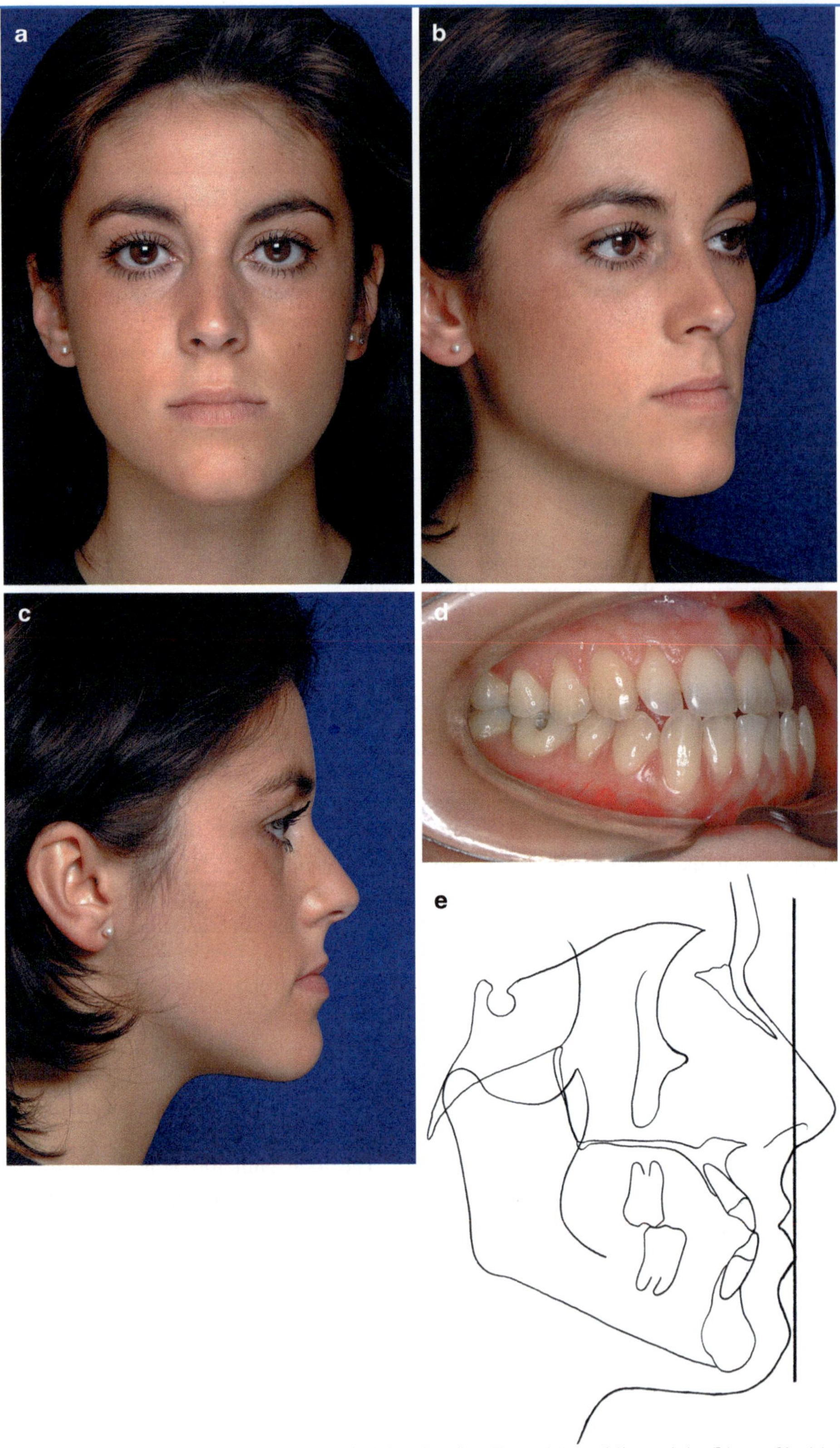

Fig. 6.21 (a–e) A clinical case of class III dentofacial deformity. Frontal (a), oblique right (b), profile (c), intraoral right oblique views (d), and cephalometric tracing (e)

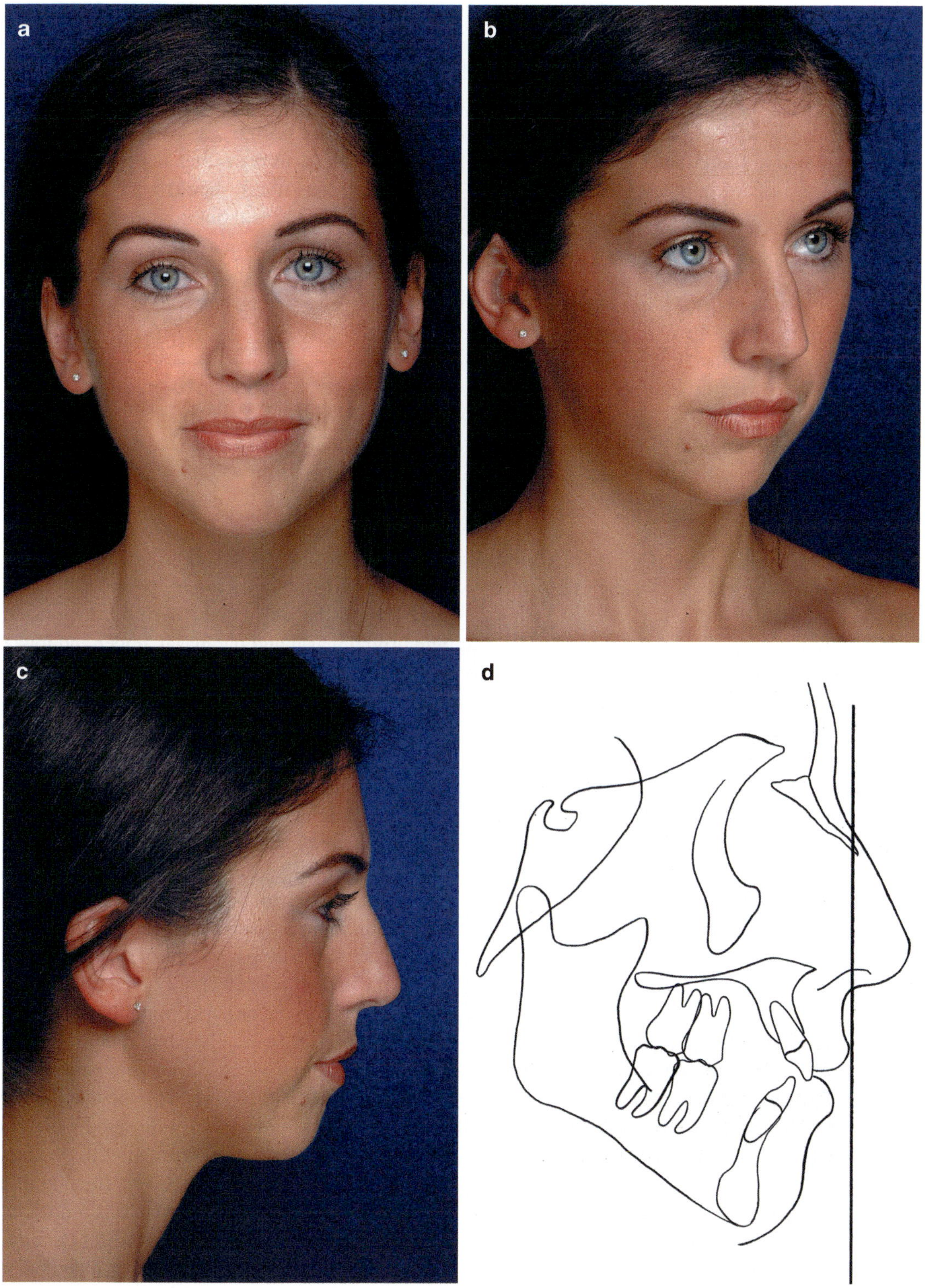

Fig. 6.22 (**a–d**) A clinical case of class II dentofacial deformity. Frontal (**a**), oblique right (**b**), profile views (**c**), and cephalometric tracing (**d**)

6.13 Transverse Discrepancies and Asymmetry of the Jaws

An asymmetric arrangement of the dental arches is frequently associated with a corresponding facial asymmetry. The clinical case presented in Fig. 6.5a–c is a clear example of that association. Analyzing the frontal and left views of the dental cast (Fig. 6.5a, b), we note these points:

- The mandibular midline is deviated on the left compared to that of the maxillary.
- Some teeth on the left side (colored in Fig. 6.5b) are in a reverse overbite relationship.
- The line connecting the two lower cuspids as well as the occlusal plane of the mandibular arch is counterclockwise rotated.

The facial frontal view (Fig. 6.5c) confirms that the facial asymmetry is coherent with the intraoral findings. In particular:

- The line connecting the two labial commissures is tilted counterclockwise.
- The chin is deviated to the left.

Figure 6.5c also shows some reference planes utilized in the assessment of the facial asymmetries, such as the lines connecting the medial canthus, the upper palpebral folds, or the apex of the eyebrows. Each of these lines must be checked in order to confirm their symmetry and therefore their reliability.

6.14 The Immense Number of Combinations of Different Types and Grades of the Basic Components of Facial Deformities

In a real clinical situation, there is almost never an isolated basic component of a facial deformity in a patient and the grade of the deformity also varies greatly.

The real cases presented for demonstration purposes have one weak point: they are without doubt a mix of these basic components, so the preoperative clinical analysis still is not finished with the understanding of the most obvious element, but must continue until a complete assessment of the case is done.

Nevertheless, in the initial steps of the analysis, any written notes should be based on the clinical assessment without taking precise metric or angular measurements. At an early stage, a rigid "computerized" method of analysis, with its normative values, must be avoided.

6.15 Direct and Photographic Clinical Analysis for Dentofacial Deformities

The biggest mistake we can make, when dealing with dentofacial deformities, is to limit our attention only to the jaw relationships. A severely retruded maxilla, for example, profoundly influences the esthetics of the lower lid, zygomatic and orbital, nasal and paranasal, upper and lower lip, mandibular and chin regions.

When dealing with dentofacial deformities, during examination and photographic documentation it is extremely important to obtain a relaxed lip position, a relaxed-rest mandibular position, and again the natural head position. In order to help the patient achieve the relaxed lip position, the examiner asks him to relax, strokes the lips gently and takes multiple pictures on different occasions; an additional assessment of the lips is obtained with successive casual observations while the patient is unaware of being observed.

Some authors favor performing the direct and photographic analysis in centric relationship or centric occlusion, which means maintaining the two dental arches in contact, with the mandibular elevator muscles contracted. I disagree with this because normally a person is only in this position while swallowing, obtaining it for a fraction of a second. Maintaining it for a minute is a difficult task for patients because of the need for continuous muscle strain and the unnatural mandibular position.

Instead, for my basic esthetic considerations, I want a relaxed position of the mandible in every

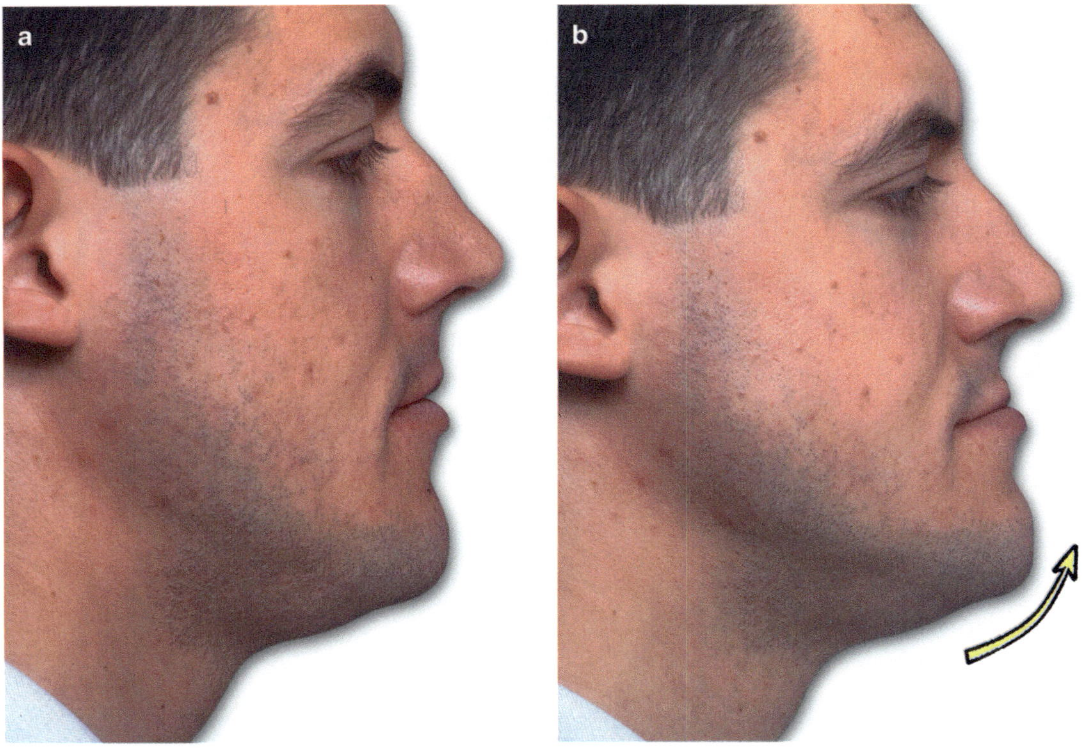

Fig. 6.23 (**a**, **b**) Differences in facial soft tissue adjustment in the same subject in his habitual posture (**a**) and in the close bite mandibular position (**b**). The patient obtains the latter condition only during the act of swallowing

case, doing a further facial examination in the close bite position only if a large difference in soft tissue arrangement exists between the two, as shown in Fig. 6.23a, b.

As a general rule, in the clinical assessment of the total and regional vertical facial heights, it is possible to highlight more or less pronounced curves and more or less acute angles. In particular, the long face in profile and oblique views can be seen as an open accordion (Fig. 6.24a) with obtuse angles and flat curves, whereas a short face can resemble a closed accordion (Fig. 6.24b) with acute angles and pronounced curves.

Particular attention should be given to the cheekbone–nasal base–lip curve contour described by Arnett and Bergman.[1] In a subject with good facial proportions, it is composed of a convex, anteriorly facing, uninterrupted line that starts just anterior to the ear, follows the zygomatic arch, passing through the cheekbone point, extending anterior-inferiorly reaching the maxilla point, which constitutes its most anterior point, and then ending lateral to the commissure of the mouth (Fig. 6.25a–c).

A maxillary retrusion is clinically related to a straight or concave cheekbone–nasal base–lip curve contour at maxilla point, a flat cheekbone point, and a clockwise rotation of the lower lid inclined in profile view, whereas the ogee profile on oblique view shows a flat outline at the level of the malar eminence (Fig. 6.26a–c).

Utilizing the frontal and oblique views, further attention should be given to the triangular area situated between the nasal base at the alar crease junction and the upper end of the nasolabial sulcus, the paranasal triangle, evaluating its depth. Again, a maxillary hypoplasia is associated with a deep paranasal triangle (Fig. 6.27a, b).

In order to visualize the relationship between the maxillary anteroposterior position, the nasal

[1]Arnett GW, Bergman R. Facial keys to orthodontic diagnosis and treatment planning, Parts I and II. Am J Orthop Dentofacial Orthod 1993; 103: 299–312 and 395–41.

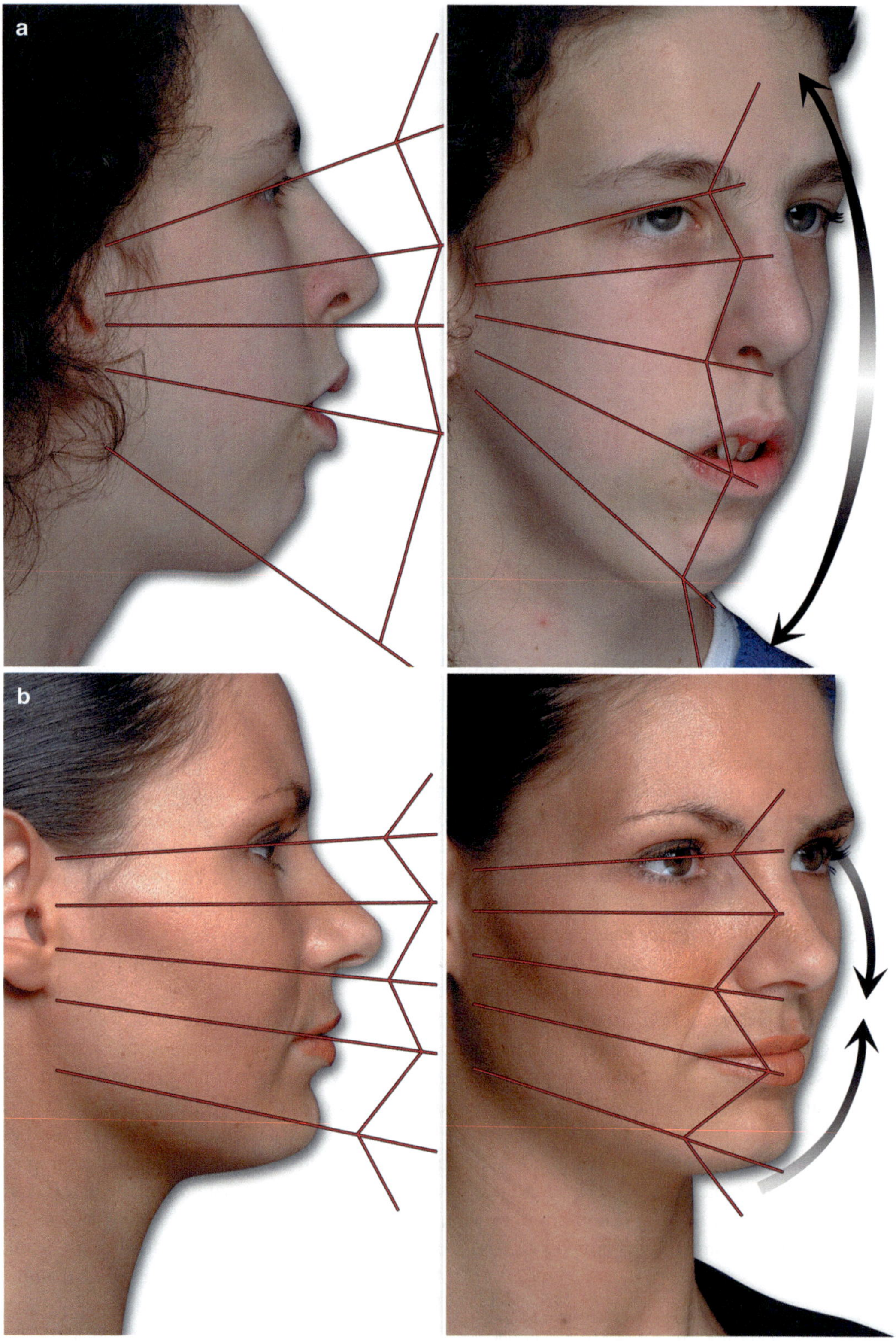

Fig. 6.24 (**a**, **b**) The long face in profile and oblique views can be seen as an open accordion (**a**) with obtuse angles and flat curvatures, whereas the short face can resemble a closed accordion (**b**) with acute angles and pronounced curves

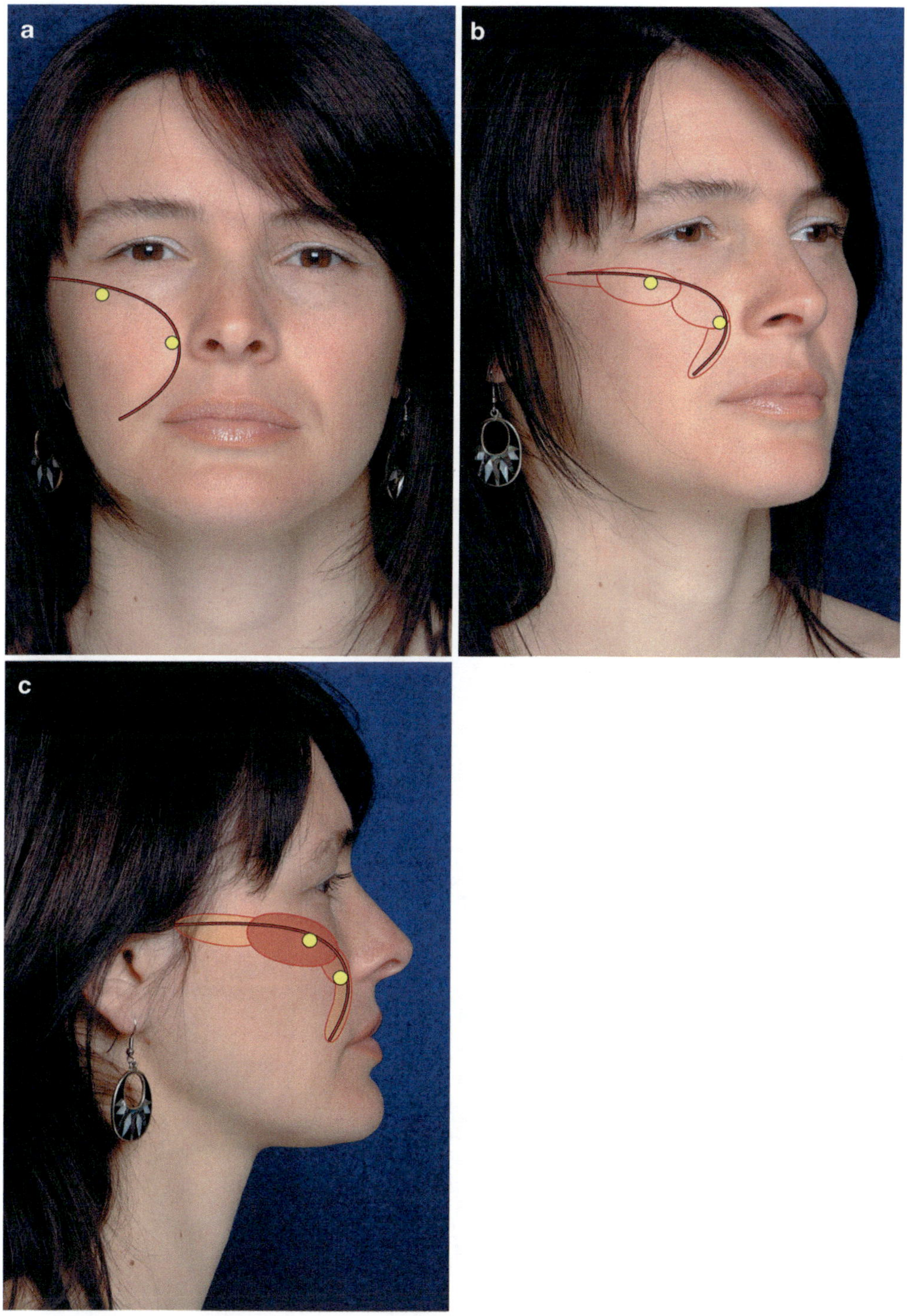

Fig. 6.25 (**a–c**) The cheekbone–nasal base–lip curve contour described by Arnett and Bergman in frontal (**a**), oblique (**b**), and profile views (**c**) of a subject with good facial proportions. The cheekbone point, in a subject with good facial proportions, is the apex of osseous cheekbone that is located 20–25 mm inferior and 5–10 mm anterior to the outer canthus of the eye when viewed in profile and is 20–25 mm inferior and 5–10 mm lateral to the outer canthus of the eye when viewed frontally. A flat cheekbone point is often associated with malar deficiency and maxillary hypoplasia. The maxilla point is the most anterior point on the continuum of the cheekbone–nasal base–lip contour described by Arnett and Bergman and is an indicator of maxillary anteroposterior position

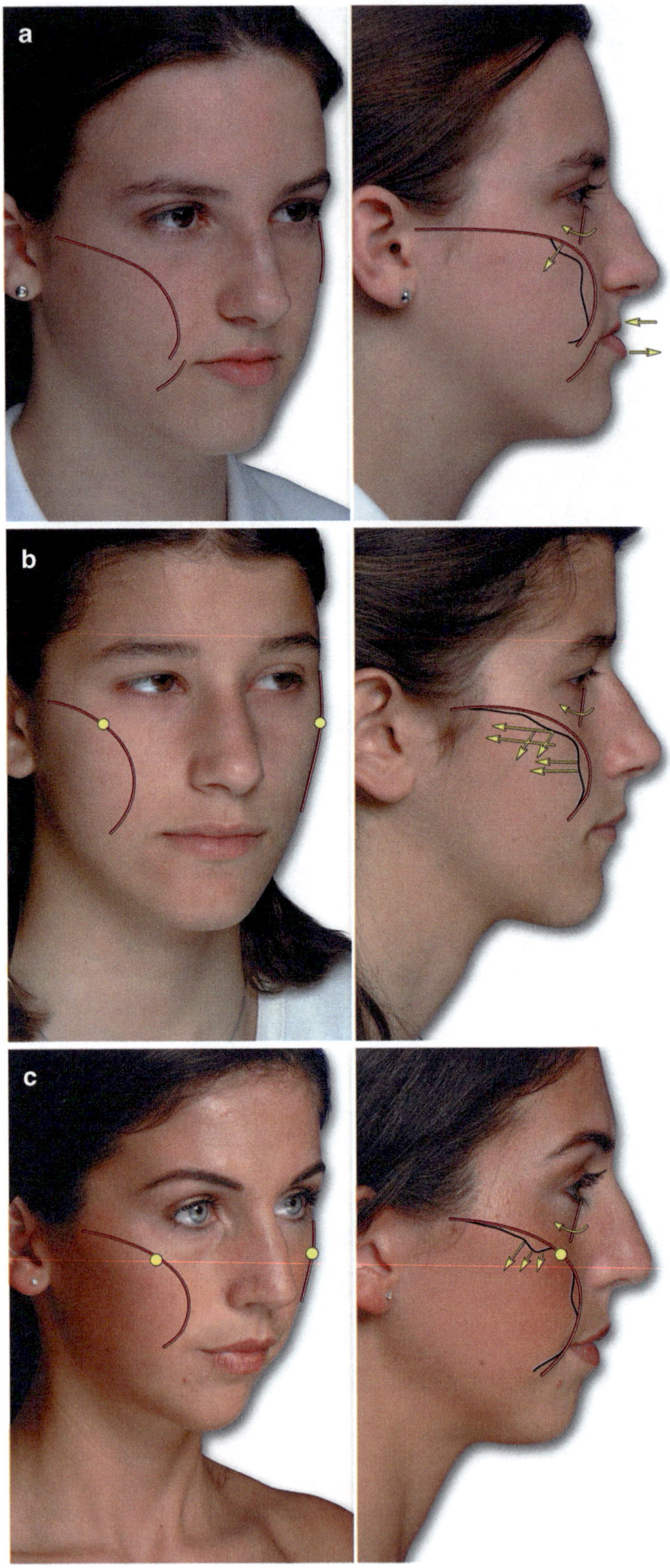

Fig. 6.26 Profile and oblique views of three subjects (**a–c**) with maxillary retrusion in which the cheekbone–nasal base–lip curve contour displays a flat cheekbone point, a posterior positioned maxillary point, and a clockwise rotation of the right lower lid incline in profile view, whereas the ogee profile on oblique view shows a flat outline at the level of the malar eminence

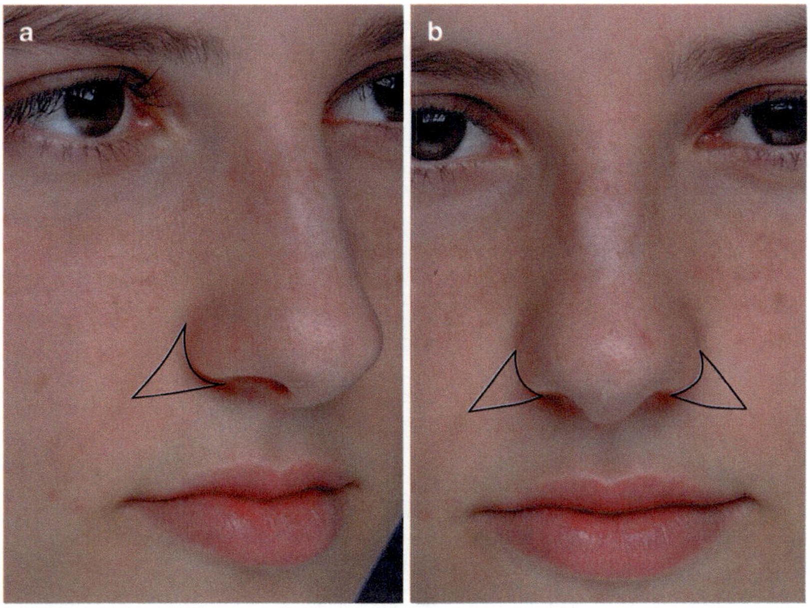

Fig. 6.27 (**a**, **b**) Assessment of the paranasal triangle. In these two cases, the maxillary hypoplasia is associated with a deep paranasal triangle, the triangular area situated between the nasal base at the alar crease junction and the upper end of the nasolabial sulcus (**a–e**)

tip projection, and the chin projection better, I suggest drawing three angles over the life-size profile view photograph. The first is the angle obtained by connecting glabella, nasal tip, and soft tissue pogonion (G′-P-Pog′), the second is the angle obtained by connecting glabella, subnasale, and soft tissue pogonion (G′-Sn-Pog′), also called the angle of facial convexity, and the third is the angle obtained by connecting glabella, alar crease junction, and soft tissue pogonion (G′-ACJ-Pog′). Even if I do not measure these angles, simple observation of the drawing helps in finding and differentiating the anteroposterior relationships of the maxilla, chin, nasal tip, and anterior nasal spine, as shown in the clinical examples in Fig. 6.28a–f.

The upper lip length should be considered in its absolute and relative values. It is the distance from subnasale and upper lip inferior should be between 19 and 22 mm. Sometimes an apparently short upper lip can be confused with vertical maxillary excess, which also produces an increased upper incisors exposure, or a clockwise rotated nasal tip, which "hides" the upper lip; in contrast, the counterclockwise rotated nasal tip makes the upper lip appear longer (Fig. 6.29).

Another important step in the analysis of dentofacial deformities is the assessment of the chin–throat–neck profile, as well as the mandibular border contour. The main points to consider are:

- Mandibular size. More than its absolute size, it is important to consider the relative dimensions, the supporting action offered to the overlying soft tissue, as well as the shape of the mandibular contour.
- Mandibular incline in profile view. Counterclockwise rotation of the mandible increases the chin projection, shortens the lower facial third height, and usually favorably affects the chin–throat–neck profile. In contrast, the mandibular clockwise rotation decreases the chin projection, increases the lower facial third height, and usually worsens the chin–throat–neck profile (Fig. 6.30).
- Mandibular border definition from angle to chin. A thin soft tissue envelope and mandibular counterclockwise rotation produce a well-sculptured border, whereas a poor definition is due to fat accumulation and mandibular clockwise rotation. The definitions of mandibular angle and posterior third of mandibular border are also variable depending on the volume of the masseter muscle.
- Chin shape at rest and chin dynamics. As reported in Sect. 6.7, the assessment of the

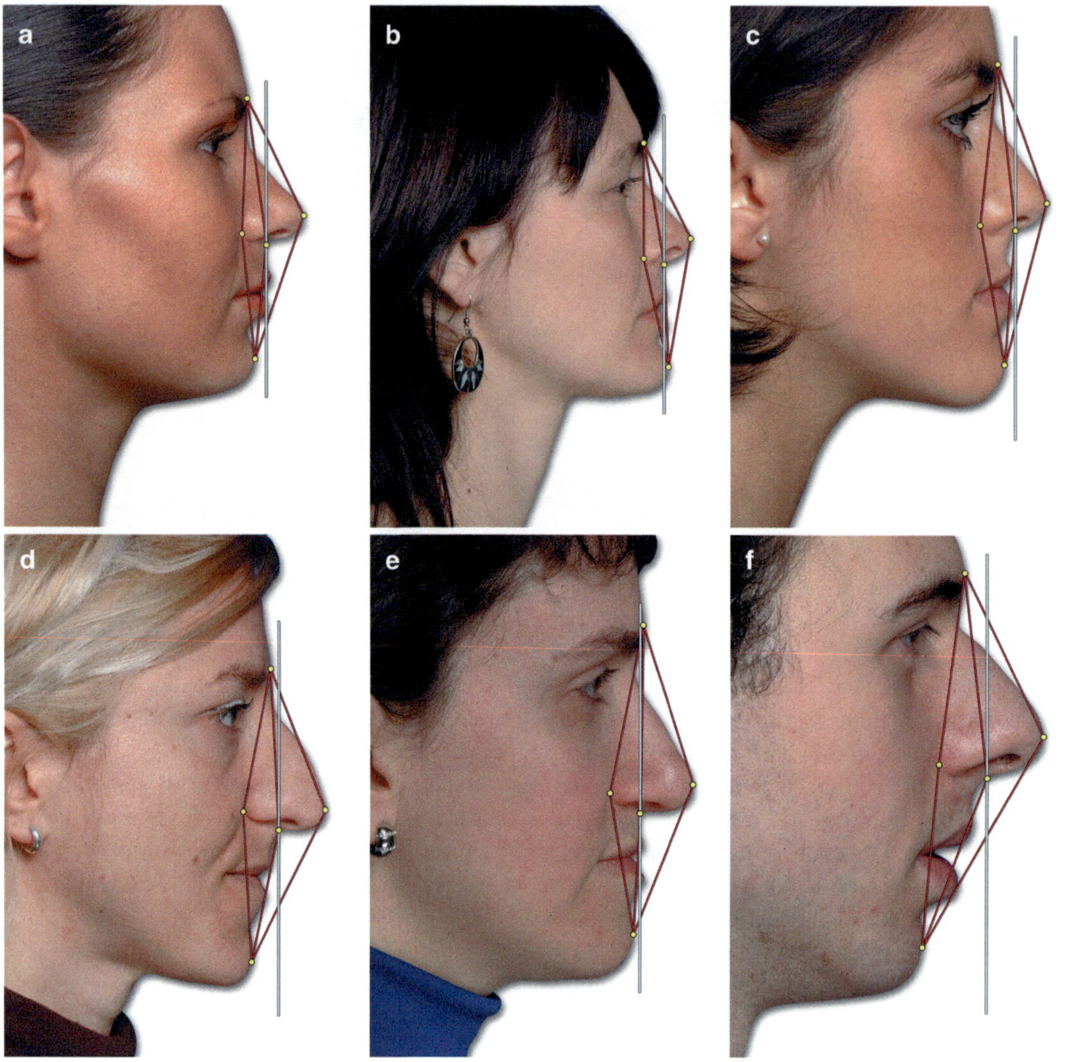

Fig. 6.28 (**a–f**) In these profile views of six different cases, three angles are superimposed. The first is the angle obtained by connecting glabella, nasal tip, and soft tissue pogonion (G′-P-Pog′), the second is the angle obtained connecting glabella, subnasale, and soft tissue pogonion (G′-Sn-Pog′), also called the angle of facial convexity, and the third is the angle obtained connecting glabella, alar crease junction, and soft tissue pogonion (G′-ACJ-Pog′). A normal maxilla may be associated with a slight over-projected nasal tip (**a**) or an over-projected chin (**b**), whereas a hypoplasic nasal base and maxilla may be associated with a normal nasal tip and chin projection (**c**), an over-projected nasal tip (**d**), an underdeveloped nasal spine (**e**), and an over-projected nasal tip and a mandibular retrusion (**f**)

bony as well as the soft tissue components that determine the external chin shape is of paramount importance. The profile assumed by the subject when sustaining the lip seal with musculature contraction should also be noted.

– The throat length (NTP-Me′). This is the distance between the neck–throat point (NTP) and soft tissue menton (Me′) on the lower facial outline (Fig. 6.31a, b). The throat length is preferably assessed clinically to be short or long and not measured instrumentally.
– The throat incline. This is the angle formed between the throat outline and the horizontal plane passing through the soft tissue menton; a favorable incline is that which remains over or near the horizontal plane, whereas an exces-

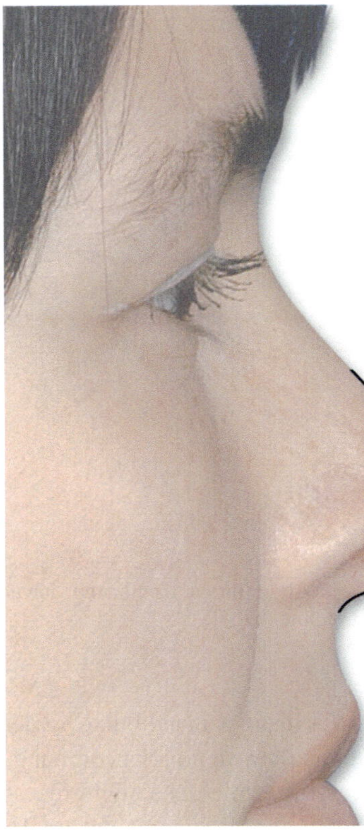

Fig. 6.29 The clockwise rotation of the nasal tip makes the upper lip appear shorter, whereas the counterclockwise rotation makes the upper lip appear longer

sively downwardly oriented incline is associated with poor esthetics of the lower face. Again, it is not measured instrumentally but only clinically assessed (Fig. 6.31a, b).

- Hyoid bone spatial position. The vertical and anteroposterior hyoid bone position greatly affects the throat length and incline and the submental–neck angle due to the need for a supero-posteriorly positioned hyoid bone for favorable esthetics. Palpation and lateral cephalograms help in differentiating a malpositioned hyoid bone from muscular bulging or true fat accumulation.
- Soft tissue thickness. The submental–throat–neck is one of the facial regions most prone to fat accumulation. Palpation helps in differentiating muscular bulging from true fat accumulation.
- Soft tissue redundancy and ptosis. Even if skin excess and platysma banding, as with many other problems, are associated with the aging process, they must also be investigated and assessed in middle-aged subjects in order to differentiate between the various causes of the esthetic problems.

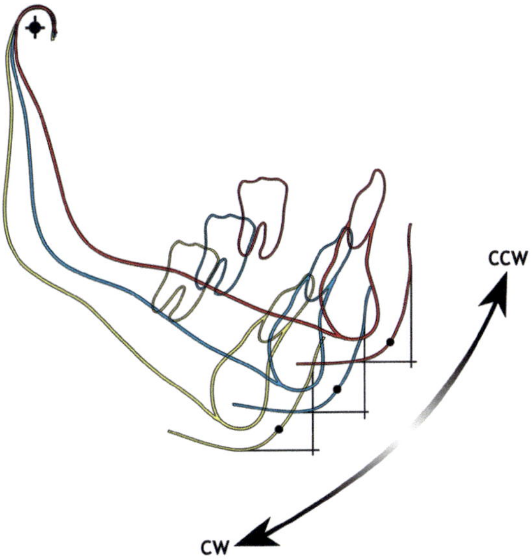

Fig. 6.30 The degree of mandibular incline is associated with many other features of the lower facial third. A mandibular clockwise (CW) rotation increases the chin projection, shortens the lower facial third height, and usually favorably affects the chin–throat–neck profile. In contrast, a mandibular counterclockwise (CCW) rotation decreases the chin projection, increases the lower facial third height, and usually worsens the chin–throat–neck profile

In the case of an esthetically poor chin–throat–neck profile, it is mandatory to separate the skeletal factors, such as mandibular dimension, shape and orientation, from the soft tissue factors related to the skin, platysma muscle, and fat.

6.16 The Youthful Neck

As for other facial regions, defining the ideal chin–neck features helps us to understand and analyze the clinical problems. Although the approach of Ellenbogen and Karlin[2] which utilizes five visual

[2]Ellenbogen R, Karlin JV. Visual criteria for success in restoring the youthful neck. Plast Reconstr Surg. 1980; 66:826–837.

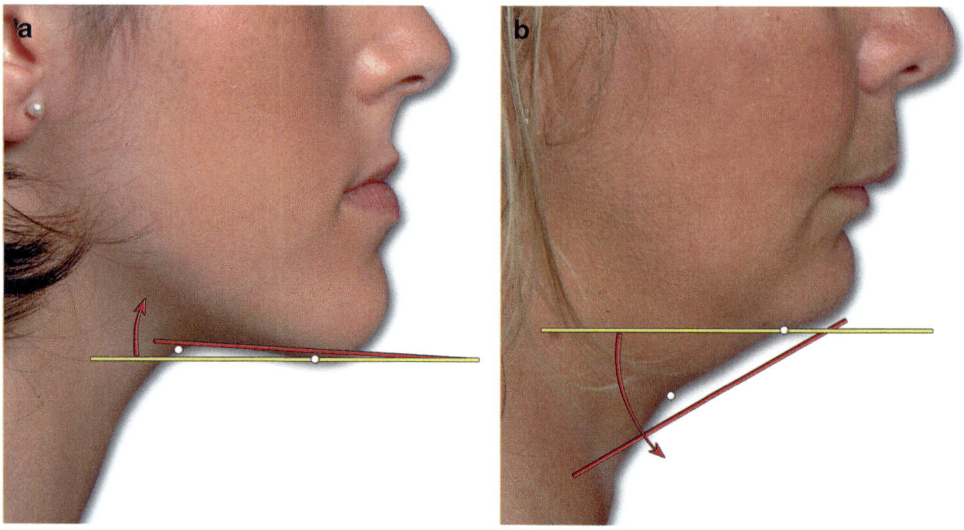

Fig. 6.31 (**a**, **b**) Clinical evaluation of throat length and throat incline. A clinical case of long throat length and upwardly rotated throat incline (**a**) compared with the converse condition of a short throat length and downwardly rotated throat incline (**b**)

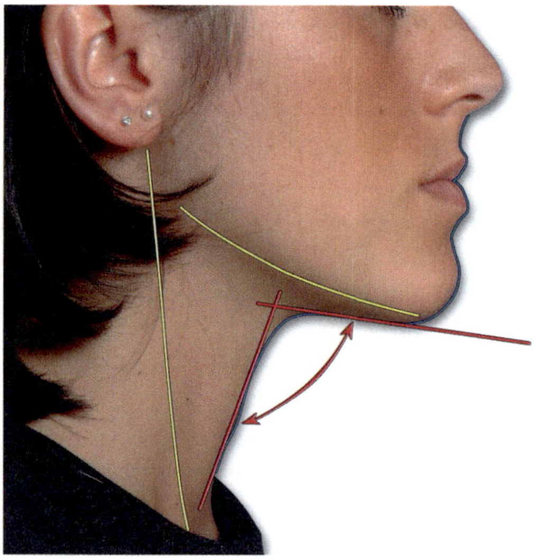

Fig. 6.32 A clinical case of a youthful neck. This shows a well-defined inferior mandibular border, cervicomental contour, and anterior border of the sternocleidomastoid muscle with a cervicomental angle of 103°

criteria in the assessment of the neck was devised for rhytidectomy patients, it is reported here because of the strong relationship between dentofacial deformities and neck problems.

The five visual criteria of Ellenbogen and Karlin characterizing the ideal youthful neck are (Fig. 6.32):

1. The presence of a distinct mandibular border from mentum to angle with no jowl overhang.
2. Subhyoid depression, which is a slight recess below the apex of the cervicomental angle. We can utilize the radius of curvature of the cervicomental angle for the second visual criteria. The ideal radius is rather small to give a well-defined cervicomental angle, whereas a long radius is related to an obtuse angle and poor esthetics.
3. Visible thyroid cartilage bulge.
4. Visible anterior border of sternocleidomastoid muscle distinct in its entire length from the mastoid to sternum.
5. Cervicomental angle between 105 and 120°.

6.17 A Personal View on Radiographic Cephalometry

Orthodontics applied to jaw surgery was one of my earliest professional interests and, as a consequence, over a couple of years, my library was full of books and articles on cephalometrics and every day at least one new head film was in my viewbox for tracing and analysis. The head of the department often gave me the cephalograms from his clinical cases and during 1989 I was in Milan every Friday attending the orthodontic section of the dental school, where the then chief was famous for his cephalometric analysis.

Cephalometrics is a demanding form of analysis, many points of reference are hidden in the depths of the face and others are simply nonexistent (artificially constructed); it also requires anatomical, dental, and radiological knowledge and it is a time-consuming activity.

To complicate this field further, hundreds of different cephalometric analyses have been published, giving clinicians an immense number of different parameters and a correspondingly difficult technical language.

After years of daily clinical experience, I am sure that I need less data from cephalometrics and more data from other sources in order to give better treatment to my patients. However, I still recommend that my young colleagues spend a regular part of their time studying and practicing it because:

- One of the largest groups of specialists working with the face, orthodontists, uses cephalometrics to classify, define, treat, and follow up their clinical cases and we all need to communicate with one another.
- The comparison of serial tracing is one of the best methods of studying what has happened to the facial profile and skeletal structure in a given clinical case, not only with orthodontic treatment but also with surgery.
- In the first years of practice, the other forms of analysis are not sufficiently developed to be utilized without an extra "cephalometric check."

In other words, we need cephalometric analysis early in our career in order to develop, whereas later we need to surpass cephalometric analysis to continue to develop.

6.18 Essential Radiographic Cephalometry

The most utilized cephalometric analyses contain a collection of parameters, which can be divided into three subgroups: dental, skeletal, and soft tissue analysis. The following sections report a limited selection of the basic cephalometric measurements obtainable from the lateral cephalometric tracing; these are included with the main purpose of encouraging the reader to discover more about cephalometric analysis in his future practice.

6.19 Dental Cephalometric Analysis

The main scope of dental cephalometric analysis is to study the spatial position of the upper and lower central incisors.

- Interincisal Angle. The interincisal angle is drawn by passing a line through the incisal edge and the apex of the root of the maxillary and mandibular central incisors. Its normative value is 130°. In the case of a more acute value, one or both of the incisors are excessively labial (anteriorly) inclined, whereas in the case of a more obtuse value, one or both of the incisors are excessively lingual (posteriorly) inclined (Fig. 6.33). The measurement of the interincisal angle does not by itself clarify which set of incisors (the upper or the lower) is abnormally inclined.

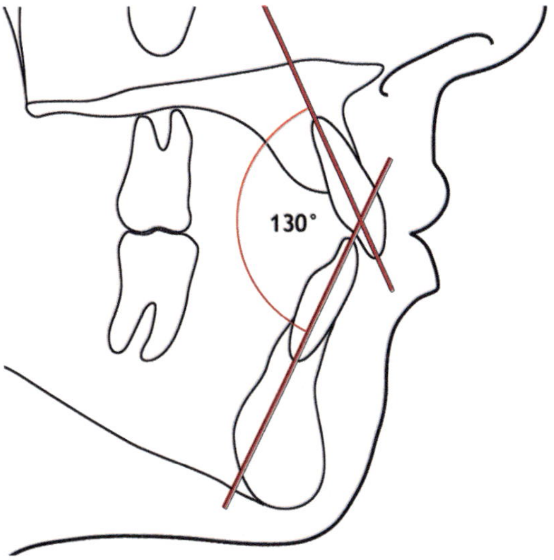

Fig. 6.33 Interincisal angle. Its normative value is 130°

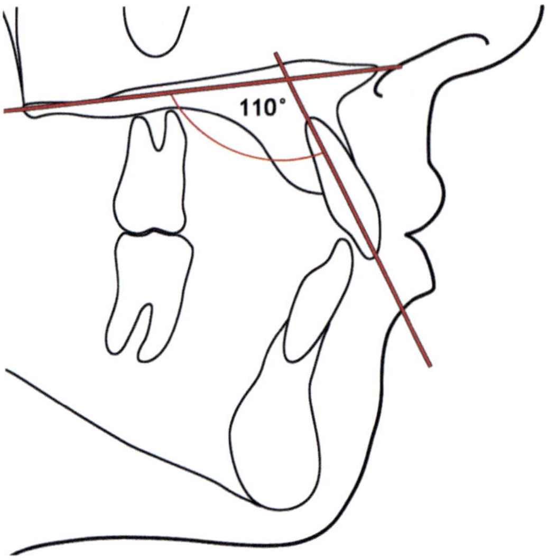

Fig. 6.34 Upper central incisors to maxillary plane angle. Its normative value is 110°

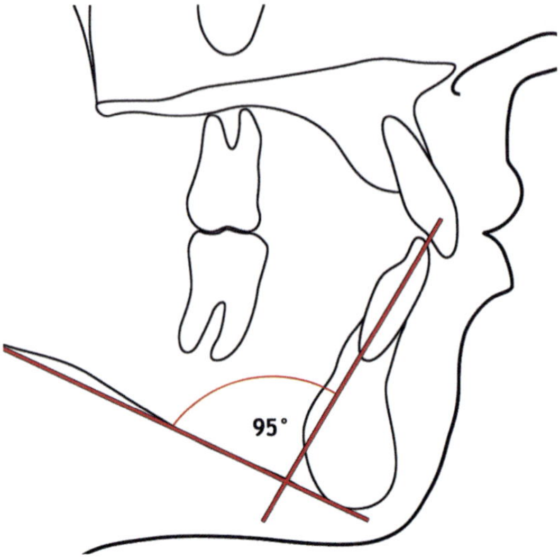

Fig. 6.35 Lower incisors to mandibular plane angle. Its normative value is 95°

- Angle Between the Upper Central Incisors and the Maxillary Plane. It helps in analyzing the incline of the upper anterior teeth. Its normative value is 110°. The maxillary plane is constructed passing a line through the anterior nasal spine and posterior nasal spine on the traced maxilla (Fig. 6.34).
- Angle Between the Lower Incisors and the Mandibular Plane. This angle helps in analyzing the incline of the lower anterior teeth. Its normative value is 95°. The mandibular plane can be constructed utilizing various methods, the simplest one is by drawing a line tangent to the lower border of the traced mandible (Fig. 6.35).
- Protrusion of Maxillary Incisors. It is measured as the distance between the incisal edge of the maxillary central incisors and the line obtained passing through the A and pogonion points (A–pogonion line). Its mean normative value is 2.7 mm anterior to that reference line and ranges between 5.0 mm anterior and 1.0 mm posterior (Fig. 6.36). This particular measurement is reliable only if the pogonion point is in its normal anteroposterior position; for example, in a case of a too posterior pogonion, this analysis can produce a false diagnosis of too protruding upper incisors.

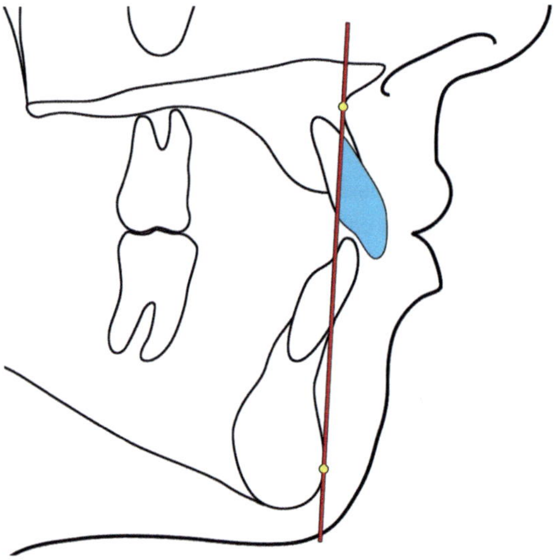

Fig. 6.36 Distance from the incisal edge of the upper central incisors to A–pogonion line. Its mean normative value is 2.7 mm anterior to that reference line and ranges between 5.0 mm anterior and 1.0 mm posterior

6.20 Skeletal Cephalometric Analysis

The vertical and anteroposterior spatial relationship between the jaws and between the jaws and other skeletal structures can be studied in depth with cephalometry. The following parameters are

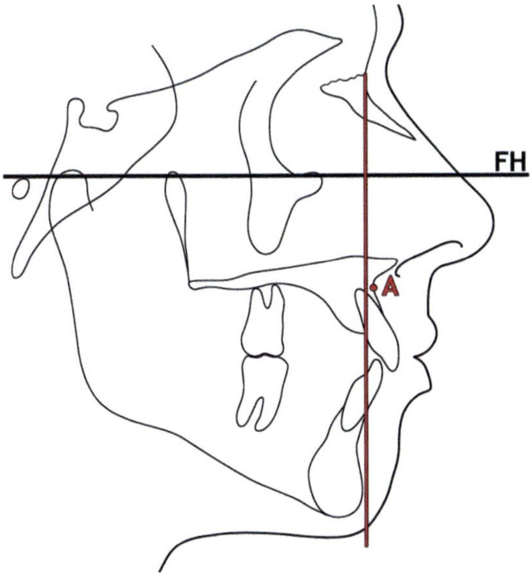

Fig. 6.37 McNamara's maxilla to cranial base anteroposterior assessment. The A point, in an ideal adult subject, should be 1 mm anterior to the reference line

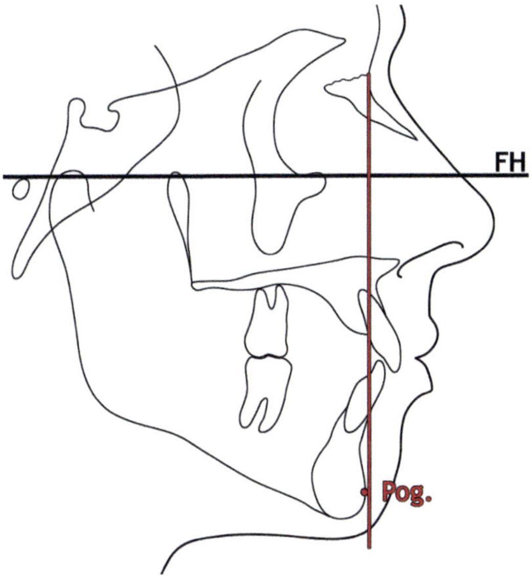

Fig. 6.38 McNamara's mandible to cranial base anteroposterior assessment. The point pogonion, in an ideal adult subject, should be comprised from 2 mm posterior to 4 mm anterior to the reference line

part of a more complex modern analysis published by James McNamara in 1984[3]:

- Maxilla to Cranial Base Anteroposterior Assessment. This measurement utilizes a vertical reference line passing through the nasion. The A point, in an ideal adult subject, should be 1 mm anterior to the reference line (Fig. 6.37). As for the possibility of discrepancy between the clinical and cephalometric observation of the maxillary anteroposterior position, James McNamara suggests that "the clinical examination should take precedence. Treating a patient only in accordance with cephalometric norms must be avoided."
- Mandible to Cranial Base Anteroposterior Assessment. This measurement also utilizes a vertical reference line passing through the nasion. In an ideal adult subject, the pogonion should be comprised from 2 mm posterior to 4 mm anterior to the reference line (Fig. 6.38).
- Mandible to Maxilla Assessment. To study the relationships between the mandible and maxilla, McNamara proposed the construction of a triangle (Fig. 6.39) consisting of the length of the mandible, measured as the distance from the condylion to the gnathion (Co-Gn), the length of midface, measured as the distance from the condylion to the A point (Co-A point), and the lower anterior facial height, measured as the distance between the anterior nasal spine and the menton (ANS-Me). Utilizing Table 6.1 it is possible to correlate, for any given midfacial length, the range of corresponding normal mandibular length and corresponding normal lower anterior facial height.

6.21 Soft Tissue Cephalometric Analysis

Many of the soft tissue cephalometric measurements can also be done on the life-size clinical photographs and directly on the subject, as anthropometric measurements. Each of the following examples of soft tissue analysis is

[3]McNamara JA. A method of cephalometric evaluation. Am J Orthod.1984; 86: 449–469 and McNamara JA, Brudon WL. Orthodontic and orthopedic treatment in the mixed dentition. Ann Arbor: Needham Press: 1993.

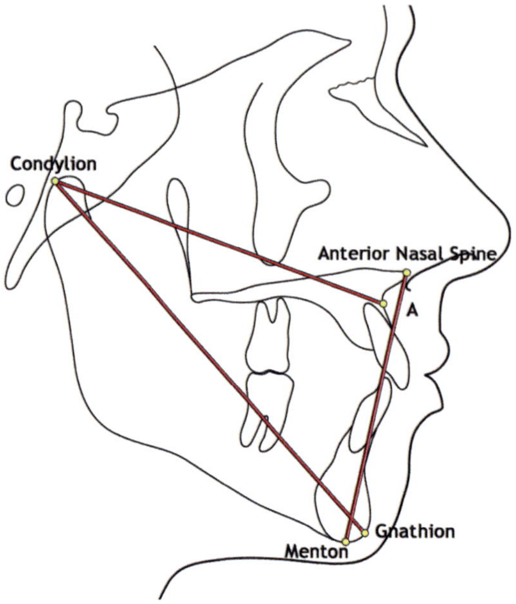

Fig. 6.39 McNamara's mandible to maxilla assessment. A triangle is constructed utilizing the length of the mandible, measured as the distance from the condylion to the gnathion (Co-Gn), the length of midface, measured as the distance from the condylion to A point (Co-A point), and the lower anterior facial height, measured as the distance between the anterior nasal spine and the menton (ANS-Me). The proportions between each of these three distances, in ideal subjects, are reported in Table 6.1

Table 6.1 McNamara's composite norms representing the relationship between the midfacial length, mandibular length and lower anterior vertical height

Midfacial length (mm; Co-A point)	Mandibular length (mm; Co-Gn)	Lower anterior facial height (mm; ANS-Me)
80	97–100	57–58
81	99–102	57–58
82	101–104	58–59
83	103–106	57–58
84	104–107	59–60
85	105–108	60–62
86	107–110	60–62
87	109–112	61–63
88	111–114	61–63
89	112–115	62–64
90	113–116	63–64
91	115–118	63–64
92	117–120	64–65
93	119–122	65–66
94	121–124	66–67
95	122–125	67–69
96	124–127	67–69
97	126–129	68–70
98	128–131	68–70
99	129–132	69–71
100	130–133	70–74
101	132–135	71–75
102	134–137	76–76
103	136–139	73–77
104	137–140	74–78
105	138–141	75–79

Co-A point condylion to the A point, Co-Gn condylion to the gnathion, ANS-Me anterior nasal spine to the menton

presented utilizing a tracing and a photograph of two different subjects for comparison.

- Vertical Proportions. The proportion of the upper and lower face can be evaluated dividing the vertical distance between the glabella and soft tissue menton at the subnasale point; the distance from glabella to subnasale should be equal to that from subnasale to soft tissue menton. The upper lip should be one-third of the subnasale to soft tissue menton vertical distance, whereas the lower lip should be about two-thirds (Fig. 6.40a, b).
- Nasofacial Angle. The nasofacial angle is formed by the intersection of the line drawn from glabella to soft tissue pogonion with a line drawn along the outline of the nasal dorsum. The average values range from 30 to 35° (Fig. 6.41a, b).
- Nasomental Angle. It is constructed by drawing a line along the outline of the nasal dorsum and a line connecting the tip of the nose to soft tissue pogonion (E-line). The average values range from 120 to 132° (Fig. 6.41a, b).
- Mentocervical Angle. It is formed by the intersection of the E-line with a tangent to the submental outline. The average values range from 120 to 132° (Fig. 6.41a, b).
- Submental–Neck Angle. It is formed by the tangents to the submental and neck outlines. The average value is 126° in men and 121° in women (Fig. 6.41a, b).
- Subnasal Vertical. A vertical line drawn through the subnasale can be used as a reference to assess the prominence of the upper

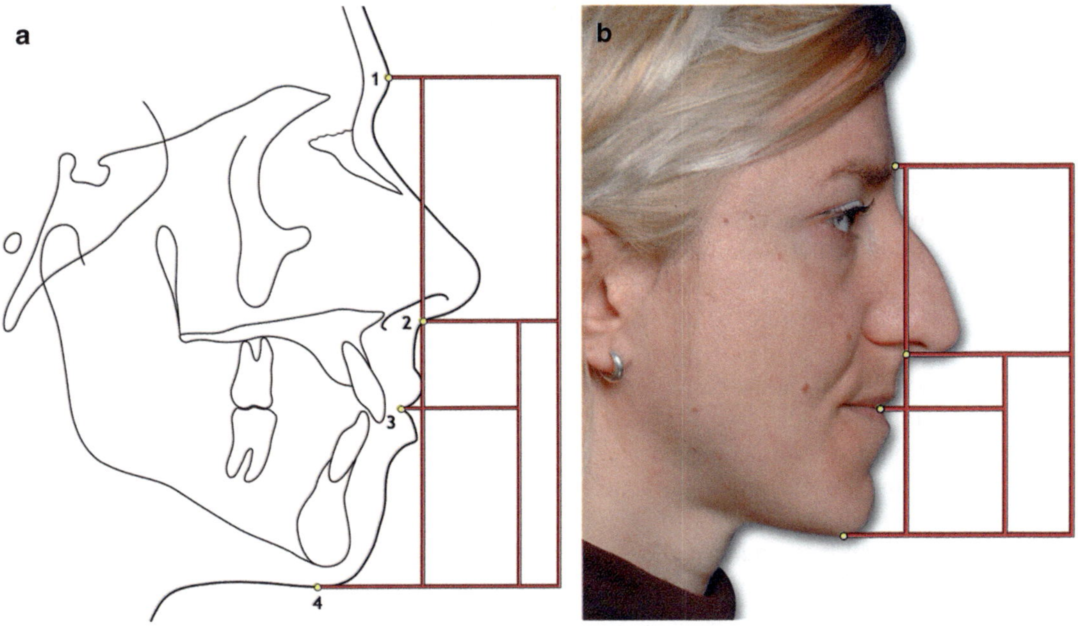

Fig. 6.40 (**a**, **b**) Vertical proportion measured over a cephalometric tracing obtained from a lateral cephalometric radiograph (**a**) and over a profile view clinical photograph (**b**) of two different subjects

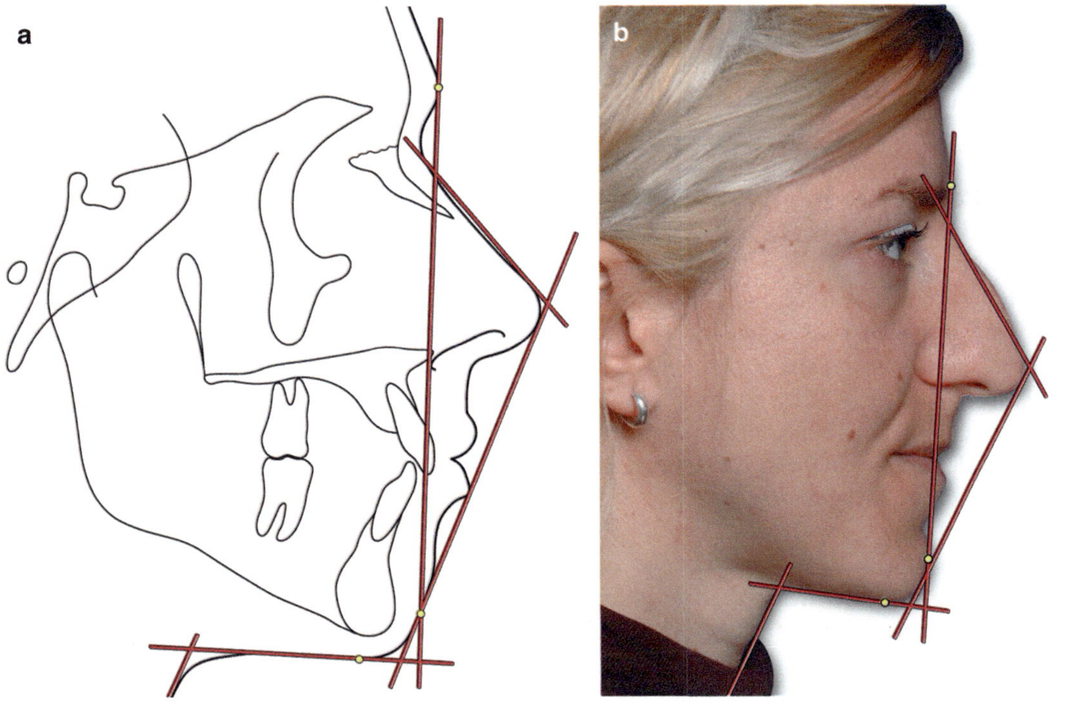

Fig. 6.41 (**a**, **b**) Nasofacial, nasomental, mentocervical, and submental–neck angles measured over a cephalometric tracing obtained from a lateral cephalometric radiograph (**a**) and over a profile view clinical photograph (**b**) of two different subjects

and lower lip as well as the chin. Before selecting the subnasale as a reference, it is essential to obtain the natural head position and to exclude a regional deformity of the subnasal region itself, such as a prominent or recessive nasal spine, an overgrowth of the caudal septum, or any other condition leading to a malposition of the subnasale point. The upper lip should be 1–2 mm in front of the subnasal vertical reference line, the lower lip should be on the line or 1 mm posterior to it, and the pogonion soft should be 1–4 mm posterior to it (Fig. 6.42a–d).

– Nasolabial Angle. It is formed by the intersection of a columella tangent and an upper lip tangent. In an adult sample with an ideal occlusion and well-balanced face, the average value was 102° with a standard deviation of 8° for both males and females. The angle can be further subdivided to assess the columella and the upper labial inclines independently utilizing a horizontal line passing through it (Fig. 6.43a, b). Also for this parameter special effort should be made to detect any abnormal position of the subnasale point before judging the incline of the columella and the upper lip.

6.22 Points, Lines, and Angles Difficult to Trace

Sometimes, one or more of the points, lines, or angles are difficult to identify and trace as a result of the subject's anatomical variability. In these cases, instead of mistakenly utilizing a cephalometric rule to obtain a linear or angular value, it is preferable to return to the direct clinical examination to assess a facial feature.

6.23 The Maxillomandibular Complex Concept

In many clinical cases, the findings obtained from the dental analysis are closely related to those obtained from the facial assessment. For example, a class II dental occlusion with a mandibular anteroposterior deficiency is usually correlated to a specific facial profile with a poor lower lip–chin–submental–neck contour, a recessive chin, and a relative over-projection of the nasal tip.

In other cases, a nearly perfect occlusion, either spontaneously developed or resulting from previous orthodontic treatment, is found in subjects with poor facial balance, subjects that at first sight can be quite similar to those with a dentofacial deformity. Unfortunately, a similar clinical scenario can also be seen after a surgical-orthodontic treatment in spite of correct dental occlusion having been achieved.

The concept of moving the maxillomandibular complex (MMC) backwards or forwards, upwards or downwards, and rotating clockwise or counterclockwise with jaw surgery is not new in the process of planning orthognathic surgery and should be extended in the future to every form of facial analysis as a basic tool.

Figure 6.44a shows the essential dental and skeletal components of the MMC obtained from a cephalometric tracing. The assessment of the spatial position of the MMC considers its anteroposterior, vertical, transverse, and the grade and point of rotation in clockwise or counterclockwise direction (Fig. 6.44b–e).

Figure 6.45 reports an example of a malpositioned MMC (the clinical case is presented in Fig. 6.19a–e). Even if the dental occlusion is acceptable, due to previous orthodontic treatment carried out in his childhood, a developmental clockwise rotation of the MMC at the level of the anterior nasal spine is responsible for the flattening of the labiomental fold, the recessive soft tissue chin, the lack of definition of the mandibular border, and the poor chin–neck profile.

6.24 Dentofacial Analysis: Preferred Terms

– **Alar crease junction.** The most posterior point of the curved line formed by the alar crease as seen in profile view; it is utilized as a landmark for measuring tip projection.

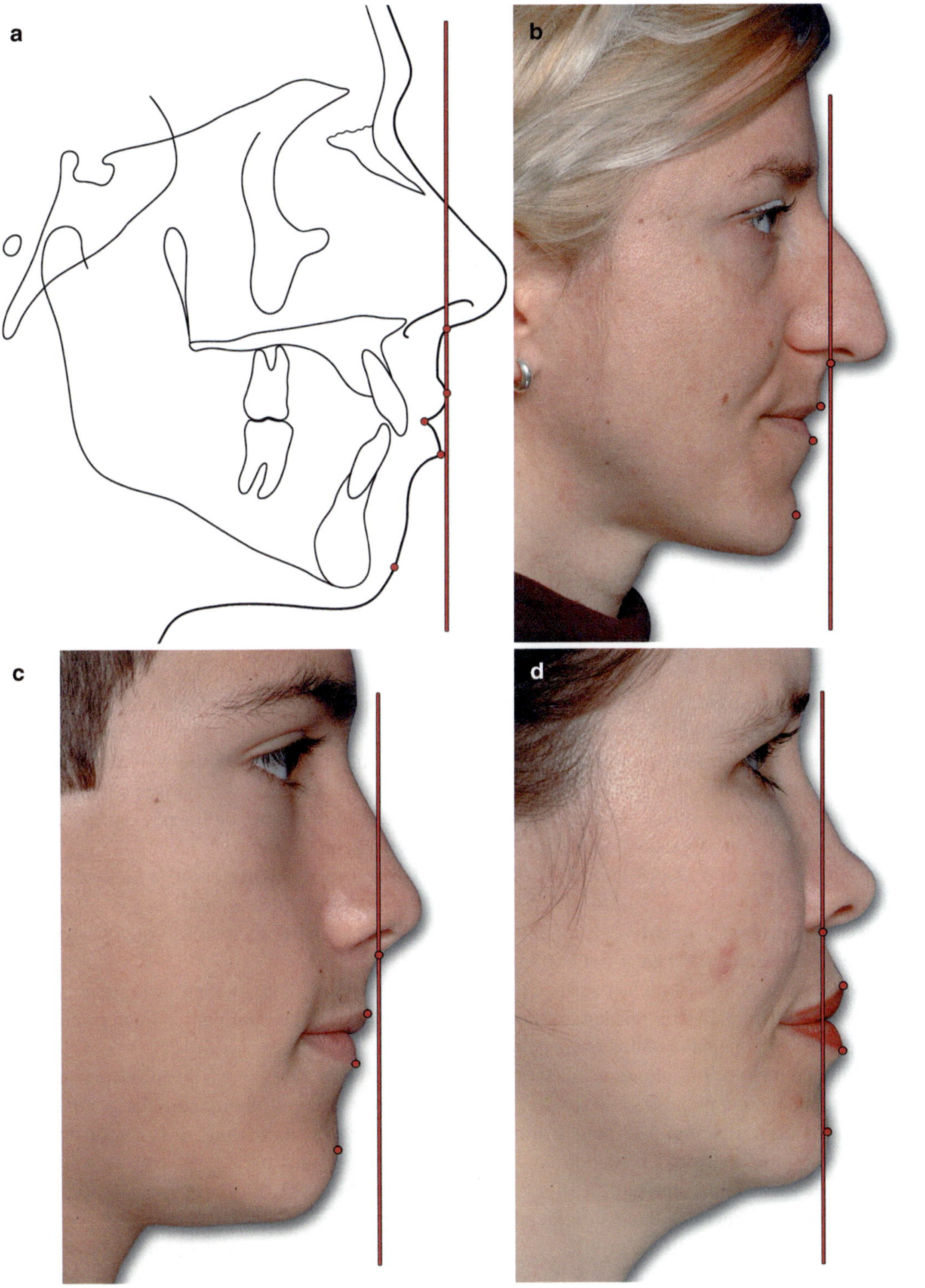

Fig. 6.42 (**a–d**) Subnasal vertical reference line measured over a cephalometric tracing obtained from a lateral cephalometric radiograph (**a**) and over a profile view clinical photograph (**b**). A too anterior (**c**) or too posterior subnasale (**d**) needs to be detected in advance to avoid errors in the construction of the reference line

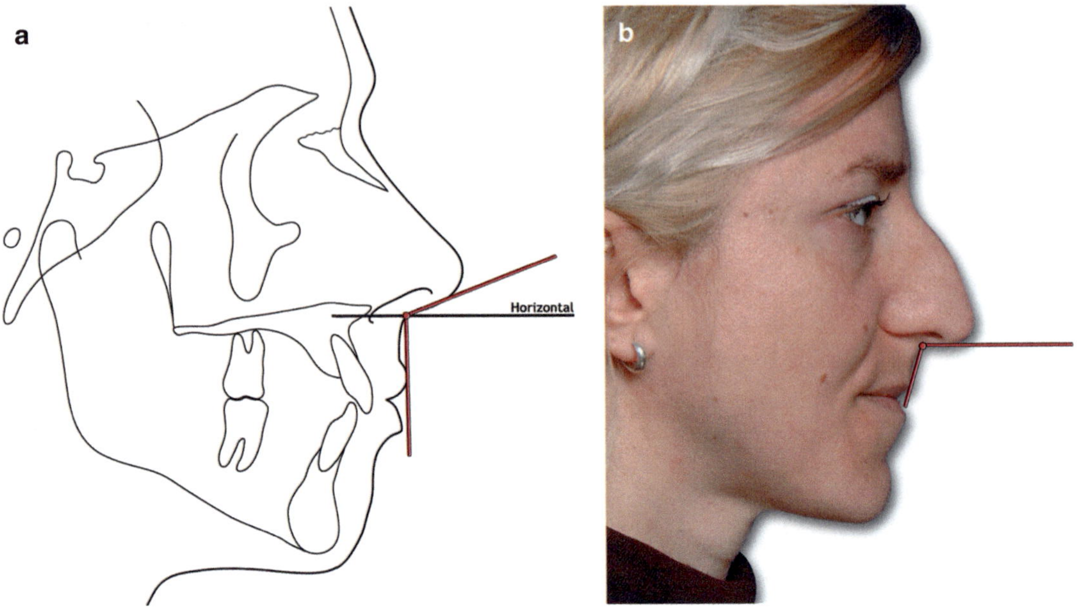

Fig. 6.43 (**a**, **b**) The nasolabial angle is formed by the intersection of a columella tangent and an upper lip tangent. The angle can be further subdivided to assess the columella and the upper labial inclines independently utilizing a horizontal line passing through it (**a**). A clinical case of maxillary deficiency in which the whole nasolabial angle measures 103°degrees but the columellar component is 0° and the upper lip component is 103° (**b**)

- **Anterior nasal spine.** The most anterior point in the traced maxilla (tip of the nasal spine). It is a cephalometric reference point.
- **Black triangle.** The presence of a dark and unesthetic triangular space, base up, between the two upper central incisors caused by midline gingival retraction and/or dental inclination.
- **Buccal corridors (negative space).** The space that is created when a patient smiles, between the buccal (vestibular) surface of the posterior teeth and the commissure of the lips. The perceived dimension of this space depends partially on the type of lighting utilized during the assessment and photographic session.
- **Cephalometric tracing.** The pencil drawing obtained by tracing from a cephalogram, onto an acetate matte paper, the outline of some of the anatomical structures like teeth, facial and cranial bones, and soft tissue profile.
- **Cheekbone point.** In a subject with a balanced middle facial third, it is the apex of osseous cheekbone that is located 20–25 mm inferior and 5–10 mm anterior to the outer canthus of the eye when viewed in profile and is 20–25 mm inferior and 5–10 mm lateral to the outer canthus of the eye when viewed frontally. A flat cheekbone point is often associated with malar deficiency and maxillary hypoplasia.
- **Chin deficiency.** Refers to a lack of anterior projection of the chin outline.
- **Chin pad.** The thick soft tissue overlying the bony chin.
- **Cleft chin.** The median depressed vertical skin line of the chin pad characterizing some subjects.
- **Condylion.** The most posterosuperior point on the outline of the mandibular condyle seen on lateral cephalograms. It is a cephalometric reference point.
- **Cross-bite.** When one or more of the maxillary teeth are lingually (internally) positioned relative to the respective mandibular teeth. The anterior cross-bite is also called reverse overjet.
- **Cupid's bow.** The central linear portion of the upper lip white roll skin relief between the

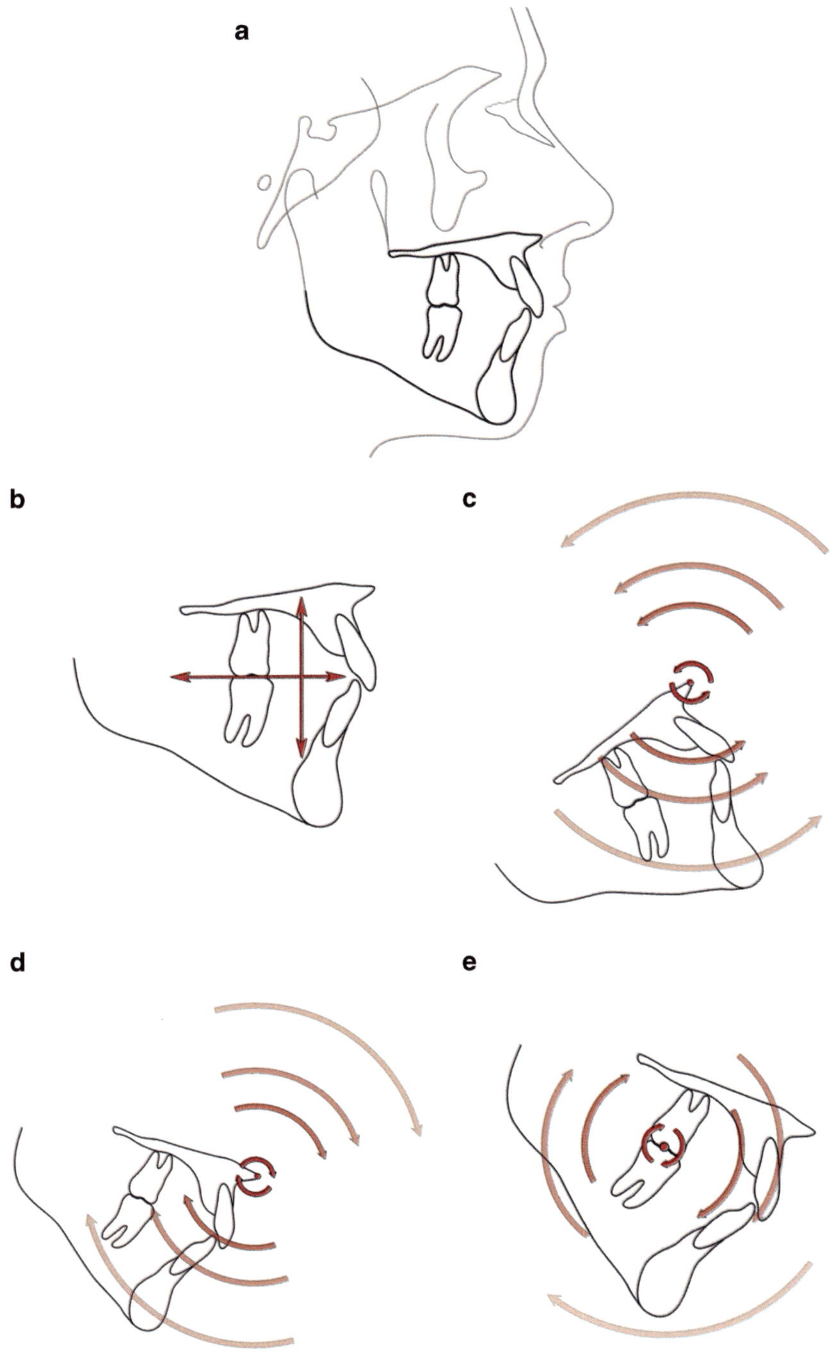

Fig. 6.44 (**a–e**) The maxillomandibular complex (MMC) traced from a subject with good occlusal relationship (**a**). The assessment of spatial position of the MMC in profile view should consider its vertical and sagittal position (**b**) as well as its grade, point, and direction of rotation. A counterclockwise rotated MMC on the anterior nasal spine produces a prominent soft tissue chin with little influence on the upper incisors (**c**), whereas the opposite rotation is responsible for a recessive chin again with little influence on the upper incisors (**d**). A clockwise rotated MMC centered on the occlusal plane at the level of first molars produces the elongation of the lower third of the face as well as an advancement of the anterior nasal spine and a setback of the chin profile (**e**)

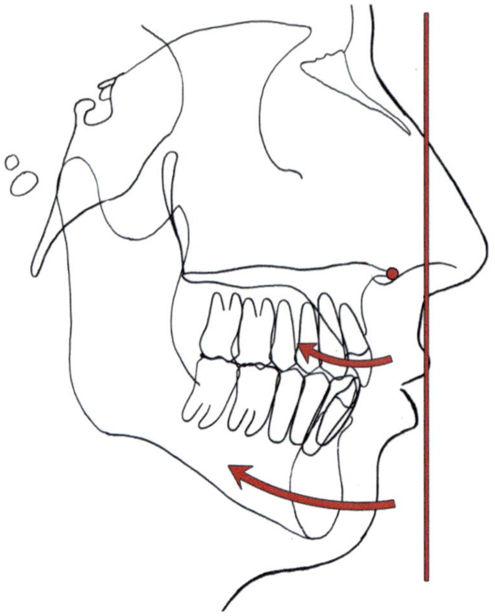

Fig. 6.45 The tracing of the MMC of the clinical case presented in Fig. 9.1. The clockwise rotation at the level of the anterior nasal spine of the MMC is responsible for the flattening of the labiomental fold, the recessive soft tissue chin, the lack of definition of the mandibular border, and the poor chin–neck profile

philtrum and the vermillion. It connects the inferior ends of the philtrum columns.
- **Dental agenesia.** The lack of development of one or more teeth.
- **Dental classes.** The classification of the sagittal relationship between the dental arches. Class I: normal posteroanterior relationship between the two dental arches. Class II: too anterior upper dental arch and/or too posterior lower dental arch. Class III: too posterior upper dental arch and/or too anterior lower dental arch.
- **Dental crowding.** The absence of alignment between adjacent teeth. It is usually graded from mild to severe crowding.
- **Dentoalveolar protrusion/retrusion.** The abnormal forward (protrusion) or backward (retrusion) position of the teeth and their alveolar bone in respect to the basal bone of the jaws. It can involve the maxillary and/or mandibular dental arches.
- **Diastema.** A space between adjacent teeth. Normally there is no space between adjacent teeth.
- **Display zone.** The area framed by the lips during the act of smiling.
- **E-line (esthetic line).** A reference line connecting the tip of the nose to the most anterior point of the chin contour (soft tissue pogonion).
- **Gingival scaffold.** The area of gingiva shown during the act of smiling.
- **Glabella (soft tissue glabella).** The most prominent anterior point in the midsagittal plane of the forehead. It is influenced by pneumonization of the frontal sinus and varies widely in posteroanterior position.
- **Gnathion.** The most anteroinferior point on the outline of the mandibular symphysis seen on lateral cephalograms. It is a cephalometric reference point.
- **High/low mandibular plane angle.** The excessive clockwise (high) or counterclockwise (low) rotation of the mandibular plane. The high mandibular plane angle is correlated with the hyperdivergent facial pattern and the long face; the low mandibular plane angle is correlated with the hypodivergent facial pattern and the short face.
- **Hyper/hypodivergent facial pattern.** The increased (hyperdivergent) and decreased (hypodivergent) anterior facial height in relation to the posterior facial height (see also high/low mandibular plane angle).
- **Labiomental fold (mandibular sulcus contour).** The horizontal skin depression that separates the chin from the lower lip. It varies from a flat curve to a deep sulcus.
- **Lip commissures.** The points at which the upper and lower lips join together. During the act of smiling, the eye of the observer can perceive the inner and the outer commissures, as delineated by the innermost and outermost confluences, respectively, of the vermillion of the lips at the corner of the mouth.
- **Labrale inferior.** A point indicating the mucocutaneous border of the upper lip. The most anterior point of the upper lip (usually). It is a cephalometric reference point.

- **Labrale superior.** The median point in the lower margin of the lower membranous lip.
- **Lip support.** The action of the anterior teeth and their surrounding alveolar bone in shaping the lips.
- **Lip white rolls.** The linear white skin relief placed around the vermillion border of both lips. It flattens and sometimes totally disappears with aging.
- **Malar eminence.** The point of maximal outer projection of the malar region.
- **Mandibular deficiency.** The hypoplasia of the whole mandible. It is the most common cause of class II dentofacial deformities.
- **Mandibular plane.** A cephalometric reference plane constructed by drawing a line tangent to the traced mandibular border.
- **Maxilla point.** The most anterior point on the continuum of the cheekbone–nasal–lip contour described by Arnett and Bergman[4]; it is an indicator of maxillary anteroposterior position.
- **Maxillary plane.** A cephalometric reference plane constructed by drawing a line passing through the anterior nasal spine and the posterior nasal spine on the traced maxilla.
- **Menton.** The lowest point on the symphyseal shadow of the mandible seen on lateral cephalograms. It is a cephalometric reference point. Soft tissue menton—The lowest point on the contour of the soft tissue chin. Found by dropping a perpendicular line through the skeletal menton. It is a cephalometric reference point.
- **Microgenia.** This term refers to an underprojected chin independently from occlusal consideration.
- **Mouth width.** The distance between the two lip commissures; it is measured by utilizing the close-up view of the lip at rest with ruler. It is not modifiable with surgery.
- **Muscle strain.** The flattening of the chin outline due to muscular contraction produced to achieve lip seal. It is a frequent finding in many dentofacial deformities (dental and skeletal open bite, dental and skeletal class II).
- **Nasion.** The most anterior point on the frontonasal suture in the midsagittal plane. It is a cephalometric reference point. Soft tissue nasion—The point of greatest concavity in the midline between the forehead and the nose.
- **Neck–throat point.** The more posterior-superior point of the submental–neck outline.
- **Occlusal plane.** The line bisecting the overlapping cusp of the first molars and the incisal overlap.
- **Overbite.** The vertical overlap of the incisors obtained when the two dental arches occlude together. Deep bite—Excessive vertical overlap between upper and lower incisors. Open bite—In this condition there is no overlap but a vertical separation.
- **Overjet.** The horizontal overlap of the upper incisors in front of the lower incisors. Normally it is 2–3 mm due to the thickness of the edge of the upper incisors. Increased overjet is the excessive horizontal distance between the upper and lower incisors. Reverse overjet (anterior cross-bite)—If the lower incisors are in front of the upper incisors.
- **Philtrum.** The central and vertically oriented portion of the upper lip situated between the two skin reliefs of the philtrum columns. There is a gentle concavity on its lower portion, the philtrum dimple.
- **Platysma bands ("turkey gobbler" effect).** The vertical skin bands, usually one for each side, of the aging submental and neck region. It is caused by platysma muscle attenuation, lengthening, and dehiscence, along with fat accumulation, skin excess, and photo-damage.
- **Pogonion.** The most anterior point of the bony chin contour. It is a cephalometric reference point. **Soft tissue pogonion**. The most prominent or anterior point of the chin contour. It is a cephalometric reference point.
- **Point A.** The most posterior midline point in the anterior concavity of the traced maxilla situated between the anterior nasal spine and the most inferior point on the alveolar bone overlying the maxillary incisors. It is a cephalometric reference point.

[4]Arnett GW, Bergman R. Facial keys to orthodontic diagnosis and treatment planning, Parts I and II. Am J Orthop Dentofacial Orthod 1993; 103: 299–312 and 395–41.

- **Posed smile.** A voluntary smile; it need not be elicited or accompanied by emotion. A posed smile can be sustained and it is reliably repeatable. **Unposed (spontaneous) smile.** An involuntary smile, induced by joy or mirth. An unposed smile cannot be sustained (it is dynamic).
- **Posterior nasal spine.** The most posterior point of the palatine bone on the traced maxilla. It is a cephalometric reference point.
- **Pronasale.** The tip of the nose. The most prominent or anterior point of the nose.
- **Skeletal classes.** The classification of sagittal relationship between maxilla and mandible. Class I: normal posteroanterior relationship between maxilla and mandible. Class II: too anterior maxilla and/or too posterior mandible. Class III: too posterior maxilla and/or too anterior mandible.
- **Scleral show (inferior scleral show).** The presence of a strip of white sclera between the iris and the lower lid margin with the subject in natural head position and straight gaze. It may be a sign of exophthalmos, previous trauma, prior surgery, lower lid laxity, or dentofacial deformities with maxillary hypoplasia.
- **Smile arc.** The relationship of the curvature of the incisal edges of maxillary incisors and canine to the curvature of the lower lip in the posed smile.
- **Stomion.** The point of contact between the two lips in profile view. In the case where contact between the lips is absent, the stomion superior can be considered to be the lowermost point of the vermillion of the upper lip, and the stomion inferior to be the upper-most point of the vermillion of the lower lip.
- **Subnasale.** The point at which the columella merges with the upper lip in the midsagittal plane. It varies widely in relation to caudal septum prominence and nasal spine morphology.
- **Throat length.** The distance between the neck–throat point and the soft tissue menton on the lower facial outline. The throat length is preferably assessed clinically as short or long and not measured instrumentally.
- **Vermillion.** The red portion of the external surface of the lips.
- **Witch's chin deformity (ptotic chin).** The flattening and ptosis of the chin pad associated with the deepening of the submental crease. It can be age-related or iatrogenic.

Further Reading

An interesting overview of dentofacial deformities and their surgical treatment can be found in the second edition of "Essentials of Orthognathic Surgery" by Johan P. Reyneke (Qintessence Publishing Co, 2019, ISBN-13: 978-0867155006).

Another book that offers in-depth coverage of the interplay between orthognathic surgery and rhinoplasty is that recently edited by Derek M. Steinbcher. Aesthetic orthognathic surgery and rhinoplasty. (Wiley-Blackwell; 2019. ISBN-13: 978-1119186977).

7 Preoperative CT Scan for Nasal Surgery

The external complexity of each nose, with its individual proportions, curves, angles, volumes, and small important details, cannot fail to have a corresponding internal complexity. The study of the supporting structures, the division of internal spaces, the discovery of anomalies and deformities as well as any sign of injury represents a fascinating world to be studied in depth in anticipation of surgery. So, the ability to analyze and obtain useful findings from the CT scan images must be cultivated daily with strong commitment by the surgeon. On the contrary, reading quickly the short report of the radiologist on the CT scans cannot represent a shortcut to avoid the surgeon's direct work on the images.

At each meeting with a new patient, after taking the clinical photos of the face, a CT investigation must always be requested, explaining that it is not possible to carry out rhinoplasty "*by looking only at the roof of the house and without inspecting its foundations and internal walls*."

In the BOR discipline, a CT scan of the paranasal sinuses is mandatory in every new patient. The main reasons are to:

- Study the septum and its frequent deformities reducing the risk of mucosal tears during flap elevation.
- Check the dimensions, thickness, and any curves of the quadrangular cartilage thinking of it as a source of available cartilage. The finding of an unknown septal perforation is not so rare also in primary cases.
- Study the nasal turbinates by evaluating separately their bone and mucous components.
- Correlate the external nasal shape with the internal supporting framework.
- Plan some additional functional and reconstructive steps as needed.
- Identify any limiting factors or contraindications to rhinoplasty.
- Exclude nasal polyposis and sinusitis.
- Ask the patient for a first personal commitment to prepare for surgery. What collaboration can we expect from a patient who is unwilling to comply with the surgeon's small requests needed to prepare him for the surgery?
- Explain precisely the limits and problems of nasal surgery to the patient. Direct sharing of CT images with the surgeon is a key part of the patient's preoperative education.
- Extend the storable electronic imaging documentation of clinical cases for further postoperative analysis and research, as is done with clinical facial digital photography.
- For any later medico-legal needs.

This chapter, consisting essentially of fairly "abstract" descriptions of images, should be read a second time after the chapters dedicated to the surgical technique in order to appreciate how useful the preoperative study of the CT scan is for conducting the surgical procedure.

F. Meneghini, *Basic Open Rhinoplasty*, https://doi.org/10.1007/978-3-030-61827-8_7

7.1 Cone Beam Computed Tomography (CBCT) and Rhinoplasty

In the past, the availability of CT scanners was limited and the radiation dose to which the patient was exposed would induce the surgeons to avoid this preoperative investigation.

The first commercial Cone Beam Computed Tomography (CBCT) was produced in Verona, Italy, in 1996. The new equipment was less expensive, fast in volumetric acquisition and the radiation dose was approximately one sixth that of traditional spiral CT. The main disadvantage was the small volume acquired.

After 20 years of technical improvements and experience in the field of oral and maxillofacial imaging, current CBCT equipment is close to perfection for the preoperative study of rhinoplasty patients thanks to good image quality, worldwide diffusion, and reduced radiation dose. Even the costs, both for the radiology center purchasing the equipment and for the individual patients who need the exam, are certainly lower if compared with conventional CT.

7.2 Nostrils and Columella Evaluation

Figure 7.1a–c shows the anterior portion of three axial section CBCT scans of a primary rhinoplasty case in which a wide base of the columella (arrows in Fig. 7.1b) is associated with protruding and divergent footplates of the medial crura (asterisks in Fig. 7.1c). This condition can be also detected clinically and should be noted in the treatment plan as one of the corrective steps of the surgery. Reducing the alar base width as well as de-projecting the nasal tip leaving untouched a wide base of the columella can reduce the nostril apertures with postoperative functional problems.

Likewise, Fig. 7.2a–c shows a primary rhinoplasty case in which a wide base of the columella and two protruding and divergent footplates of the medial crura are associated with an anterior deviation to the right of the quadrangular cartilage. The final combined effect is a clear reduction in the opening of the left nostril.

7.3 Anterior Septal Deformities

Exploration of the anterior septal cartilage looking for deformities is an important preoperative step. Frequently a visible asymmetry of the nasal tip is the first sign to suspect an underlying deviation of the nasal septum.

Figure 7.3a–d shows four axial CT scan sections of the tip of the nose in a primary case. The boxy tip presents an evident asymmetry of the dome and an anterior septal deviation to the left (arrows). Slightly more posterior, at the level of the osteocartilaginous junction, the septum appears deviated to the right side, reducing the airway (asterisk).

Figure 7.4a–f shows an unusual preoperative CBCT finding in which a symmetrical nasal tip covers a septal fracture. The two segments of the cartilaginous anterior septum are overlapped, drawing a bayonet-like shape outlined in yellow. Patient history does not reveal any previous major nasal trauma. Explaining these findings to the patient increases her understanding of the need for a reconstructive and not only "esthetic" surgery.

Figure 7.5a–c shows three axial CT scan sections of an extreme anterior septal deviation to the left side associated with contralateral tip deviation and obliteration of left airways. The coronal views (Fig. 7.5d, e) confirm the cartilaginous deformity and depict the deviation to the left by the maxillary bony crest. Also in this primary case, the patient history does not reveal any previous nasal trauma.

7.4 Midline Cartilaginous Septal Deviation

The simplest and one of the more common septal deviations is the overlapping on one side of the anterior nasal spine (ANS). Even if the ANS does

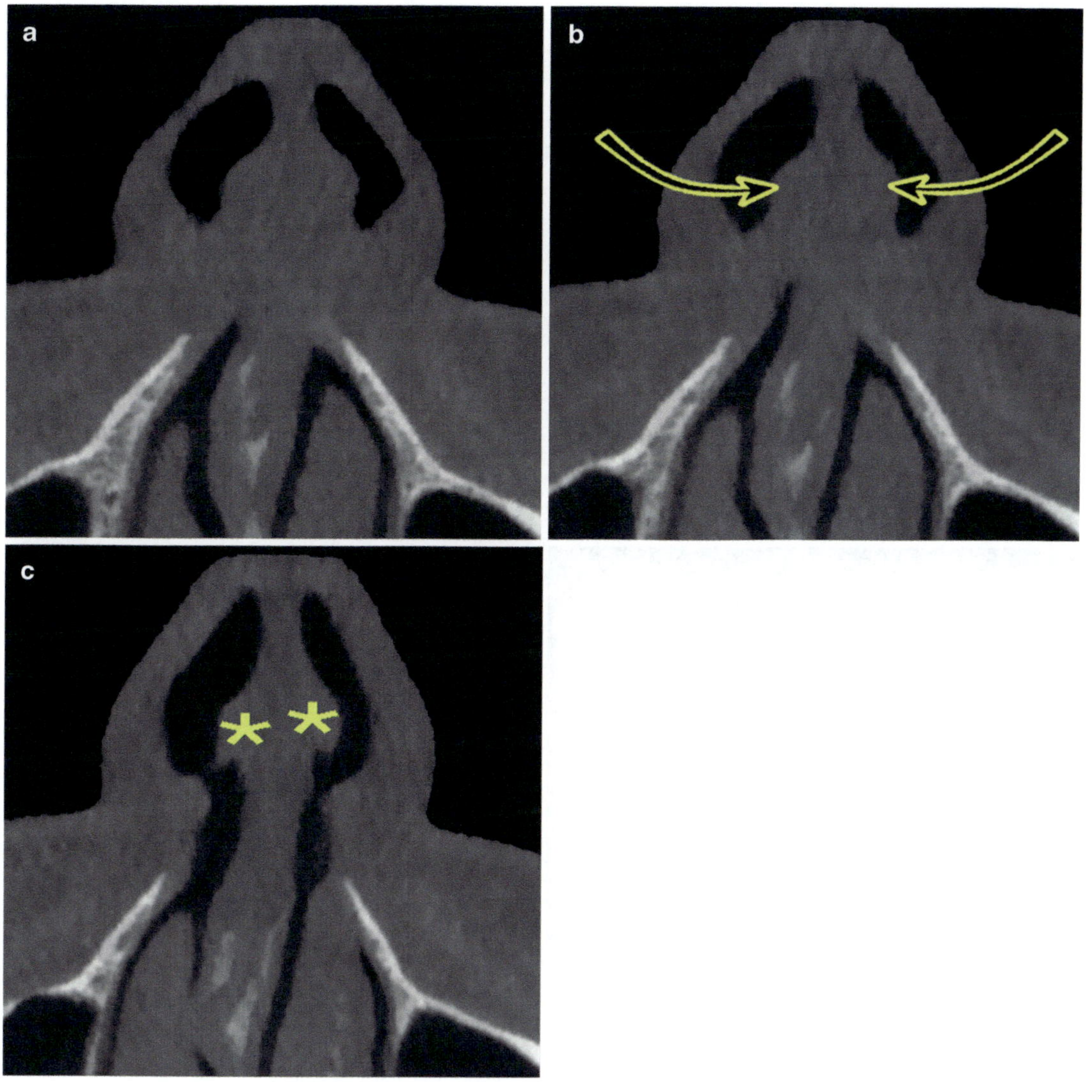

Fig. 7.1 (**a–c**) Axial CBCT views. Details of the nostril apertures in a primary rhinoplasty case. Wide base of the columella (arrows) associated with protruding and divergent footplates of the medial crura (asterisks)

not always lie in the midline, often the deviated component is the caudal quadrangular cartilage. With a coronal CT scan reconstruction passing through the ANS the caudal septum position is easily identified. Figure 7.6a, b shows the excessive length of the quadrangular cartilage tilted and located on the right side of the ANS of a primary rhinoplasty case.

Figure 7.7a–f shows a series of coronal CT scan reconstructions in which all of the caudal septum lies centered along the ANS and the maxillary crest but presents a strong curvature (straight arrows) that causes an important obstruction of the right nasal cavity. In the same clinical case (Fig. 7.7a–d), the nasal valves are asymmetric with an evident width reduction of the left valve (curved arrows). Knowledge of these details is very important in the definition of the operative steps of straightening and reconstructing the nasal septum.

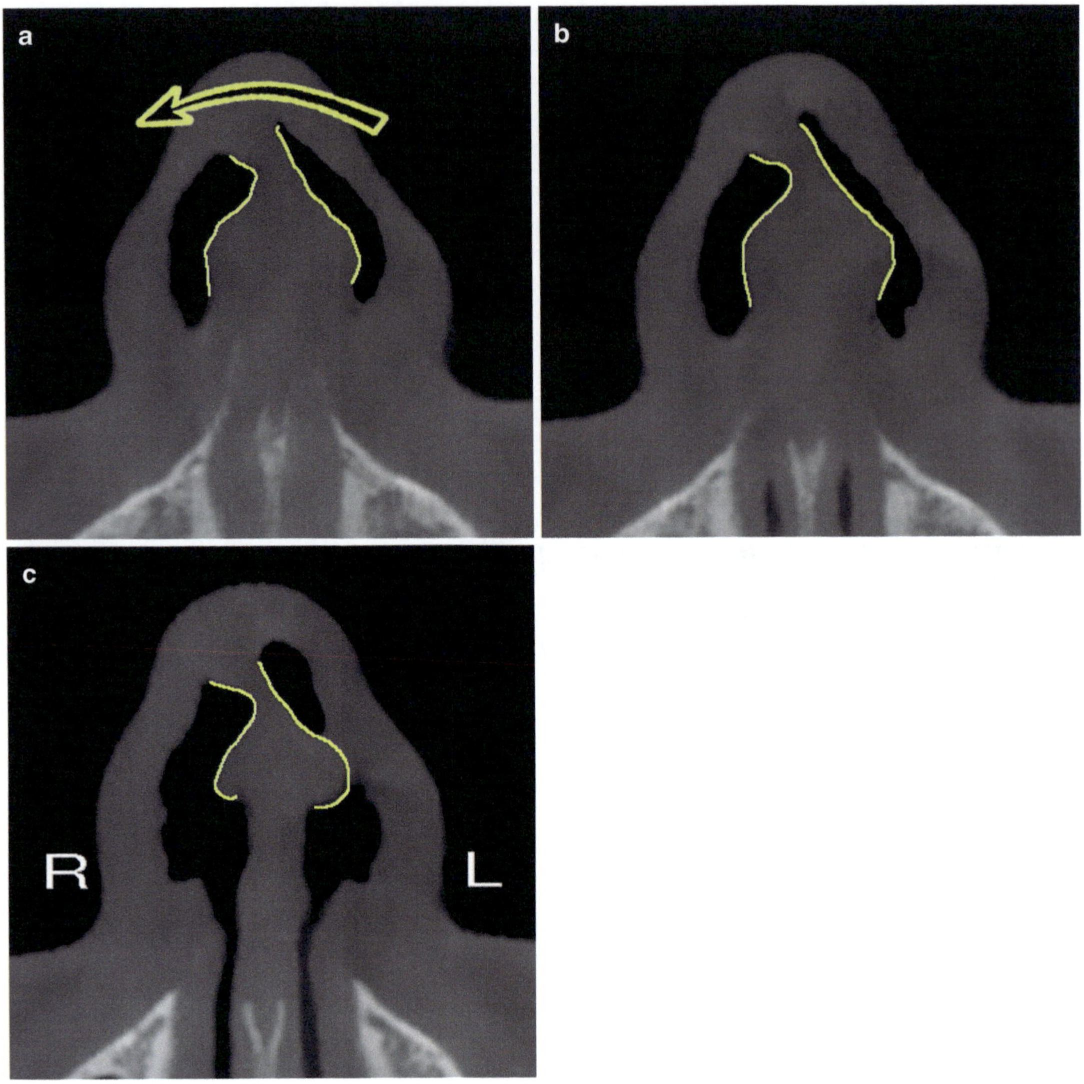

Fig. 7.2 (a–c) Axial CBCT views. Details of the nostril apertures in a primary rhinoplasty case. Wide base of the columella and protruding and divergent footplates of the medial crura (outlined in yellow) associated with an anterior deviation to the right of the septal cartilage (arrow)

7.5 Nasal Valve Analysis

The study of CT images allows finding the narrowing of one or both nasal valves even in subjects with straight and balanced noses who have never undergone surgery and have no previous nasal trauma in the clinical history. In other words, it can be said that the nasal valves deserve a closer preoperative look even when there is no sign to indicate a problem.

Figure 7.8a–c clearly depicts a narrowed right nasal valve despite a cartilaginous dorsum that is straight and free of deformity.

Figure 7.9a–d illustrates four CBCT axial sections of another clinical case. Moving from caudal to cranial, despite the wide and symmetric nasal tip, a progressive shift to the right side of the quadrangular cartilage associated with a minimal grade of septal convexity reduces unilaterally the width of the nasal valve. Reducing the

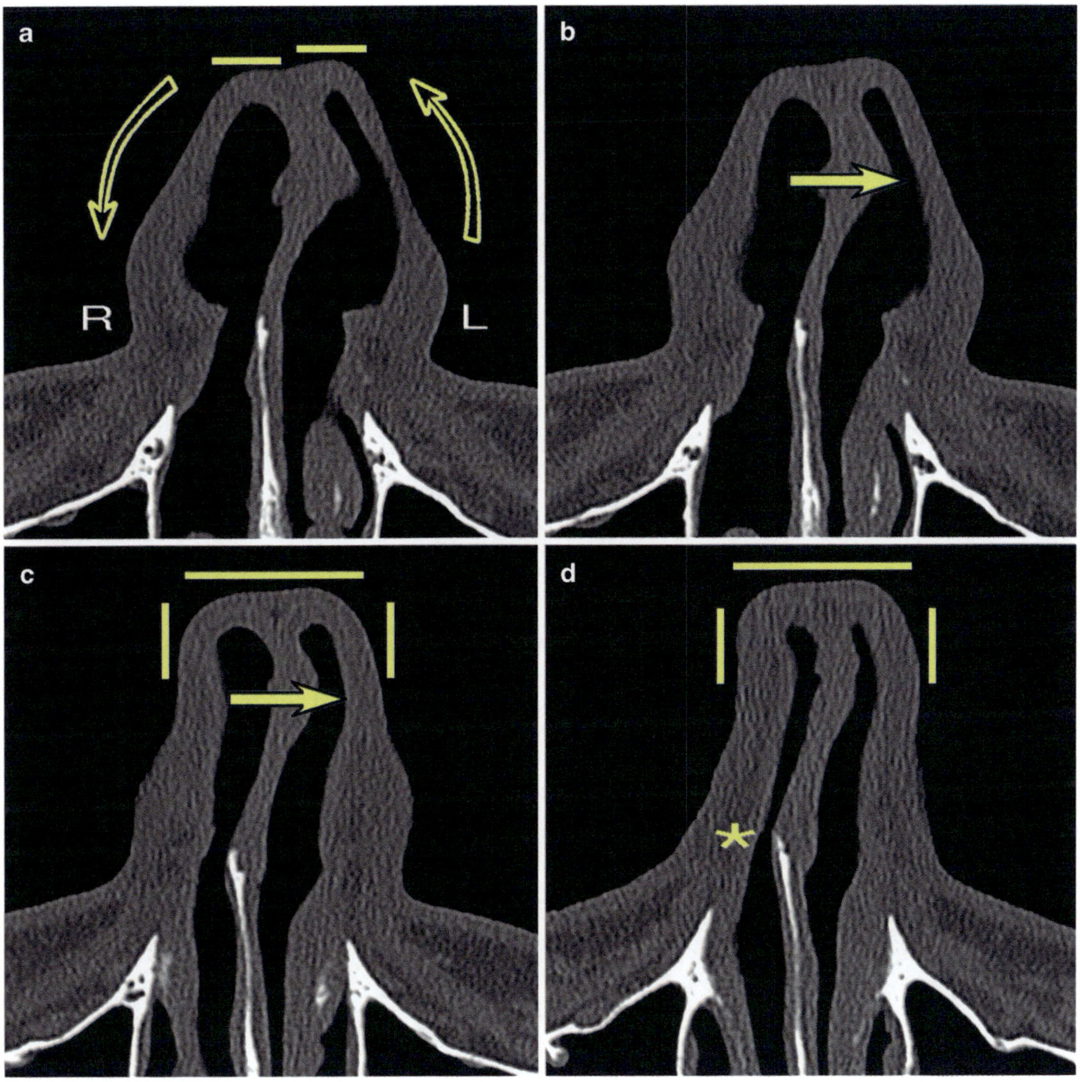

Fig. 7.3 (**a–d**) Axial CBCT views. A boxy nasal tip with asymmetrical domes. The cartilaginous septum is deviated to the left (arrows) whereas its osteocartilaginous junction is deviated to right, reducing the airway (asterisk)

bulbous tip, as requested by the patient, without treating the right nasal valve can create a major functional impairment.

Figure 7.10a–c shows a more severe case of right nasal obstruction from valve collapse in a primary rhinoplasty patient.

7.6 Complex Septal Deviation

The first phase (one of the most important) of septoplasty consists of bilateral flap elevation. Avoiding or minimizing mucosal tears is the main goal of the surgeon. So, a good rule in flap elevation is to proceed first with the less deformed area and then approach the more deformed ones. Exploring the septum with CT images in the case of complex septal deviation is mandatory to prepare this important initial phase of rhinoplasty.

Figure 7.11a–d shows a central septal deformity in a posttraumatic case. The complexity arises both from the angulation between the two septal segments, with lack of continuity, and from the extreme thinness of the mucous layers. This particular condition exposes the surgeon to a high risk of mucosal tearing during flap elevation

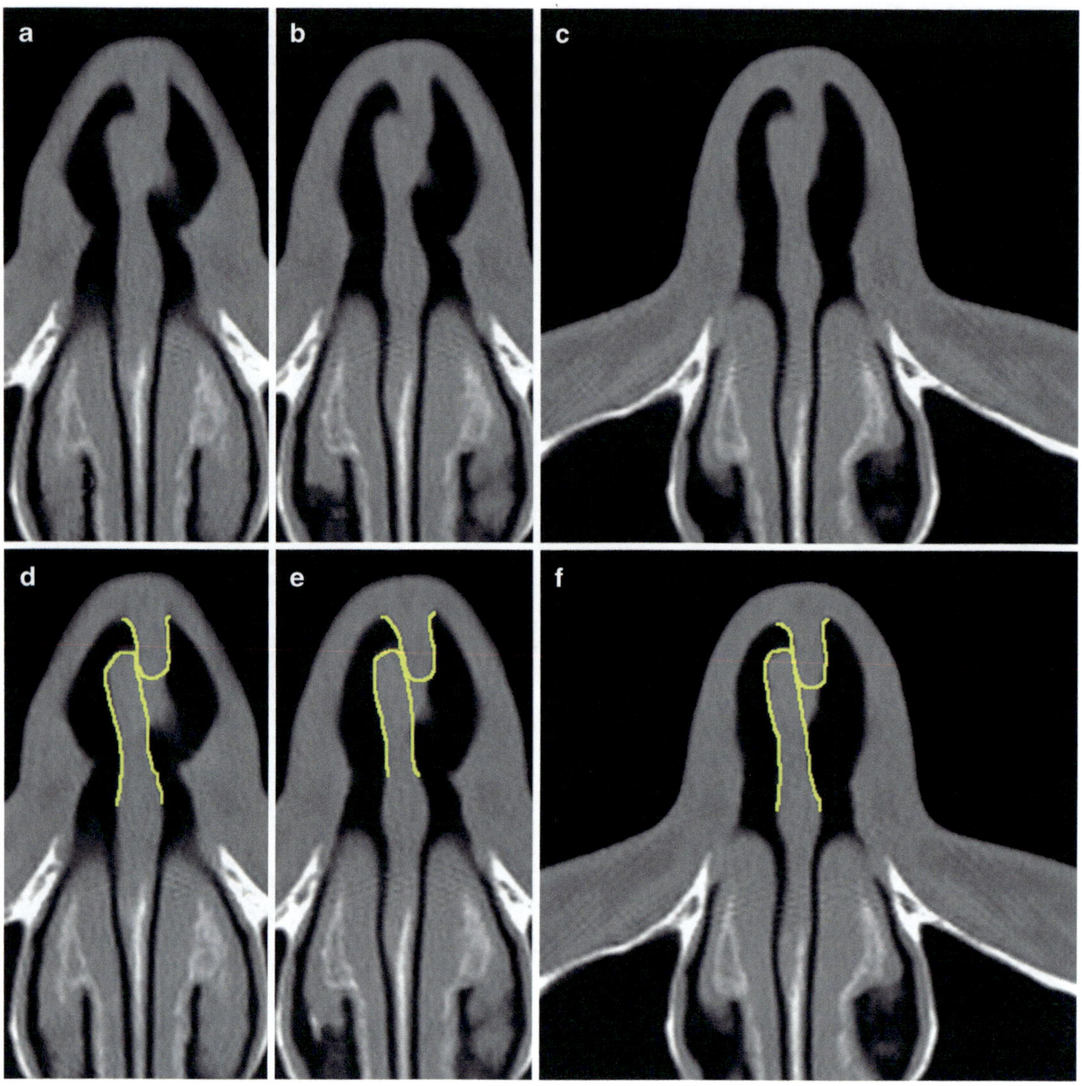

Fig. 7.4 (**a–f**) Axial CBCT views. Anterior septal fracture with overlapping of the two cartilaginous segments (outlined in yellow in **d–f**)

as well as to a difficulty in obtaining adequate harvesting of septal cartilage fragments for the next steps of reconstructive grafting. The coronal section (Fig. 7.11d) offers an example of anterior high septal deviation from the midline, which will be discussed in the next section.

The four axial sections of Fig. 7.12a–d show a clinical case in which all the three septal segments (membranous, cartilaginous, and osseous) taken individually are quite straight. Unfortunately, the inclinations between them create a "zigzag" inside the nose. An in-depth examination reveals many interesting points to know preoperatively:

- The membranous and the cartilaginous septum are not connected in a straight manner but angulated (see dots in Fig. 7.12b). This condition creates some difficulties during the septal caudal access after splitting apart the two medial lateral crura.
- Also the cartilaginous and the bony septum are not connected in a straight manner but angulated (see dots in Fig. 7.12b). This condi-

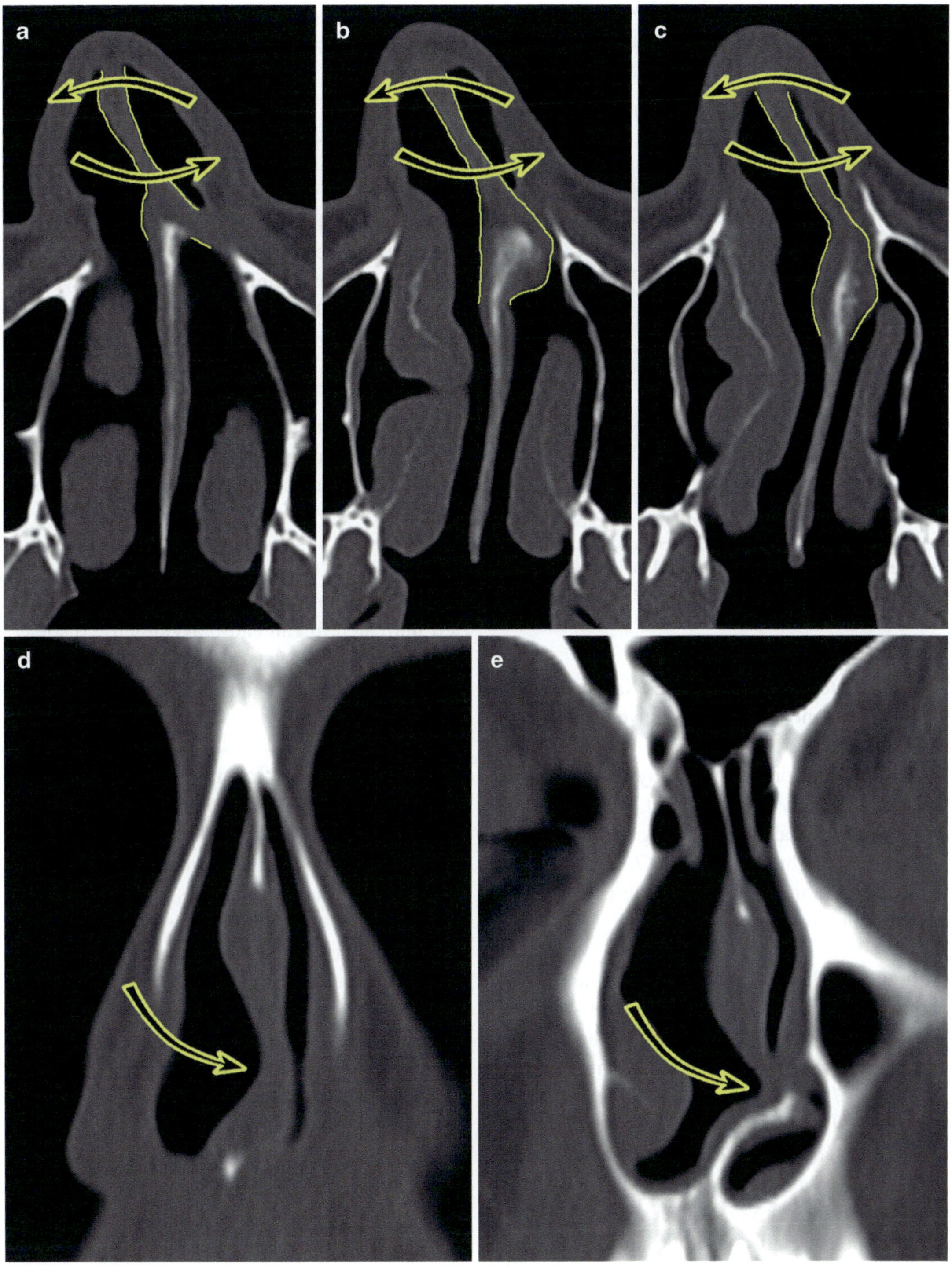

Fig. 7.5 (**a–e**) Axial (**a–c**) and coronal (**d**, **e**) CBCT views of an extreme anterior left septal deviation associated with contralateral tip deviation and obliteration of the left airways in a primary rhinoplasty case

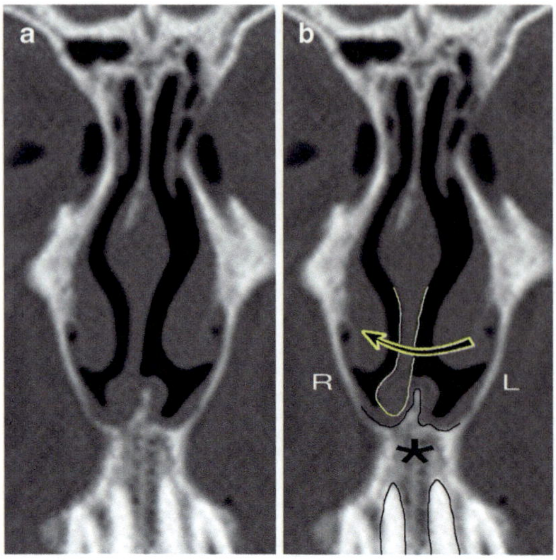

Fig. 7.6 (**a**, **b**) Coronal CBCT view at the level of anterior nasal spine (ANS). The cartilaginous caudal septum lies at the right of the ANS. The asterisk between the ANS and the root apex of the upper central incisors (outlined in black) marks the midline, whereas the caudal septum is outlined in yellow (**b**)

tion creates some difficulties during mucosal elevation, mostly on the convex side of the deviation.

- The left inferior turbinate is hypertrophic (outlined in yellow in Fig. 7.12b).
- The right septal spur touching the inferior turbinate (straight arrow in Fig. 7.12d).
- The deviation to the left of the external nose (straight arrow in Fig. 7.12d).

Figure 7.13a–e shows a reverse situation. The septal deformity resembles a bayonet shape but does not affect the external shape of the nose and probably does not cause functional impairment.

Figure 7.14a–c shows an S-shaped septal deformity. In this case, the complex shape is composed of curves instead of angles. Sometimes this deformity creates difficulty in harvesting a straight cartilage fragment necessary for carving the columellar graft and other similar structural grafts. Figure 7.14a–c also clearly depicts the narrowness of the right valve, outlined in yellow (a–c) and the hypertrophy of the head of the right inferior turbinate (pale yellow dots in Fig. 7.14c).

7.7 Anterior High Septal Deviation

In rhinoplasty, a very common step consist of reshaping a wide nasal dorsum as well as closing the so-called "open roof" after hump removal. To do this, the lateral bone walls of the nose, made up of the nasal bones and the frontal process of the maxilla, are osteotomized and symmetrically approached. Maintaining or obtaining a symmetric dorsum is obviously the main goal of this surgical maneuver that requires:

- Perfect control of the movements of the osteotomized lateral bone walls.
- A stable, straight and midline centered anterior high bony septum as a guide and support.

Figure 7.15a–e shows a coronal (a–c) and axial (e–f) CT views of a typical anterior high septal deviation to the left. If unrecognized and left untreated, it can cause asymmetric displacements of both the lateral bone walls on the left side of the nose after the osteotomies.

7.8 Nasal Cycle and Inferior Turbinate Hypertrophy

The nasal cycle is the spontaneous congestion and decongestion of the nasal mucosa, where congestion of one side is accompanied by reciprocal decongestion of the contralateral side. It is present in the majority of healthy adults. So, it is a normal phenomenon and must be suspected during CT scan analysis in order to differentiate it from the causes of unilateral structural nasal obstruction such as septal deviation and inferior turbinate (IT) hypertrophy.

Figure 7.16a–e shows axial and coronal CT scans of a young healthy adult suggestive for the presence of a normal nasal cycle. The osseous component of both IT, outlined in yellow in Fig. 7.16c, e, is quite symmetrical and equidistant from the septum. The only obvious difference between the two airways concerns the thickness of the mucosa. In particular, the medial

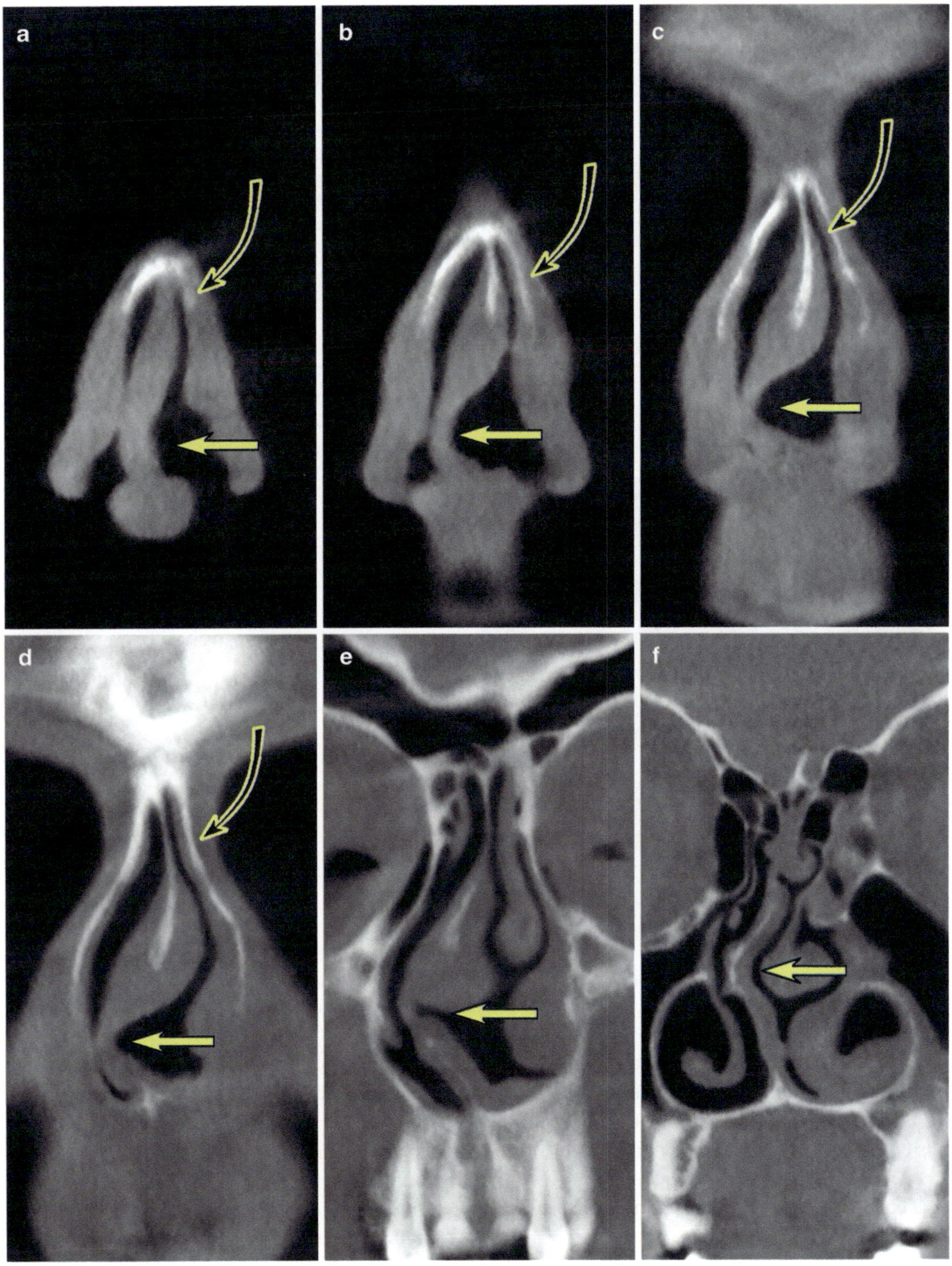

Fig. 7.7 (**a–f**) Multiple coronal CBCT views. The caudal septum is centered on the ANS and along the maxillary crest but presents a strong curvature that causes an important obstruction of the right nasal cavity (straight arrow). The nasal valves are clearly asymmetric with an evident reduction of the left one (curved arrows)

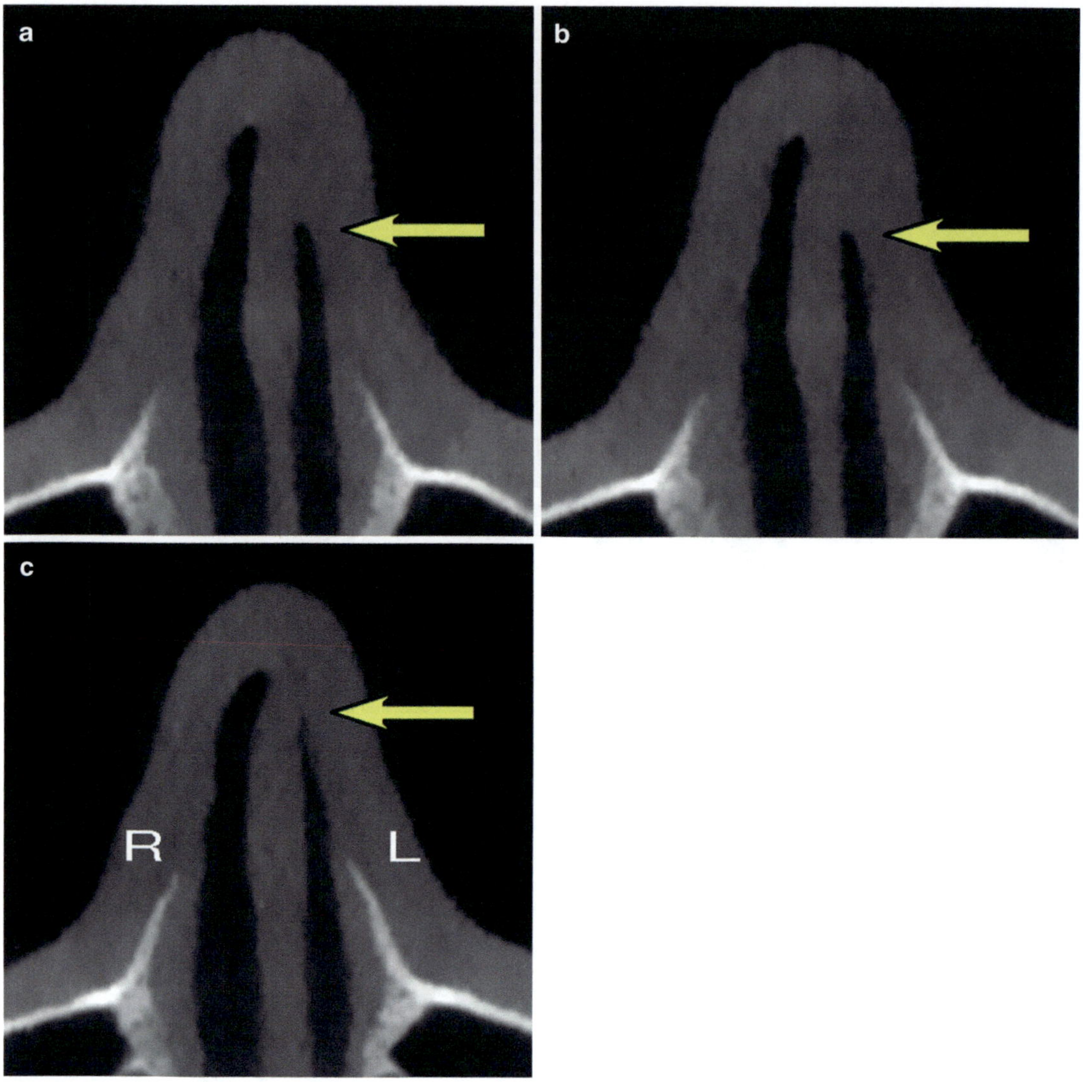

Fig. 7.8 (**a–c**) Axial CBCT views at the level of the cartilaginous dorsum in a primary rhinoplasty case. The straight arrow indicates the narrowed left nasal valve present in all of the three CT sections

layer of the right IT is almost two to three times thicker than the left (dotted area in Fig. 7.16c, e).

The architecture of IT depicted in Fig. 7.17a, b is completely different from the previous one:

- The marked airway obstruction is bilateral and symmetrical.
- The IT osseous component is very close to the septum in its central portion (wide yellow lines).
- The anterior and posterior portions of the IT hypertrophy are constituted by mucosa (fine yellow lines).
- The space comprised between the head of the IT and the septum can be imagined as the narrowest tract of an hourglass (yellow asterisk) and so the main objective of the functional surgical treatment.

Figure 7.18a–c shows another variation of IT hypertrophy:

- The bony component maintains a relative distance from the septum and does not appear to contribute to nasal obstruction.

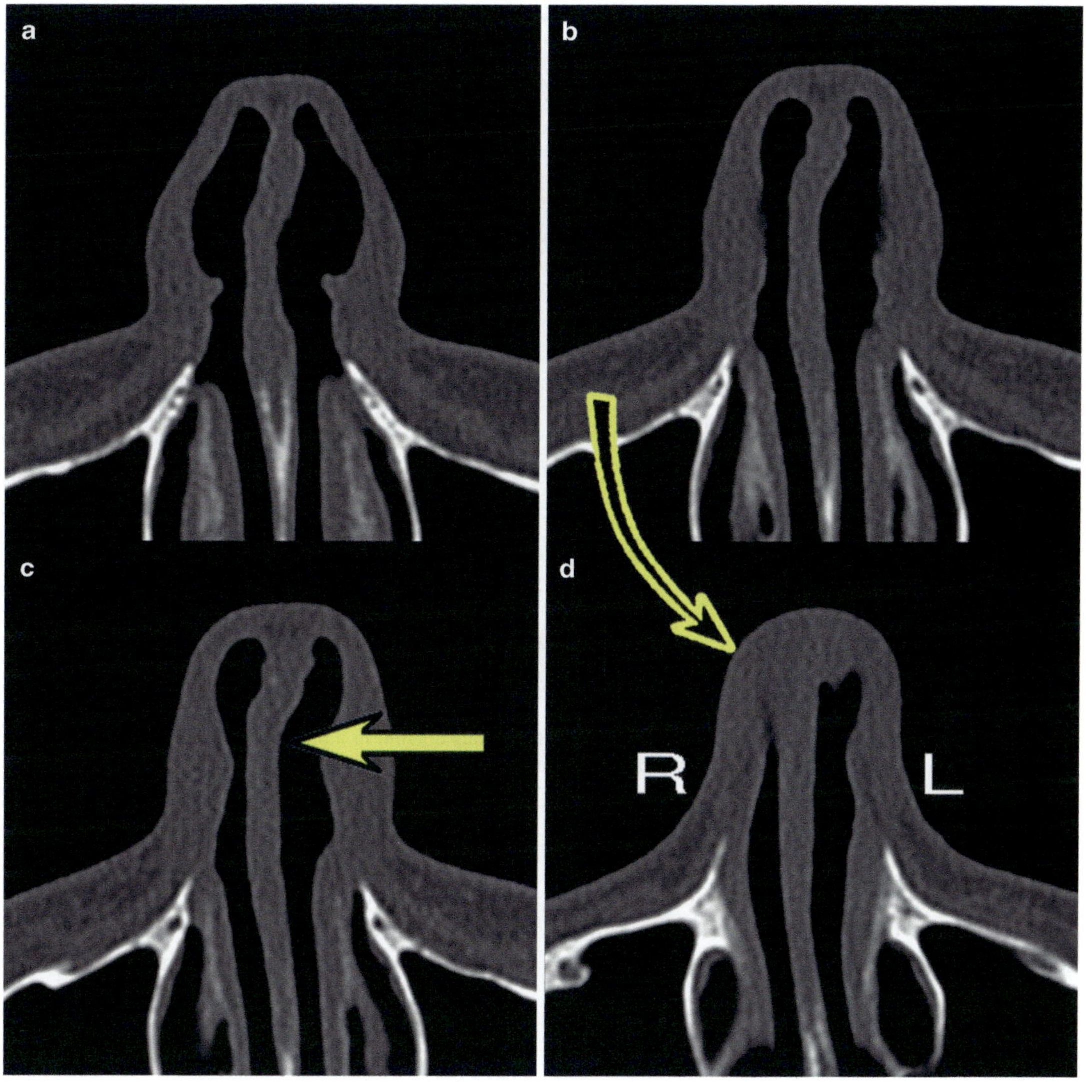

Fig. 7.9 (**a–d**) Axial CBCT views at the level of the tip and the cartilaginous dorsum. From caudal to cranial, the progressive curvature of the septum (straight arrow) and the narrowing of the right nasal valve (curved arrow) are evident

- The hypertrophic mucosa affects the entire length of the turbinate.
- The extremely long tails of the IT exceed the choana (straight arrow) and invade the nasopharyngeal space, which appears reduced (asterisk).
- The two tails of the IT lie in contact with each other (curved arrows).

Figure 7.19a–c shows a frequent preoperative condition in which nasal obstruction is characterized by the combination of IT hypertrophy and septal central deviation. Here are the main analysis points:

- Bilateral IT mucosal hypertrophy.
- Both IT tails exceed the choana margins (asterisk).
- The central septum is deviated to the left (fine yellow line) and the presence of an osseous spur contributes to reduce the right airway.
- The bony left IT (pale yellow line) must be reduced or fractured and laterally luxated to gain space for septal straightening.

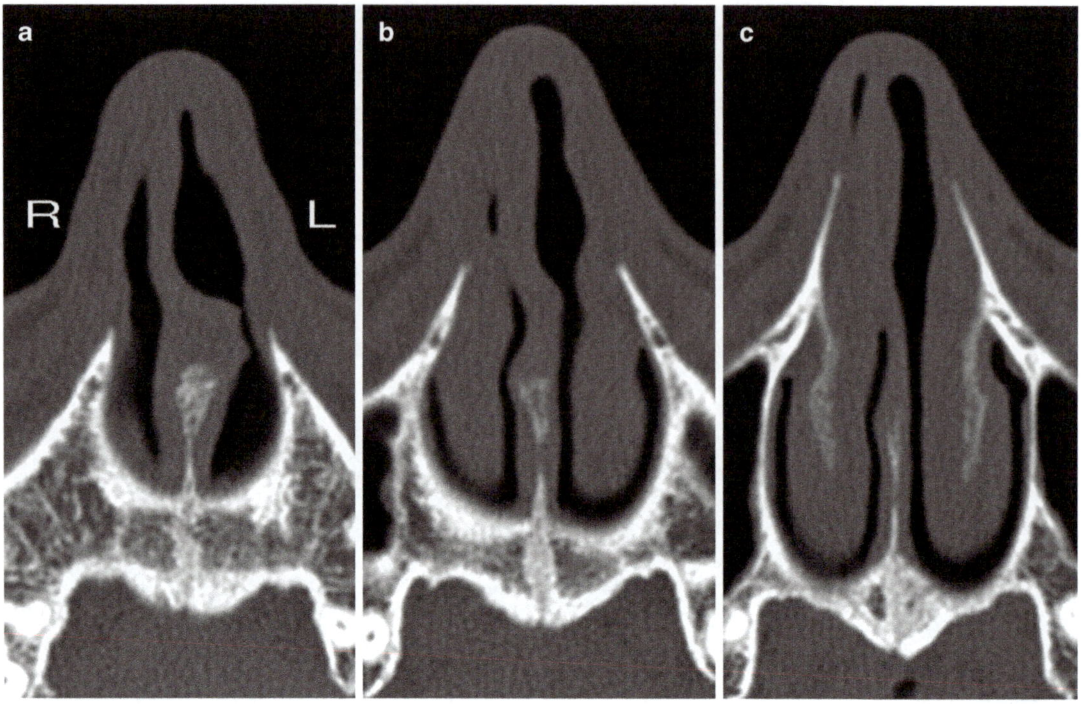

Fig. 7.10 (**a–c**) Axial CBCT views at the level of the cartilaginous dorsum in a primary rhinoplasty case. The three sections depict a severe right-sided obstruction due to valvular collapse

For surgical purposes, the preoperative CT analysis of IT hypertrophy can be divided into three areas (head, body, and tail). So, the hypertrophic right IT depicted in Fig. 7.20a–c can be schematically divided into:

- Head, mucosal hypertrophy (curved arrow).
- Body, osseous hypertrophy (straight arrow).
- Tail, mucosal hypertrophy (asterisk).

7.9 Nasal Bony Vault and Walls

Nasal bone structures, such as the bony dorsum, are easy to study with CT. General shape, thickness and asymmetry of the nasal bone and frontal process of the maxilla should be assessed preoperatively. Figure 7.21a–d shows three axial and one coronal CT scan of a wide and asymmetric bony vault. The main findings are:

- The right nasal wall is more anteriorly projected in comparison with the left one (straight arrows in Fig. 7.21b). This creates an evident asymmetry of the bony dorsum even if the soft tissue envelope partially hides this deformity (fine yellow lines in Fig. 7.21c).
- The left nasal wall is thicker than the left one.
- The coronal view (Fig. 7.21d) shows also the recurvature of the lateral crura of the alar cartilages (asterisks) that reduce the airway mostly on the right side (curved arrow).

An unusual case of weak right nasal wall is clearly visible in the CBCT sections shown in Fig. 7.22a–d. The bony hole, indicated with curved arrows, is evident both in axial and in coronal reconstructions (Fig. 7.2a–c) and it measures, in its superior-inferior dimension, about 10 mm (Fig. 7.22d). Performing nasal osteotomies unaware of this anatomical detail is at high risk of postoperative functional impairment and esthetic deformities.

In preparation of nasal radix deepening with electric bone burs or ultrasonic bone surgery, the thickness of the bony vault, the radix and the

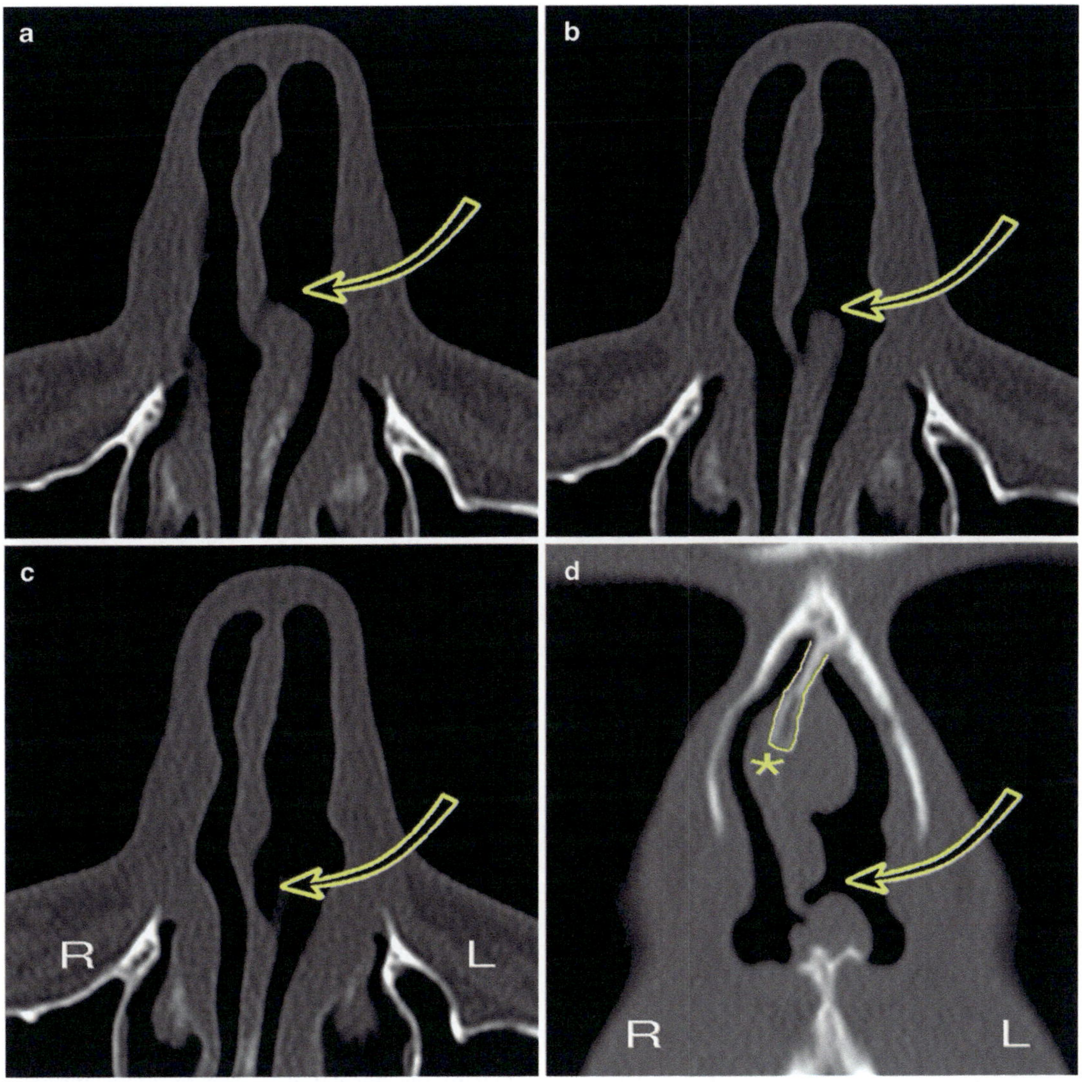

Fig. 7.11 (**a–d**) Axial (**a–c**) and coronal (**d**) CT views of a posttraumatic case. The central cartilaginous septum is clearly angulated with a lack of structural continuity and presence of extremely thin mucosal layers. The coronal section (**d**) depicts an anterior high septal deviation outlined in yellow and marked with an asterisk

dimension of the frontal sinuses must be analyzed with CT including also a midline sagittal section (Fig. 7.23a–e). The dotted area depicts (Fig. 7.23e) the safe quantity of bone to be removed at midline to avoid penetration of the instrument into the nasal cavities or frontal sinus.

The outcomes of previous nasal bone fractures should also be studied with CT in preparation for reconstructive surgery. Figure 7.24a–d shows a clinical case at 1 year from the trauma. The multiple fragments under the skin (curved arrows) are responsible for the clinically evident deformities of the upper third of the nose.

7.10 Evaluation of Secondary Cases

CT imaging of secondary cases can help to find two main kinds of problems: stable deformities, such as bony irregularities, and irreversible lesions, such as inferior turbinate amputation.

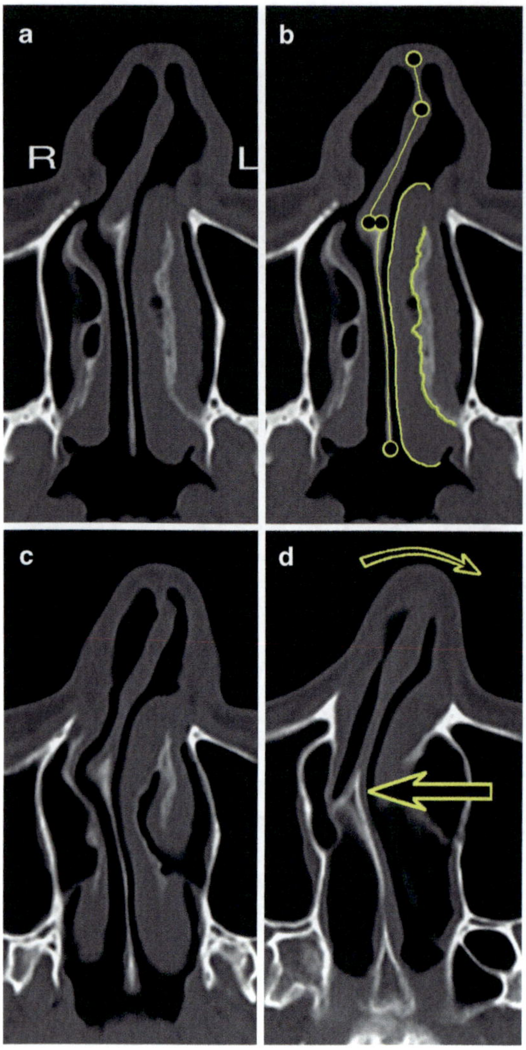

Fig. 7.12 (**a–d**) Axial CT views. Angled septal deformity (**b**) and a central spur touching the right inferior turbinate (straight arrow in **d**). A hypertrophic left inferior turbinate (outlined in yellow in **b**) and a clear deviation to the left of the external nose (curved arrow in **d**) are also part of the complex deformity

Figure 7.25a, b shows a right-displaced nasal wall due to an incorrect osteotomy; the couple of curved arrows help to imagine the rotational movement of the bony segment. The final result is a palpable and high deformity close to the right-side nasal radix (straight arrow) in a thicker bony area, known as Rocker deformity. On the contrary, the osteotomy on the left side appears more regular and without steps (asterisk). The osteotomy line is lower and placed in a thinner area.

The following CBCT images represent an in-depth study of a patient 5 months after an aggressively performed rhinoplasty. The documented outcomes are serious from both a functional and esthetic point of view. Figure 7.26a–d shows three axial sections at the level of the middle third of the nose (between the tip and the caudal margin of the nasal bone). The dotted areas show the bilateral loss of airway collapse between the cartilaginous septum and the paired triangular cartilages at every level considered (Fig. 7.26a–c). Figure 7.27a–d shows three axial sections at the level of the nasal bone. The right bony wall osteotomy line lies too anterior creating a small fragment. Its medial displacement is exaggerated creating a step deformity and losing any bone contact at the osteotomy site (straight arrows in Fig. 7.27a–d). The left wall osteotomy line appears at a correct anteroposterior level but the osteotomized fragment slips completely inside the nasal fossa and partly penetrates the anterior cells of the ethmoidal labyrinth (curved arrows in Fig. 7.27a–c). What happens can be considered one of the major complications of nasal osteotomies: the complete loss of control of the spatial position of the bone fragment by the surgeon. Also in these CBCT images both the anterior airway spaces are reduced, as depicted by the thin yellow lines in Fig. 7.27a. Figure 7.28a–d shows three axial sections at the level of the nasal radix. The previous findings are confirmed (see straight and curved arrows in Fig. 7.28a) and another fractured fragment of thick bone appears clearly collapsed at the level of the left nasal radix. A further study with a coronal reconstruction (Fig. 7.29a, b) confirms the presence of a displaced radix fragment connected with the perpendicular plate of the ethmoid (bright yellow in Fig. 7.29b) and the extreme medialization of the left lateral wall (pale yellow in Fig. 7.29b). Fracture of the nasal radix is quite unusual due to the strong bone structure of this region compared with the surrounding ones and it must be considered a major complication of nasal surgery.

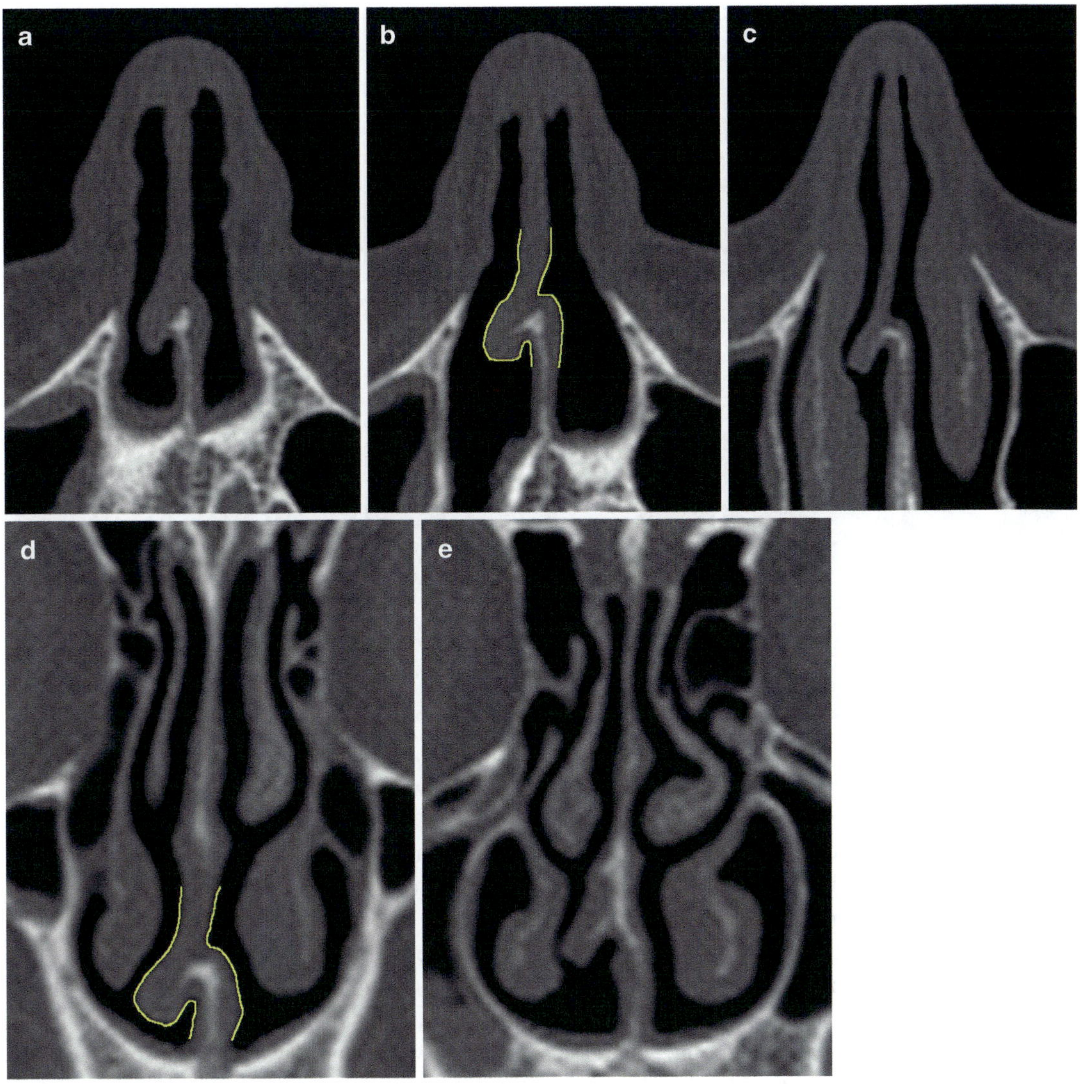

Fig. 7.13 (**a–e**) Axial and coronal CT views. The septal deformity resembling a bayonet shape (outlined in yellow in **b** and **d**)

An evident external deformity of the nose, such as a pinched nose, should also be examined with CBCT in order to:

- Document the obstruction.
- Illustrate with images the functional problem to the patient.
- Make possible a postoperative comparison after reconstructive surgery.

Figure 7.30a–c shows a pinched tip deformity secondary to aggressive surgery. The nasal valves are severely narrowed and the tip is deviated to the left.

Investigating the presence of a septal perforation or an inferior turbinate secondary lesion is a mandatory step in the preoperative study for rhinoplasty. Recognizing the etiology of the lesion, changing the treatment plan, and sometimes declining further nasal surgery are some of the additional issues in these patients.

Figure 7.31a–d presents two axial and two coronal reconstructions of a secondary case. The patient with a small "multi-operated" nose strongly

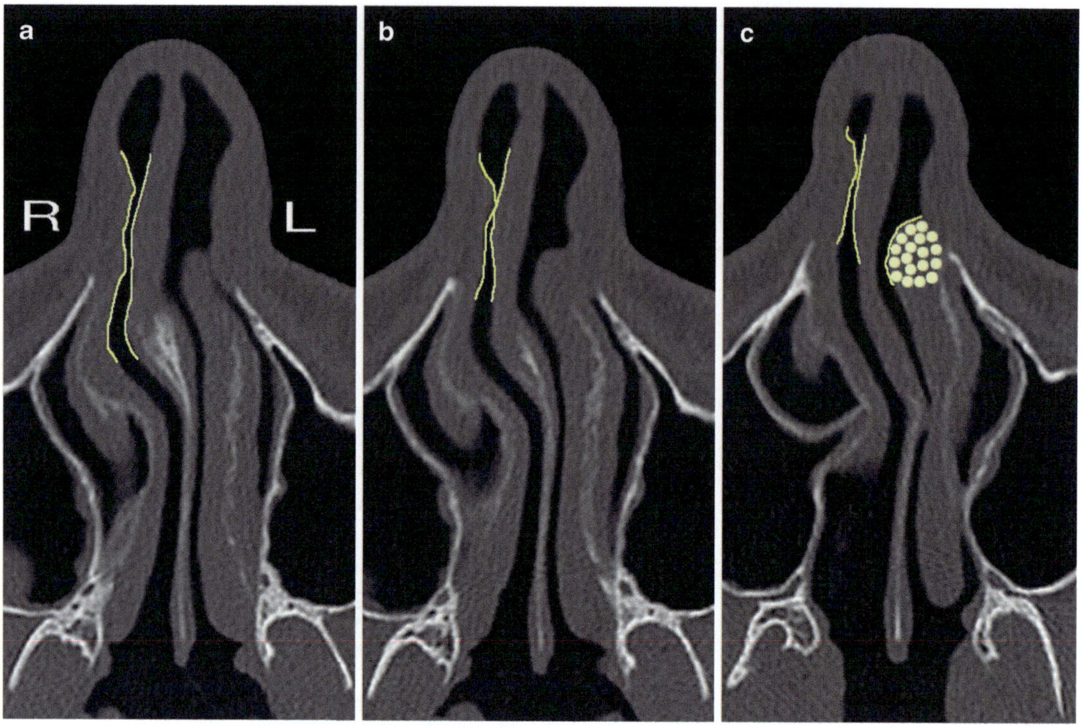

Fig. 7.14 (**a–d**) Axial CT views. S-shaped septal deformity with narrowness of the right valve, outlined in yellow (**a–c**), and hypertrophy of the head of the right inferior turbinate (pale yellows dots in **c**)

requested a smaller nose and, during the three preoperative visits, seemed unconcerned by her nasal obstruction and evident mouth breathing. The image analysis revealed the combination of a bilateral valve collapse with the absence of both inferior turbinates suggestive of previous aggressive surgery. From a medical standpoint, the case needed a nasal reconstruction with some degree of enlargement of the framework requiring an obvious increase of nasal size. Due to the opposing opinions between surgeon and patient, the only solution was to decline further surgery.

Figure 7.32a–d shows four axial CT views of a patient requesting a visit for rhinoplasty. His major complaint was the drooping tip. On history taking he reported a previous turbinate surgery many years earlier. His septum presents two small septal cartilage perforations, one placed anteriorly and inferiorly close to the anterior nasal spine of maxilla (single asterisk) and another more central (double asterisks).

Figure 7.33 shows an axial CT view depicting a small central septal perforation secondary to a previous rhinoplasty and Fig. 7.34a, b shows another case in which a fairly similar septal lesion coexists with a nasal valve collapse. These last three cases have many common points and suggest some considerations:

- All patients were unaware of their septal perforation.
- All radiologists failed to describe the presence of small septal perforations in their reports but they wrote and signed that the nasal septum was "straight."
- All these lesions are small and not easily identified with anterior rhinoscopy utilizing a nasal speculum.

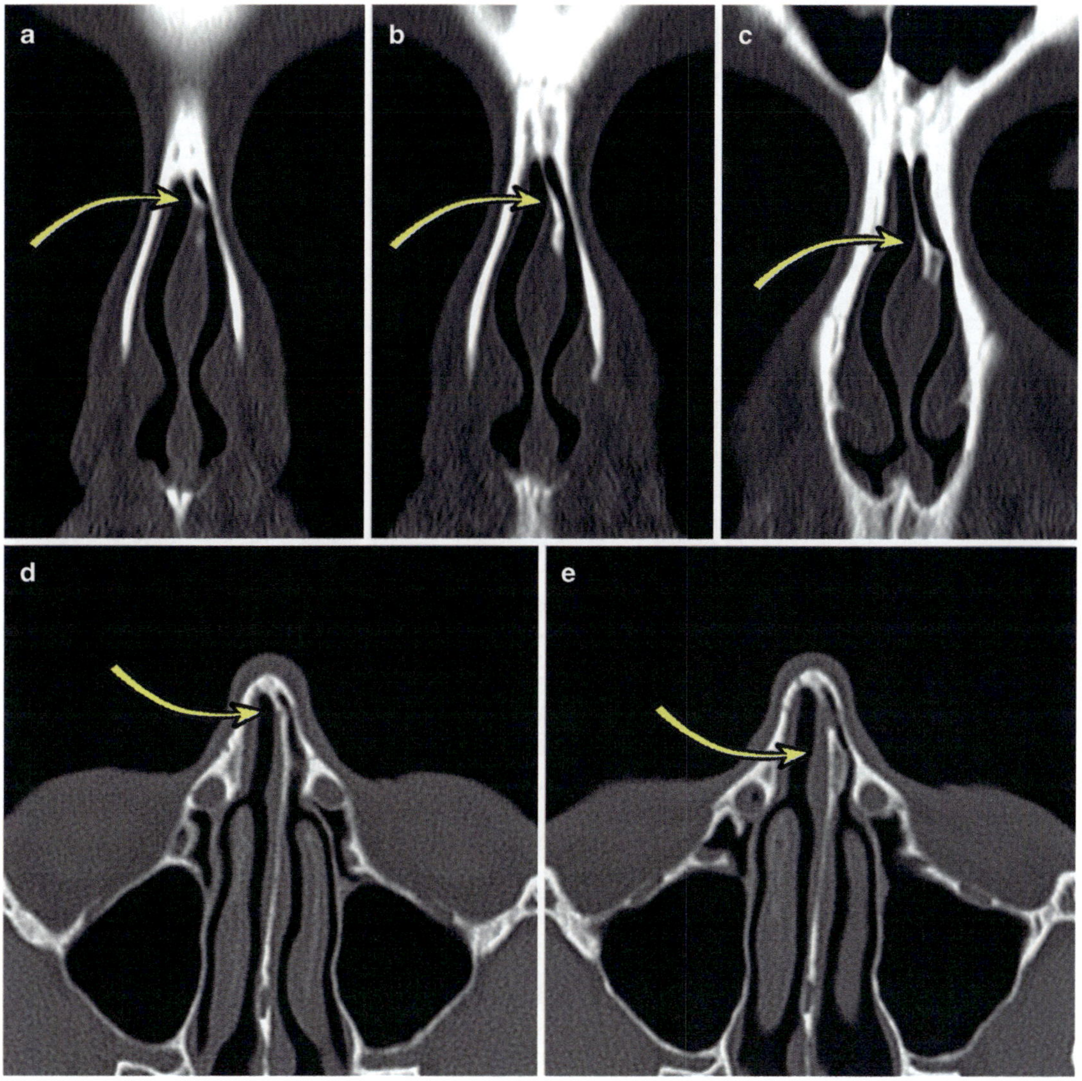

Fig. 7.15 (**a–e**) Axial and coronal CT views. Anterior high bony septal deviation to the left (curved arrows)

- All these patients require a nasal framework reconstruction with autologous cartilage grafts.
- All these patients require a septal reconstruction.

In conclusion, showing a CT image is the best way for the surgeon to inform patient of the presence of the septal lesion and of the possible need to harvest autologous cartilage from an extranasal site during surgery.

Finally, Fig. 7.35 shows a CT axial scan of a patient some year after a Le Fort I maxillary osteotomy done for the correction of a class III dentofacial deformity. The image confirms the presence of titanium screws and plates at the level of frontal process of the maxilla. These internal osteosynthesis devices must be removed by an intraoral approach in a single surgical session immediately before starting rhinoplasty to permit safe osteotomies of the nasal pyramid.

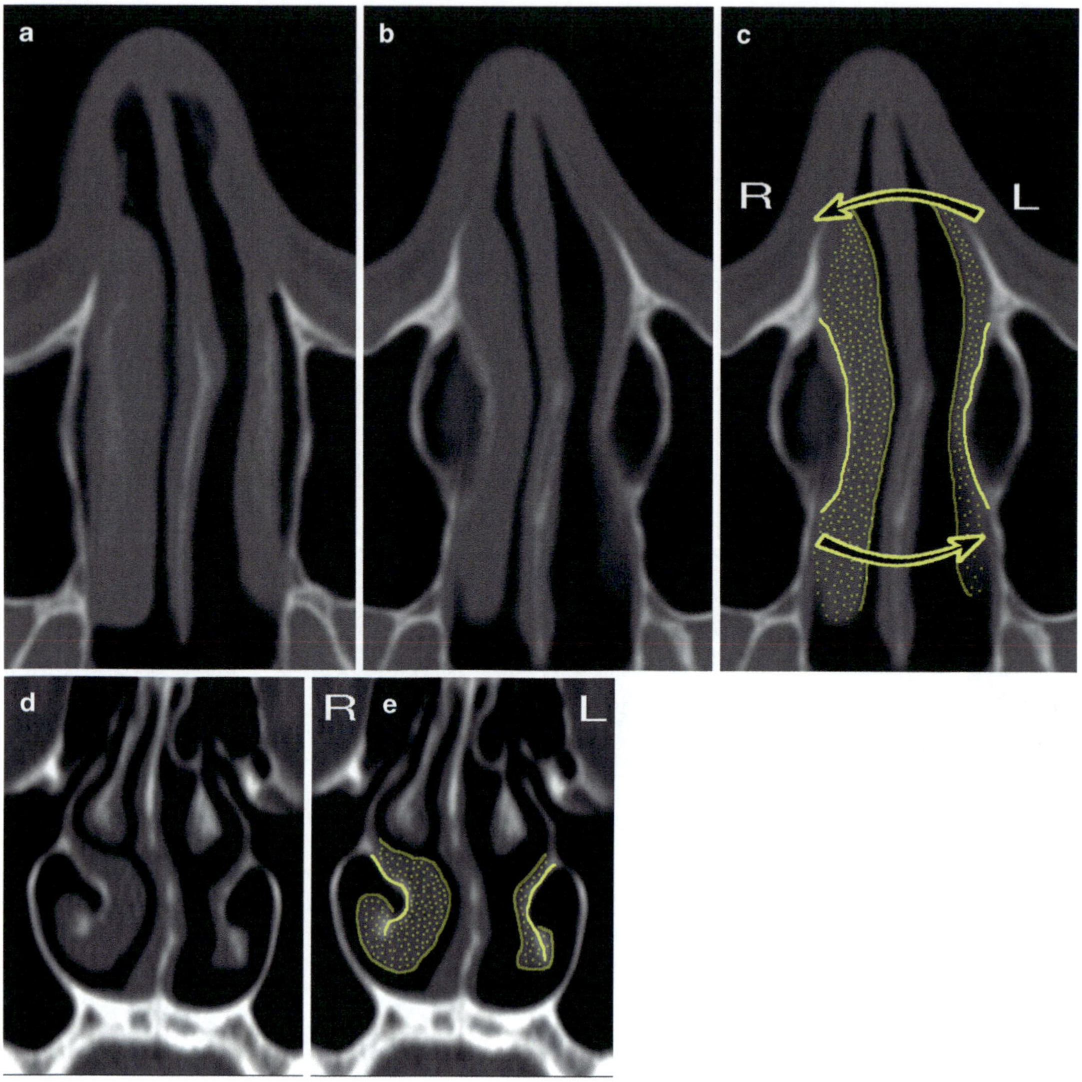

Fig. 7.16 (**a–e**) Axial and coronal CT views showing a case of normal nasal cycle. The osseous component of both IT (yellow line in **c** and **e**) is quite symmetrical and equidistant from the septum. Unilateral enhanced thickness of the right IT mucosa (dotted area)

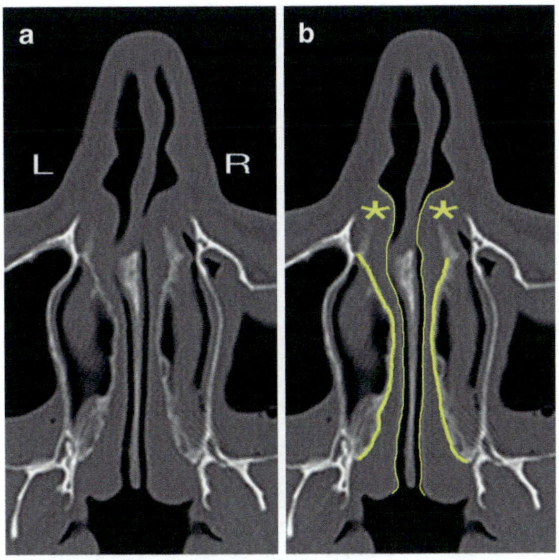

Fig. 7.17 (**a**, **b**) Axial CT view in a case of bilateral IT hypertrophy. The osseous component (wide yellow lines) and mucosa (fine yellow lines) are both hypertrophic. The asterisks mark the head of the IT

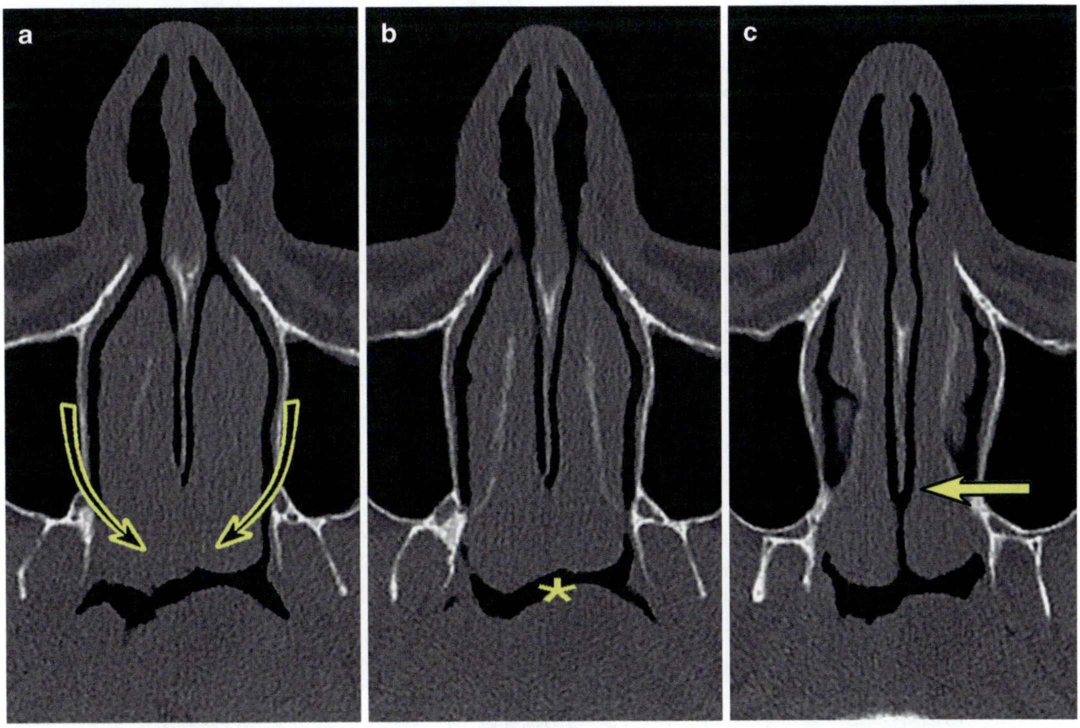

Fig. 7.18 (**a–c**) Axial CT views in a case of bilateral IT hypertrophy. The extremely long tails of the IT exceed the choana margins (straight arrow) and invade the nasopharyngeal space, which appears reduced (asterisk). The two tails of the IT lie in contact with each other (curved arrows)

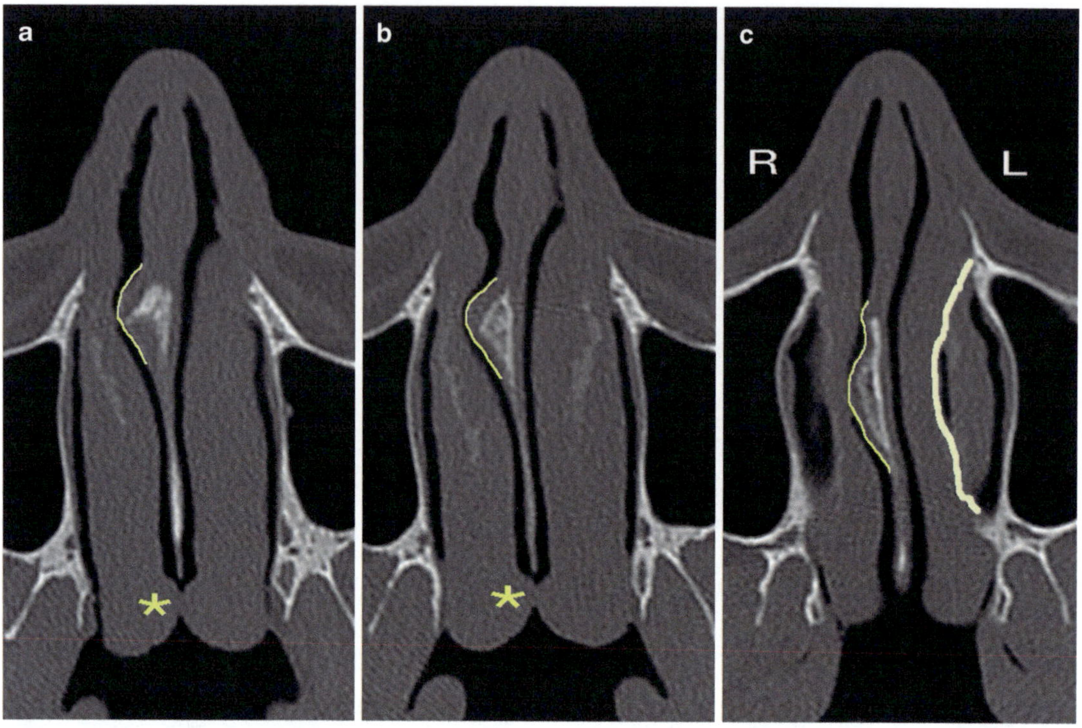

Fig. 7.19 (a–c) Axial CT views in a case of septal deviation and bilateral IT hypertrophy. The osseous component of the left IT (pale yellow line) and septal osseous spur (fine yellow lines). The two tails of the IT are long and lie in contact with each other (asterisk)

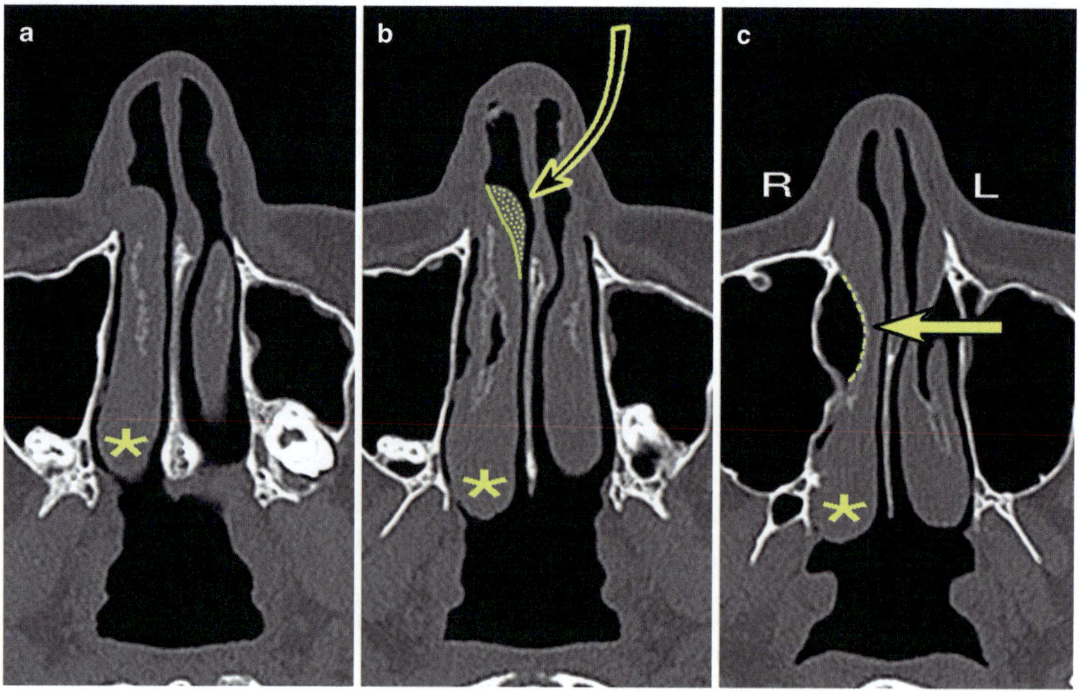

Fig. 7.20 (a–c) Axial CT views in case of bilateral IT hypertrophy involving the head (mucosal hypertrophy—curved arrow), the body (osseous hypertrophy—straight arrow) and the tail (mucosal hypertrophy—asterisk)

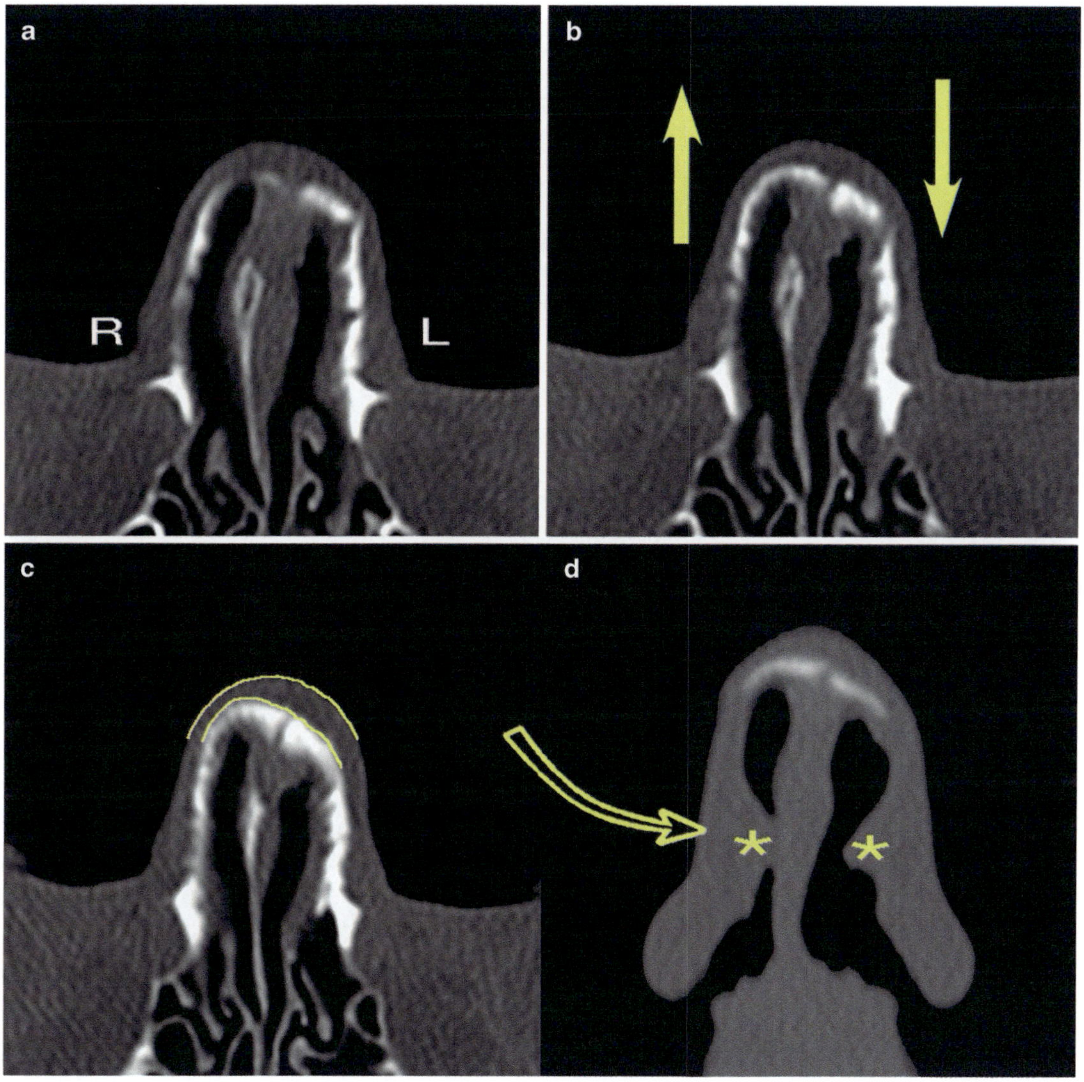

Fig. 7.21 (**a–d**) Axial and coronal CT scans. Wide and asymmetric bony vault due to different anterior projection between the nasal walls (see straight arrows in **b**). The soft tissue envelope partially hides the deformity (fine yellow lines in **c**). The coronal view (**d**) shows also the recurvature of the lateral crura of the alar cartilages (asterisks) that reduce the airway especially on the right side (curved arrow)

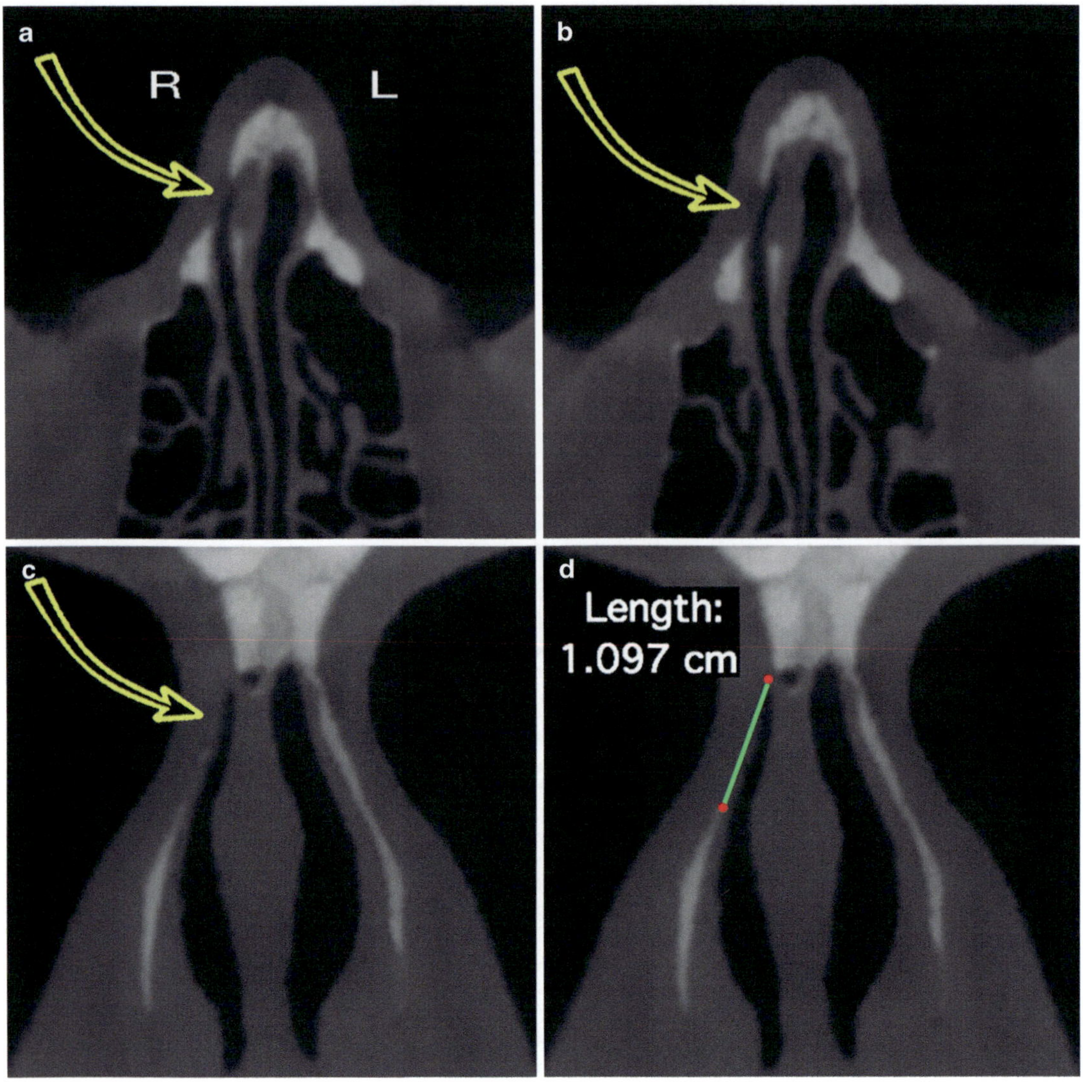

Fig. 7.22 (**a–d**) Axial and coronal CBCT scans. A bony hole in the lateral nasal wall is evident both in the axial and in coronal reconstructions (**a–c**). It measures, in its superior-inferior dimension, about 10 mm (**d**)

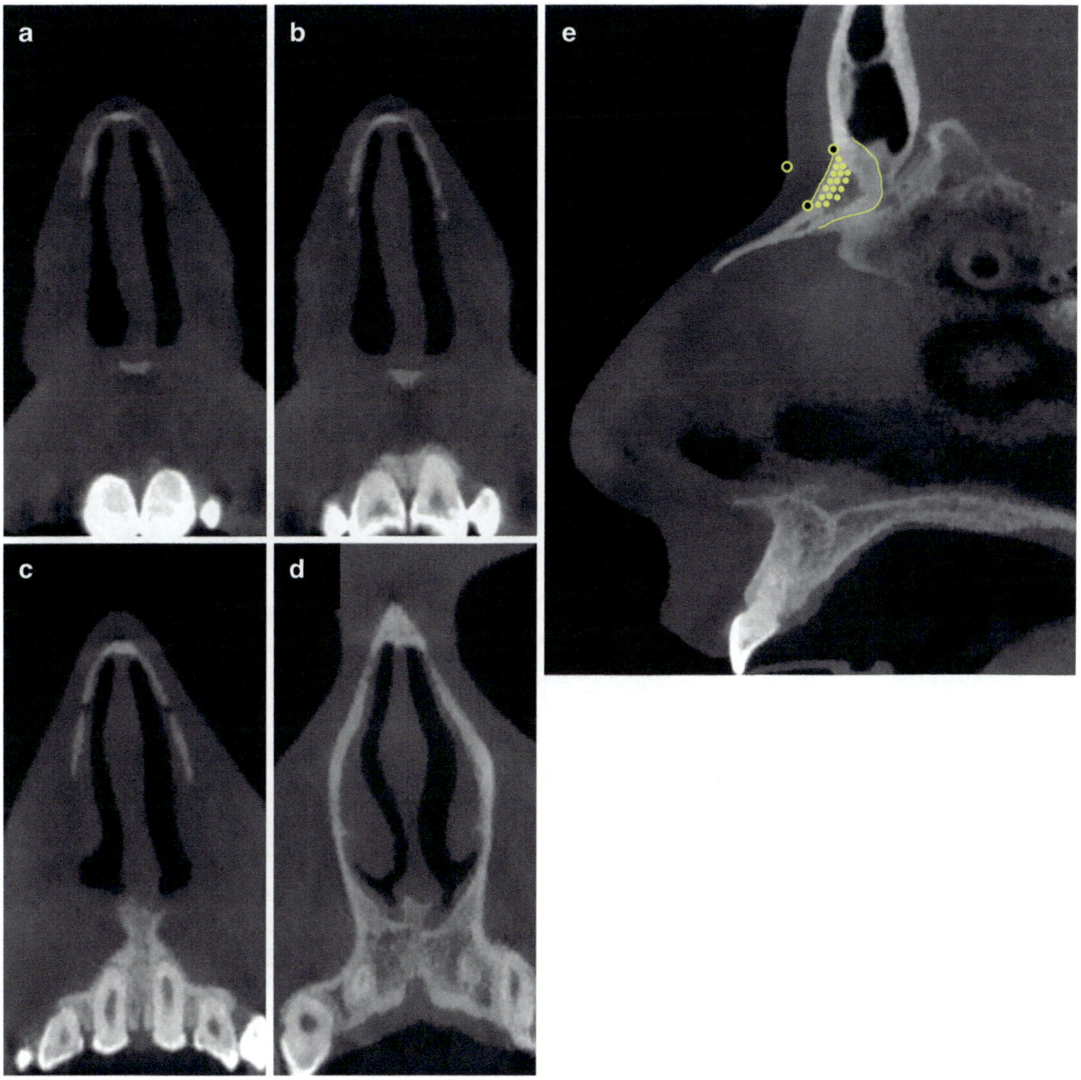

Fig. 7.23 (**a–e**) Axial and midline sagittal CBCT scans. The dotted area (**e**) shows the safe limits of bone removal at midline when radix deepening is planned

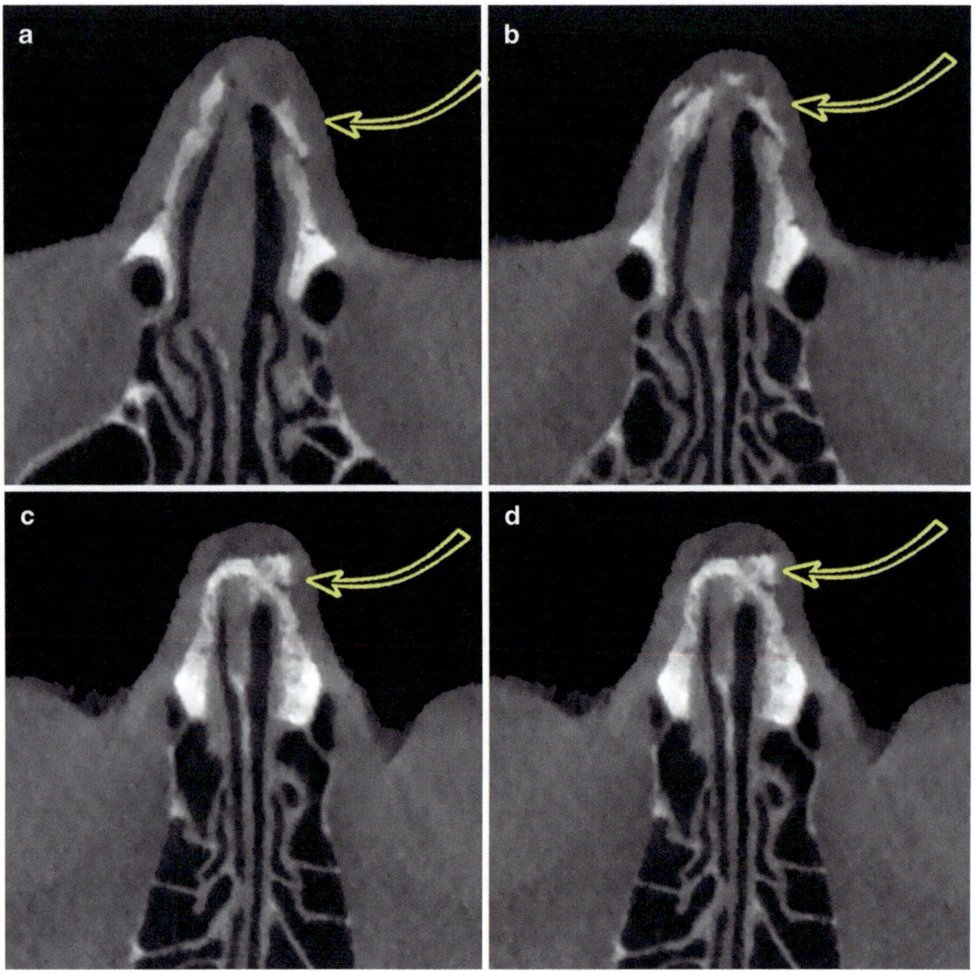

Fig. 7.24 (**a–d**) Axial CBCT scans. Multiple bony fragments under the skin (curved arrows) secondary to a previous nasal fracture

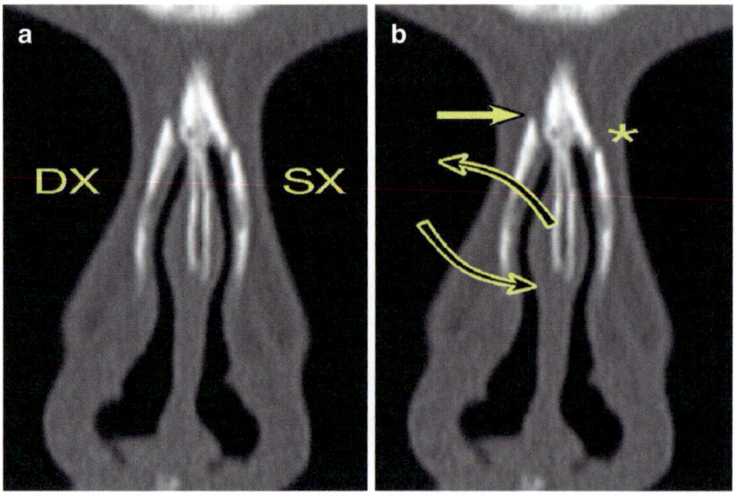

Fig. 7.25 (**a**, **b**) Axial CBCT scan. Incorrect right nasal bone osteotomy with high deformity close to the right-side nasal radix (straight arrow) in a thicker bony area (the so-called Rocker deformity). The couple of curved arrows help to imagine the rotational movement of the bony segment necessary to produce this deformity. The osteotomy on the left side appears more regular and without steps (asterisk)

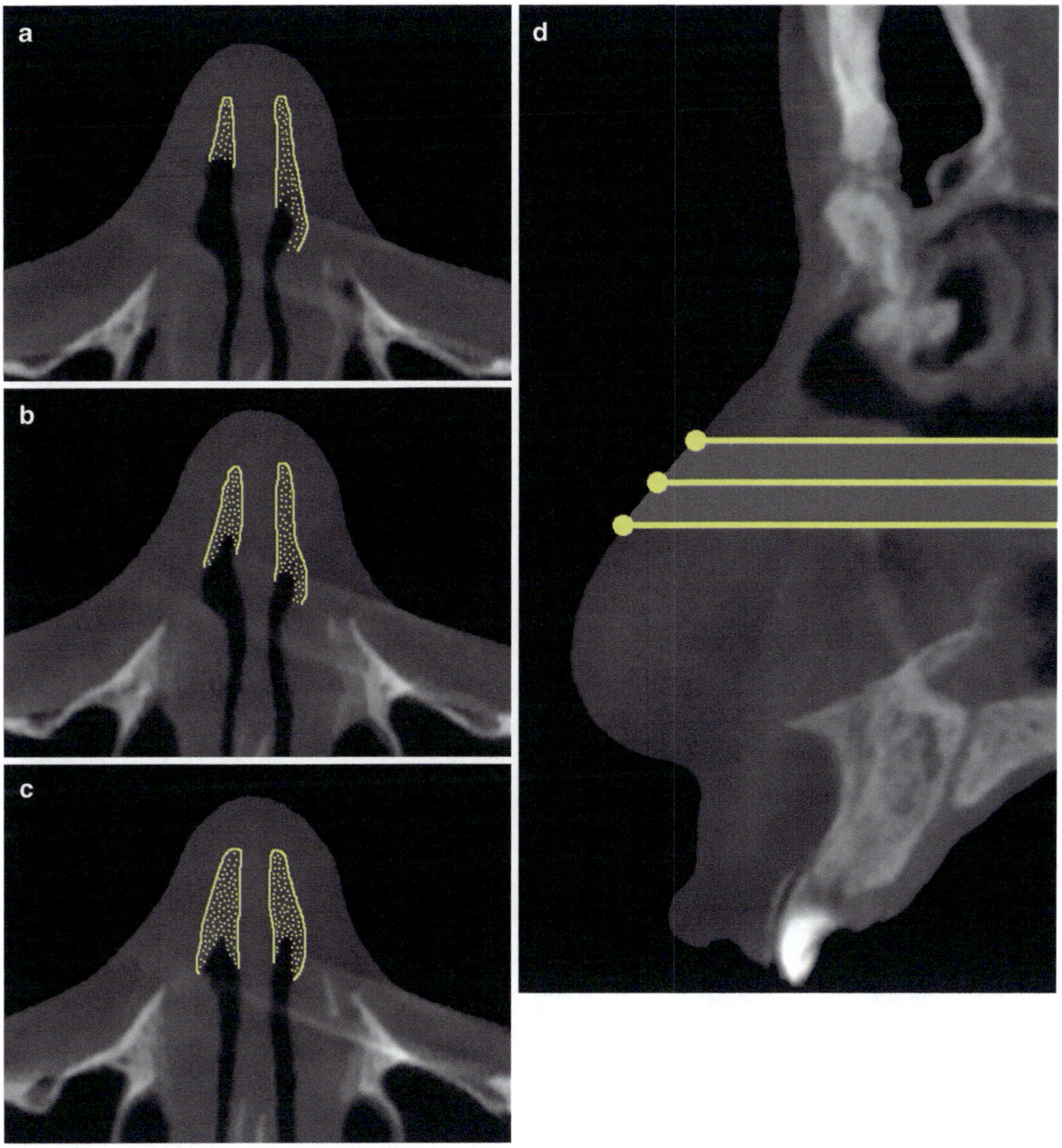

Fig. 7.26 (**a–d**) Three CBCT axial scans of the middle third of the nose (**a–c**) plus a sagittal midline reconstruction (**d**) that helps to identify the planes of the study. Bilateral loss of airway collapse between the cartilaginous septum and the paired triangular cartilages (dotted areas in **a–c**)

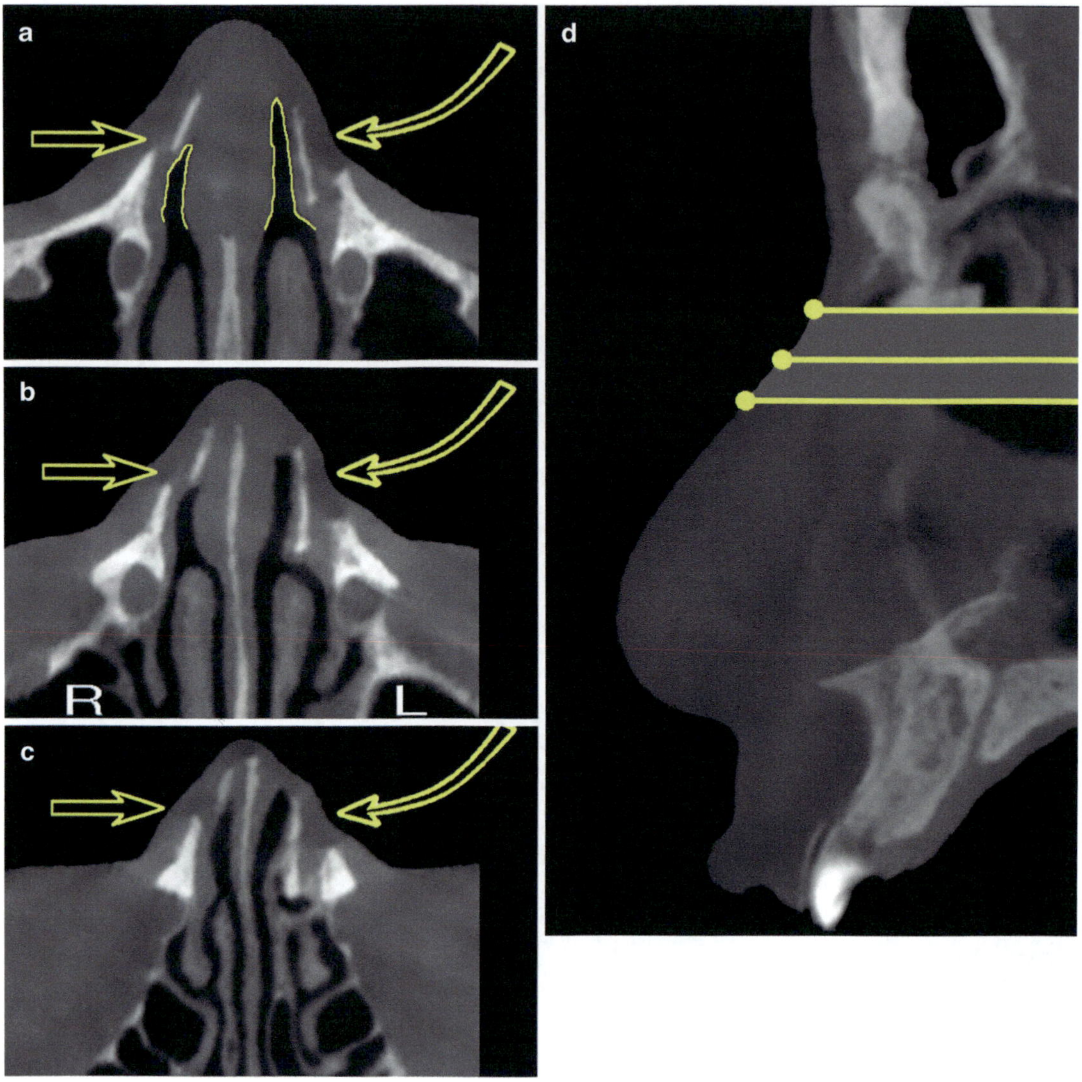

Fig. 7.27 (**a–d**) Three CBCT axial scans of the bony vault of the nose (**a–c**) plus a sagittal midline reconstruction (**d**) that helps to identify the planes of the study. Excessively anterior right osteotomy line (straight arrows) and a major displacement of the left-side osteotomized bony fragment that slips inside the nasal fossa (curved arrows in **a–d**). Bilateral anterior airway collapse (thin yellow lines in **a**)

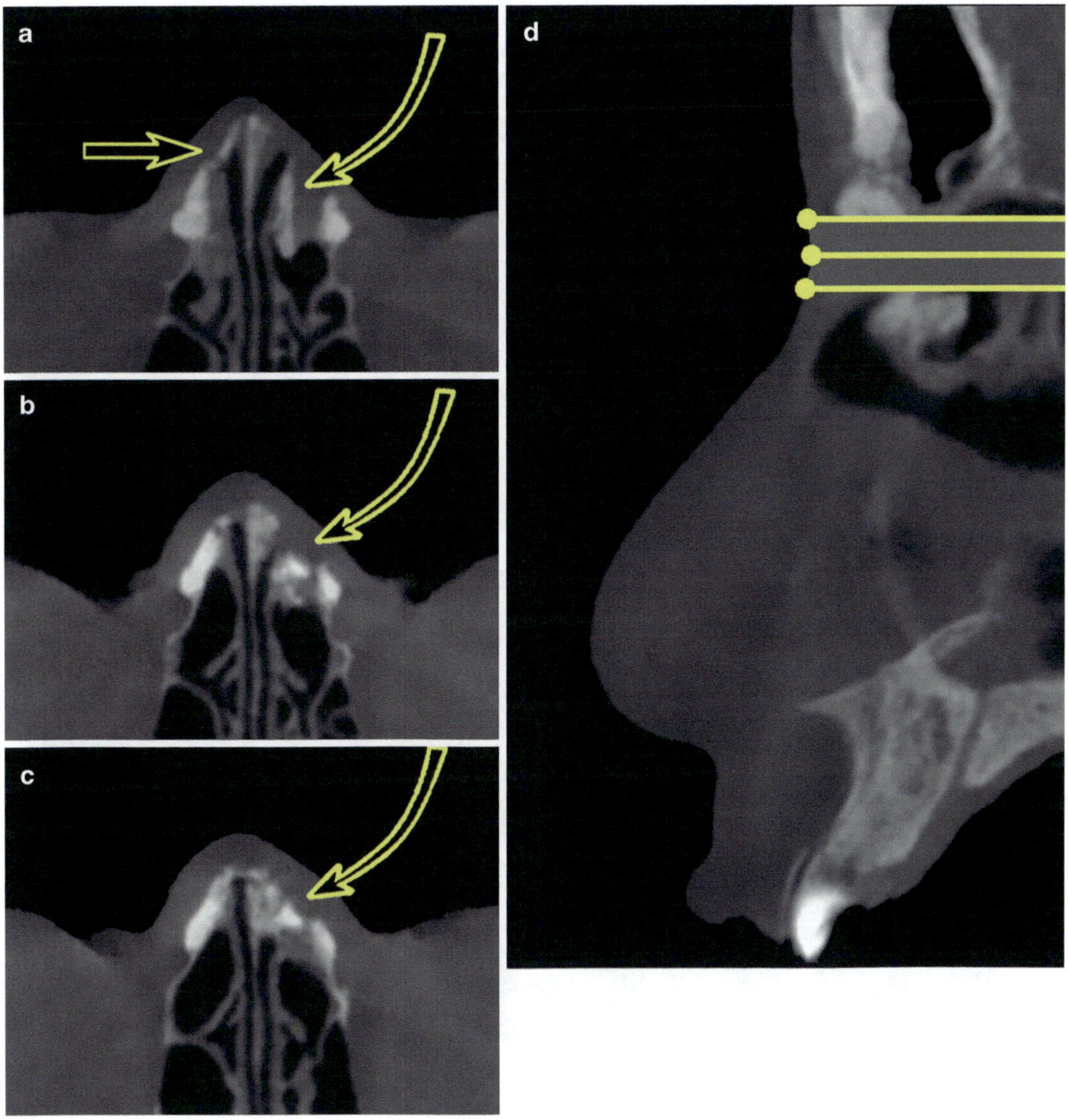

Fig. 7.28 (**a–d**) Three CBCT axial scans of the radix of the nose (**a–c**) plus a sagittal midline reconstruction (**d**) that helps identify the planes of the study. Too anterior right osteotomy line (straight arrows) and a major displacement of left-side osteotomized bony fragment slip inside the nasal fossa (straight and curved arrows in **a**). A fractured fragment of thick bone is clearly collapsed at the sidewall of left nasal radix (curved arrows in **b**, **c**)

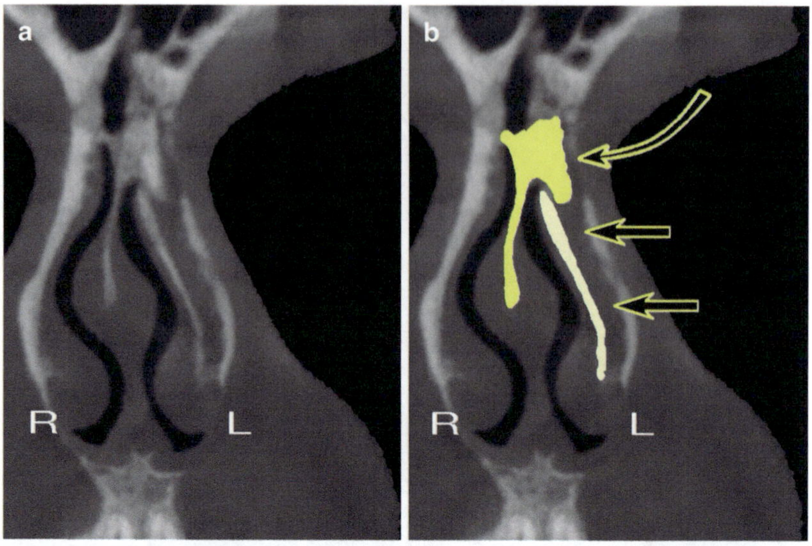

Fig. 7.29 (**a**, **b**) CBCT coronal reconstruction of the same clinical case presented in the previous figures. Displaced nasal radix fragment connected with the perpendicular plate of the ethmoid (bright yellow in **b**) and extreme medialization of the osteotomized left lateral wall (pale yellow in **b**)

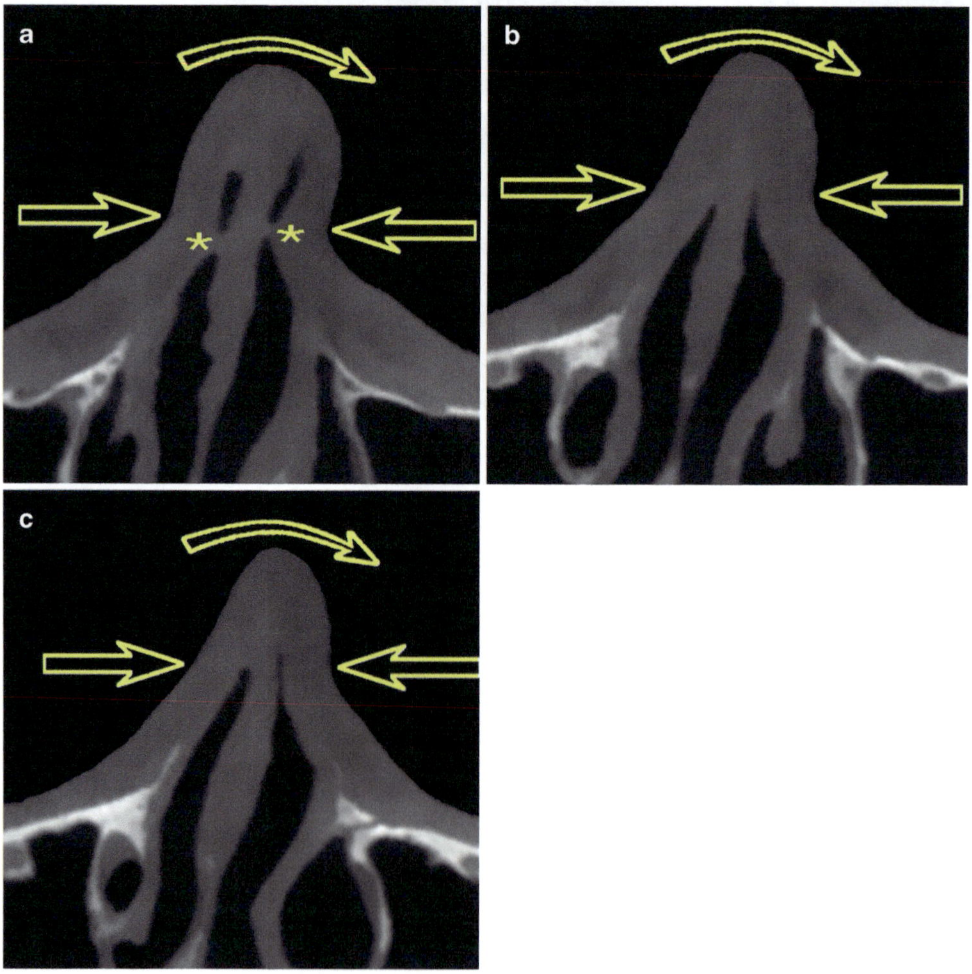

Fig. 7.30 (**a–c**) CBCT axial scans of a "pinched" nose in a secondary case with severely narrowed airways and deviation to the left of the tip

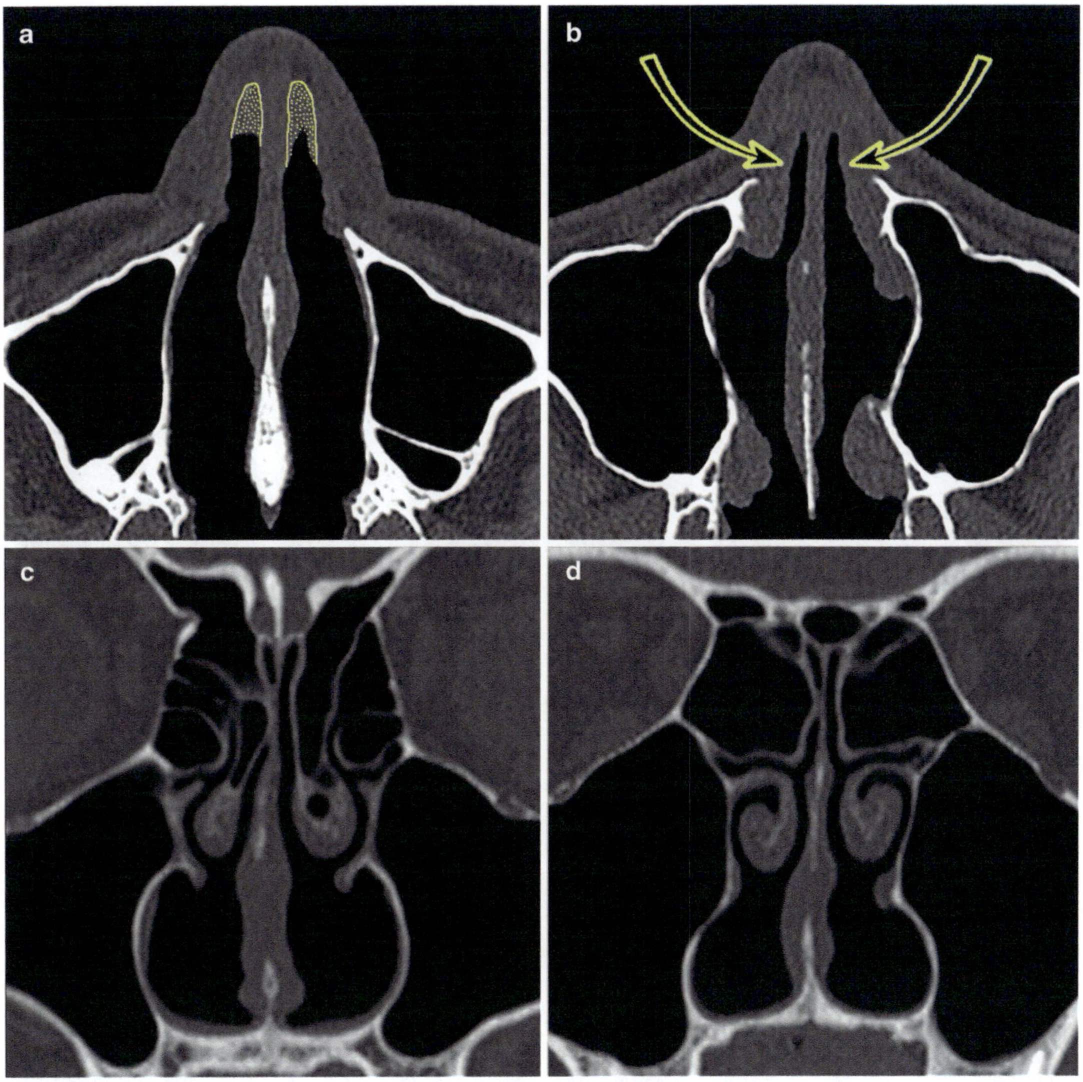

Fig. 7.31 (**a–d**) Axial (**a**, **b**) and coronal (**c**, **d**) CT reconstruction of a secondary case. Bilateral nasal valve collapse (dotted areas and curved arrows in axial views) associated with the absence of both inferior turbinates suggestive of previous aggressive surgery

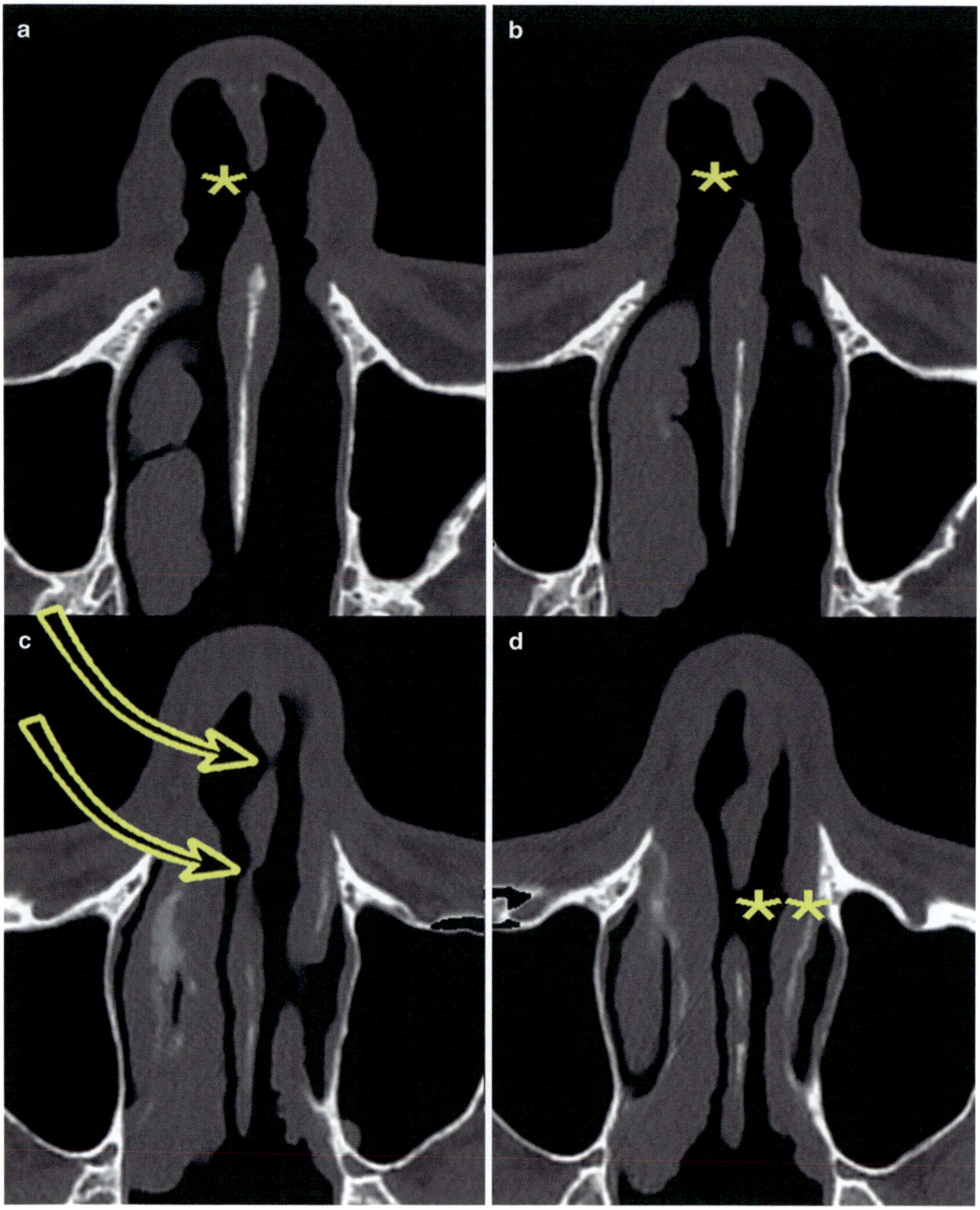

Fig. 7.32 (**a–d**) Axial CT scans show the presence of two septal perforations. The anterior one is marked with one asterisk and the central one with two asterisks

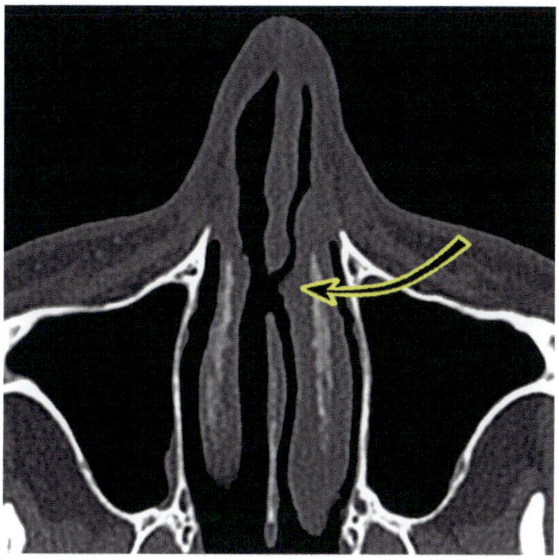

Fig. 7.33 Axial CT scan shows the presence of a central small septal perforation in a secondary case

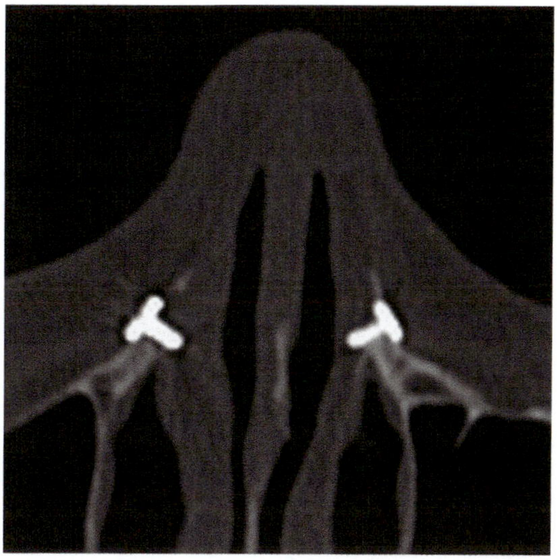

Fig. 7.35 Axial CT scan shows the presence of bilateral titanium screws at the level of the frontal process of the maxilla

Fig. 7.34 (**a**, **b**) Axial CT scan shows the presence of a central small septal perforation (single curved arrow) associated with bilateral nasal valve collapse (couple of curved arrows and dotted areas) in a secondary case

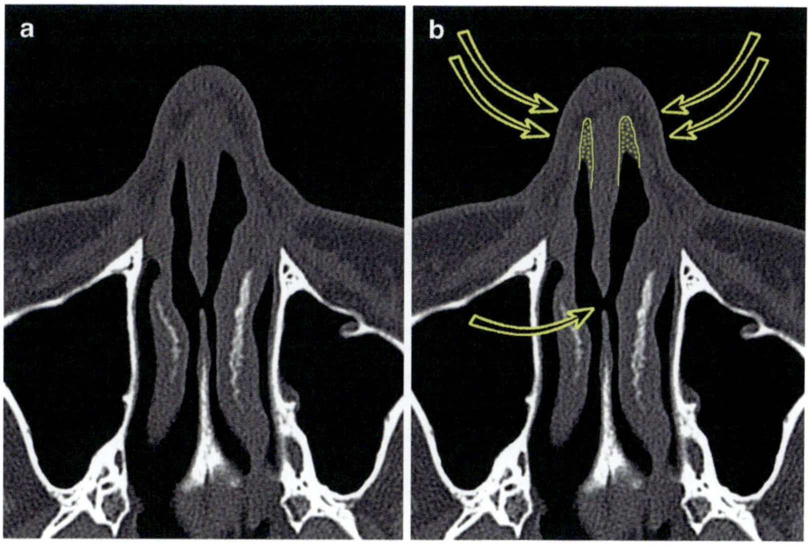

Further Reading

Many books are available on head and neck imaging, but unfortunately the chapters dedicated to the nasal and paranasal sinuses are very generic and of little value for a rhinoplasty surgeon. This is unsurprising given that most of the books on rhinoplasty seldom, if ever, recommend a standard preoperative study with CT. One of the consequences is that there is an editorial void in this particular field, which lacks a radiological atlas dedicated to rhinoplasty.

Should the readers want to deepen their knowledge about CBCT, the recent book edited by Scarfe WE and Angelopoulos C titled "*Maxillofacial Cone Beam Computed Tomography: Principles, Techniques and Clinical Applications*" (Springer International Publishing AG, 2018, ISBN-13: 978-3-319-620-596) is a good overview, even though it covers a broad range of topics (mostly centered on oral and maxillofacial surgery) and only few pages are dedicated to the nose.

8 The Rationale of Basic Open Rhinoplasty for Young Surgeons

In everyday practice there are no "easy noses" that need a simple and unique corrective surgical maneuver such as removing the hump or narrowing the tip of the nose. Performed at state-of-the-art levels, every single rhinoplasty is a complex, unique, and unrepeatable procedure carried out on a unique and unrepeatable patient at a particular moment in his life. Sometimes, during surgery, unpredictable situations can arise.

For a young surgeon the choice of the basic surgical approach, the surgical techniques to master, the variables to be considered, and the general rules to be respected in rhinoplasty are real difficulties to face. The versatility and reliability of the approach are two major qualifying elements of any functional, reconstructive, and esthetic nasal surgery.

In this chapter, we will describe the general aspects that make Basic Open Rhinoplasty (BOR) not a mere "incisional" approach to nasal surgery but a broad and articulated surgical discipline where fundamental principles and rules allow one to tackle the great majority of clinical cases.

8.1 Why Start with the Open Approach?

There are several reasons for a young surgeon to start the practice of nasal surgery focusing on the open approach. First of all, the current historical period, which is very different if compared with some years ago.

The first surgeon who approached the nasal tip through a small columellar incision was Dr. **Aurel Réthi** of Budapest (Fig. 8.1). His work dates back to 1921 and the sole objective of his technique was the correction of nasal tip deformities as he approached the nasal dorsum through an endonasal incision.

It took almost three decades for the next logical evolution of Réthi's idea to be realized: in 1954, Dr. **Ante Šercer** of Zagreb not only modified the Réthi incision (Fig. 8.1b) but also explored and treated both the dorsum and the tip of the nose through the same access. In 1957 he published his experience naming his technique "Nasal Decortication." At that time the most influential nasal surgeon of the twentieth century, Dr. Maurice Cottle of Chicago, was strongly opposed to the "decortication approach" and the work of Dr. Ante Šercer went largely unnoticed.

The third surgeon to make some fundamental steps forward was Dr. **Ivo Padovan**, an assistant of Dr. Šercer. He, for the first time, corrected septal deformities and not only the superficial structures of the nose utilizing a similar incision (Fig. 8.1c). He continued to call the surgical approach "Nasal Decortication." The other contribution of Dr. Padovan was a lecture entitled "External Approach to Rhinoplasty (Decortication)" presented at the First International Symposium of Plastic and Reconstructive Surgery of the Face and Neck held in New York in 1971. Approaching the nose through an outside incision appeared, at that time, a heretical idea and Dr. Padovan's presentation

F. Meneghini, *Basic Open Rhinoplasty*, https://doi.org/10.1007/978-3-030-61827-8_8

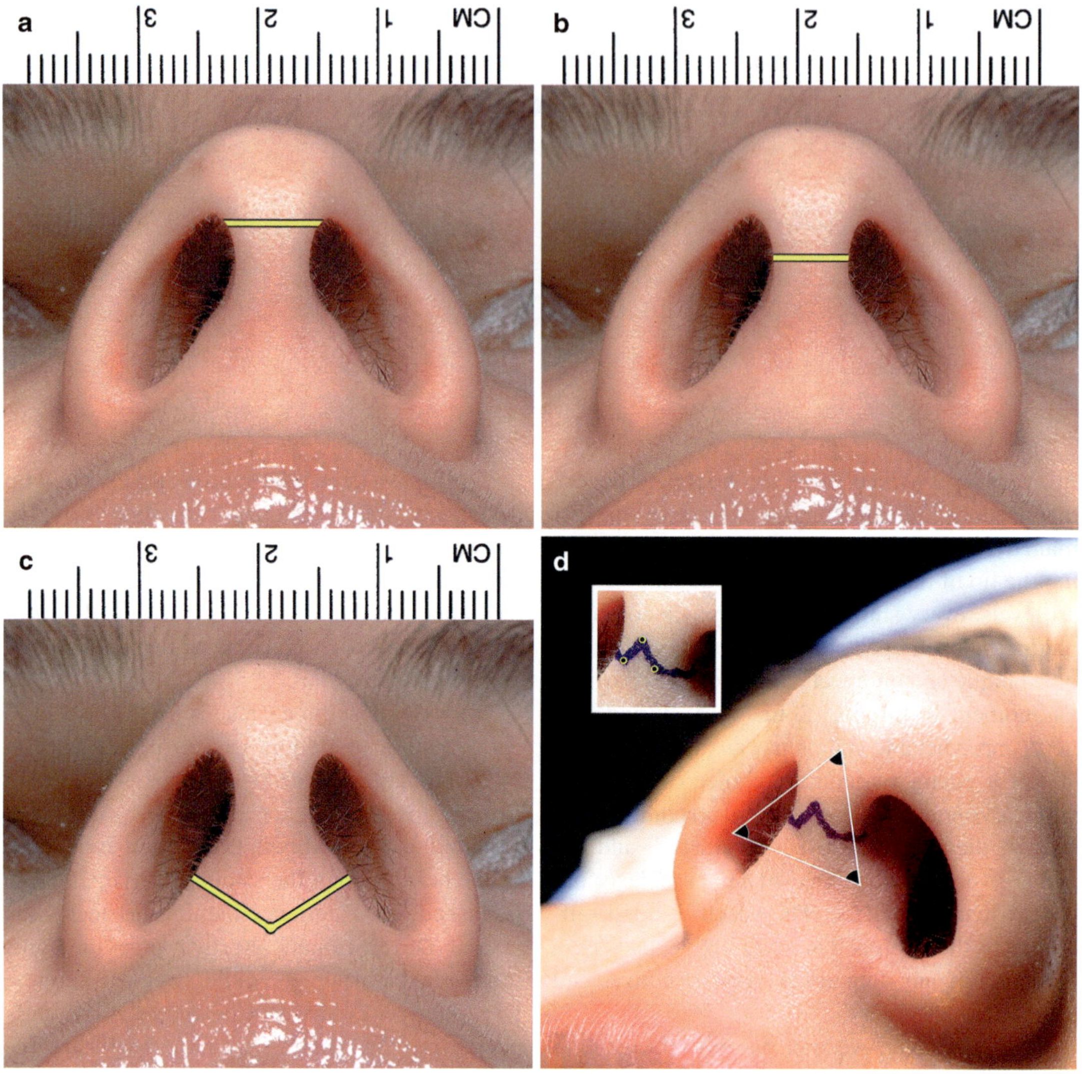

Fig. 8.1 (**a–d**) Historical columellar incisions: Aurel Réthi (**a**), Ante Šercer (**b**), Ivo Padovan (**c**), and Wilfred S. Goodman (**d**). Goodman's incision is probably the most utilized today

received mostly negative comments with the exception of Dr. Wilfred S. Goodman from Toronto. Goodman changed the terminology, avoiding "Decortication Approach" and using only "External Approach," introduced his columellar line incision (Fig. 8.1d), one of the most used until now, and presented his experience at various meetings in Canada and in the Unites States. But the climate did not change much, given that a senior staff surgeon to Dr. Goodman during a grand rounds presentation on External Rhinoplasty at the Toronto General Hospital in 1977 commented: "*I think it is malpractice to make that scar in the columella.*"

But it was only a matter of waiting a few more years.

A famous authority on rhinoplasty, Dr. Jack R. Anderson of New Orleans, once decided to "try" and since then there has been no serious voice in the field of rhinoplasty which denies the value of the external approach. The abstract written by Dr. Anderson in his article published in 1982 states: "The senior author (J.R.A.), having taught endonasal rhinoplasty for more than 25 years, felt obligated to evaluate so-called open rhinoplasty. His experience, and that of his co-authors, indicates that, on balance, this technique offers more advantages than disadvantages; in fact, there is no reason why it should not be used routinely if the surgeon desires. However, while open rhinoplasty permits the surgeon to approach the correction with more confidence, visualization of the structures of the nose does not, of itself, guarantee a good result."[1]

Today, a century after Aurel Réthi's first clinical experiences, is the best time ever for a young surgeon to take his first steps in the field of rhinoplasty by studying the open approach. Today, as never before, the open approach is widely diffused and taught throughout the world. Today, as never before, there is an abundance of specific didactic books and videos. Even the free scientific resources available on the web are remarkable. Meetings and courses dedicated to open rhinoplasty are held every month around the world. And, most important, today, as never before, it is easy for the young surgeon to find a mentor for a guided, one-to-one direct experience in open rhinoplasty.

8.2 The Fourth Surgeon and the Missing Link in the Logical Evolution of the Open Approach

In recent years, the practical revolution of the open approach has been finally completed. Schematically we can summarize it like this:

- First surgeon, Dr. **Aurel Réthi**, Budapest, 1921, nasal tip surgery.
- Second surgeon, Dr. **Ante Šercer**, Zagreb, 1954, nasal tip and dorsum surgery.
- Third surgeon, Dr. **Ivo Padovan**, Zagreb, 1970, nasal tip, dorsum, and septal surgery.
- Fourth surgeon, Dr. **Olivier Gerbault**, Paris, 2013, nasal tip, dorsum, septum, and lateral walls surgery.

Dr. Gerbault has shown us that also the frontal process of maxillary bone can be safely skeletonized and treated under direct vision without further skin or mucosal incisions. With this final progress, today every part of the osteocartilaginous nasal framework can be directly analyzed, shaped, cut, moved, rotated, grafted, and stabilized.

8.3 A Single Skin Incision Surgery

One of the major goals of the BOR discipline is to start rhinoplasty with a single skin incision and perform all the subsequent steps through that incision alone. In particular, it is possible to:

- Study directly the osteocartilaginous framework, its deformities, and any structural deficiencies in order to confirm or change the treatment plan if necessary.
- Achieve all surgical objectives avoiding other surgical incisions.
- Offer the surgeon ample surgical flexibility.
- Address the most frequent and sometimes inevitable intraoperative problems by allowing safe alternative solutions.
- Photographically document the surgery for clinical research and medical-legal purposes. It is not strange that books dedicated to the closed approach utilize intraoperative photographs of clinical cases treated with the open approach for demonstration purposes.

The BOR method uses a single skin incision that incorporates three segments: the right and left marginal incisions and the transcolumellar one. The only possible variant is the design of the columellar tract that is chosen based on the conformation of the central portion of the columella. The incision is started and completed by seeking symmetry.

[1]Anderson JR, Johnson CM, Adamson P. Open rhinoplasty: An assessment. Otolaryngol Head Neck Surg. 1982;90(2): 272–274. Abstract presented at the 1981 Annual Meeting of the American Academy of Otolaryngology—Head and Neck Surgery, New Orleans, Sept 20–24.

Only for surgery on the inferior turbinate and for some osteotomy techniques of the lateral wall, small stab incisions of about 2 or 3 mm will be made to allow the insertion of surgical instruments in direct contact with the bone.

Those surgical sequences that start with a septoplasty performed through a mucosal incision with the goal of removing part of the quadrangular cartilage for a later grafting step are no longer acceptable. There is no reason to make additional incisions, removals and manipulations of the septal cartilage before a first complete surgical exploration of the entire nasal framework. The need to perform one or more cartilage grafts, for example, cannot be decided in advance and therefore it is not correct to start by cutting or altering the main source of cartilage: the septum.

8.4 A Graduated Logical Approach to Surgical Steps

Mainly, the steps of the rhinoplasty sequence must respect certain time pairs that can be summarized as follows:

- First, surgically EXPLORE and then TREAT the nasal structures.
- First do the REVERSIBLE SURGICAL STEPS and then, only if there is no alternative, do the IRREVERSIBLE STEPS.
- First do the more PREDICTABLE steps of the work and then do the less PREDICTABLE steps.
- First do the HARD WORK and then do the DELICATE WORK.
- First treat the DEEP structures and then the EXTERNAL ones.
- First approach the MACRO areas and then approach the DETAILS.
- First try to obtain the MAIN GOALS of the treatment plan and then the SECONDARY ones.
- First PRESERVE and then RECONSTRUCT/REINFORCE the nasal structures.
- First do the STRUCTURAL INVISIBLE GRAFTS and then do the SUPERFICIAL GRAFTS.

8.5 How to Communicate Your Surgical Approach to Patients

The previous principles, even though purely related to the surgical phases, also influence the communication between doctor and patient as they must be concisely explained during the preoperative visits and, sometimes, they must be recalled later when evaluating the clinical outcomes. There are no perfect approaches to nasal deformities and obstruction and it is part of preoperative communication to describe the surgical principles followed by the surgeon and clearly discuss the pros and cons.

Here is an example. The treatment of the hypertrophy of the lower turbinate can vary from a small reduction in volume, often at the level of the anterior third, to removal of a large part of the structure. The BOR discipline clearly indicates a conservative approach and the way to communicate it to the patient in plain words is: “In the case of recurrence of hypertrophy we are always able to treat it again with a minor surgical procedure while if we completely remove the turbinate its essential functions are lost and there is no method to reconstruct it.”

In other words, it is better to make the mistake of not finishing the job than to make the mistake of compromising the job. One should remind the patient that a secondary procedure to finish the job is usually less invasive than the procedure needed to reconstruct the nose.

Usually, if the logic of an approach is good in the eyes of the surgeon it will also be good in the eyes of the patient.

8.6 The Relationship Between What a Surgical Approach Offers and How Much a Surgeon Take Advantage of It

In our everyday life, we use books, electronic appliances, cars, cameras, smartphones, computers, and many other objects. As we well know, we only take advantage of a small part of what they can offer us. Since these are objects, there is perhaps nothing wrong with that. On the other hand, if we talk about a medical practice and even more for a particular surgical approach, a similar condition is morally deplorable.

The open approach in rhinoplasty, as represented in the BOR discipline, must be used to obtain full advantages both for the patient and for the surgeon. For the latter, my advice is to exploit all the esthetic, functional, and reconstructive possibilities. Not to stop at the most obvious aspect, the single problem that the patient or the radiological investigation highlights. As surgeons, we must avoid the so-called "Tunnel Vision."

"Tunnel Vision" in our field is the fact that the surgeon, the patient, or both consider only one part of the multiple problems of the nose rather than having a more general understanding. Initially it may happen that the patient sees only his nasal hump and concentrates his requests to the surgeon on removing the hump only. Even the surgeon can forego the overview and focus only on his patient's hump. For them hump removal is the solution—clean and plausible (but wrong).

It is clear that a surgical technique that allows the correction of most of the problems of a nose requires the patient and the surgeon to share an equally broad vision of the problems that must be studied and understood together in preoperative meetings.

8.7 The Continuous Intraoperative Analysis

Continuous thinking and evaluation of the situation during the surgery and the necessary pauses to review what has been done and what remains to be done have always been part of rhinoplasty. This intraoperative analysis is the best defense for the surgeon to avoid falling into the "Tunnel Vision" during the most important moments of the surgery.

8.8 Working Under Direct Vision

Returning to the initial question of why to start with the open approach, rhinoplasty has changed considerably in the last three decades and probably will continue to change rapidly. A versatile approach offers the best possibility for the young surgeon to add, over time, new techniques, new instruments, and new technologies to his surgery.

In such a changing and vast field, open rhinoplasty can also be helpful in reducing the learning curve. Direct vision of the bone and cartilaginous structures is fundamental to understand the cause and effect relationship of the surgical actions.

Other valuable merits of working under direct vision on the nasal framework are that it allows the surgeon to:

- Easily reach and maintain a perfect anatomical plane of flap elevation (You see where you are!).
- Evaluate the strength and weakness of the cartilages.
- Reduce the margin for error in shaping the cartilages and bones.
- Evaluate the symmetry of the framework more easily.
- Avoid the risk of losing control over the position of the osteotomized bones.
- Find and remove small superficial irregularities more easily.
- Perform more precise and gentle sutures of the lower lateral crura.
- Fix the grafts with multiple sutures.
- Check the cleanliness of the surgical field from small bone fragments and dust.
- Document the surgical steps with photos and videos.
- Discover in time a previously undetected problem or an unexpected event.

And most importantly, it helps the surgeon evaluate at any moment what is "insufficient," what is "enough," and what is "too much."

8.9 A Still Valid Concept

In 1998, JB Tebbetts reported this concept in his book:

> *Reserving open rhinoplasty for more 'difficult' cases is illogical. Every primary rhinoplasty is 'difficult' and maximizing control and available techniques*

minimizes risks of secondary operation. The primary indications for open rhinoplasty are control, predictability, and maximal technique options. These indications are as important in a primary case (if not more important) than in reoperations. If used initially, a reoperation is less likely.

Following the same logic, there is no reason why a doctor should start studying and using a technique other than the open one at the beginning of his career.

Further Reading

JB Tebbetts' works are fundamental to understand the origin, the principles, and the recent evolution of the open approach. The reader should read at least these three: Tebbetts JB. Open rhinoplasty: more than an incisional approach. In: Daniel RK, editor. Aesthetic plastic surgery: rhinoplasty. Boston: Little, Brown; 1993. p. 525–53; Tebbetts JB. Shaping and positioning the nasal tip without structural disruption: a new systematic approach. Plast Reconstr Surg. 1994;94:61–77; Tebbetts JB. Primary rhinoplasty. A new approach to the logic and techniques. St Louis: Mosby; 1998.

More information on the historical origins and systematic application of the open technique can also be found in the milestone volume by Slobodan J. Surgical atlas of external rhinoplasty. Edinburgh: Churchill Livingstone; 1995.

The article that describes the fourth (and final) step of the practical evolution of the open approach is: Gerbault O, Daniel RK, Kosins AK. The role of piezoelectric instrumentation in rhinoplasty. Aesth Surg J. 2015; 36(1):21–34.

9 Rhinoplasty Treatment Plan: Basic Principles

One of the fundamental steps in the preoperative activity prior to rhinoplasty is the creation of a detailed and personalized treatment plan. The ideal treatment plan must respect:

- The wishes expressed by the patient.
- The morphology of the patient's face and nose (initial conditions).
- Nasal function.
- The abilities of the surgeon himself, who must feel comfortable carrying out the procedure that he is doing for the good of his patient.

It is necessary to address the patient's questions and needs, the complexity of the deformities to be corrected, the technical difficulties of the surgery as well as the instruments at our disposal, the limits imposed by the anatomy, the recognition of the risks that must be minimized, the need not to extend excessively the surgical times, and the degree of collaboration that the patient can offer after surgery. All these points, without exception, must be respected in the treatment plan.

So, in defining the treatment plan the aspects to be taken into consideration are many, complex, and interrelated. Without forgetting that most of the details that make up the nasal deformities are difficult, if not impossible, to measure. This activity of the surgeon has been compared by many colleagues to the decisions and anticipations of a chess player during the course of a difficult game.

Preoperative time spent with the patient is never wasted and much of this time devoted to building the treatment plan has to do with reading images: direct reading of the face as well as the clinical facial portraits and the axial and coronal CT scan reconstructions. Face reading has something in common with reading books. Each of you will have experienced those moments when we would like to read but do not succeed, in which we persist in leafing through the pages of a book but it literally falls from our hands. Something similar can happen when you approach the profession of nasal surgery. The main solution is practicing, practicing, practicing and once again practicing.

In this chapter, we have attempted to differentiate by points some of the aspects that come into play in reading faces and drafting the treatment plan; most of these points are flexible, self-contradictory, even conflicting and not applicable to every patient. It is a difficult task which requires a mental exercise that cannot be framed in a fixed scheme or geometric rule. Also a computer simulation or a pencil drawing on the photographs cannot completely describe the objectives of a rhinoplasty treatment plan. Especially for the esthetic goals of rhinoplasty, it is necessary that the surgeon mentally visualize the form to be realized by answering some questions, most of them reported in this chapter.

This mental process was described by Jack Sheen like this: "*Visualization is a more difficult concept to capture but no less more important. It*

F. Meneghini, *Basic Open Rhinoplasty*, https://doi.org/10.1007/978-3-030-61827-8_9

is the process by which a mental image is formed, in the same way that our architect visualizes the remodelled building, anticipating the effects of structural changes before technically implementing them. In rhinoplasty, this process takes the form: "This is how the nose would look if…"".[1]

9.1 Think in Terms of Angles

The simplest example concerns the modification of the nasolabial angle. In clinical practice, there is no habit of measuring the nasolabial angle in degrees while it is almost inevitable to ask whether with surgery the angle should be kept stable or whether it should be opened or closed.

The study of the patient profile of Fig. 9.1 shows how a slight increase in the nasolabial angle would be favorable to the esthetics of the nose. It should also be noted that the flattening of the upper lip is a partial contraindication. A useful compromise to optimize the upward rotation of the tip without negatively affecting the esthetics of the lip is to move the rotation point forward leaving the posterior part of the curve between the profile of the nose and the lip unchanged, as simulated in Fig. 9.2.

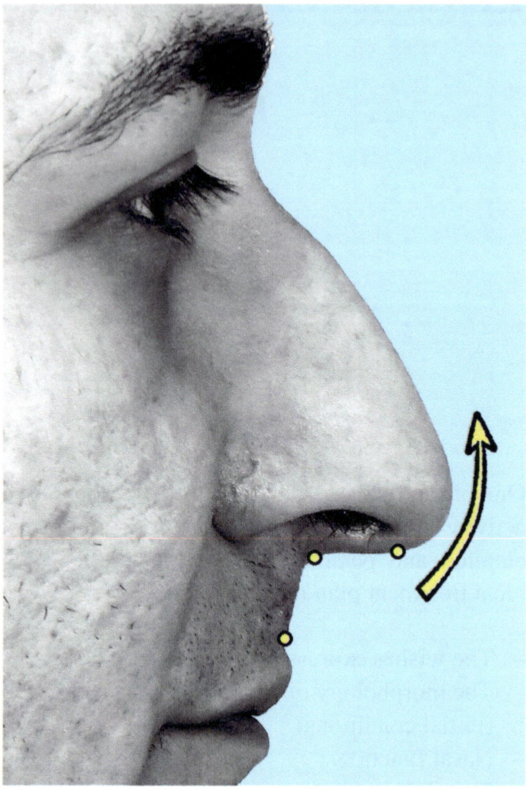

Fig. 9.1 Nasolabial angle. A slight increase in the nasolabial angle would improve the esthetics of the nose (curved arrow)

9.2 Think in Terms of Millimeters

The question the surgeon asks himself has to do with the linear dimensions of the nose such as width, height, and projection. In the nose, the linear unit of measurement is the millimeter since adding or removing a millimeter in some points of the nose outline or shape can change the esthetic judgment from beautiful to unacceptable.

Also in this case instrumental measurements are rarely used and instead the evaluations are expressed through direct clinical examination and the analysis of photographic images.

An example is the nasal tip width and the alar base in the basal projection of the nose. Figure 9.3a, b shows a case where both the alar base and the tip require a transverse narrowing and the two linear measurements visually confirm it.

9.3 Think in Terms of Vectors

When analyzing a photograph or a CT image of the nose, a very useful mental exercise is to identify a specific point and move it to a new position with a vector. The vector also helps to evaluate the need for reductive procedures with removal of bone or cartilage, or reconstructive ones with cartilage grafts, to obtain the desired result.

In cases of a position asymmetry of the nasal domes associated with their different projection, as in the case of Fig. 9.4, the surgical correction can be visualized by two vectors, each of which indicates the direction to improve the symmetry of the tip of the nose.

[1]Sheen JH, Sheen AP. Aesthetic Rhinoplasty. St. Louis, Missouri: Quality Medical Publishing, Inc.; 1998. p. 68.

9.4 Think in Terms of Volume (Volume Gain or Loss in One or More Specific Nasal Areas)

During the first visit with a new patient, it is sometimes helpful to ask this simple question: "*Do you want a smaller or larger nose?*".

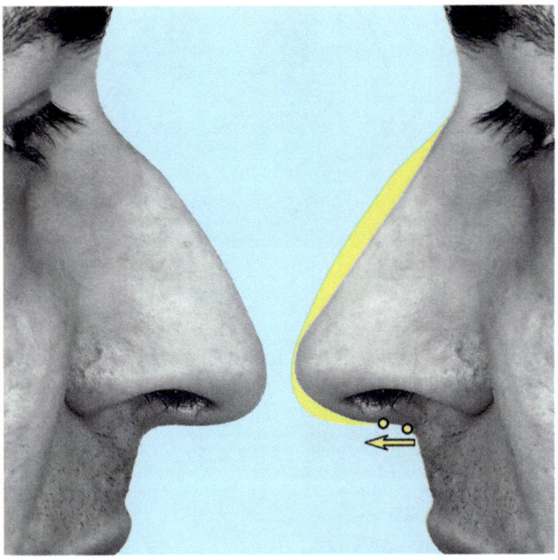

Fig. 9.2 Mirror simulation with increasing of the nasolabial angle. The posterior segment of the curve between the profile of the columella and the upper lip is left unchanged moving forward the rotation fulcrum (straight arrow)

Almost always the answer is "*I would like a smaller one!*". In reality, the volume change obtained with surgery, with the exception of special anatomical conditions, is now very small compared to the past, both for functional reasons and to maintain adequate support for the skin. This conservative approach should nonetheless aim to achieve a natural and proportionate nasal shape. One of the ways to predict the result is therefore to decide which areas of the nose will be reduced and which will be increased in volume.

Figure 9.5a, b is a simulation with only an increase in volume of the nasal tip region in a case of evident hypoprojection of the nasal tip; the yellow area shows the difference between the two oblique profiles of the patient (Fig. 9.5b). Although the simulated result shows an improvement, having acted only on a specific area of the nose fails to give a sense of balance and optimal proportion. Figure 9.6 compares the clinical result obtained in the same subject by combining a small reduction of the hump to the obviously needed reconstruction of the tip. As a general rule, a treatment plan that provides a combined increase and decrease of volumes in areas close to each other of the nose may represent the best solution in a good percentage of clinical cases.

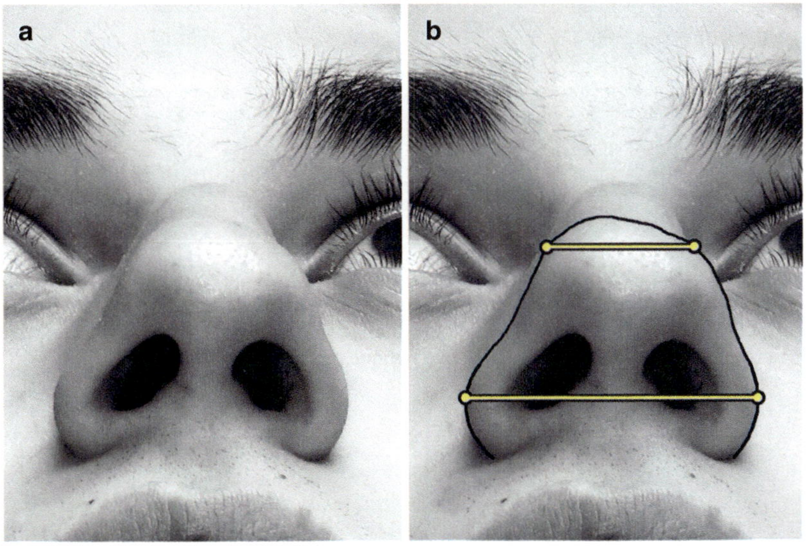

Fig. 9.3 (**a**, **b**) Nasal base view. The nasal tip as well as the alar base requires a transverse narrowing and the two linear measurements visually confirm it (**b**)

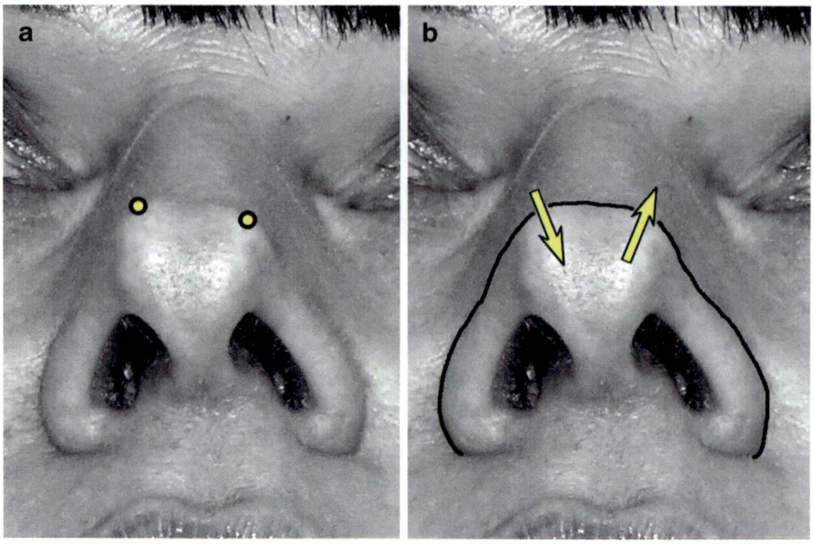

Fig. 9.4 (**a**, **b**) Nasal base view. The asymmetry of the nasal domes is clearly depicted by the two dots (**a**). The two vectors indicate the direction needed to obtain a symmetric nasal tip (**b**)

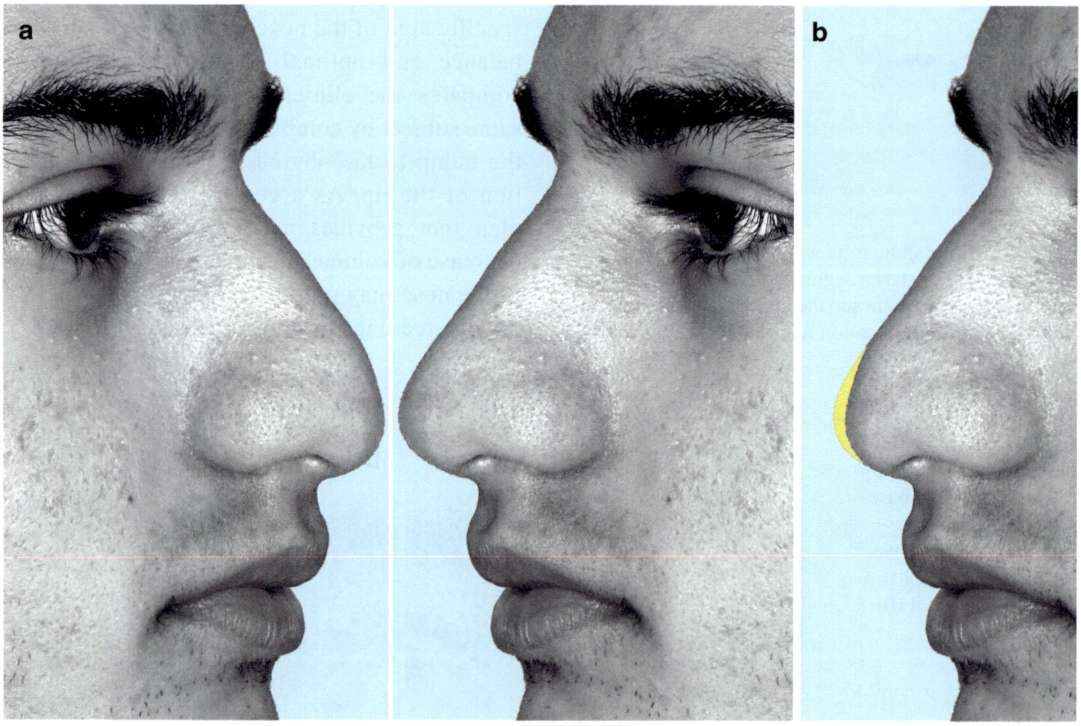

Fig. 9.5 (**a**, **b**) Right oblique view. Mirror simulation of a clinical case with under-projected nasal tip (**a**). The yellow area shows the difference between the two oblique profiles (**b**)

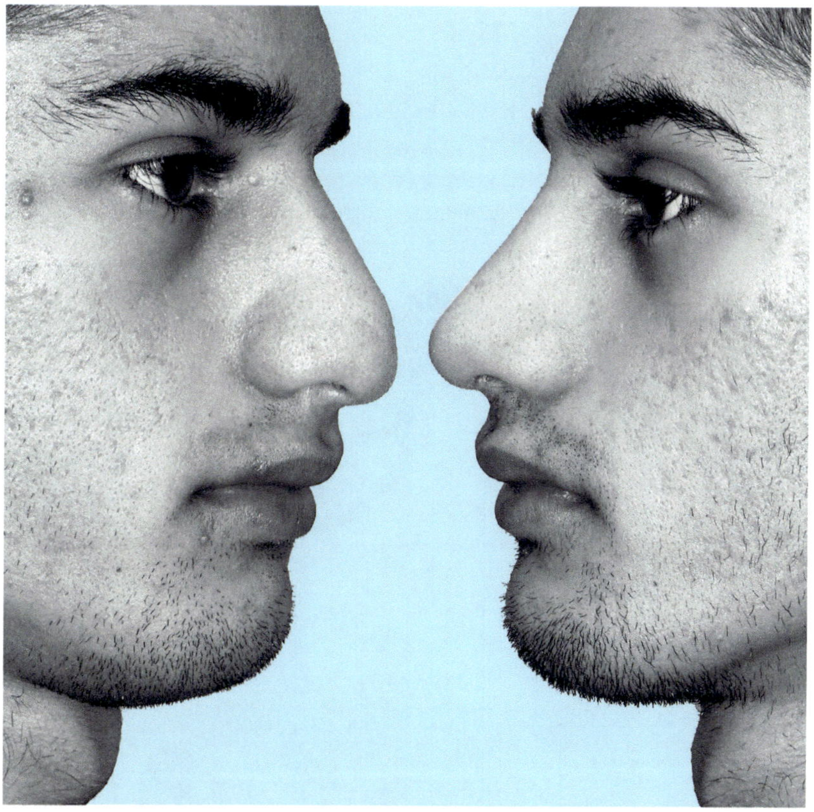

Fig. 9.6 Right oblique views of the same patient as Fig. 9.5a, b before and after surgery

9.5 Think in Terms of Shapes

Imagining a new shape is perhaps the most artistic approach to the rhinoplasty treatment plan. Modeling a new nose is easier starting from oblique projections and from the profile as it is a matter of creating a new outline; in Fig. 9.7 the new shape of the nose was traced with a black pen.

In any case, trying to describe the shape of the nose and the deformity to be corrected is also fundamental in the dialogue with the patient. Figure 9.8a shows a trilobate nasal tip in basal projection; the goal of surgery is to modify it and obtain a more triangular shape, as shown in Fig. 9.8b.

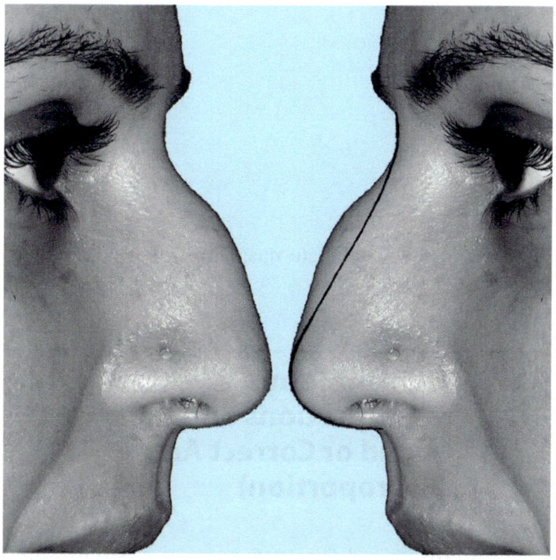

Fig. 9.7 Oblique right view. Mirror simulation traced with a black pen

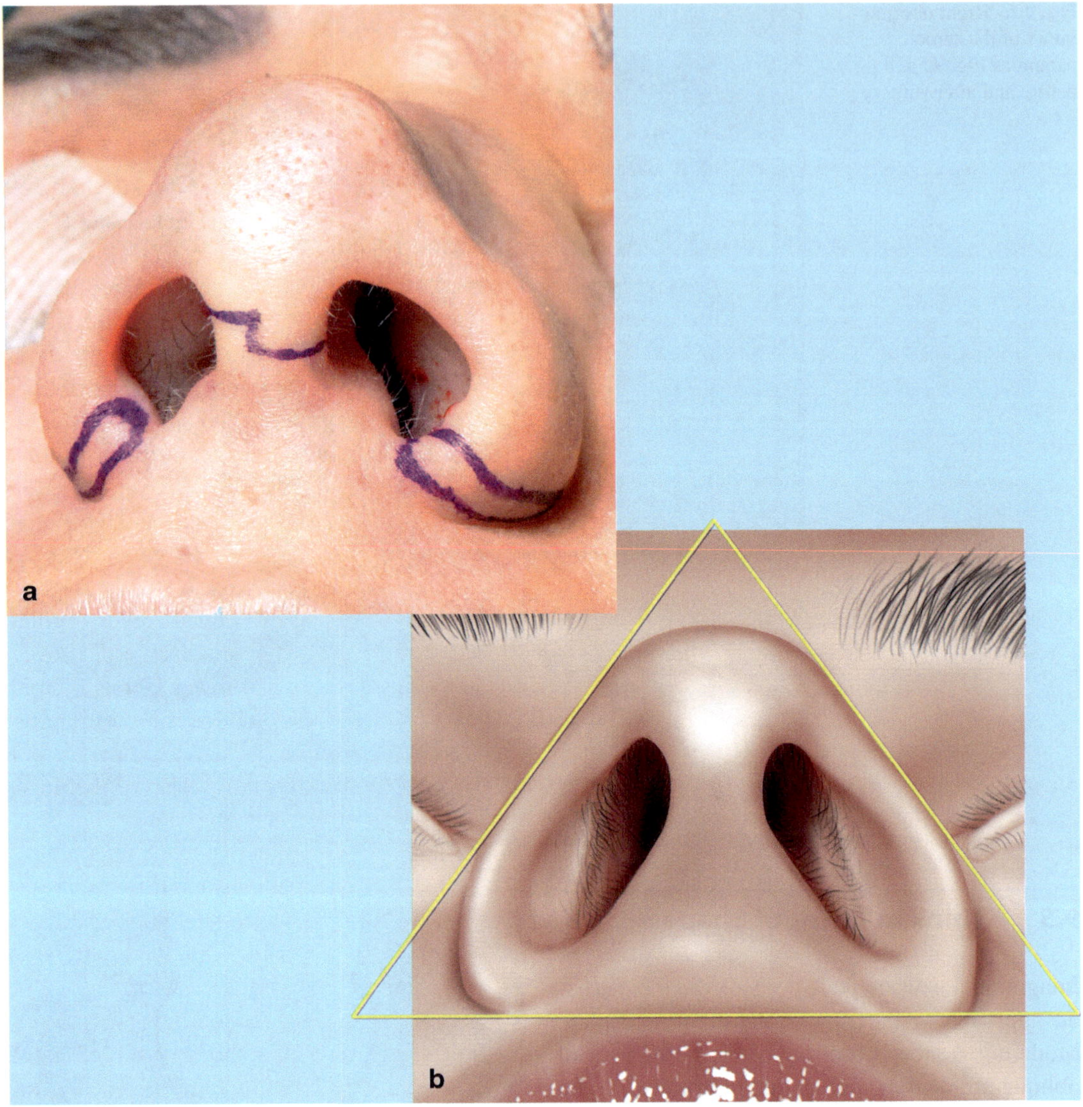

Fig. 9.8 (**a**, **b**) A trilobate nasal tip in basal projection (**a**). The surgical objective is to obtain a more triangular shape (**b**)

9.6 Think in Terms of Proportions and Balance (Avoid or Correct Any Disproportion)

Once again it is difficult to give a mathematical rule and even less a tool like a caliper, a compass, a ruler, or even a plastic template with which to determine the perfect nose.

When studying a face and nose clinically by looking at proportions, Jack Sheen suggests thinking about the balance of the various components:

> *A SENSE OF PROPORTION.*
> *... The word sense is used advisedly to distinguish it from the application of numerical proportions...*
> *But without calipers and indices, how can you assess? Think balance.*[2]

Again Jack Sheen on proportion:

[2]Sheen JH, Sheen AP: Aesthetic Rhinoplasty. St. Louis, Missouri: Quality Medical Publishing, Inc.; 1998. p. 114.

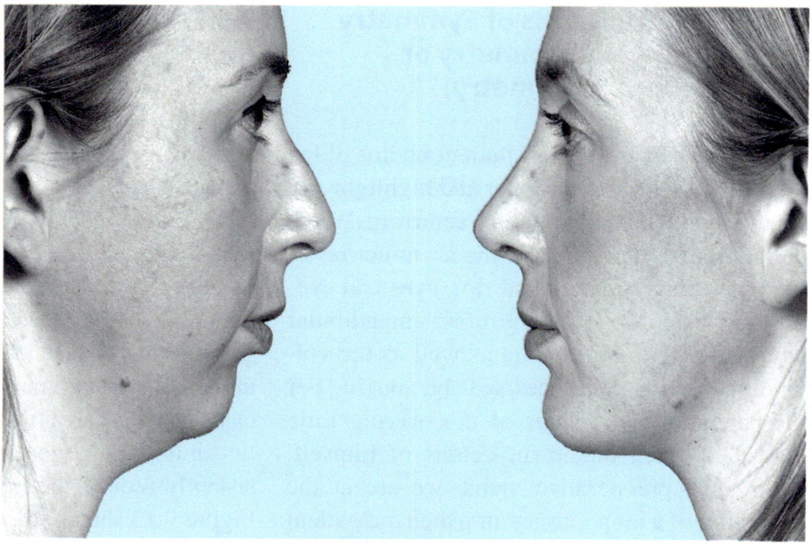

Fig. 9.9 Right profile views. Before and after multiple surgical procedures combined with orthodontic treatment

Proportion, not measuring millimeters, is what matters.[3]

Figure 9.9 shows an example of a treatment plan guided by thinking in terms of proportion and balance. The main steps of the treatment were as follows:

- Preoperative orthodontic treatment.
- One-stage surgery composed of four distinct procedures: sagittal mandibular ramus osteotomies with mandibular advancement, chin implant, submental liposuction, and open approach septorhinoplasty.
- Postoperative orthodontic treatment.

In this case, the orthodontic treatment and the four surgical steps have produced small local changes but the overall result is impressive.

9.7 Think in Terms of Disproportions (Maintain, Enhance, or Produce a Specific Disproportion)

Many attractive faces do not have perfect proportions and so, sometimes, we need to change our previous way of thinking and visualize a "particular" nose for a "particular" face.

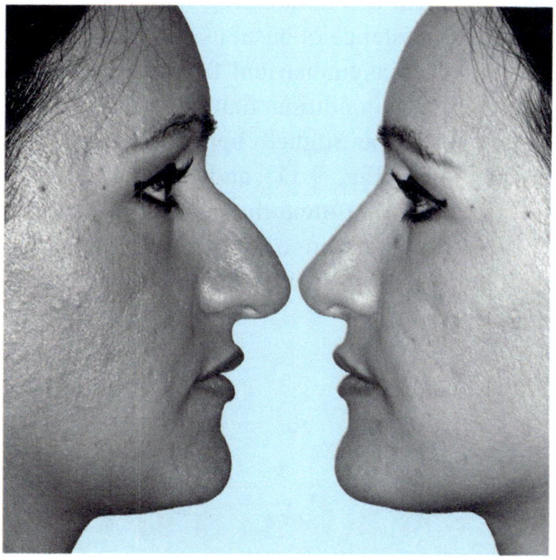

Fig. 9.10 Right profile views. Views before and after 8 months, in which the nose fits the face despite its shape and dimension being far from the ideal proportion for a feminine nose

Figure 9.10 shows the before and after right profile at 8 months of a young female patient with strong chin, broad forehead, and thick skin, in whom the nose fits the face despite its shape and dimensions being far from the ideal proportion for a so-called feminine nose.

[3]Sheen JH, Sheen AP. Aesthetic Rhinoplasty. St. Louis, Missouri: Quality Medical Publishing, Inc.; 1998. p. 126.

9.8 Think in Terms of Symmetry (Maintain Symmetry or Reduce Asymmetry)

When illustrating to a new patient photos of his face, it is essential to discover and highlight any small asymmetry. Through a centrifugal path on the frontal view portrait, the asymmetries of the nose (radix, dorsum and tip), eyes and eyelid grooves, lip commissures, mandibular angles and dental occlusion as well as the volume of the two hemifaces will be sought. For the patient it is a matter of discovering little known, or even unknown, details of himself. During the preoperative visits, we are at the beginning of a long journey in which the patient will gradually become more and more experienced, critical and demanding with his appearance. The existence of nasal asymmetries in the context of an asymmetrical face is a very frequent clinical condition that requires a treatment plan to be studied both on frontal and basal photos (Fig. 9.11) and on the CT scan (Fig. 9.12a, b). Often the results achievable with nasal surgery are only partial and must be thoroughly discussed with the patient.

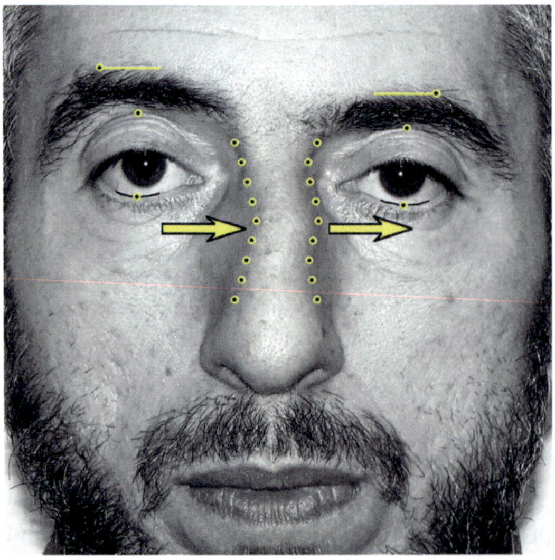

Fig. 9.11 Frontal view. Multiple facial asymmetries combined with nasal deviation to the left

9.9 Think in Terms of Surgical Feasibility and Realistic Goals

Perhaps the simplest and most direct phrase to define surgical feasibility is this: "*It's a matter of reconciling the ideal with the real.*", written by Jack Sheen.[4]

For surgical feasibility and realistic objectives in rhinoplasty we frequently need septal cartilage for grafting but, in a planned volume reduction, we may initially think that grafts are unnecessary and conclude that there are no surgical feasibility problems.

An infrequent goal of nasal surgery is to consistently reduce the projection of the nasal tip. Figure 9.13 shows some intraoperative steps:

- Interruption and removal of a segment of about 5 mm of the right medial crus and comparison with the original height still present in the left dome (Fig. 9.13a, b).
- Similar interruption and removal of a segment from the left medial crus.
- Symmetric reconstruction of the nasal tip with columellar strut and modified Sheen's shield tip graft sutured in place with 5/0 polydioxanone (Fig. 9.13c, d).

This is a volume and projection reductive procedure which requires the availability of septal cartilage to shape, reconstruct, and stabilize the alar cartilages in a new spatial position. It might seem strange that to reduce considerably the nasal tip projection we need to add cartilage fragments more than remove them.

9.10 Think in Terms of Surgical Preferences and Abilities

A surgeon can only have a relatively small number of surgical techniques at hand and a frequent mistake is to further simplify or adapt the surgical steps

[4]Sheen JH, Sheen AP. Aesthetic Rhinoplasty. St. Louis, Missouri: Quality Medical Publishing, Inc.; 1998. p. 124.

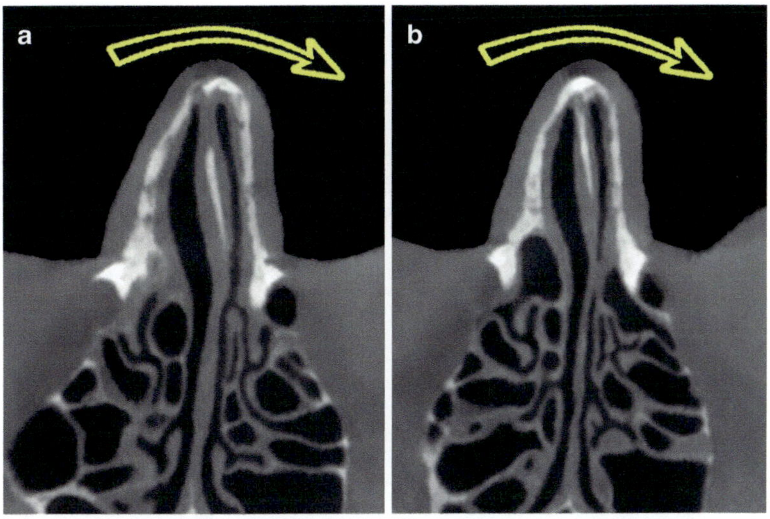

Fig. 9.12 (**a**, **b**) CBCT axial scans of the same patient as Fig. 9.11

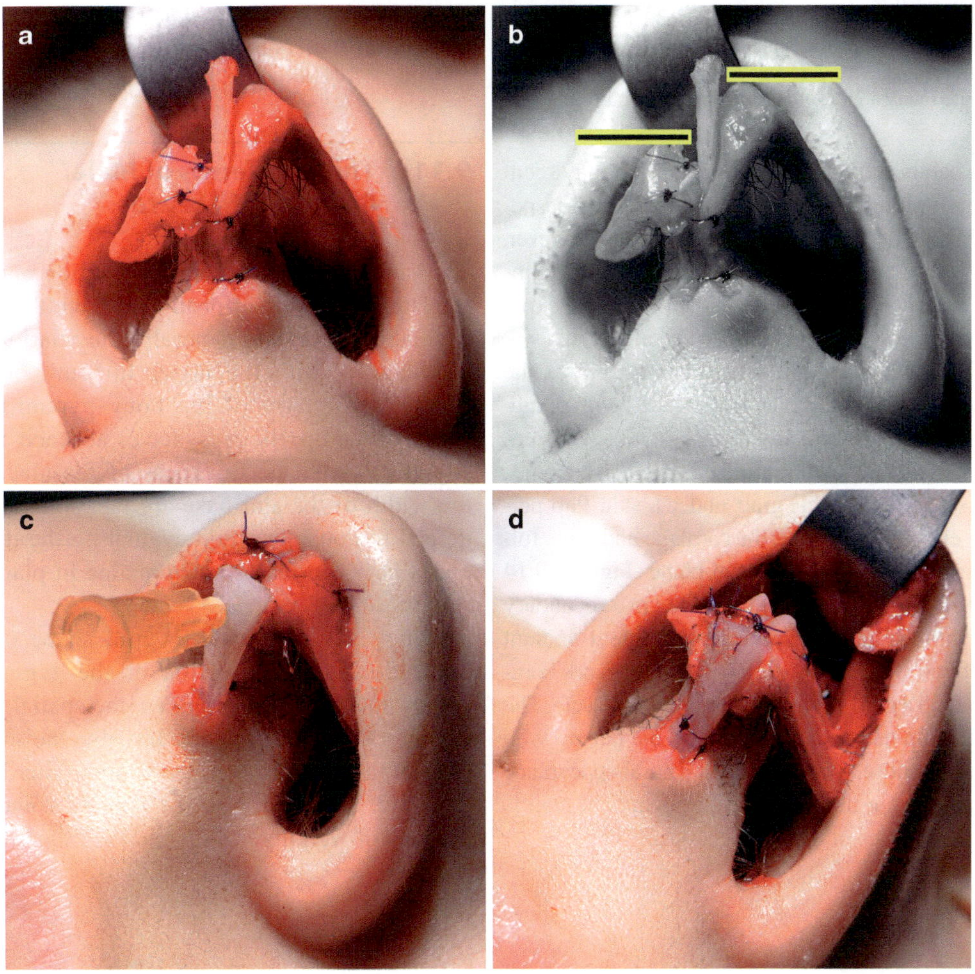

Fig. 9.13 (**a–d**) Intraoperative views of a procedure to reduce nasal tip projection. Interruption and removal of a segment of about 5 mm of the right medial crus and comparison with the original height still present in the left dome (**a**, **b**). Symmetrical reconstruction of the nasal tip with columellar strut and modified Sheen's shield tip graft sutured in place with 5/0 polydioxanone (**c**, **d**)

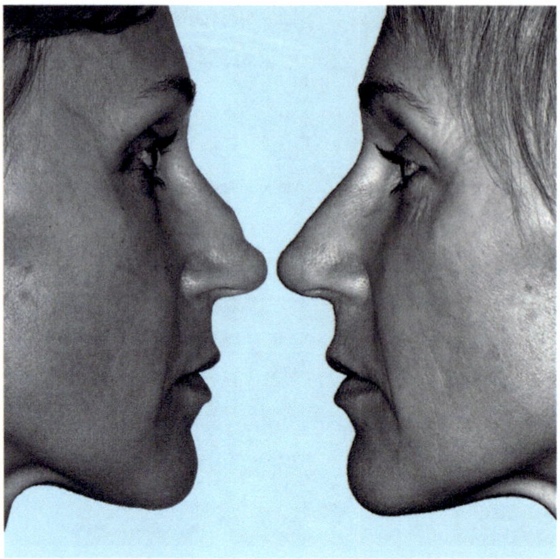

Fig. 9.14 Right profile views. Before and after images of a secondary case with evident deformities of the nasal dorsum treated with a reconstruction of the framework associated with a graft of autologous temporal fascia

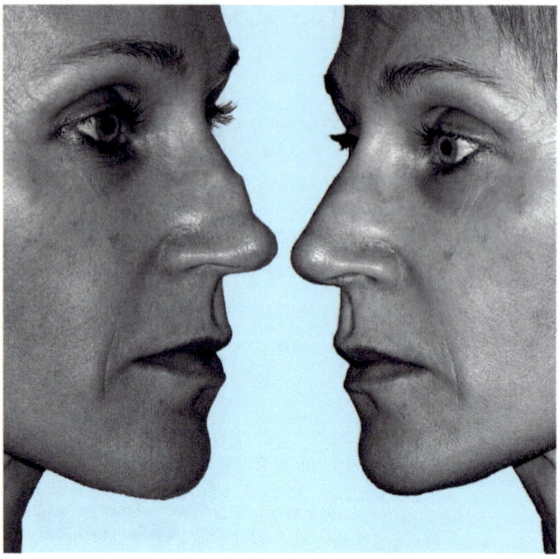

Fig. 9.15 Right oblique views. Before and after images of the same patient as Fig. 9.14

to his habits and laziness. This condition may seem to be a limiting factor for the treatment plan, especially when dealing with a complex case. However, there is also a logical solution to the surgeon's limits: it is sufficient to extend the team to a more experienced professional or one with specific skills.

There are few nasal surgeons who utilize the autologous temporal fascia but, in cases with particularly thin skin where any irregularity of the osteocartilaginous framework could be visible, it becomes necessary to insert this graft under a skin flap perfectly elevated just above the cartilage and bone following the deep areolar tissue plane. Figures 9.14 and 9.15 illustrate the result obtained in a secondary case with evident deformities of the nasal dorsum treated with a reconstruction of the framework combined with a graft of autologous temporal fascia. The small hump had been requested by the patient who wanted her nose to have the most natural appearance as possible, but this aspect of her treatment plan is dealt with in one of the next sections.

9.11 Think in Terms of Male/Female Differences

The nasal radix depth, the inclination and silhouette of the dorsal profile, the width of the nasolabial angle and generally the relationship of the nose with the upper lip outlines, the width of the base of the bony pyramid, the shape of the tip, the presence or absence of the supratip break, the thickness of the alae, and the width of the alar base are just some of the details to consider when evaluating the differences between males and females in planning rhinoplasty.

Other aspects are the overall shape of the face, the lateral projection of the zygomatic arches and mandibular angles, the spatial position and shape of the chin, but also the weight and height of the person, the width of the shoulders and, I believe, also the tone of voice and the way of walking.

9.12 Think in Terms of Simplicity/Complexity of the Treatment

Rhinoplasty rarely is a simple procedure.

The easiest and fastest way to increase the profile of the nasal dorsum is to insert a preformed alloplastic material, such as solid silicone or PTFE. This can be done through a small incision of the nasal mucosa and a limited soft tissue elevation along the midline of the nose, just above the cartilage and bone. This procedure takes minutes and not hours.

Unfortunately, this simple shortcut cannot be recommended due to the high rate of infection and extrusion of the implant through the skin or mucosa and, eventually, the need for an urgent implant removal. Afterwards the skin progressively scars and contracts producing a new and evident nasal deformity with a complete loss of the initial result.

Probably the best choice to increase the profile of the nasal dorsum is to engage in a more complex, difficult, demanding and time-consuming procedure that requires many surgical steps such as:

- Autologous cartilage harvesting (sometimes at an extranasal surgical site to obtain conchal or rib cartilage).
- Meticulous carving and beveling of the graft margins to adapt it to the desired result and lower the rate of visible irregularities.
- Careful soft tissue elevation avoiding asymmetries and excessive enlargement of the pocket for the dorsal graft.
- Insertion in place and stabilization of the graft with multiple small sutures.
- Acceptance, and sometimes later repair, of the frequent minor irregularities that may be evident after months or years postoperatively.

Rhinoplasty rarely is a simple procedure.

9.13 Think in Terms of Minimally Invasive Surgery

Different treatment plans mean different surgical approaches with different skin and mucosa incisions, different area of exposure of the nasal framework, different reduction and/or reconstruction of the nasal framework, and so on. This immense variability offers the surgeon the choice to select from many surgical solutions. Here are two examples:

- If the treatment plan includes a full rhinoplasty and septoplasty, a unique "long" skin incision giving access to all nasal structures is often preferable and considered safe and *less invasive* compared with multiple mucosa and skin incisions with small and fragile flaps interrupting or reducing the vasculature of the mucosal soft tissue envelope.
- If the planned hump reduction exceeds 2 mm at the keystone, a dorsal reconstruction with bilateral spreader grafts or spreader flaps becomes mandatory but spreader flaps should be considered a better choice in terms of minimally invasive surgery, because it is a *more conservative* approach with the triangular cartilages themselves as well as for the reduced amount of harvested septal cartilage.

In rhinoplasty, the concept of "minimally invasive surgery" does not exist in the light of the intrinsic complexity of this surgery and so this simple and reductive little phrase, perfect for the marketing man, is considered inacceptable for a surgeon. Probably we should talk of "highly conservative surgery" and therefore this section should be titled: "Think in Terms of Highly Conservative Surgery".

9.14 Think in Terms of the Patient's Wishes

The reason that leads the person to contact the surgeon is central to the decision whether or not to perform the surgery; if the surgeon deems it futile, useless, unfeasible, or inappropriate, it is better to stop and refuse to proceed.

If the requests are realistic and detailed, at every preoperative meeting, the list of priorities expressed by the patient should be discussed, updated and entered in the treatment plan.

As early as the first visit, the list must be completed with the words used by the patient himself, and the surgeon must resist translating this simple fundamental message into medical language.

9.15 Think in Terms of the Patient's Convenience

If the previous point focused on the patient's main requests, here we concentrate on capturing those aspects that the patient does not feel important or perhaps even ignores, but that the surgeon points out and aims to include among the objectives of the treatment.

Adjusting the treatment plan by including small additional procedures is a matter of completeness and finishing. Here are some examples:

- Reduce the width of the columella base with multiple readsorbable monofilament sutures.
- Reduce the volume of one or both anterior thirds of hypertrophic inferior turbinates.
- Put a small sheet of fine morselized cartilage into the radix area to soften a hollow radix.
- Cover the dorsal framework with autologous temporal fascia in the case of thin skin.

It is a matter of completeness.

9.16 Think in Terms of the Patient's Psychological Status

The surgeon's idea of interpreting and changing the shape of a nose based on the patient's personality may seem overwhelming and pretentious.

Generally speaking, the deformed nose should be made more natural, regular and less present in the person's face to bring out the person's mimicry that expresses the feelings of joy, happiness, coldness, contrast, anger, pain, tiredness, and attention. However, a "neutral" perfect nose, a straight nose, neither large nor small, neither tall nor short, is not always desirable.

To further complicate the planning, there is a possible psychological instability of the patient that makes it difficult to identify a shared and stable morphological objective. A possible solution to this problem is to postpone the date of the surgery and give the patient a basic set of photographic printed portraits asking her to work with a pencil.

Any extra time spent preparing for the surgery is always useful to answer the question: Should I or shouldn't I go to the operating room?

9.17 Think in Terms of Long-Term Results and Structural Support

An exaggerated reduction of the nose support structures with generous removal of bone and cartilage, disregard of surgical dissection planes, failure to stabilize the nasal structures with slow reabsorbing sutures, failure to use autologous structural support grafts to the nasal frameworks are all aspects of the same problem: a lack of attention to the long-term stability of the result.

However, there is another point not to be overlooked. A small and thin nose, pleasant in the face of a young girl, might risk appearing ridiculous and inappropriate when the same person is 60 years old, has a greater body weight and the soft tissues of the nasal back will have slowly reduced in thickness and atrophied as a result of the inevitable aging processes.

9.18 Think in Terms of Functional or Esthetic Outcome

Sometimes, after a frank discussion on the treatment objectives, the patient still stubbornly demands to pursue his or her single goal. More rarely, the request is exaggerated and incomprehensible. One example of this patient category is the young tall boy, a sportsman who every day goes the gym or rides miles by bike to keep fit but wants to persuade the surgeon that a small feminine nose with an elegant low dorsum and a narrow tip is perfect for him.

The fundamental priorities of a rhinoplasty treatment plan are both functional and esthetic and any extreme requests must be rejected firmly by the surgeon.

9.19 Think in Terms of Avoiding Surgical Stigmata (Natural, Not-Operated on Look)

A good method for communicating the goals of rhinoplasty to the patient is based not only on the simulation of the desired result but also on the description of the postoperative deformities to be avoided. In the author's personal experience, it has proved useful to draw on the photo of the patient's real profile, in addition to the planned outline, also a deliberately exaggerated correction in order to explain the limits within which a natural appearance result is obtained.

Even adding to the treatment plan a procedure with low impact on the final overall result but having a great chance of visible postoperative problems should be considered carefully. An example of this is smoothing of a deep nasal radix by inserting a solid graft. Sometimes it is a very interesting step of the surgery that can help to realize a balanced nose with a straight dorsum avoiding too aggressive an approach to an osteocartilaginous hump; unfortunately, it is at a high risk of visible postoperative irregularities in the radix area.

9.20 Think in Terms of Small Incremental Adjustment

Most frequently this principle should be reserved for secondary nasal surgery, as in the case of small skin depressions to be filled with cartilage onlay grafts. However, even in primary rhinoplasty this approach can be useful to carry out some apparently difficult treatment plans.

Figure 9.16 shows the pre- and postoperative profile view of a primary rhinoplasty clinical case characterized by a masculine nasal shape, profile deformities, and very thick skin. A small volume increment was done with "autologous cartilage gel" at the end of the procedure when almost all skin stitches were in place. The soft graft, less than 1 cc in volume, was inserted with a syringe both over the domes and the cartilaginous dorsum (small dots) through a small opening of the right marginal incision. As a final touch, before nasal taping and splinting, the graft was molded under the skin with delicate pressure of the fingers.

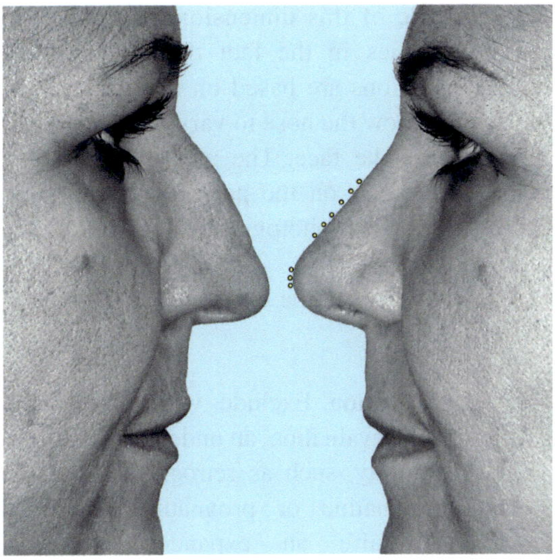

Fig. 9.16 Right profile views. Before and after images of a primary rhinoplasty case. A small volume increment was done with "autologous cartilage gel." The soft graft, less than 1 cc in volume, was inserted both over the domes and over the cartilaginous dorsum (small dots)

9.21 Think in Terms of Geometry

The author does not use, in his clinical practice, a standard approach for drawing a new nasal outline on a patient's preoperative profile view photograph. However, having a standardized method is useful for several purposes such as teaching, research and, most important, for self-training.

In 1993, H. Steve Byrd and P. Craig Hobar published a useful nasal analysis method for planning rhinoplasty.[5] The main purpose was to determine the esthetically proportioned nasal length, tip projection, and radix projection. The

[5]Byrd HS, Hobar PC. Rhinoplasty: a practical guide for surgical planning. Plast Reconstr Surg. 1993; 91:642–654.

Byrd HS, Burt JD. Dimensional approach to rhinoplasty: perfecting the esthetic balance between the nose and chin. In: Gunter JP, Rohrich RJ, Adams WP (eds) Dallas rhinoplasty. Nasal Surgery by the Masters. St. Louis: Quality Medical Publishing; 2002.

characteristic of this dimensional approach to rhinoplasty lies in the fact that the planned nasal dimensions are based on facial measurements that allow the nose to vary in size proportionally with the face. The measurements can be made directly on the patient or, better, by utilizing life-size photographs in frontal and profile views.

The main steps of the Byrd and Hobar method are as follows:

- Check occlusion. Exclude, with the intraoral and general evaluation, an underlying dentofacial deformity, such as retrognathic maxilla and retrognathic or prognathic mandible, which require an expanded analytical approach.
- Identify the soft tissue glabella (Gs), the alar base plane (ABP), the soft tissue menton (Mes), the stomion (S), the alar crease junction (ACJ), the corneal plane (CP), the superior palpebral fold (SPF), the R point, and the T point. Figure 9.17 illustrates all these anatomical and constructed landmarks.
- Measure the midfacial height (MFH) and the lower facial height (LFH). The first is the linear distance from the Gs to the ABP, the second is the linear distance from the ABP to the MEs (see Fig. 9.17b). In a vertical balanced face, the LFH should be equal to or 3 mm greater than the MFH.
- Measure the chin vertical (SMes). This is the distance from the stomion (S) to the soft tissue menton (Mes) (Fig. 9.17b).
- Measure the actual nasal length (RT) (Fig. 9.17b).
- Calculate and draw the ideal nasal length (RTi) utilizing two different procedures: RTi = 0.67 × MFH or RTi = SMes.
- Choose between these two measurements the one that is closest to the actual nasal length (RT).
- Measure the actual tip projection (ACJ–T) (Fig. 9.17c).
- Calculate the ideal tip projection, deriving it from the ideal nasal length: ideal tip projection = RTi × 0.67.
- Measure the actual radix projection, the distance from the corneal plane to the radix plane (CP–RP) (Fig. 9.17c).
- Calculate the ideal radix projection, deriving it from the ideal nasal length: ideal radix projection = RTi × 0.28. The range is from 9 to 14 mm.
- The ideal radix projection, the ideal tip projection, and the ideal nasal length are used to draw the ideal R point and the ideal T point on the profile view. In this way it is possible to envision the "boundaries" of the ideal nose.
- Plan, in agreement with the patient, the desired dorsal profile. As reported by the authors, variation may include a slight dorsal convexity, a straight dorsum between the radix and the tip, and a straight dorsum reduced to a level of 1–2 mm below the tip, creating a retroussé nose with a supratip break.

In the same papers the authors presented a further step dedicated to the assessment of chin projection.

9.22 Think in Terms of Other Specialties

In some complex clinical cases, being able to make a treatment plan can be difficult and even more difficult is being able to complete the planned surgery in all its details. In these cases, the best option is to surround yourself with experts. Sharing doubts, solutions and part of the work together with colleagues from other specialties can enrich both you and them. I have tested this precious piece of advice many times and have found that it works exceptionally well. Avoid professional loneliness!

9.23 Think in Terms of Revision Rate

Statistical factors sooner or later must enter into the compilation of the treatment plan. The three most common reasons for patient dissatisfaction following rhinoplasty are:

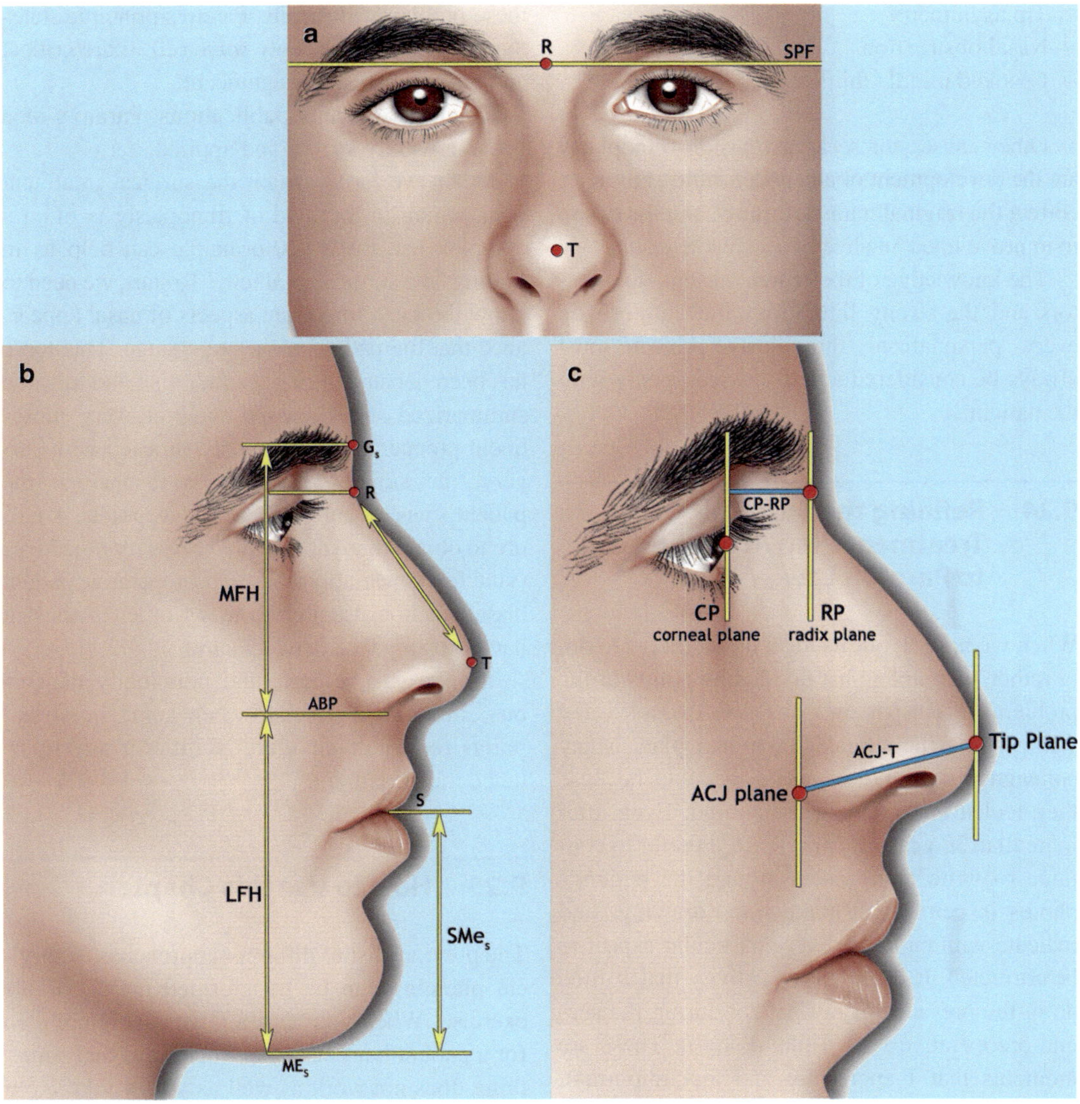

Fig. 9.17 (**a–c**) The landmarks utilized in the Byrd and Hobar method on frontal (**a**) and profile views (**b**, **c**). *Gs* soft tissue glabella, the clinically palpable and usually visible anatomic midline point in the lower forehead; this is the most prominent point on the curve of the frontal bone before the nasal-frontal junction. *ABP* alar base plane, is a plane running through the alar base and utilized as a division between the midface and the lower face. *S* stomion, is the midline point at the junction of the upper and lower lip vermillion. *Mes* soft tissue menton, is the most inferior midline point on the inferior border of the chin. *ACJ* alar crease junction, is the most posterior point of the curved line formed by the alar crease as seen in profile view; it is utilized as a landmark for measuring tip projection. *CP* corneal plane, is a coronal plane tangential to the surface of the cornea in profile view; it is utilized as a landmark for measuring the radix projection. *SPF* superior palpebral fold, is the vertical reference landmark utilized to identify the R point in the midline of the nasal dorsum (the R point is constructed and may differ with the existing radix break-point). The T point is the midline point on the nasal tip taken at the level of the dome projecting points of the lower lateral cartilages

- Tip asymmetry
- Nasal obstruction
- Crooked middle third

Other causes for seeking revision rhinoplasty are the development of a new deformity, failure to correct the original main deformity, and the desire to improve upon an already acceptable result.

The knowledge of these general statistical factors and the strong limitations they impose on every personalized rhinoplasty project must always be considered and discussed openly with the patient.

9.24 Refining the Surgical Treatment Plan According to Pareto's Law

When we have in our hands a list of things to do, or rather, a complete list divided by points of the problems of our patient's nose, we can relax and start writing the surgical treatment plan. Many colleagues do not even write the plan because they feel it is written in their mind. Even after more than 30 years of experience, I prefer to continue to write many notes around the patient's photos in pen. I still make some drawings and indicate with an arrow every particular aspect to be corrected. It is a creative activity that I often do in the presence of my patient during the second preoperative visit. I like doing it. These are moments that I appreciate and feel important. There is, however, something better to be done if we look back at our list of things to do following the 80/20 Pareto's principle.

In 1897, the Italian economist Vilfredo Pareto noticed a regular pattern in the distribution of wealth or income, no matter the country or time period examined. The pattern was so reliable that Pareto was eventually able to predict the distribution of income accurately before looking at the data. In 1941, Joseph Moses Juran, an engineer and management consultant began to apply the Pareto principle to quality issues. This is also known as the "Rule of the Vital Few." Juran separated the "vital few" from the "trivial many" showing how quality problems could be largely eliminated cheaply and quickly, by focusing on the vital few causes of these problems. Basically, Pareto's principle states that in any situation, only *some* (20%) are critical and *many* (80%) are insignificant.

Thanks to Juran's publications, Pareto's idea became widely known and applied.

When we have written the surgical treatment plan, which in the field of rhinoplasty is often a complex list, the 80/20 principle can help us in finding "the surgical vital few." To start, we need to know the most important aspects of nasal appearance that the patient wishes to change. This topic has been debated during the first visit and must be summarized and discussed again at every subsequent preoperative meeting. To proceed with surgery, the surgeon must agree to include the patient's wishes among the vital few points. A failure to obtain these absolutely necessary objectives (vital few) invariably leads to postoperative patient dissatisfaction despite the many other goals that have been reached (trivial many).

Similarly, a reverse, and potentially dangerous, situation can occur when some important points for the surgeon are of little or no importance for the patient.

9.25 How to Use this Chapter

The previous list of different approaches to surgical planning can be transformed into a simple exercise. When you have a written surgical plan for a patient but your inner voice says that something does not work as well as you would like it to, read this chapter again. You will be surprised at the productivity of rethinking a treatment plan.

Further Reading

For every surgeon who is approaching the analysis and planning of rhinoplasty cases, I recommend the fundamental articles written by Dr. Guyuron: Guyuron B. Precision rhinoplasty. Part I: the role of life-size photographs and soft-tissue cephalometric analysis. Plast Reconstr Surg. 1988;81:489–99; Guyuron B. Precision rhinoplasty. Part II: prediction. Plast Reconstr Surg. 1988;81:500–5; Guyuron B. Dynamics of rhinoplasty. Plast Reconstr Surg. 1991;88:970–8.

By the same author: Guyuron B. Patient assessment for rhinoplasty. In: Guyuron B, editor. Rhinoplasty. Edinburgh: Elsevier Saunders; 2002.

Individual Treatment Plan for Rhinoplasty

10

An individual treatment plan for rhinoplasty consists of two elements:

- A detailed written list of objectives to be achieved.
- A standard series of photographic images printed on paper where, with a pen or pencil, the nasal deformities are identified. Also one or more simulations of the profile must be realized and printed on paper.

The completion of the treatment plan is carried out in front of the patient during the second preoperative visit. The patient takes an active part with clarifying questions, advice, considerations, and personal requests.

In particular, the list of objectives must be written by hand in the form of a series of numbered points around the printed frontal projection photo of the patient. In this way, even taking back the document after some time, there can be no doubt that this list of objectives relates to that patient and to no one else.

The required materials for carrying out the treatment plan are the following:

- A computer with Photoshop application installed, for processing digital images of the patient's face acquired during the first visit, and an application for displaying and processing paranasal sinuses CT images stored in DICOM format.
- A complete series of preoperative patient photographs in the following projections: frontal, right and left oblique, right and left profile, basal face-up, face-down, frontal and right profile during smiling. The pictures must be printed on sheets of A4 paper with the patient's full name at the top, one sheet for each projection.
- One or more simulations of the facial profile processed with Photoshop and printed on sheets of A4 paper with the patient's full name at the top. The mirror version and the addition/subtraction version must be printed in separate sheets to maintain large-scale dimension.
- CT images of paranasal sinuses.

10.1 Images Selection and Preparation

During the first visit with a new patient, face portraits are taken in the standard projections. For every projection, two or three shots should be done. This material must be processed and printed in preparation for the second visit. For each projection the best image must be selected for brightness, focus, and position of the subject. If possible, also the images with blinking eyes or eyes not looking ahead should be discarded. Utilizing Photoshop, the chosen images must therefore be centered, framed, adjusted for size and resolution and improved for brightness and contrast.

F. Meneghini, *Basic Open Rhinoplasty*, https://doi.org/10.1007/978-3-030-61827-8_10

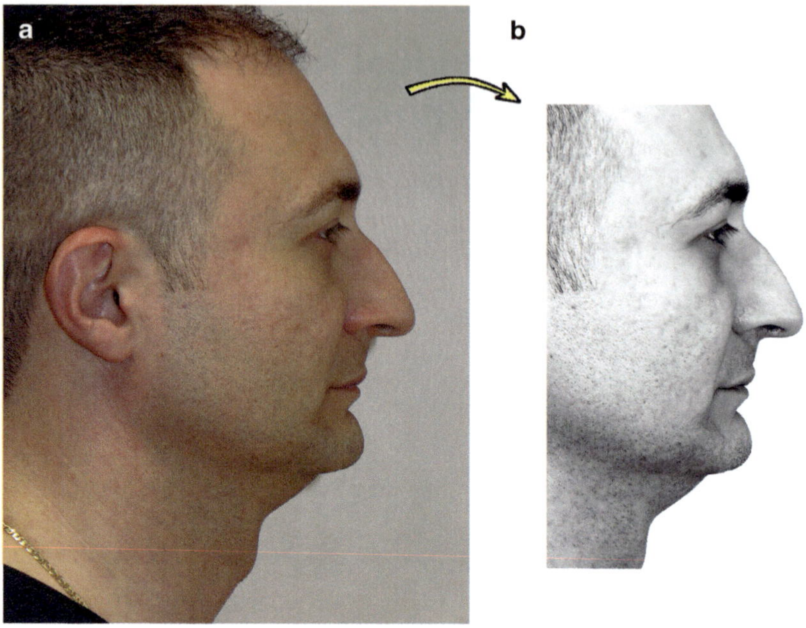

Fig. 10.1 (a, b) Right profile view. Original (a) and processed image (b). The irregular background, too dark below the nasal angle and the neck, has been replaced by a uniform white increasing the legibility of the facial and nasal profile details

Figure 10.1a illustrates an original image taken with a small portable camera during the first visit without an adequate background and with the only illumination of the camera flash. The patient's head tilt and his forward gaze are correct. Also the orientation and distance of the camera with respect to the subject is ideal as described in Chaps. 3 and 4. With Photoshop the irregular background, too dark below the nasal angle and the neck, has been replaced by a uniform white increasing the legibility of the facial and nasal profile details. The subject was then transformed into black and white and the contrast and brightness were increased. Finally, the subject was framed removing all the excess areas (Fig. 10.1b).

10.2 Realize One or More Simulation of the Nasal Profile

Always in preparation for the second visit, it is necessary to carry out a simulation of the new nasal profile starting from the right profile image. The starting image, to which the background has been removed for better readability, must be modified using the "Liquify" filter of Photoshop. The purpose is to help the patient understand what could be a natural result and without deformity. Probably a test with small changes, without great variations in the overall size of the nose, is the best approach.

A simulation with an "ideal or perfect" profile could be mistakenly judged by the patient as an easy to obtain result or constitute a convincing factor in an individual who is still in doubt whether or not to undergo surgery. For this reason it must always be specified that the simulation does not represent a promise of achieving the result but a help to the patient to understand the desirable changes to the nasal shape.

For each simulation, two versions must be created and printed:

– The "Overlap" simulation. In this image the modifications of the nasal profile point by point are clear. This version of the simulation may not be pleasant for the patient due to its abstract or artificial appearance. For the surgeon, on the other hand, this version is very important because it represents a precise guide, perhaps irreplaceable, to some surgical maneuvers.

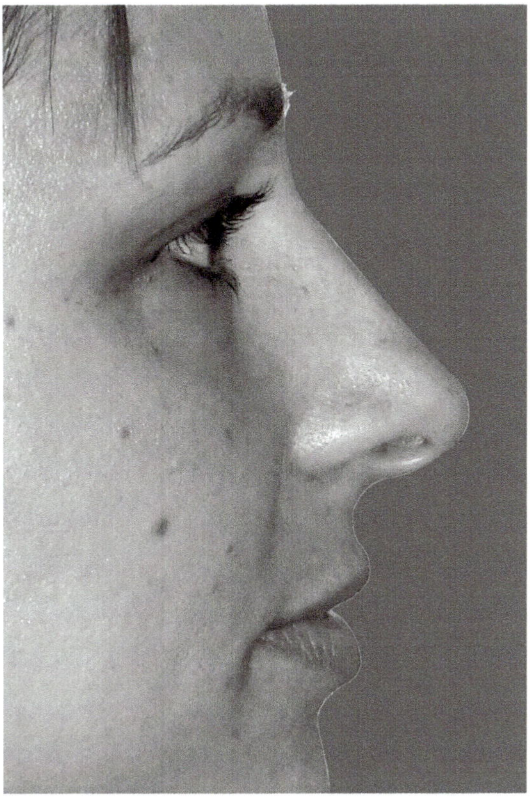

Fig. 10.2 Right profile view. "Overlap" simulation in case of a planned dimensional reduction of the nose

Figure 10.2 illustrates an example of overlap between the patient profile and the simulation. It was created with Photoshop selecting the background of the real profile with the "magic wand" tool (Fig. 10.3a) and painting it with a fairly dark and uniform gray (Fig. 10.3b). This background (Fig. 10.3c) was then selected and superimposed on the white background of the profile simulation (Fig. 10.3d) realizing the variation of silhouette. In this specific case, as often happens, the simulation involved surgery of nasal reduction only. With some variations in using the same Photoshop tools, it is also possible to highlight the incremental areas, as in reconstructive rhinoplasty.

- The "Mirror" simulation. Figure 10.4 illustrates the previous simulation rotated horizontally and placed in front of the original image. The patient often prefers this version, as it is perceived as simpler to read and realistic.

10.3 Realize a Printable File Containing the Standard Set of Photography for Rhinoplasty and Profile Simulations

The images of the face and the two versions of the simulation, one for each page, must be inserted in a Word template that will present the patient's data in the header and, in the footer this writing:

> Facial photographs help the surgeon to inform the patient about the objectives of the surgery. The photographic simulations serve the same informative purpose but do not ensure in any way that the result obtainable with the surgery will correspond to them.

During setting the layout of the document, it is essential to leave a large white space around the images. At the second visit, this white space will allow the surgeon to write the points of the treatment plan, the requests, of the patient, any possible considerations and to draw sketches or diagrams related to the treatment plan.

If the CT scan images of the paranasal sinuses have already been acquired, it is advisable to insert some of these in axial or coronal projection in order to have, in a single document, all the useful pre-operative iconographic material.

Once the layout is finished, the file is saved in PDF format and printed on standard A4 paper. Figure 10.5a–l shows the final document of a clinical case ready for printing.

This work of the surgeon on photographs done in the physical absence of the patient is clearly an important time spent with the patient. Preparing the images and elaborating a new profile represents a further and important process of knowledge of the clinical case and cannot be delegated to a close collaborator or to a professional photographer. To get the most value from this preoperative step it is advisable to be alone, not to have other commitments or appointments neither to be disturbed by phone calls or messages. Obviously, we should not do work in a hurry. It is a meditative moment in which we apply some of the basic principles listed in Chap. 9.

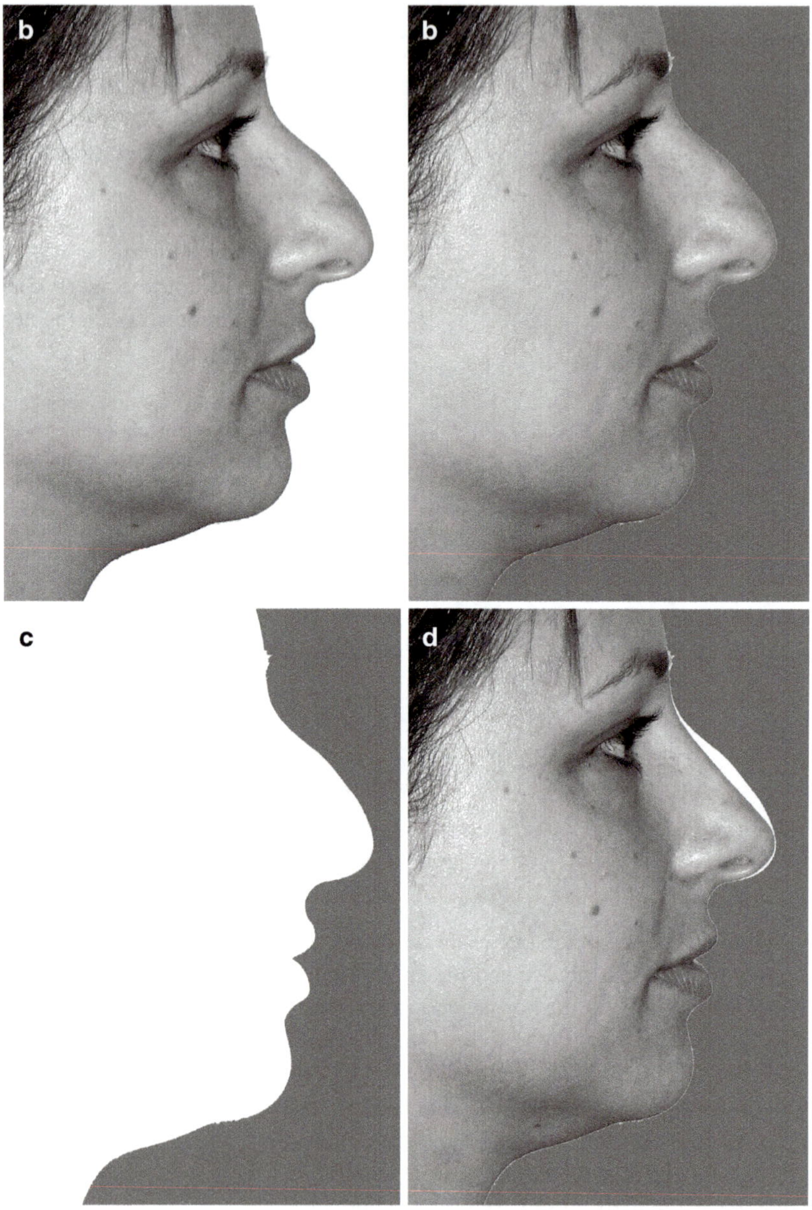

Fig. 10.3 (**a–d**) Main steps of the "Overlap" simulation process

It is not appropriate to think at this preparatory phase as at the time to take all the surgical decisions that will make up the final treatment plan. In a correct relationship with our patient, it is better to postpone this moment, the moment of conclusions, to the second visit. Getting help from the patient, in the form of a joint dialogue, is an essential aspect of the first meeting and became a mandatory one during the second. Any decisions, written in the form of a series of points, must be debated and shared. They should not be confused with the initial clinical photographic analysis and its expected surgical findings, carried out by the surgeon even if, statistically, they are often very similar.

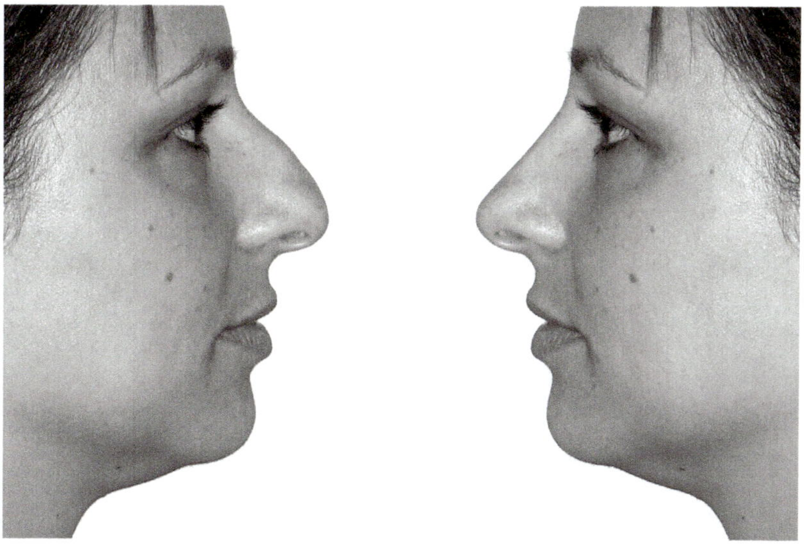

Fig. 10.4 The "Mirror" simulation

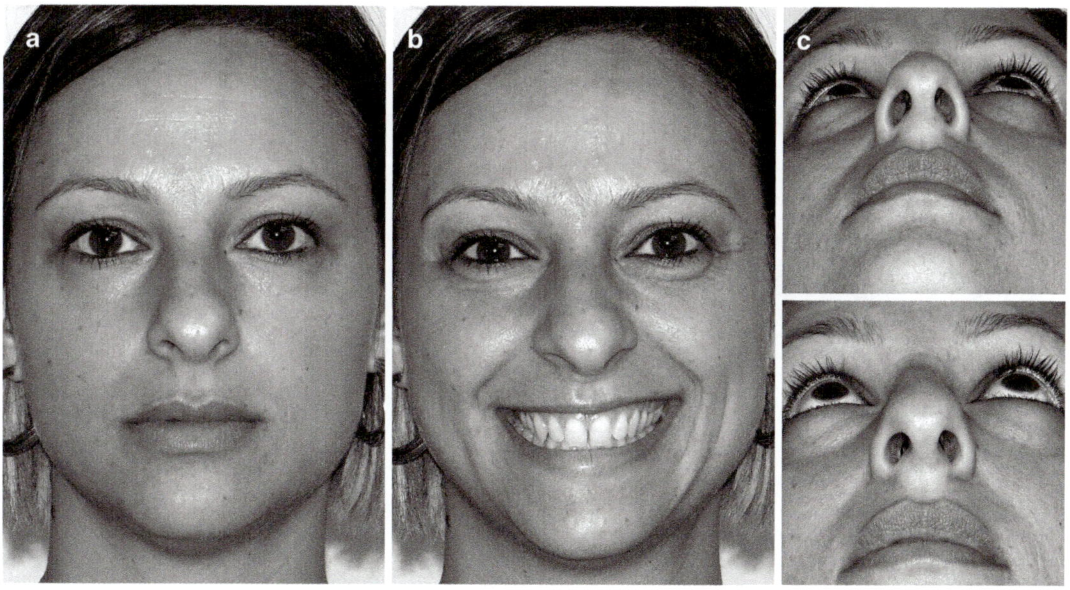

Fig. 10.5 (**a–l**) A complete set of processed images ready for the second preoperative visits: clinical portraits (**a–i**), profile simulation (**j**, **k**) and CT scan (**l**)

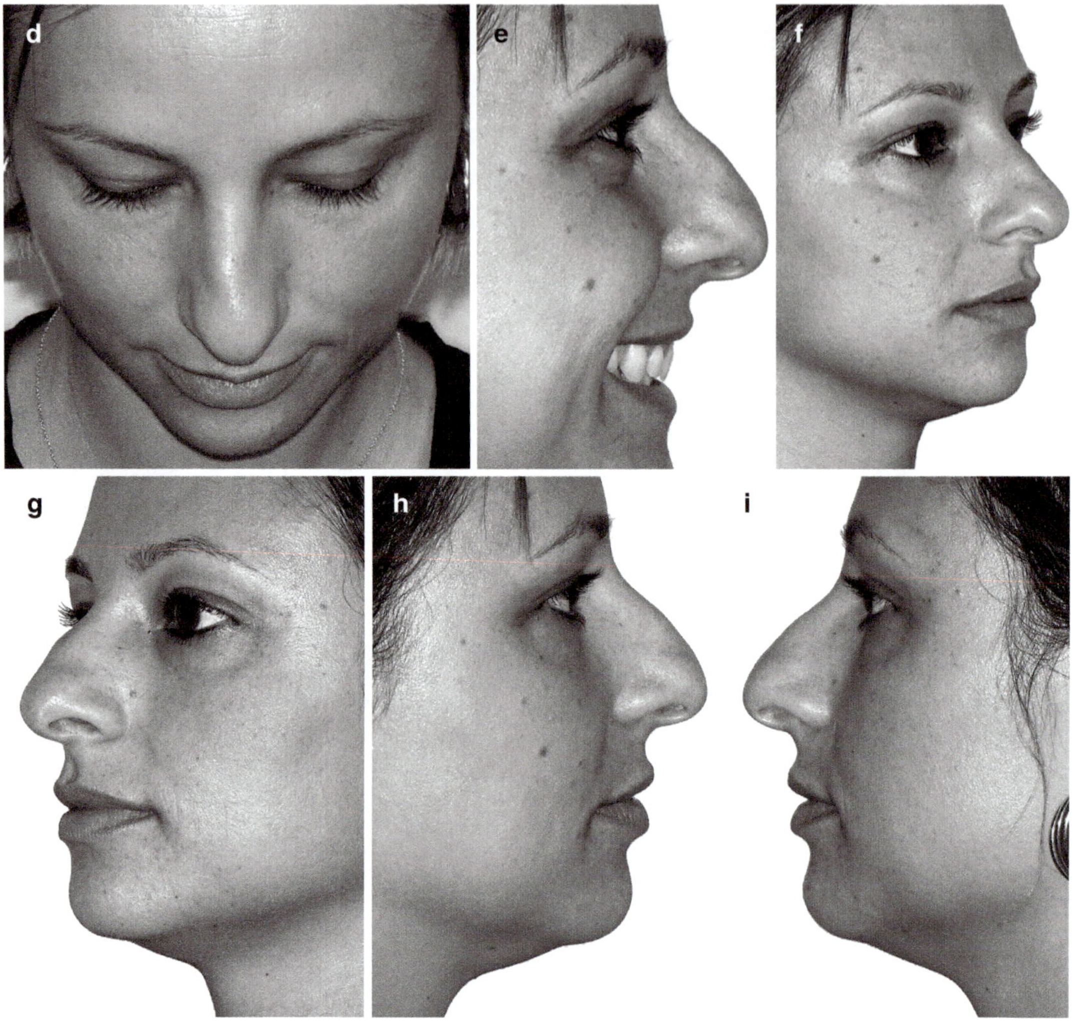

Fig. 10.5 (continued)

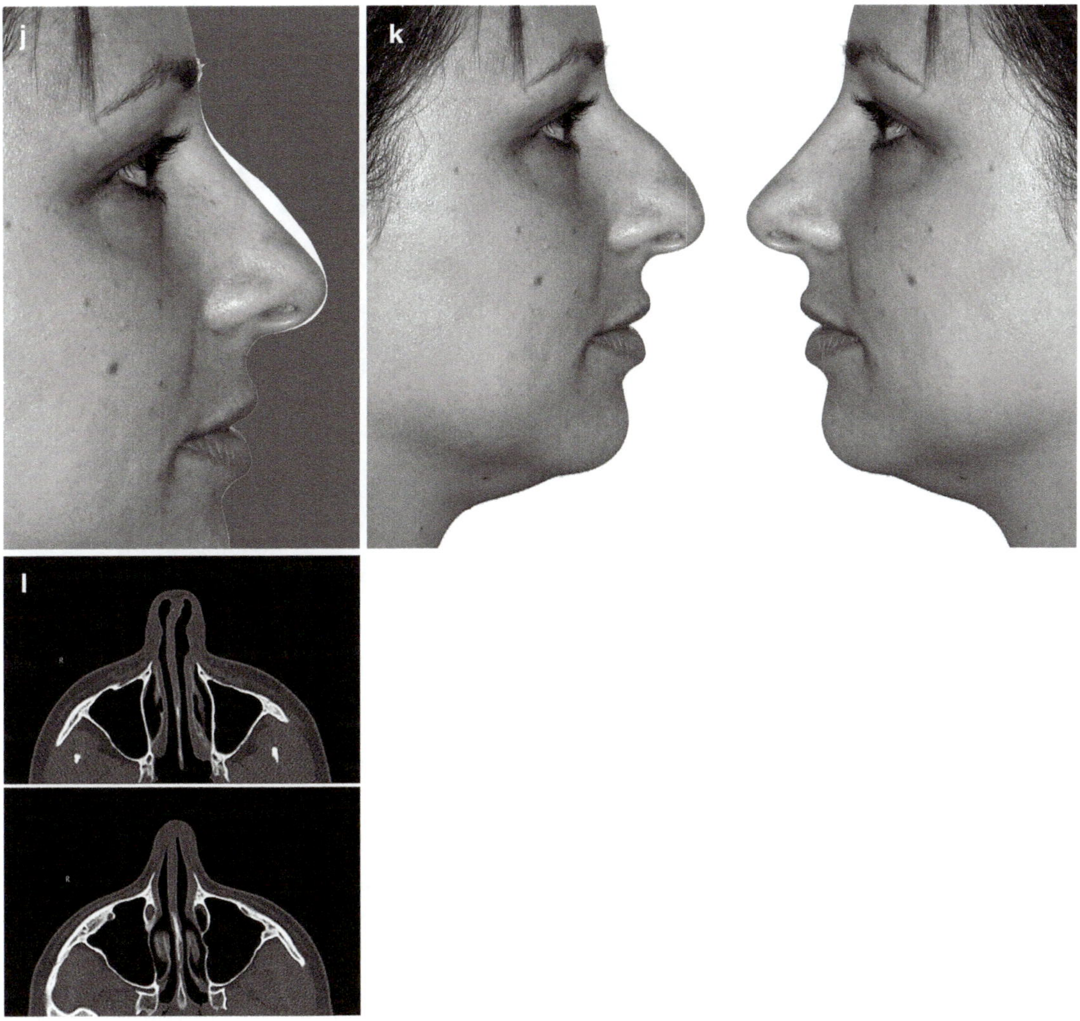

Fig. 10.5 (continued)

10.4 Realize the Best Individual Treatment Plan

Compiling the treatment plan alongside the patient is an extraordinary and challenging act, always unique and mutable every time. Each patient has different problems, different questions, and different needs. Each patient will use different languages. Even his reactivity, resilience, and collaboration are unique and special.

Adapting, for the surgeon, means looking for the necessary personalization of the relationship.

After 30 years of clinical experience, readings, and debates with colleagues, we identified some conditions and rules to be respected to work together with the patient in drawing up the best possible treatment plan:

- Refrain from work in deep at the treatment plan during the first visit.
- Best prepare for the second visit by creating and printing high-quality materials. The quality of the images to be shown to the patient is a clear indication of attention and professionalism.
- Reserve at least 30 or 40 min of time for the second visit.
- Sit near the patient when working on the printed photos and CT images (Fig. 10.6a, b).
- Use the computer screen to view CT scan images if there was no time to print them on paper.

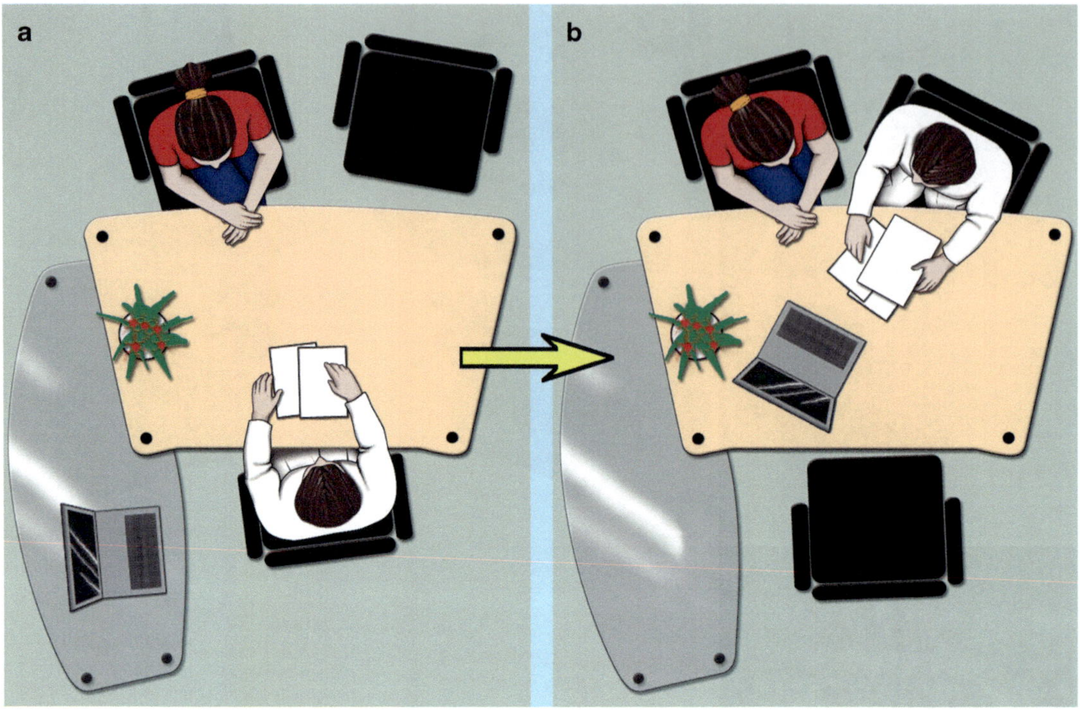

Fig. 10.6 (**a**, **b**) When working on the printed photos and CT images, the surgeon sit near the patient to facilitate communication and drawing over the images

- Use the photos printed on standard A4 paper to write every note.
- Describe the photos and CT images using the simplest words, without haste, making equally simple examples.
- Make sure the patient understands a detail or a point before moving on to the next.
- Write the treatment plan in the form of a list of points. Each point corresponds to a problem to be solved and sometimes even to a reference to the workable solution.
- All the points composing the treatment plan must be written and numbered on the sheet with the image in frontal projection. This is a perfect opportunity to summarize every detail with the patient in one single sheet.
- During the dialogues with the patient and in the compilation of objectives, always use the term "improvement" and never "correction." For example, the "correction" of nasal asymmetry implies obtaining a symmetrical nose, which is desirable but difficult to reach. It is better to speak of "improvement" of the asymmetry, which implies that the result will be obtained even without reaching a perfect symmetry.

When the patient sits next to the surgeon to look at the photos, a good start is to ask the patient if he wants to start commenting on them, to express ideas and judgments, or if he prefers to leave the task of analyzing the nose and face to the surgeon. The goal is to help the patient to express, in simple words, everything that comes to mind about his nose and his face.

The surgeon must recognize if the patient's requests are appropriate and converging towards an esthetic result proportionate to the rest of the face, achievable and compatible with the respiratory function.

10.5 An Example of Handwritten Individual Treatment Plan

Figure 10.7 shows an example of a treatment plan written down on the printed sheet with the preoperative frontal view. During the second visit, five unpleasant points to be corrected were identified together with the patient:

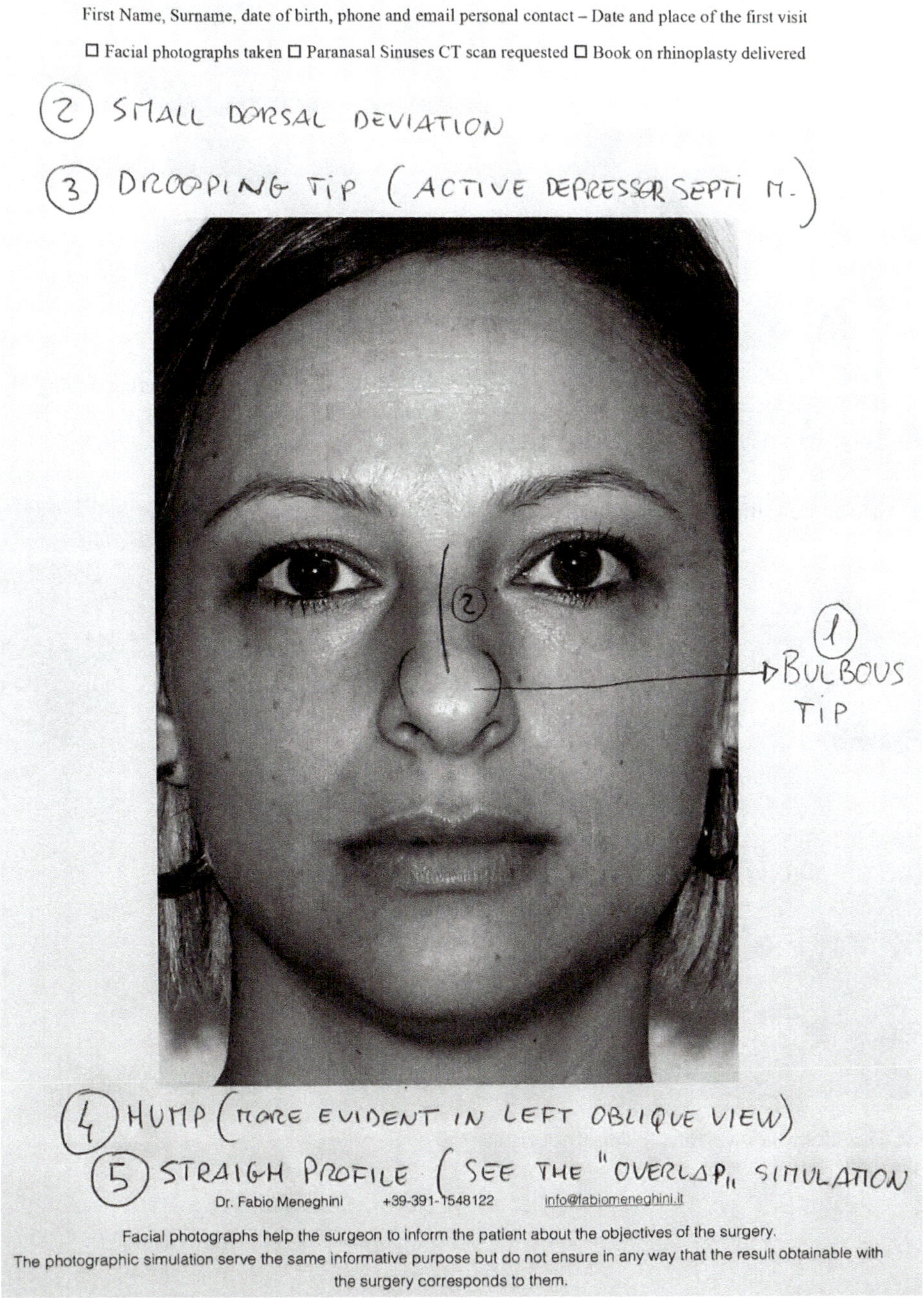

Fig. 10.7 Preoperative frontal view. The white space around the portrait is useful for writing down the main points of the treatment plan

- Bulbous nasal tip, evident on the frontal and face-up views (Fig. 10.8).
- Small dorsal deviation towards the right side visible in face-down view (Fig. 10.9).
- Hyperactive depressor septi muscle documented on profile view during smiling (Fig. 10.10).
- Dorsal hump, more evident on the left oblique view (Fig. 10.11).

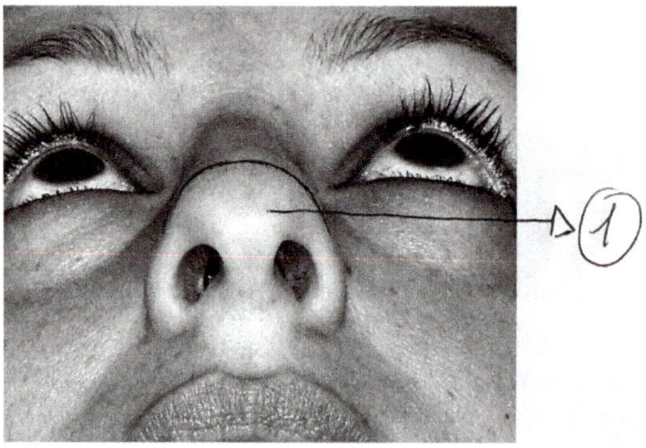

Fig. 10.8 Face-up view. Bulbous nasal tip

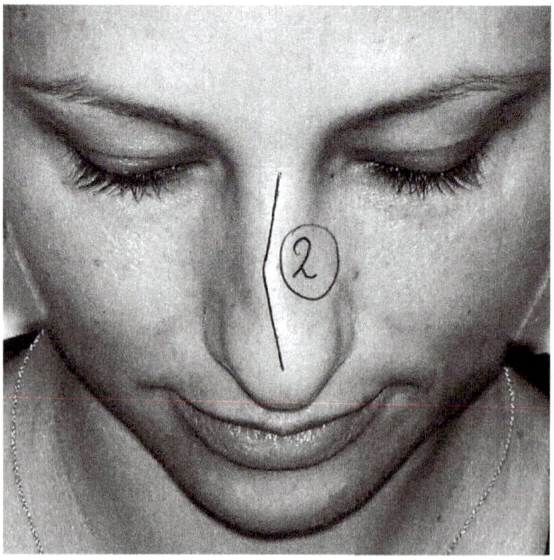

Fig. 10.9 Face-down view. Small dorsal deviation towards the right side

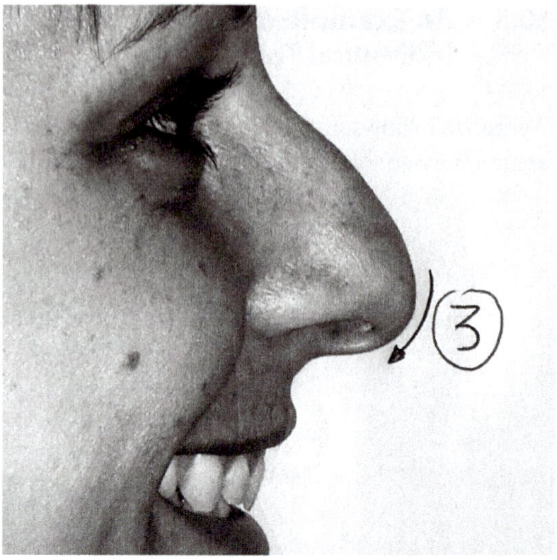

Fig. 10.10 Right profile view during smiling. Hyperactive depressor septi muscle

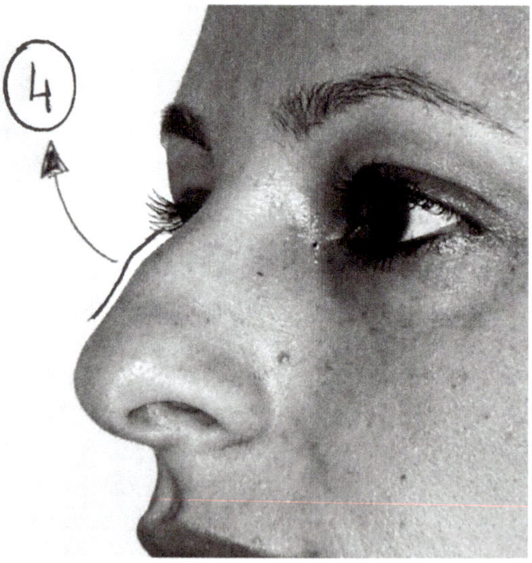

Fig. 10.11 Left oblique view. Dorsal hump

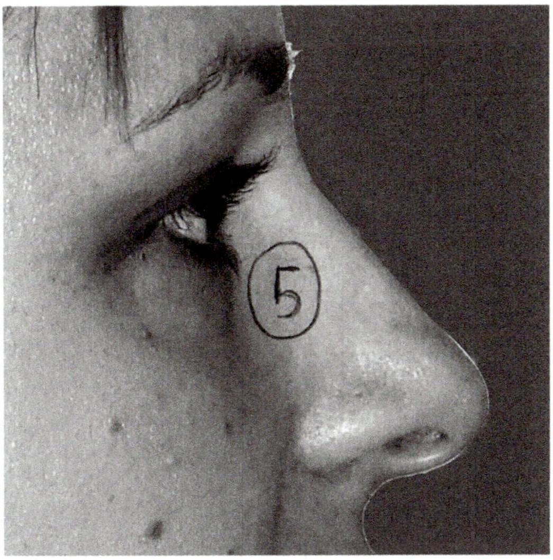

Fig. 10.12 Right profile view. The "Overlap" simulation shows the desired nasal profile with highly conservative nasal tip projection reduction and straight dorsum

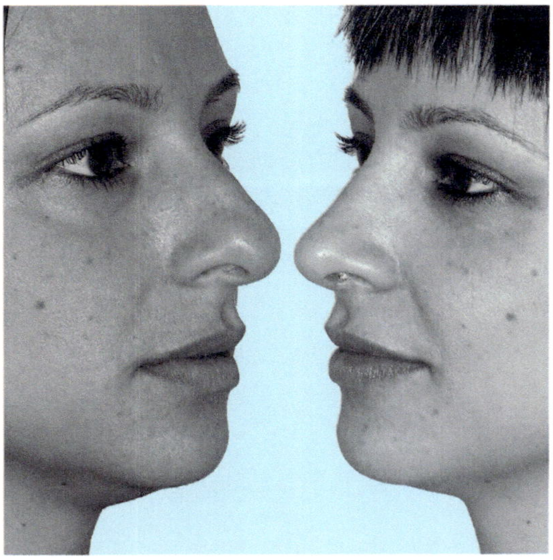

Fig. 10.13 Right oblique view. Pre- and postoperative right oblique view at 4 months in the same clinical case of the previous figures

– Desired nasal profile with highly conservative nasal tip projection reduction and straight dorsum studied with an "Overlap" simulation (Fig. 10.12).

Figure 10.13 shows the pre- and postoperative right oblique view at 5 months in the same clinical case.

Further Reading

One of the authors that dedicated himself to the preparation of photographic images to study and predict the new profile is certainly Dr. Bahman Guyuron. His studies and suggestions are published in these works:

Guyuron B. Rhinoplasty. Edinburgh: Elsevier Saunders; 2012.

Guyuron B. Precision rhinoplasty. Part I: the role of life-size photographs and soft-tissue cephalometric analysis. Plast Reconstr Surg. 1988;4:489–99.

11 Patient Preparation for Rhinoplasty

This chapter describes the sequential steps between deciding to program the rhinoplasty and beginning the actual surgical operation.

After the second visit with the patient it is possible to fix the place and date of the intervention. To take this decision it is important for the surgeon to have had confirmation in previous meetings that the patient is a good candidate for rhinoplasty from all points of view and that mutual esteem has developed.

Sometimes, both the patient and the surgeon decide to reconsider and to let time pass before proceeding towards surgery or planning a further meeting to review once more the objectives and the pros and cons of the intervention.

If both agree to proceed, the surgeon fixes the date and location of the surgery, requires a series of standard preoperative blood tests and an electrocardiogram, organizes the preoperative visit with the anaesthesiologist and provides a checklist with some useful information.

11.1 The Preoperative Checklist

In preparation for the operation, it is useful for the patient to have a list they can check from time to time. Like any information provided to the patient, a written list with few clear points is preferable.

Here's one example:

- Do not take aspirin or other drugs containing acetylsalicylic acid within 15 days prior to surgery.
- Do not smoke.
- If you are a man, remember to shave your beard and mustache the day before the surgery.
- Do not forget to bring the reports of your preoperative exams (blood tests and electrocardiogram) with you to the clinic.
- Do not forget to bring your preoperative imaging tests (CT scan).
- Remember to avoid eating or drinking any solid or liquid foods (even water) in the 6 h prior to the operation.
- Remember to obtain the prescribed medications you need to take during the postoperative period.
- On the day of the operation and the following ones, wear a loose shirt or top with buttons or zips (that can be put on and removed without pulling them over your head).
- Remember that when you have been discharged, you must NOT drive.
- Remember that you cannot remain alone during the first 24 h following the operation.

A good idea is to leave an extra space on the sheet for a series of additional suggestions and prescriptions to add to the standard list based on the preoperative conditions of the individual patient.

F. Meneghini, *Basic Open Rhinoplasty*, https://doi.org/10.1007/978-3-030-61827-8_11

11.2 Preoperative Visit and Exams

As with any other surgery, it is necessary to request some standard preoperative blood tests and an electrocardiogram and share all data emerging from the anamnesis with the anesthesiologist. The patient will email the reports of preoperative exams to the surgeon a few days before the date of the intervention. If any alterations of the clinical and instrumental data emerge, the last days before the intervention will be dedicated to consultations and instrumental investigations to confirm the patient's operability.

11.3 Meet the Patient Immediately Before Entering the Operating Room

Meeting the surgeon once more, a few minutes before entering the operating room, is very important for the patient.

On this occasion as well it is necessary to have with you the printed photos with the notes on the treatment plan as this confirms the importance that the surgeon reserves to the preoperative steps done with the patient. It only takes a few minutes to summarize the fundamental and shared goals of surgery to reassure the patient.

Once again it is necessary to ask the patient if he has allergies, if he has taken aspirin or other medicines in the previous days, if he has been fasting for at least 6 h, etc.

11.4 In the Operating Room

Patient photos, with written details of the treatment plan, as well as the most significant CT images, should be hung up in the operating room on a wall or on a special panel close to the first surgeon (Fig. 11.1).

The preferred anesthesia for a complete rhinoplasty operation is general anesthesia with con-

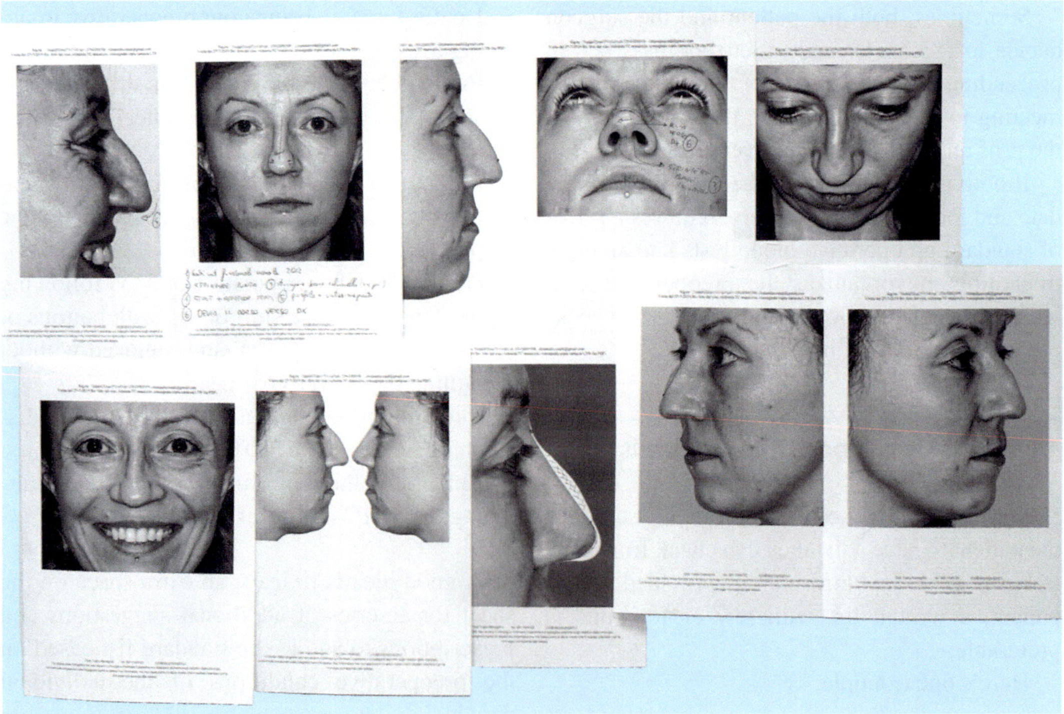

Fig. 11.1 Patient photos, with written details of the treatment plan, should be hung up in the operating room close to the first surgeon

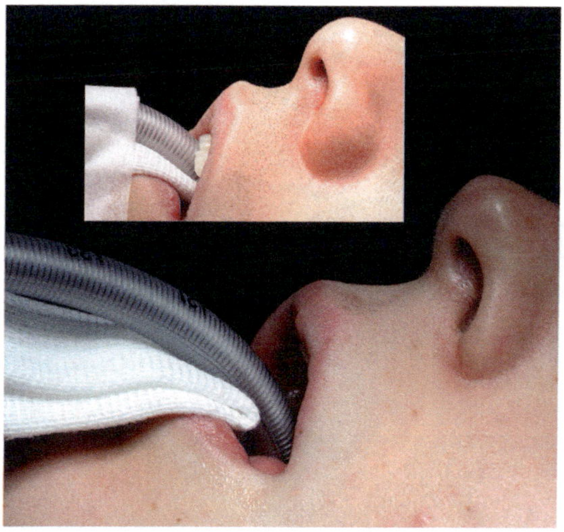

Fig. 11.2 Interposition of a small gauze between the endotracheal tube and the lower lip to protect the latter

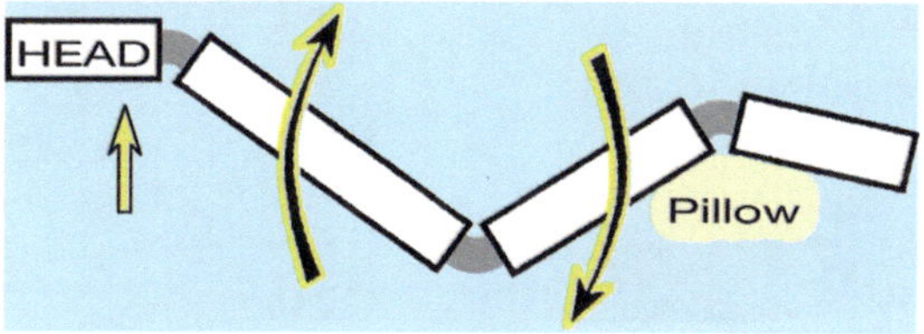

Fig. 11.3 The patient is placed in a slight reverse-Trendelenburg position on the surgical table. A pillow should be placed under the knees

trolled hypotension and oral-tracheal intubation. The positioning and fixation of the endotracheal tube must be central, without distortion of the soft facial tissues around the nose and without excessive pressure on the lower lip.

Figure 11.2 shows the interposition of a small gauze between the endotracheal tube and the lower lip to protect the latter and to avoid any traction to the upper lip.

The patient is placed on the surgical table in a slight reverse-Trendelenburg position (Fig. 11.3) with the head resting stably in slight hyperextension on a gel head positioner. A pillow should be placed under the knees.

To prevent ingestion of blood, the anesthesiologist places a 5 cm wet gauze throat wrap.

Skin disinfection is performed with half-strength (5%) povidone-iodine solution; this concentration of antiseptic solution is also used

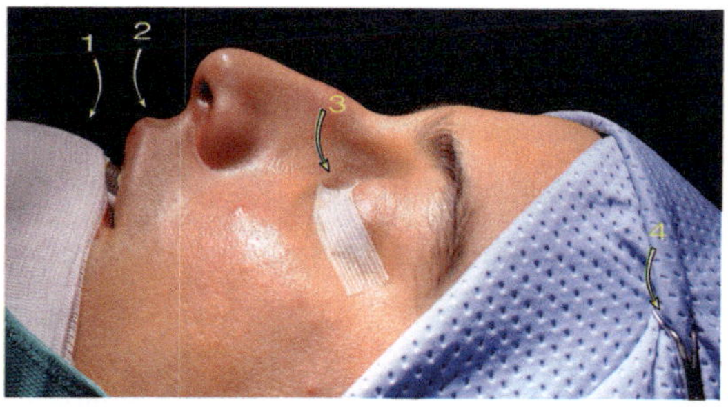

Fig. 11.4 Operative field preparation (see text)

in ophthalmology in the preparation for conjunctival surgery and therefore can be considered safe.

After drying the skin with sterile gauze, eye protection is obtained by applying ophthalmic ointment to the conjunctiva and closing the eyelids with one or two Steri-Strips 12 mm wide and cut to half their length.[1]

To prepare the operative field for rhinoplasty, disposable tissue drapes with adhesive margins should be avoided. These adhesive bands risk deforming the skin of the face with a distortion of the nasal tip and the nasal base. At the end of the operation, the removal of the adhesive bands can cause the stripping of hair or irritate the skin.

Soft sterile drapes are still preferable for a proper preparation of the operative field. A sterile gauze will always be placed between the endotracheal tube and the drape to avoid pulling on the facial skin.

Figure 11.4 summarizes the main points of a correct preparation of the operative field:

1. A sterile gauze covers the endotracheal tube.
2. The upper lip and the nasal base are absolutely free and undistorted by the sterile drapes.
3. The eyes are protected by closing the lids with a half-length 50 × 12 mm Steri-Strip.
4. The cheeks and forehead are covered with a soft and non-adhesive sterile drape fixed in place with a Backhaus forceps leaving the facial skin completely undeformed.

[1] 3M Steri-Strip, ½ in ×4 in, R1547.

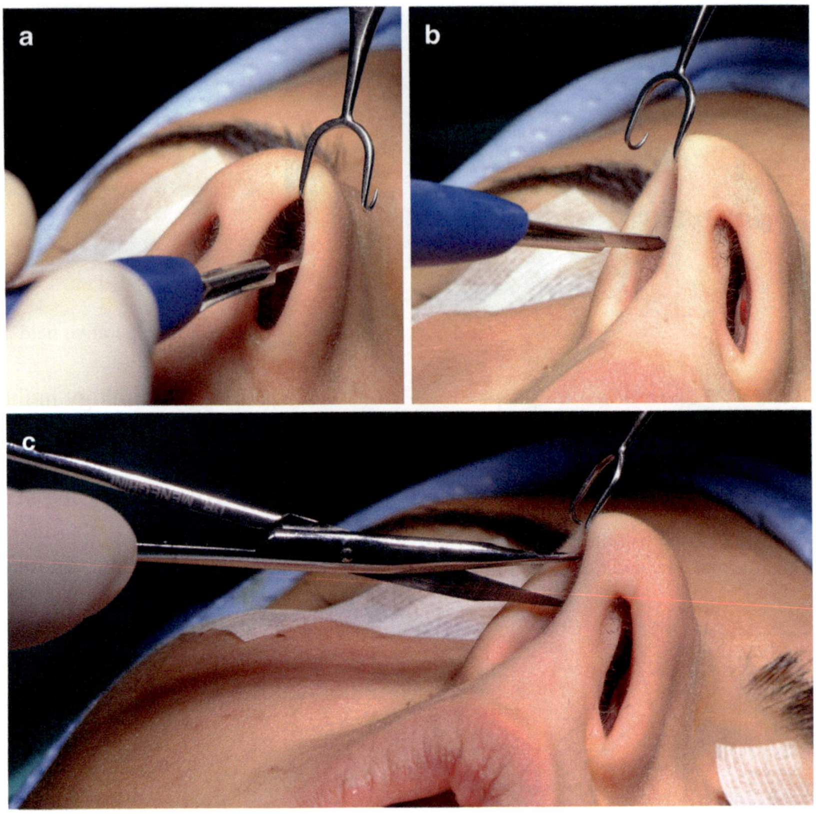

Fig. 11.5 (**a–c**) Nasal vibrissae shaving with a No. 15 scalpel blade (**a**, **b**) or small scissors (**c**)

The nasal vibrissae are then shaved with the use of a double hook, with which we support and expose the nasal vestibule, and a No. 15 scalpel blade (Fig. 11.5a, b). As an alternative to the No. 15 blade, we can trim the vibrissae with small scissors (Fig. 11.5c). A further disinfection of the nasal cavities with povidone-iodine solution completes the preparation of the operative field.

11.5 Nasal Local Anesthesia: Initial Steps

The three main objectives of infiltration with local anesthetic are all necessary in nasal surgery:

- The sensory block, which must be maintained during and beyond the operative time.
- Vasoconstriction, necessary for reducing intraoperative bleeding.
- Hydrodissection of specific areas, which helps in finding and maintaining the right dissection plane during flap elevation.

The infiltration of tissues with local anesthetic requires several steps.

Preferably we use "carpule" dental vials containing each 1.8 mL of mepivacaine hydrochloride 2% solution with 1:100,000 epinephrine mounted in an Aspiject syringe (Fig. 11.6a). The use of dental carpule cartridges has many advantages:

- Each vial contains only 1.8 mL of anesthetic and therefore it is possible to perform micro-infiltrations even in mucous areas that are not very distensible, as in the septal cartilage. Every single infiltration must be very small in order not to deform the soft tissues too much and change the original shape of the nose.
- Very thin and flexible, but not fragile, long and short dental needles are available. Even when bent they do not break. These characteristics are ideal for infiltrating very thin soft tissues such as the nasal mucosa atraumatically. The most commonly used is the 30G 0.3 × 21 mm needle.

- The solution is already diluted and ready for use; no preparation or dilution is necessary for the surgical nurse.
- By reducing the injection pressure, a suction effect is created in the vial which allows the surgeon to recognize if the tip of the needle is inside a blood vessel.
- The Aspiject dental syringe is light and autoclavable; its duration in time is excellent.
- The costs of the solution and the needles are low and the availability on the market, as for many dental products, is excellent.

Infiltration of the local anesthetic also requires a nasal speculum and a double wide skin hook (Fig. 11.6b, c). Injection of local anesthetic starts along the lateral wall of the nose over the nasal bone and upper lateral cartilage. The needle enters the mucosa between the upper and lower lateral cartilages reaching the nasal bone at the level of the interchantal line, remaining parallel to the midline (asterisk in Fig. 11.7). The solution is injected by slowly retracting the needle. A total amount of 0.6 mL of local anesthetic is injected on each side.

The radix area is instead infiltrated with a direct transcutaneous approach. Ideally, 0.4 mL of solution is injected deeply keeping the needle in close proximity to the periosteal plane (Fig. 11.8).

After these injections, the swelling produced is reduced by massaging the nasal radix and the lateral walls of the nose with the thumb and forefinger of the non-dominant hand.

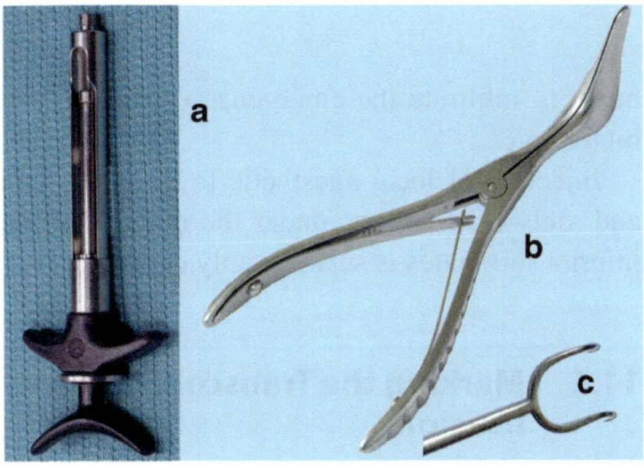

Fig. 11.6 (**a–c**) Instruments utilized for local anesthetic infiltration: Aspiject dental syringe (**a**), nasal speculum (**b**), and a double wide skin hook (**c**)

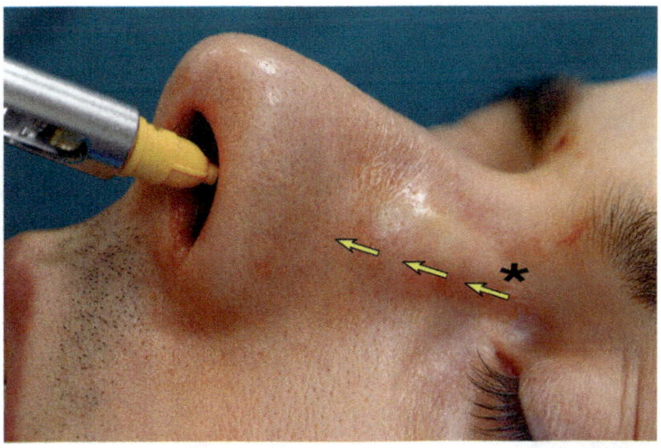

Fig. 11.7 Injection of local anesthetic along the lateral wall of the nose over the nasal bone and upper lateral cartilage. The asterisk shows the most superior point reached by the needle before starting injection. The injection is performed by slowly retracting the needle (straight arrows)

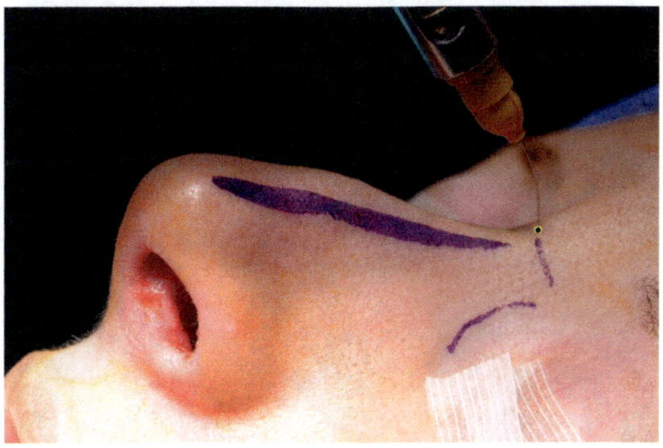

Fig. 11.8 Radix area infiltration

With the help of a nasal speculum, the caudal septum and the mucous membrane of the cartilaginous and bony septum are then infiltrated bilaterally (Fig. 11.9). The posterior extension of the infiltration depends on the necessity to later perform a septoplasty or harvest a piece of septal cartilage for grafting. The amount of solution utilized for septal infiltration on the two sides is comprised between 1.0 and 1.8 mL.

The area of the anterior nasal spine and the inferior margin of the pyriform aperture is then infiltrated with 0.6–0.9 mL of solution. The needle can be inserted through the skin of the nasal vestibule with the aid of the nasal speculum (Fig. 11.10a) or, alternatively and more simply, through the oral mucosa (Fig. 11.10b–d).

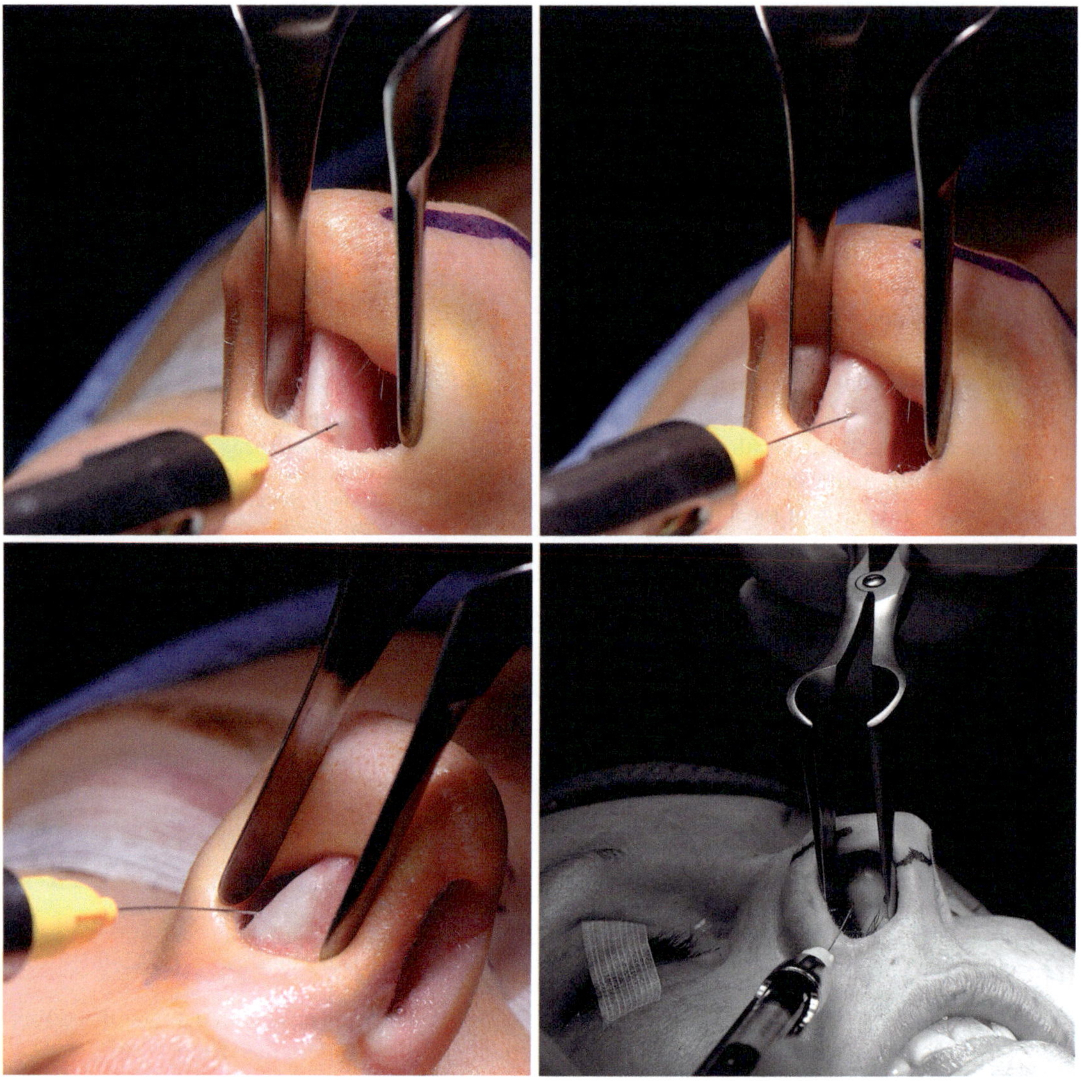

Fig. 11.9 Bilateral caudal septum infiltration

With the help of a double hook or the nasal speculum, a series of small amounts of local anesthetic are therefore infiltrated along the caudal margin of the lateral crus of the lower lateral cartilage to guarantee adequate vasoconstriction at the site of the marginal incision (Fig. 11.11). The amount of solution injected is minute.

Finally, entering from the lateral area of the nasal vestibule, the anterior maxilla close to the infraorbital foramen can be injected with 0.9 mL of solution on each side. Figure 11.12 shows how the length of the 30G 0.3 × 21 mm needle is adequate to infiltrate the emergence of the infraorbital nerve.

Injection of local anesthetic to the columella and, only if necessary, under the mucosa of the inferior turbinates is subsequently carried out.

11.6 Marking the Transcolumellar Incision

The transcolumellar incision must be perfectly drawn before injecting the columella.

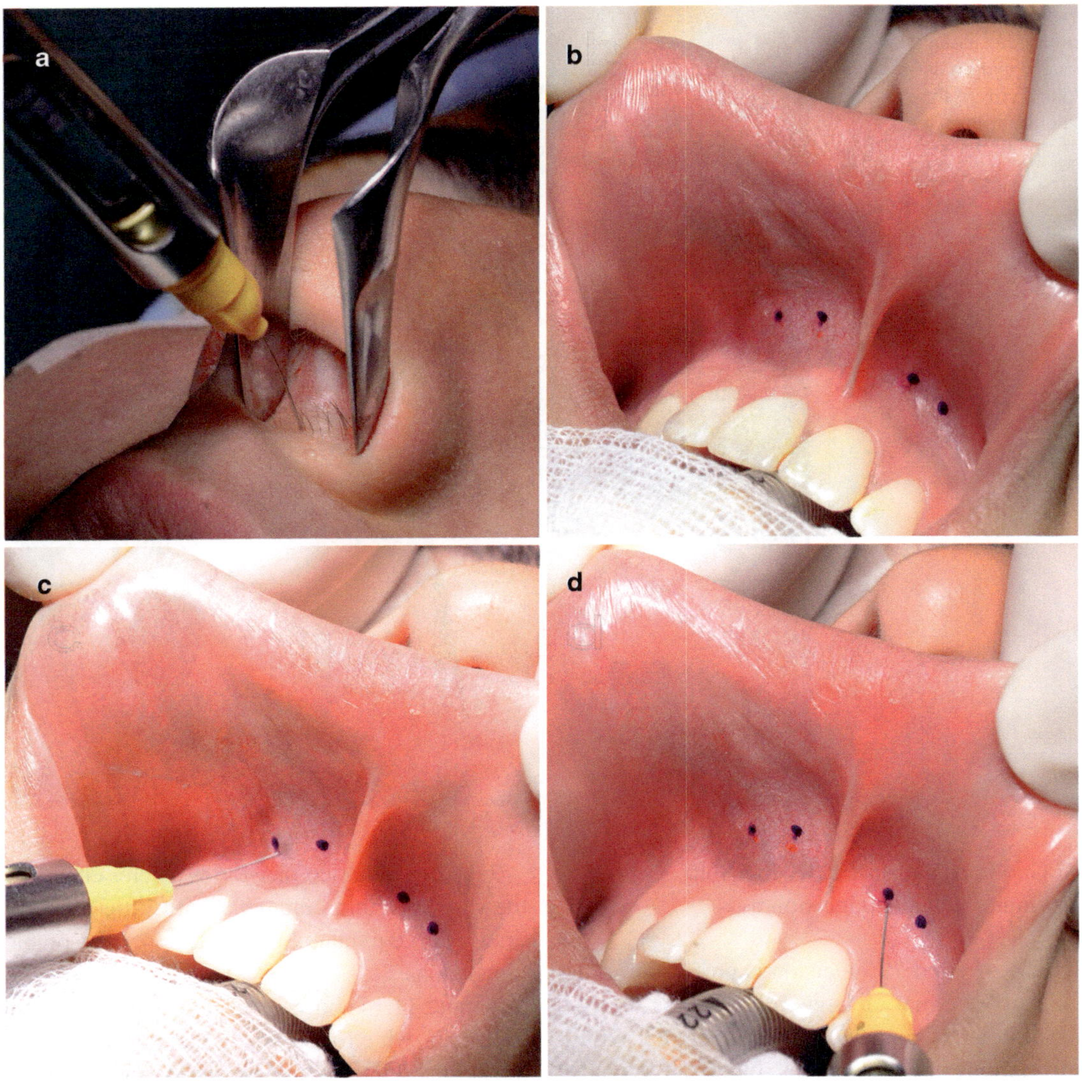

Fig. 11.10 Transnasal (**a**) and transoral (**b–d**) infiltration close to the anterior nasal spine and inferior margins of the piriform aperture

The best location for the incision is the narrowest central portion of the columella. In basal view, this area is below the columellar breakpoint and above the base of columella.

What configuration should the incision have?

The linear incisions proposed by Rethi and later by Sercer now have merely historical interest and are no longer used (Fig. 8.1 in Chap. 8). For many decades now, the insertion of small notches which interrupt the incision is preferred. Interrupting the incision line serves as a marker to guide the subsequent alignment of the flap during suturing and to give a better esthetic result by reducing tension and preventing retraction of the scar. Moreover, a retracted scar resulting from a linear incision can be evident in profile view, whereas "V" or "Z" pattern retracted scars camouflage it.

Among the many variants proposed, it is advisable to limit the choice to one of these two versions:

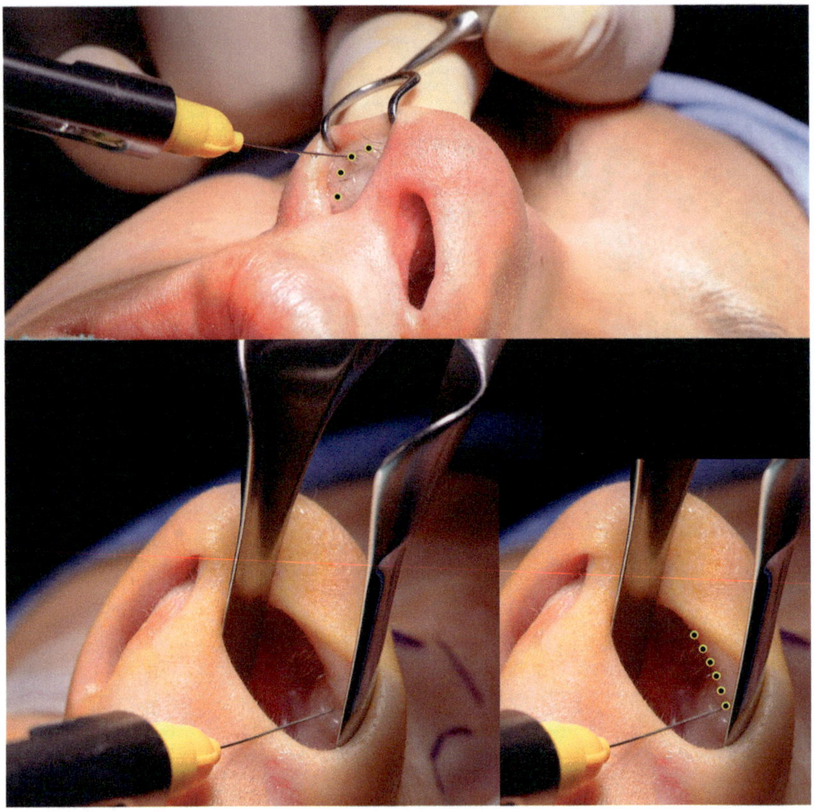

Fig. 11.11 Bilateral infiltration along the caudal margin of the lateral crus of the lower lateral cartilage

- Goodman's inverted "V" incision.
- Gunter's stairstep incision.

The inverted "V" incision is preferable in the case of a normal or large columella as the two small central incisions must be included within the margins of the cartilages. Indeed, if the latter are close to each other or even superimposed and twisted, there would be a risk of damaging them with the scalpel during the initial phase of the transcolumellar incision.

Figure 11.13a–d shows how to draw, with a fine-point skin marker, the inverted V-shaped incision starting from three small dots represented by an equilateral triangle with a lower base. The two basal points of the triangle must be included in the space between the edge of the cartilages and at the narrowest and most central point of the columella. The sides of the triangle measure about 2.5 mm.

Gunter's stairstep incision is a safer choice in the case of a thin columella with little space to draw an equilateral triangle of acceptable dimensions.

Figure 11.14 shows a basal view of a thin columella in which the two horizontal portions of the stairstep incision are centered in the narrowest area of columella with a small vertical 2 mm medial line forming a 90° angle.

In conclusion, as a general rule, the location of the transcolumellar incision is more important than the configuration.

11.7 Columellar Local Anesthesia

The last step immediately before starting the skin incision is an infiltration of about 1.8 mL of local anesthetic into the columella. The logic behind this rule lies in the need to have an effec-

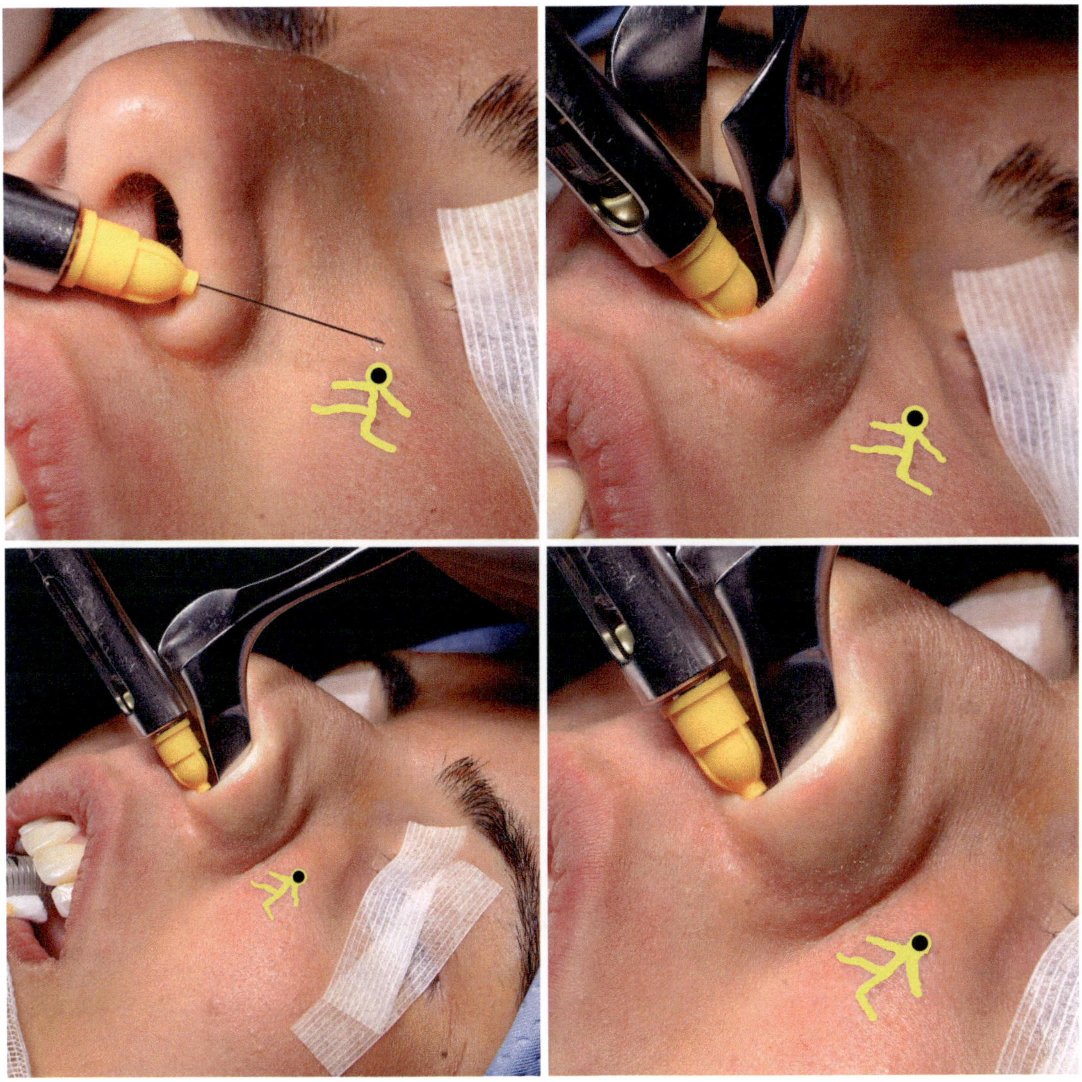

Fig. 11.12 Infiltration of the emergence of the infraorbital nerve through the nasal vestibule with a 30G 0.3 × 21 mm needle

tive hydrodissection of columellar soft tissues in order to reduce the risk of damaging the underlying cartilage with the scalpel blade during the transcolumellar skin incision.

Figure 11.15a–c shows the point of entrance of the fine needle, whereas the asterisk indicates the area reached by the tip of the needle. Figure 11.15d shows the small injection done on the lateral aspect of the columellar skin.

11.8 Directional Terminology

In the next chapters, the intraoperative images are related to patients in the supine position. A commonly accepted directional terminology, reported in Fig. 11.16 and independent of the patient's position, will be used in all descriptions. Figure 11.17 shows an intraoperative view in which the same directional terminology is applied to the lower lateral crus.

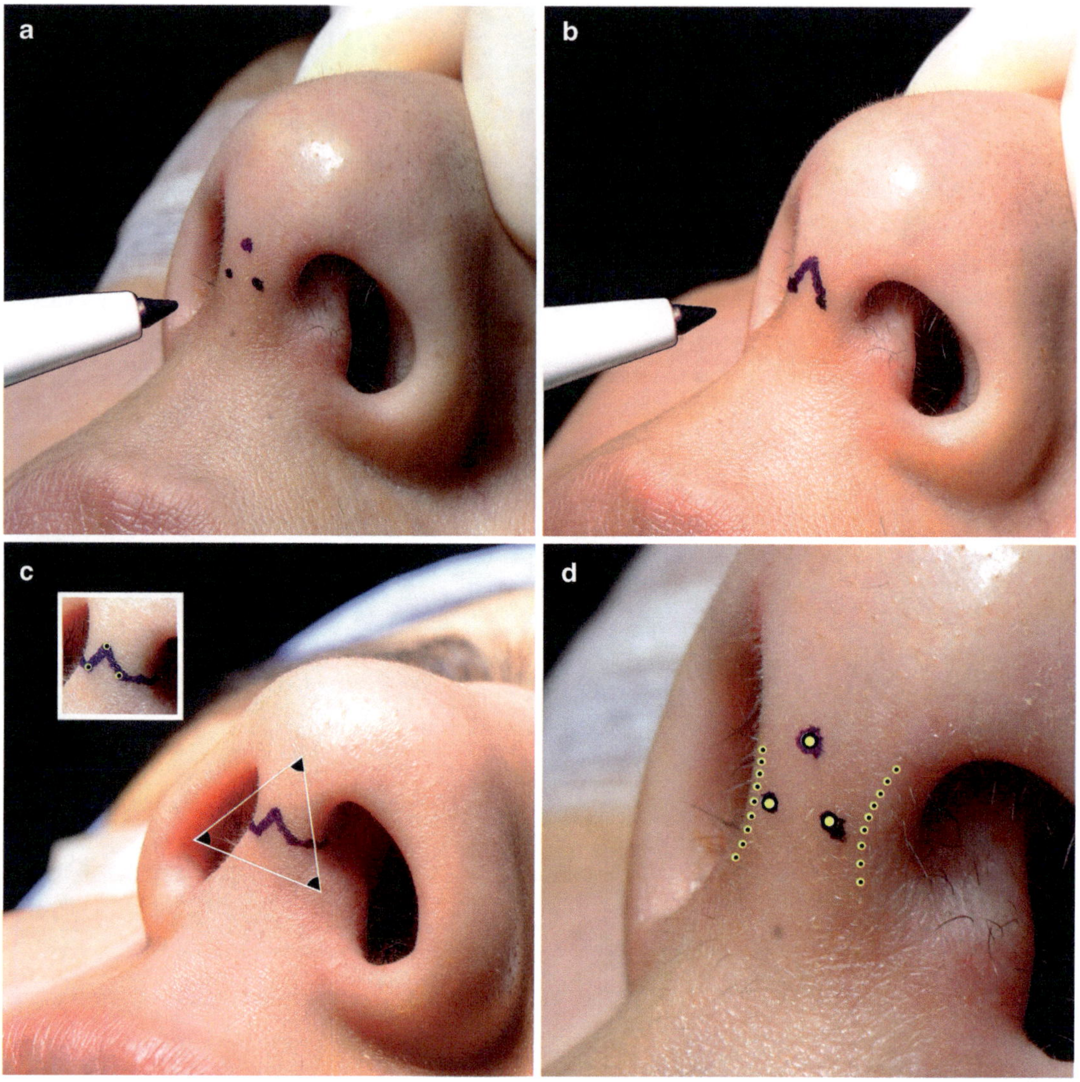

Fig. 11.13 How to draw Goldman's inverted V-shaped incision (See text)

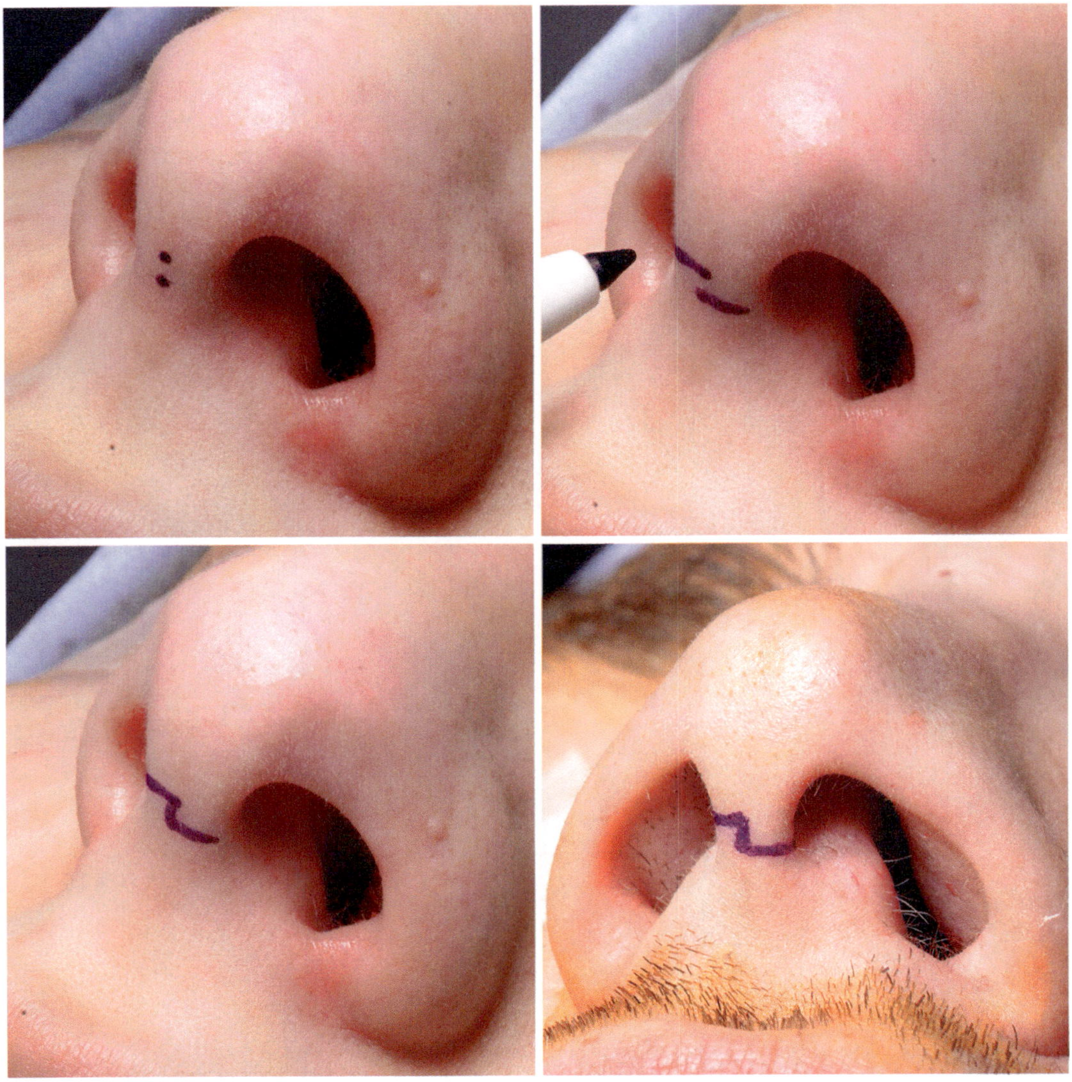

Fig. 11.14 How to draw Gunter's stairstep incision

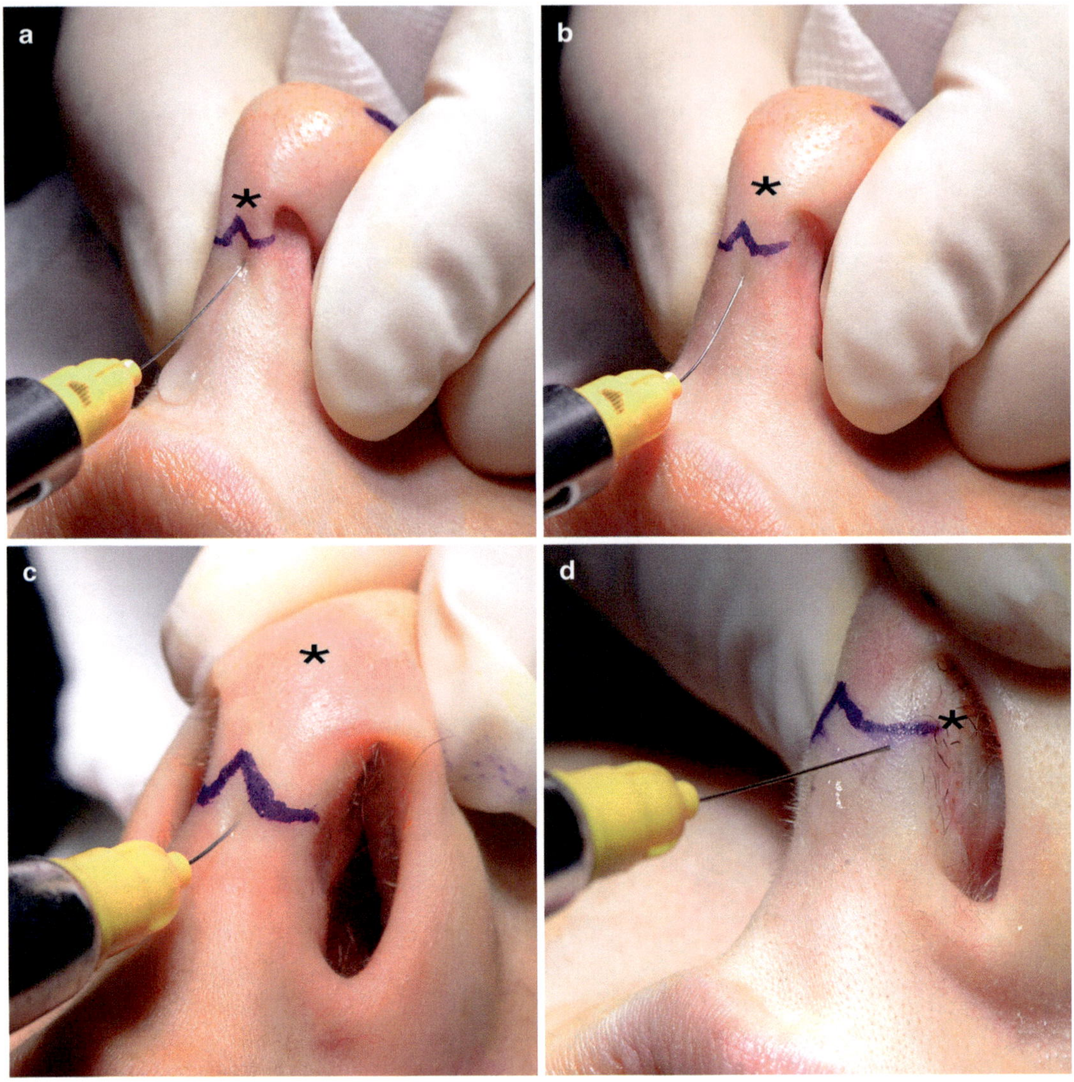

Fig. 11.15 (**a–d**) Columellar infiltration. The asterisk shows the three levels of small central injections (**a–c**). Also the lateral aspect of the columella is injected with a drop of local anesthesia (asterisk in **d**)

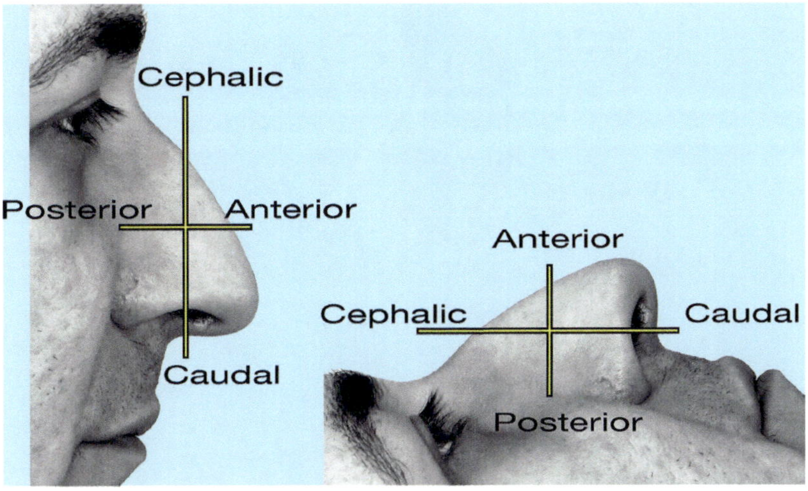

Fig. 11.16 Accepted directional terminology that is independent from the position of the patient

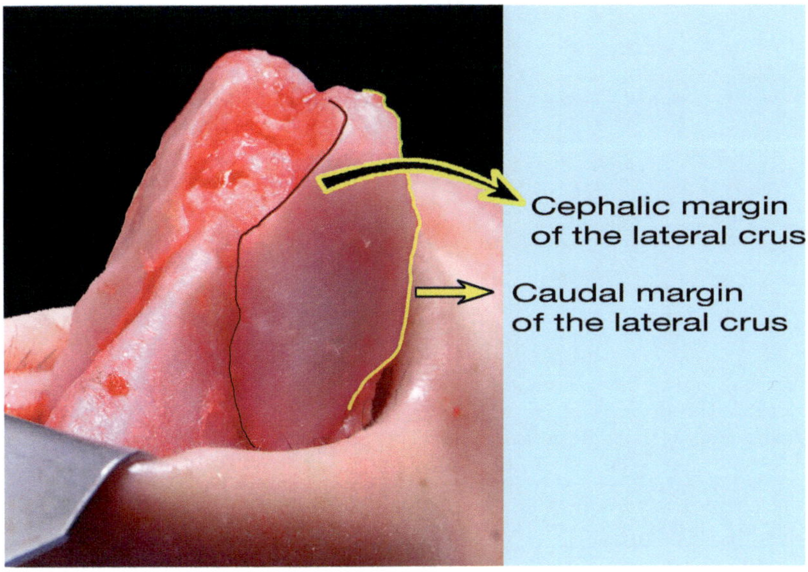

Fig. 11.17 Nasal tip intraoperative view. Accepted directional terminology applied to lower lateral crus

Further Reading

Proper local anesthesia is critical to allow for atraumatic dissection and reduction of intraoperative bleeding. An interesting reading on this topic is chapter 3, "Injection," of a classic book written by Toriumi DM, Becker DG. Rhinoplasty dissection manual. Philadelphia: Lippincott Williams & Wilkins; 1999.

12 Basic Open Rhinoplasty: An Overview

Basic Open Rhinoplasty (BOR) can be divided into successive phases and is inspired by the work of many authors who consider important the logic that governs the sequence of surgical acts in a complex procedure that is rich in variables.

RM Millard Jr. in his classic "Principlization of Plastic Surgery" described the general importance of the surgical sequence. Instead, the most important and in-depth text on the sequence in open rhinoplasty we owe to JB Tebbetts. In his 1998 book, Tebbetts describes basic operating times, presents a complete set of algorithms needed to make intraoperative decisions and describes various conditions that lead the surgeon to modify the standard operating plan.

In 2002 he wrote: "*The sequence in which surgical techniques are applied in rhinoplasty can affect the result as much as the specific techniques chosen.*"

Although the operating sequence should not be considered a rigid cage for the surgeon, generally respecting it is of great help, and any limits of the method are well outweighed by the advantages. Here are the main groups of sequential steps of BOR:

- T1—Initial exploratory steps.
- T2—Conservative corrections.
- T3—Non-conservative corrections.
- T4—Reconstructive work.
- T5—Finishing steps.

Some general principles have been considered in the evolution of the BOR sequence:

- Continuously verify the treatment plan intraoperatively.
- Give priority to maximum preservation of nasal tissues.
- Carry out the procedure symmetrically.
- Avoid making any irreversible decisions until the intraoperative exploration and analysis have been completed.
- Perform the obvious and essential maneuvers for the clinical case first.
- Correct the deep and roughly deformed components of the nasal framework first.
- Correct deformities preferably with small incremental changes rather than with a single maneuver.
- Harvest the septal cartilage only after defining the size and number of structural grafts.
- Finish the cartilage sutures and the fixation of the structural grafts before thinking about camouflage (structure first).

12.1 Initial Exploratory Steps

During skin incisions and flap elevations, the surgeon has the opportunity to explore and confirm the findings obtained during the preoperative studies.

Initially, any temptation to correct some details or harvest cartilage should be avoided. This step is not yet dedicated to correcting or act-

F. Meneghini, *Basic Open Rhinoplasty*, https://doi.org/10.1007/978-3-030-61827-8_12

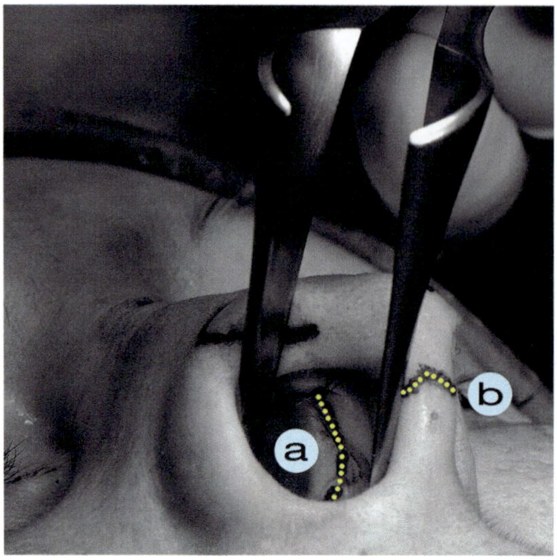

Fig. 12.1 Transfixion (**a**) and transcolumellar inverted-V incision (**b**) highlighted with small yellow dotted lines

ing on the nasal structures but rather it aims to obtain new information and confirmation of the treatment plan, reserving for later the right to make the changes that are deemed necessary.

Some authors, such as Johnson and Toriumi, Johnson and To, begin the operation by harvesting a piece of septal cartilage through a transfixion incision. Once the transfixion incision has been closed, the rhinoplasty starts with the open approach (Fig. 12.1). This sequence implies:

- An unnecessary mucosal incision (transfixion incision).
- The illogical decision that we are sure to need septal cartilage grafts.
- An excessive removal of septal cartilage in some cases and the reverse in others.
- A potential risk of structural instability of the cartilaginous framework.
- A small lengthening of the surgical times.

Other authors such as Tebbetts and Daniel perform a resection of the cephalic portion of the alar cartilage immediately after skin flap elevation. Tebbetts called this step "Creation of Structurally Symmetrical Rimstrip Elements." This sequence implies:

- Weakening of the lateral crus in an early phase of the surgery.
- Foregoing the use of a more conservative technique such as the "turn-in flap" which allows the volume of the lateral crus to be reduced without loss of cartilaginous substance. At the time of Tebbetts' publications the "turn-in flap" had not yet been described but today surgical logic suggests that it is wrong to forego an opportunity just for the haste to reduce the lateral crura.

So, in the BOR discipline, there are no indications to anticipate tissue removal, even though this is very common in nasal surgical practice; similarly, given the very wide individual variability of nasal anatomical structures, there are no reasons to act routinely.

12.2 Conservative Corrections

An example of conservative correction is the repositioning in the midline of a deviated quadrangular cartilage with minimal resection and suturing it to the anterior nasal spine. Figure 12.2 shows a typical anterior septum deviation demonstrated with coronal CT scan; only the dotted area shown on the CT scan will be removed during surgery. Once removed the small cartilage excess (Fig. 12.3), the surgeon obtains the so-called "swinging door" effect in which the quadrangular cartilage is freely moved laterally without interference with the maxillary crest and the anterior nasal spine indicated with the asterisk in Fig. 12.4.

A further detail from Fig. 12.3: the surgeon removed the cartilage excess in one solid piece without disrupting or damaging it. Later, during the reconstructive phase of rhinoplasty, this solid piece can be shaped and used as a columellar strut without any need to further harvest other pieces of cartilage from the septum.

The strategic optimization of resources and the conservation of structures is a peculiar point of the BOR discipline.

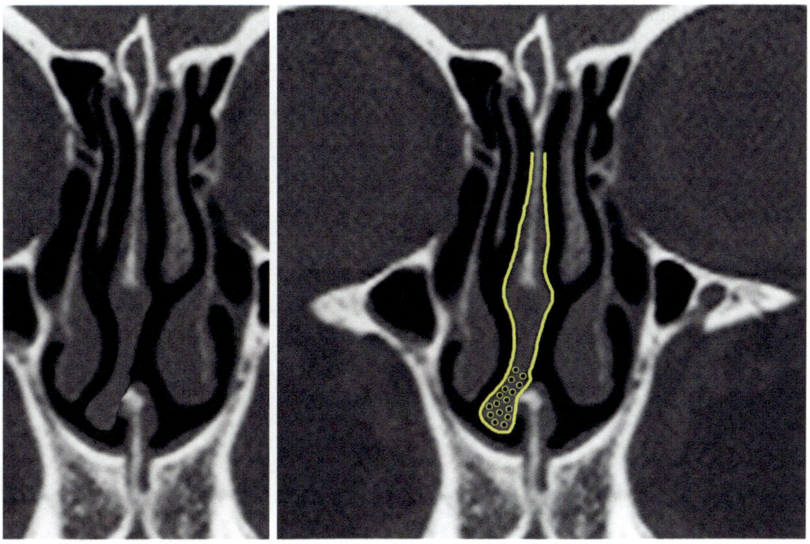

Fig. 12.2 Coronal CT scan reconstruction. Anterior deviation of the caudal septum to the right of the maxillary crest

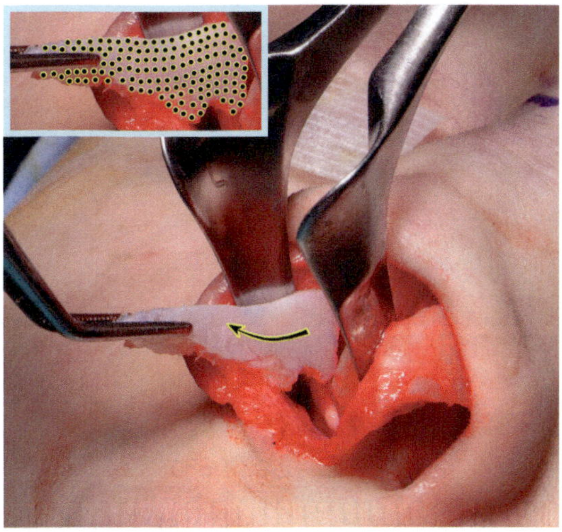

Fig. 12.3 One-piece removal of the septal cartilage excess near the maxillary crest

12.3 Non-conservative Corrections

The BOR discipline provides that any non-conservative correction is made when it is no longer deferrable and using, among the various practical solutions, those least aggressive for anatomical structures and the easiest to reconstruct.

En bloc nasal hump removal can be considered a typical non-conservative step of rhinoplasty. Figure 12.5 shows the constitutive anatomical elements of the hump: part of the nasal bones, the junction between nasal bones and triangular cartilages or K area, part of the triangular cartilages and a more or less high strip of cartilaginous septum. The partition between the cartilaginous and bone components can also be noted: the latter measures one-third of the total length of the removed hump.

To reduce the aggressiveness and potential risks of the removal of the osteocartilaginous hump en bloc, it is advisable to subdivide this step into different and more accurate surgical steps (component dorsal hump reduction) replacing also some surgical instruments:

- **T1**—With a piezosurgery saw, a bone rongeur or a small 2 mm osteotome, removing only the horizontal portion of the bony hump retains the portion of cartilage that is always present below these bones. Figure 12.6a illustrates a small piezoelectric saw in ultrasonic resonance. Thanks to ultrasonic vibrations under copious irrigation of sterile saline solution, it is possible to perform precise, clean, and limited osteotomies of small bones without dangerous tissue heating. The dotted area in Fig. 12.6b shows the horizontal portion of the bone hump to be removed.
- Before starting the osteotomy, the bone hump (bony cap concept) should be separated from the underlying septal cartilages along the

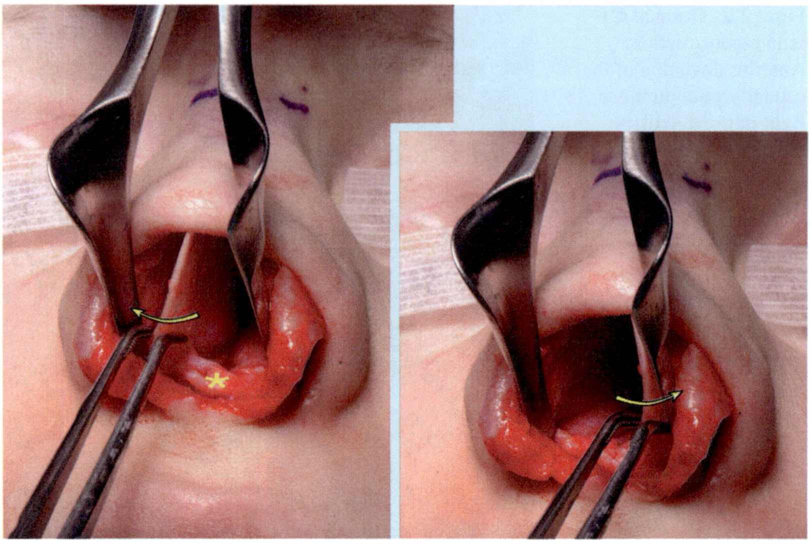

Fig. 12.4 "Swinging door" effect. The quadrangular cartilage is free to move laterally without contact interference with the maxillary crest and anterior nasal spine (the asterisk indicates the anterior nasal spine)

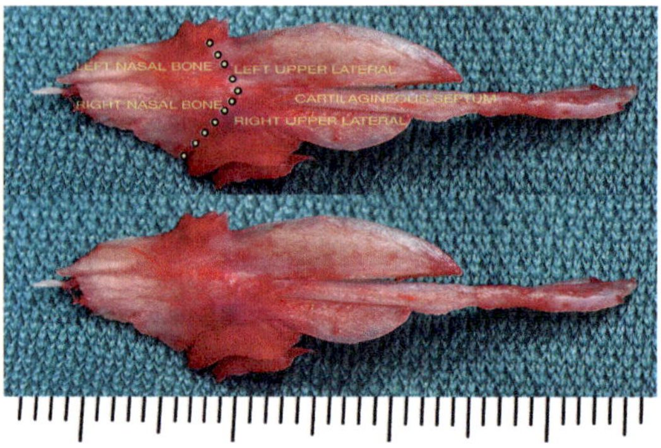

Fig. 12.5 En bloc nasal hump removal. The bone component amounts to one-third of the total length of the removed hump

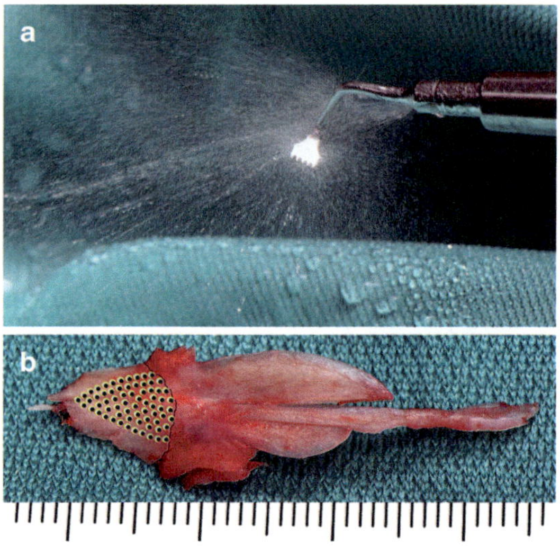

Fig. 12.6 (**a**, **b**) A small piezoelectric saw in ultrasonic resonance (**a**). The dotted area (**b**) shows the horizontal portion of the bone hump to be removed with component reduction

median line with an elevator or scissors with sharp points (Fig. 12.7a). Completion of the osteotomy under direct vision takes 2–3 min with a piezosurgery saw (Fig. 12.7b). The lines should be traced, checked and finally completed without any risk of bone over-resection (Fig. 12.7c).

- **T2**—Under direct vision the entire dorsal profile of the cartilaginous septum is reduced with Fomon scissors leaving intact the two triangular cartilages (Fig. 12.8).
- **T3**—Later, after having performed the osteotomies of the nasal bones, the nasal dorsum is reconstructed by folding the excess of the triangular cartilages on themselves and suturing them to the septum with absorbable sutures (spreader flap). Figure 12.9 shows how the two nasal bones are also sutured to the cartilaginous septum to further stabilize the new nasal dorsum.

12.4 Reconstructive Work

The BOR discipline envisages, for each nasal structure, the application of the principles of reconstructive surgery. The two main categories that apply to rhinoplasty are:

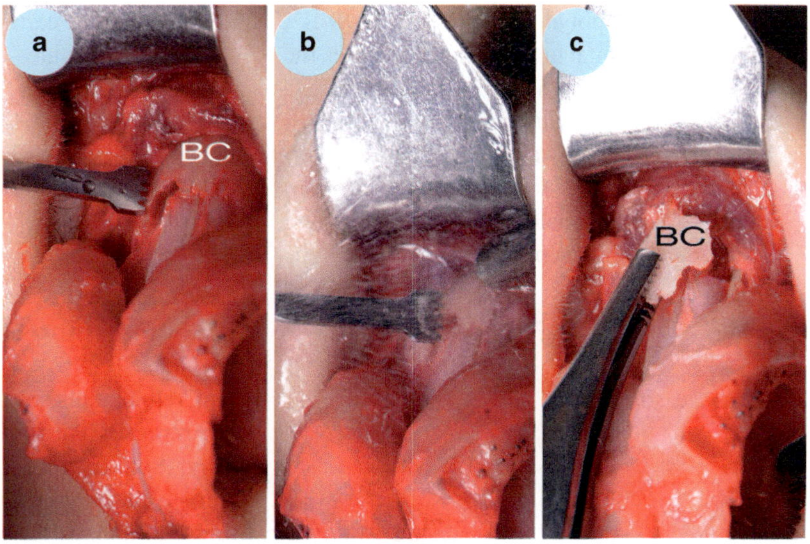

Fig. 12.7 (**a**–**c**) Dorsal hump reduction intraoperative views. Before starting the osteotomy, the bone hump (*BC*—bony cap) should be separated from the underlying septal cartilage along the median line (**a**). Osteotomy with ultrasonic saw (**b**). Removal of the thin horizontal portion of the bone hump (*BC*—bony cap) leaving intact the underlying cartilaginous hump (**c**)

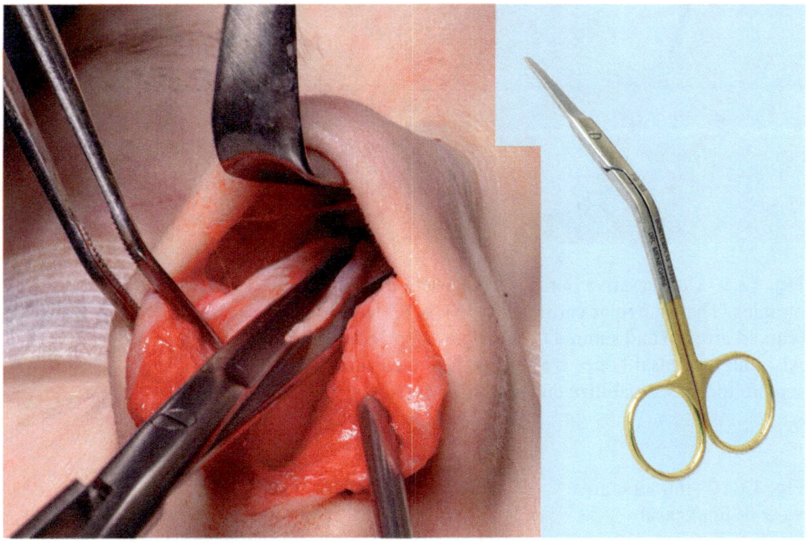

Fig. 12.8 Lowering of the entire septal dorsal profile with Fomon angulated scissors leaving intact the two triangular cartilages

- Suture techniques, with long-lasting absorbable polymer and, rarely, nonabsorbable materials.
- Structural "solid" autologous cartilaginous grafts sutured in place.

Figure 12.10 can be seen as a characteristic and fairly frequent example of this reconstructive work divided into five points:

- A—Two polydioxanone (5–0 PDS® II, Ethicon) stitches reconstruct the columella width and incorporate, between the medial crura, the posterior portion of the columellar strut (columellar sutures).
- B—A columellar strut is fixed in place and shaped in order to remain a little posterior and superior with respect to the middle crura and dome profiles.
- C—A polydioxanone (5–0 PDS® II, Ethicon) stitch reconstructs the interdomal ligaments, maintains the divergence between the two domes with a posterior contact point and also maintains them at the same height (domal equalization suture).

- D—A bilateral polydioxanone (5–0 PDS II®, Ethicon) horizontal mattress suture creates the domal definition (domal creation suture).
- E—An inferior polydioxanone (5–0 PDS® II, Ethicon) stitch and two or three superior poliglecaprone (5–0 Monocryl® II, Ethicon) stitches fold the bilateral spreader flaps and suture them to the septum, reconstructing the integrity of the cartilaginous dorsum (horizontal mattress sutures).

The combination of all these reconstructive steps should ensure an adequate and stable bilateral airway patency and a pleasant external esthetic nasal shape.

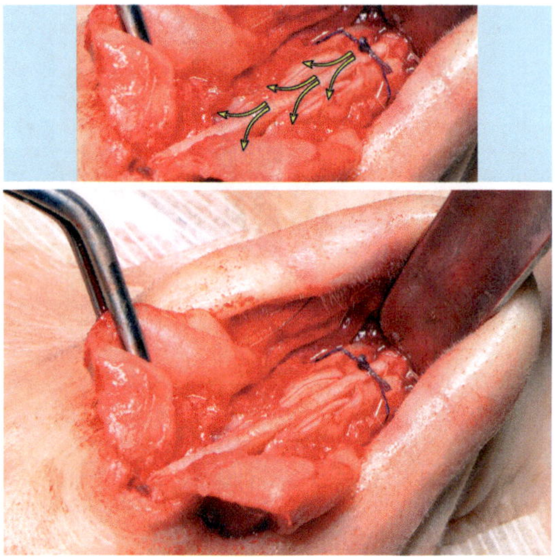

Fig. 12.9 Conservative dorsal reconstruction after osteotomies. The triangular cartilage excess is folded inward (curved arrows) and sutured to the septum (spreader flap). Also the two nasal bones are sutured to the cartilaginous septum to further stabilize the new nasal dorsum

12.5 Finishing Steps

Final refinements, although not always necessary, represent an important moment in rhinoplasty. Some of these micro-adjustments are made just before starting to suture the incisions. Sometimes, however, further refinements can be done later and take advantage of the fact that the suture of the incisions "close" the nose and permit another visual and tactile analysis step.

So, the BOR discipline requires that the surgeon be prepared for these final optional steps.

A typical example is the need only to increase the nasal tip projection. This is often a variation of less than 1 mm. Figure 12.11 shows how this little increment of tip projection can be obtained with a small quantity of autologous cartilage reduced in such fine pieces as to obtain a "cartilage gel" that can be inserted under the skin with a syringe.

Fig. 12.10 Intraoperative view of final nasal framework reconstruction (see text)

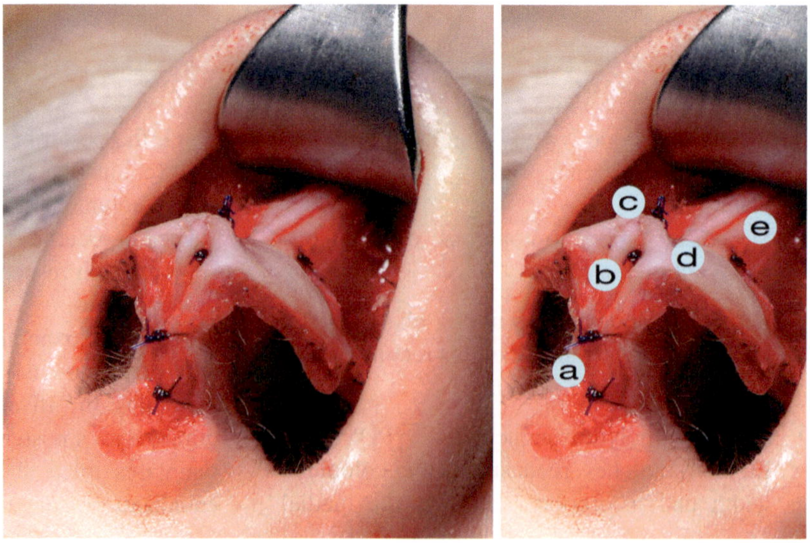

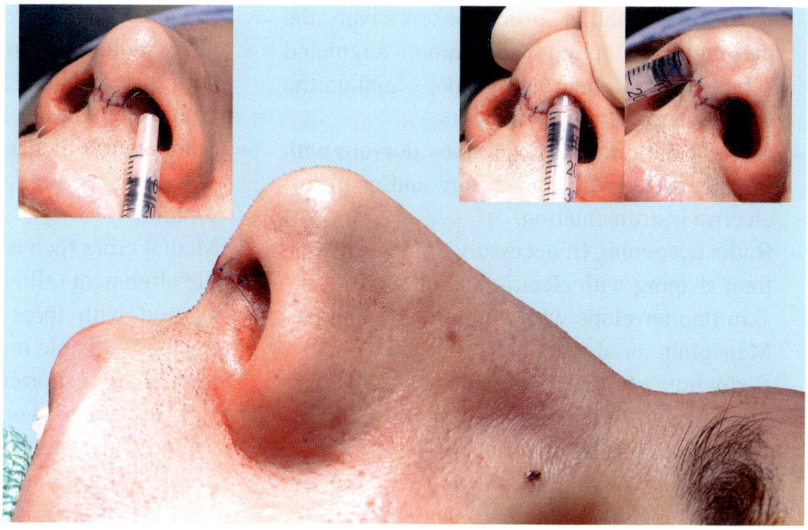

Fig. 12.11 Final nasal tip shape adjustment with "cartilage gel"

12.6 The BOR Sequence

In the following chapters, the complete BOR sequence will be described and illustrated with clinical examples. Although many variables and limitations need to be addressed on an individual basis, the following list provides a fairly faithful summary:

- Incision sequence: inverted "V" → marginal right → marginal left.
- Tip skeletonization: columella → domes → lateral crus (laterally limited or extended in the case of subsequent bone surgery with piezoelectric instrumentation).
- Tip skin flap control → conservative defatting of the tip and supratip undersurface (depending on needs).
- Dorsum skeletonization (laterally limited or extended in the case of subsequent bone surgery with piezoelectric instrumentation).
- Holding the skin flap with the Meneghini self-retained nasal retractor, irrigation and cleaning of the surgical field.
- Septal skeletonization: septal cartilage → inferior and posterior bony septum (depending on the.
- depth of the deformity that needs resection).
- Creation of a small bilateral tunnel of elevated mucosa under the junction between the upper lateral cartilages and the dorsal margin of the cartilaginous septum (preserving an intact nasal mucosa).
- Separation of the upper lateral cartilages from the septum (with a 15c blade) maintains intact the underlying nasal mucosa.
- First review of the surgical treatment plan based on the bony and cartilaginous deformities encountered.
- Depressor septi muscle work utilizing fine-needle-tip electrocautery (preferably with a nasal approach).
- Septal work, part I: submucous resection of the deviated posterior (septal spur) and inferior (overlapping redundant maxillary portion of the septal cartilage) components.
- Obtaining the "swinging door"-type free movement of the cartilage with respect to the nasal crest of the maxilla.
- Removing residual septal bony spur and maxillary crest deviation (preferably with piezoelectric instrumentation).
- Conservative inferior turbinate work.
- Anterior nasal spine work: midline repositioning with osteotomy, shaping by remodeling or resection with piezoelectric instrumentation.
- Dorsal work, part I: dorsal hump reduction: removal of the horizontal portion of the nasal bones (bony cap) preferably with piezoelec-

tric instrumentation → cut conservatively the cartilaginous septum with Fomon angulated septal scissors or surgical blade. Maintain the upper lateral cartilages intact.
- Incremental refining of the bony dorsum with rasp or better with power burr and/or piezoelectric instrumentation.
- Radix deepening (if necessary) and nasal bone final shaping with electric burr protecting the skin flap envelope with a modified Maliniac-Meneghini nasal retractor.
- Reduction of transverse dimension of large bony vault preferably with piezoelectric instrumentation (if necessary).
- Septal work, part II: harvesting cartilage for grafting maintaining an L-shaped strut for dorsal and columellar support.
- Straightening the dorsal septum with scoring of the concave side of the deviation plus unilateral or bilateral spreader graft (if necessary).
- Suture fixation of the cartilaginous septum to the anterior nasal spine.
- Caudal septal elongation with septal extension graft (if necessary).
- Quilting suture of the septal mucosa.
- Temporary bilateral anterior nasal packing with Merocel soaked with tranexamic acid solution.
- Osteotomies of bony nasal walls preferably with piezoelectric instrumentation.
- Dorsal work, part II. Reconstruct the cartilaginous dorsum with one of the following three options: (1) lowering the upper lateral cartilages by trimming the excess and suturing them to the new margin of septal cartilage with at least three 5/0 polydioxanone monofilament stitches; (2) in the case of previous placement of a spreader graft, lowering the upper lateral cartilages by trimming the excess and suturing them to either the spreader grafts or the new margin of septal cartilage with at least three 5/0 polydioxanone monofilament stitches; (3) rotating inward the excess of the upper lateral cartilages bilaterally realizing a so-called "autospreader flap" and suturing them to the new margin of septal cartilage with at least three 5/0 polydioxanone monofilament stitches.
- Stabilization of nasal bone osteotomies with at least one simple suture to the cartilaginous septum.
- Medial crura reconstructive work: caudal profile alignment utilizing a long columellar strut sutured with three 5/0 polydioxanone synthetic absorbable monofilament stitches.
- Medial crura shortening (if necessary).
- Lateral crura work, part I: conservative cephalic excision (utilizing for support the Meneghini Delicate Alar Clamp) or reinforcement with a lateral crura turn-in flap.
- Lateral crura shortening by overlapping (if necessary).
- Middle crura work, part I: tip sutures (interdomal, transdomal suture) utilizing a 5/0 polydioxanone monofilament.
- Lateral crura work, part II: lateral crura spanning suture and other sutures or grafts.
- Middle crura work, part II: visible graft (onlay tip graft, long shield graft) sutured with 5/0 polydioxanone and final "in place" refinements.
- Radix graft (if necessary).
- Dorsal work, part III: onlay grafting; solid cartilage piece sutured in place or crushed cartilage wrapped in Spongostan (if necessary).
- Autologous temporal fascia grafts (if necessary).
- Opening up an acute nasolabial angle with plumping graft (if necessary).
- Closure of the skin incisions with a 6/0 polypropylene monofilament or 6/0 polyglactin braided suture.
- Tip and dorsal final adjustment with cartilage gel moldable graft.
- Footplate work: excision and/or sutured together.
- Alar base work.
- Removal of bilateral packing (based on the presence of mucosal septal and turbinate tears

and the need to prolong the hemostatic effect of the packing).
- Nasal taping and splinting.

Further Reading

These books are classics for those who want to deepen the study of the various surgical steps as well as the general and specific guiding principles of open rhinoplasty. They are listed in order of citation in the chapter: Millard RM Jr. Principlization of plastic surgery. Boston: Little, Brown; 1986; Tebbetts JB. Primary Rhinoplasty. A new approach to the logic and the techniques. St. Louis: Mosby; 1998; Tebbetts JB. The next dimension: rethinking the logic, sequence and technique of Rhinoplasty. In: Dallas Rhinoplasty. Nasal surgery by the masters. St. Louis: Quality Medical; 2002. p. 219–49; Johnson CM, Toriumi DM. Open structure Rhinoplasty. WB Saunders: St. Louis; 1990; Johnson CM, To WC. A case approach to open structure Rhinoplasty. Philadelphia: Elsevier Saunders; 2005; Daniel RK. Rhinoplasty. An atlas of surgical techniques. New York: Springer; 2002.

13 Basic Open Rhinoplasty: Incisions and Skeletonization

The incisions and the subsequent skeletonization of the cartilage and bone nasal structures, in the great majority of rhinoplasty cases, must be carried out symmetrically and with extreme precision. Achievement of the correct dissection planes must be immediate and maintained throughout the operation. Any wrong gesture and any error in flap elevation can cause complications such as nasal stenosis, visible irregularities, and residual asymmetries.

The extent and depth of the dissection should be assessed in relation to the objectives of the individual treatment plan to avoid unnecessary trauma or loss of completeness of the intervention.

These initial exploratory phases of basic open rhinoplasty also aim to review the objectives of the intervention and deepen the preoperative studies without, however, making irreversible decisions such as the removal of cartilage or bone.

13.1 Columellar Skin Incision

Where to start the skin incision? Start laterally with one marginal incision, do the contralateral one and then leave the columellar sections last? Or do the opposite? Every surgeon has his preferences but logic suggests starting from the region that requires the greatest precision and accuracy: the central columellar incision. In this case the skin will not be distorted and the incision made by the blade will have a better chance of being perfect.

The objectives are to:

- Obtain a linear and perpendicular full skin incision.
- Avoid any damage to the caudal margin of the medial crus of the lower lateral cartilage.
- Create perfect skin angles of 60 to 90° to help later realignment and suture of the incision.

For nasal surgery the ideal blade configuration is a 15c blade mounted in a light elastic silicone-coated surgical handle (Fig. 13.4b). Compared to the other blades, the 15c has a shorter cutting edge (Fig. 13.1) and, if it is made to penetrate perpendicularly in the tissues, it produces a skin cut only 2.9 mm in length (Fig. 13.2a, b).

The 15c blade is used in oral surgery and is readily available on the market at low cost. The shape of the cutting end varies a little depending on the manufacturer (Fig. 13.3) but its small size and the semi-pointed tip are safe and advisable for nasal surgery.

Figure 13.4a shows how the width of the 15c surgical blade is proportionate to the dimension of Goodman's inverted "V" columellar incision.

For the same tract of skin incision, the blade number 15 has too wide a shape and the depth of skin incision could be too superficial or, with an exaggerated penetration, too dangerous for the caudal margin of the lower lateral cartilage.

F. Meneghini, *Basic Open Rhinoplasty*, https://doi.org/10.1007/978-3-030-61827-8_13

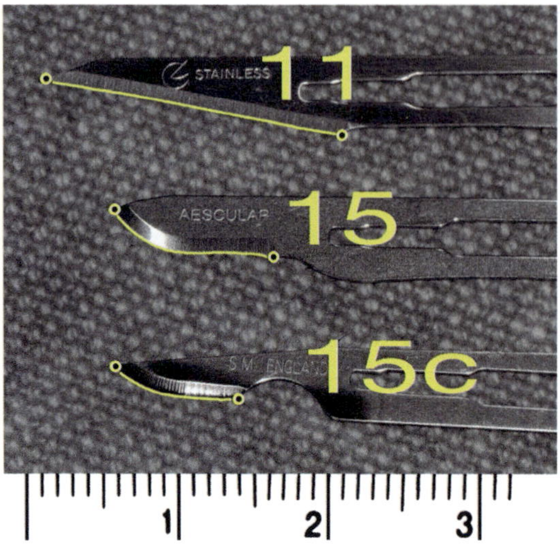

Fig. 13.1 Comparison between different types of surgical blades. The 15c blade has a shorter cutting edge, ideal for nasal surgery

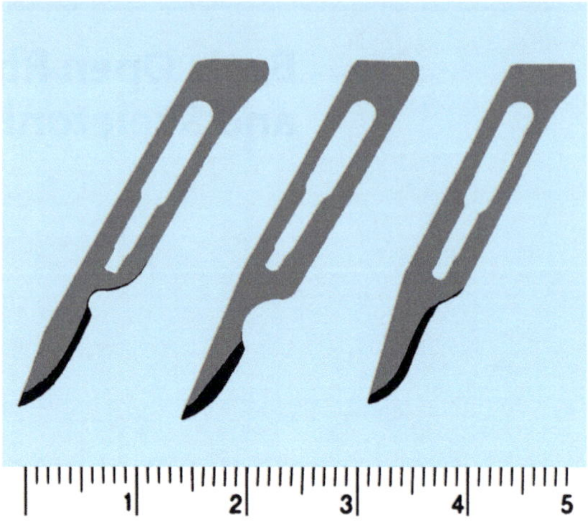

Fig. 13.3 Comparison of 15c surgical blades from different manufacturers

Fig. 13.2 (**a**, **b**) Comparison between different types of surgical blades. The 15 blade (**a**) is wider than the 15c (**b**)

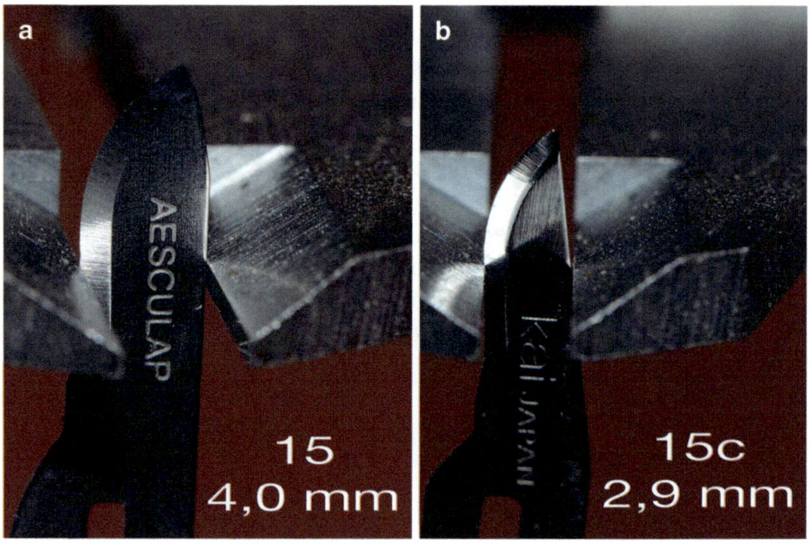

An alternative, if the 15c blade is not available, is to use a blade 11 wrapped with a Steri-Strip, leaving only the tip exposed by 3 or 4 mm, as shown in Fig. 13.5.

Figure 13.6 shows how the index and thumb of the non-dominant hand grasp the columella, stabilizing its position. The blade penetrates perpendicularly, going from laterally to medially, until it "fills" the entire right line of the inverted "V" incision. In this way the risks of cartilage damage are reduced and the cutting depth is adequate. Immediately after that, the left incision is performed (Fig. 13.7).

The lateral horizontal right and left incisions are then performed taking care to maintain a

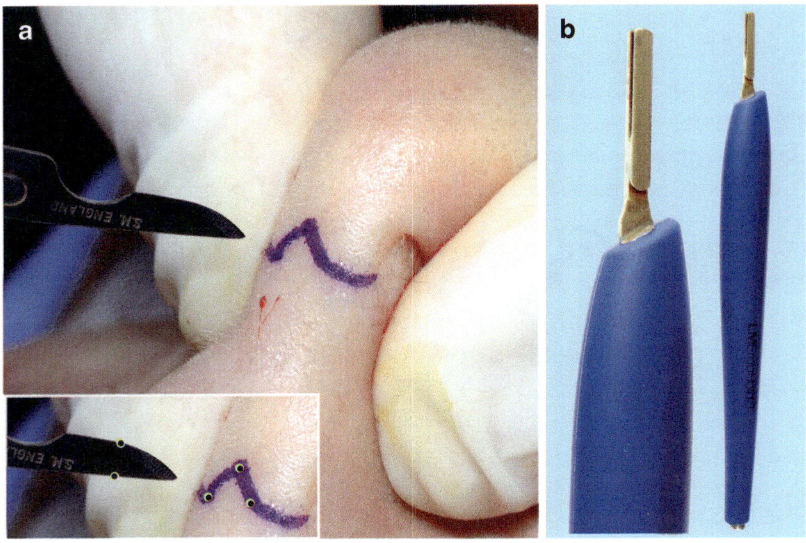

Fig. 13.4 (**a**, **b**) The width of the 15c surgical blade is proportionate to the dimension of Goodman's inverted "V" columellar incision (**a**). Light elastic silicone-coated surgical handle (**b**)

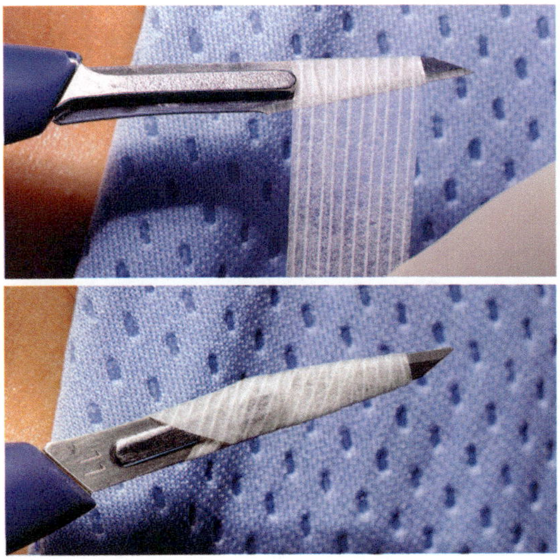

Fig. 13.5 A number 11 surgical blade wrapped with a Steri-Strip, leaving only the tip exposed by 3 or 4 mm, can be used as an alternative to the 15c surgical blade

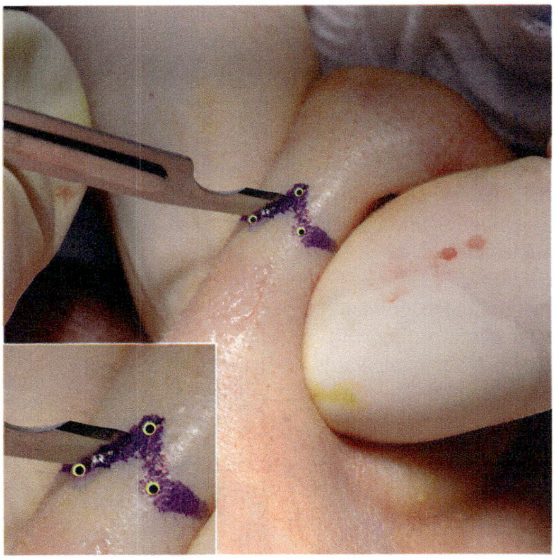

Fig. 13.6 Goodman's inverted "V" columellar incision. The index and thumb of the non-dominant hand grasp the columella, stabilizing its position, while the blade penetrates perpendicularly, going from laterally to medially, until it "fills" the entire right line of the inverted "V" incision

superficial plane. Sometimes, in the case of very thin skin, the scalpel blade is held facing outwards to avoid unwanted penetration into the cartilage (Fig. 13.8).

For safety, also the junction 90-degree angle between the columellar and marginal incisions can be made with the blade face up (Fig. 13.9a–c). The connection between the two incisions is only started due to the risk of not following exactly the cartilage margin.

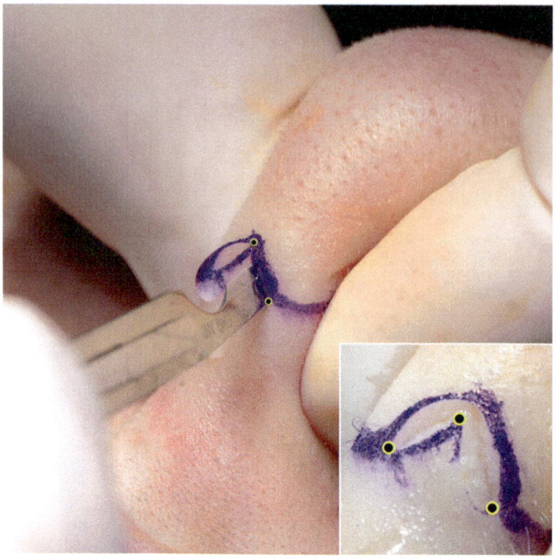

Fig. 13.7 Goodman's inverted "V" columellar incision. Symmetrical left line incision

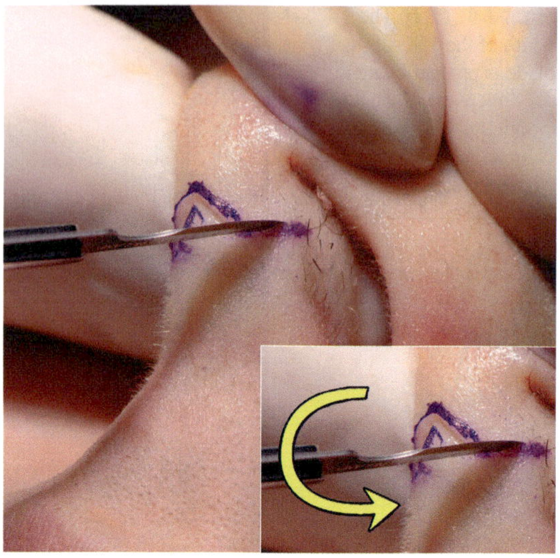

Fig. 13.8 Goodman's inverted "V" columellar incision. Lateral horizontal right left incision. The scalpel blade is held facing outwards to avoid unwanted penetration into the underlying cartilage (rounded arrow)

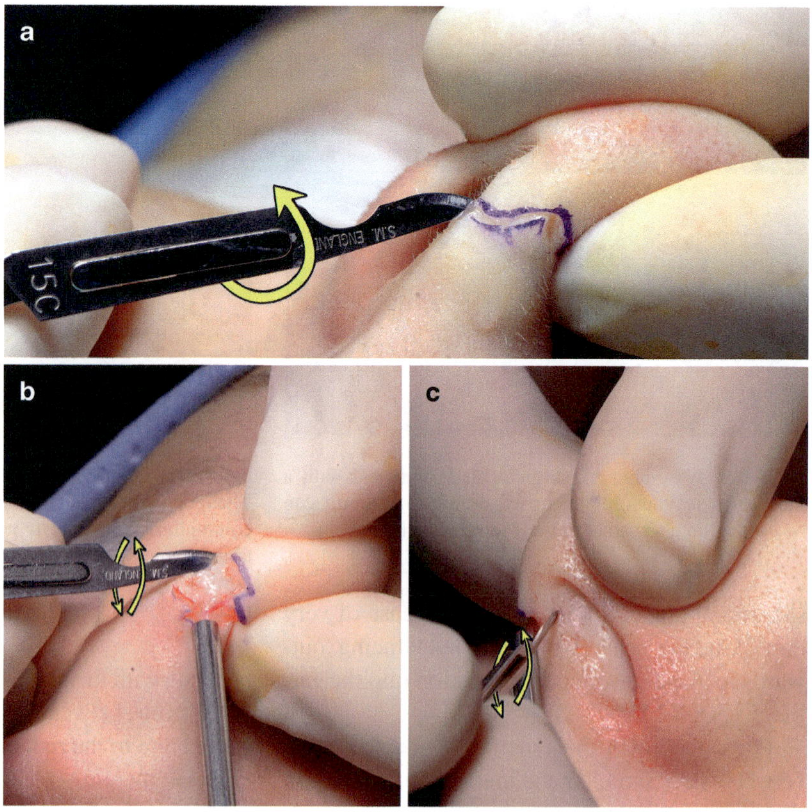

Fig. 13.9 (**a**–**c**) Goodman's inverted "V" (**a**) and stairstep columellar incisions (**b**). The junction 90-degree angle between the columellar and the marginal incisions can be made for safety with the blade facing upwards

13.2 Finishing the Columellar Skin Incision

The columellar incision is then perfected with the aid of small Converse scissors (Fig. 13.10). This instrument is invaluable in finding the right dissection plane by keeping the inclined tips of the instrument always directed in depth.

The index and thumb of the non-dominant hand hold and stabilize the columella in the proper position and the scissors create, with a delicate pressure from lateral to medial and limited spreading movements, a tunnel over the cartilage and under the horizontal portion of the columellar incision (Fig. 13.11a, b).

Figure 13.11c shows the tunnel, whereas Fig. 13.11d shows the soft tissue cut, performed maintaining the scissor blades perpendicular to the skin plane.

At this point, the simple pressure of the index and thumb diverge the skin margins (Fig. 13.12). Frequently a little bleeding from the columellar arteries at the inferior margin of the incision needs to be coagulated. The electrosurgical unit is adjusted to 15 on a scale of 100 and the ends of the small vessels are grasped with a fine-tip Micro Adson forceps or similar instrument (Fig. 13.13). Electrocoagulation on the superior margin and to the skin flap must be avoided.

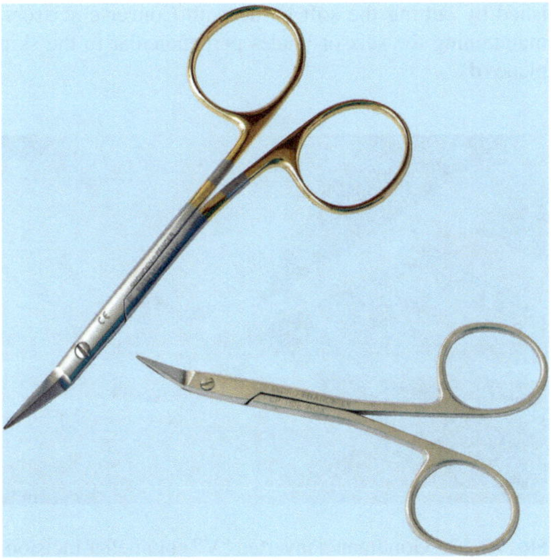

Fig. 13.10 Converse scissors

13.3 Initial Flap Elevation

To reduce total surgical time, a good rule is to change the instrument you are using as little as possible. D. Ralph Millard was interested in this aspect: "Speed in surgery is not frantic, jerky action but sure, steady progress and efficiency of never having to repeat the same thing twice."[1]

With the same Converse scissors used so far it is possible to carry out a delicate and safe detachment of the columellar soft tissues from the cartilage. Holding the scissors with the tips closed and adhering to the cartilage, it is possible to lift the flap at full thickness. Only the perichondrium remains adherent to the cartilage. The lifting movements are delicate and directed upwards (Fig. 13.14).

The columellar flap is then supported by the surgeon's assistant with a delicate double hook applied centrally in the subcutaneous tissues (Fig. 13.15).

An important general rule: in all surgical phases much attention must be paid not to apply the hooks directly to the cartilaginous structures due to the risk of tearing them.

The flap elevation continues superiorly with the aid of Converse scissors, or other fine-tip scissors, and a micro Adson tissue forceps. Figure 13.16 shows how the tips of the scissors, with small spreading movements, elevate the flap close to the medial crus of the left lower lateral cartilage.

The skin incision is performed with small scissor bites only when the cartilage margin is clearly visible; Fig. 13.17 shows the intact margins of the cartilages, marked with two dotted lines, during right flap elevation.

[1]Millard DR Jr. Principle 18: Invoke a Scot's Economy. In: Principlization of Plastic Surgery. Boston/Toronto: Little, Brown and Company; 1986. p. 275.

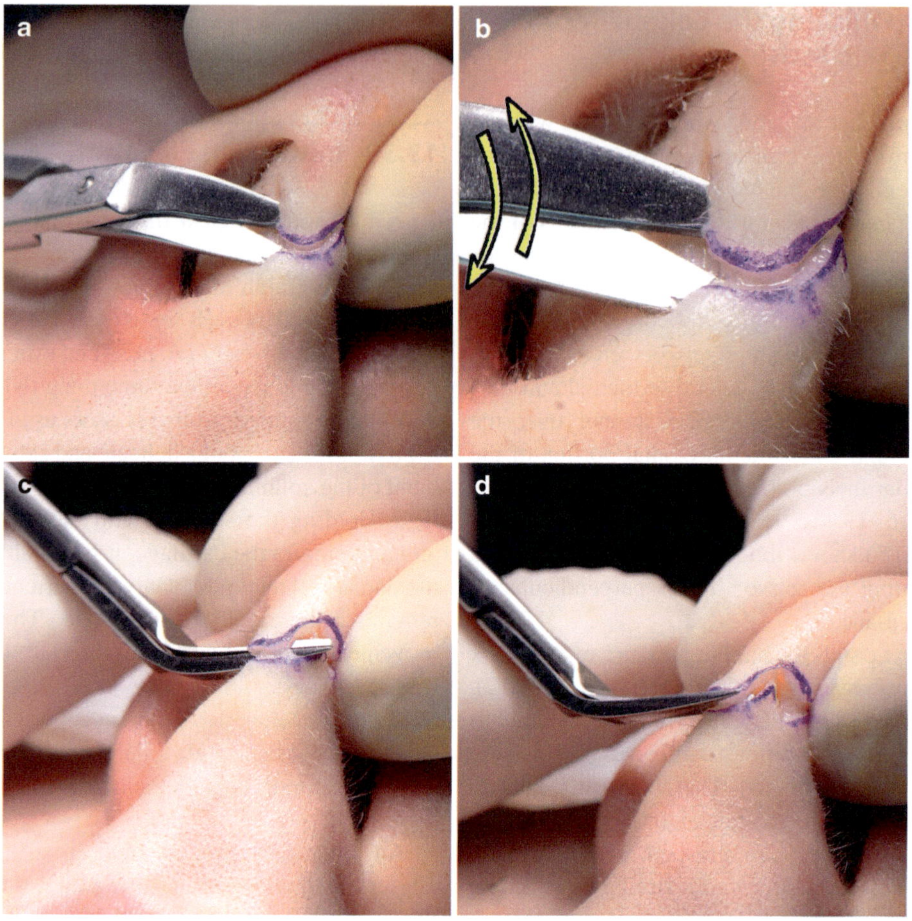

Fig. 13.11 (**a**–**d**) Goodman's inverted "V" columellar incision. Small tunnel creations over the cartilage and under the skin envelope flap (**a**–**c**). The incision is finished by cutting the soft tissue with Converse scissors, maintaining the scissor blades perpendicular to the skin plane (**d**)

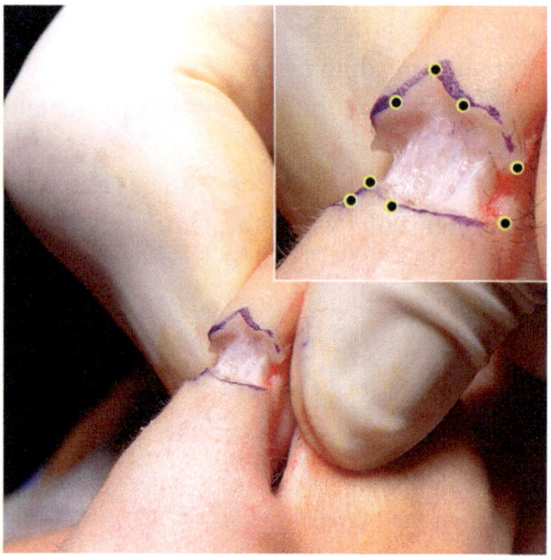

Fig. 13.12 Goodman's inverted "V" columellar incision. With simple pressure of the index and thumb the divergence of the skin margins is obtained

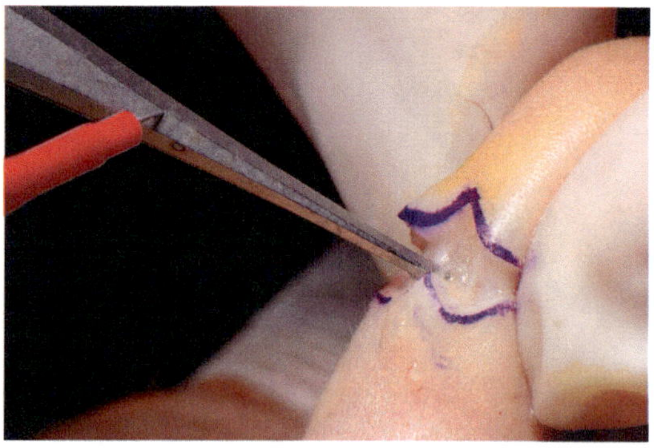

Fig. 13.13 Goodman's inverted "V" columellar incision. Electrocoagulation of the columellar arteries

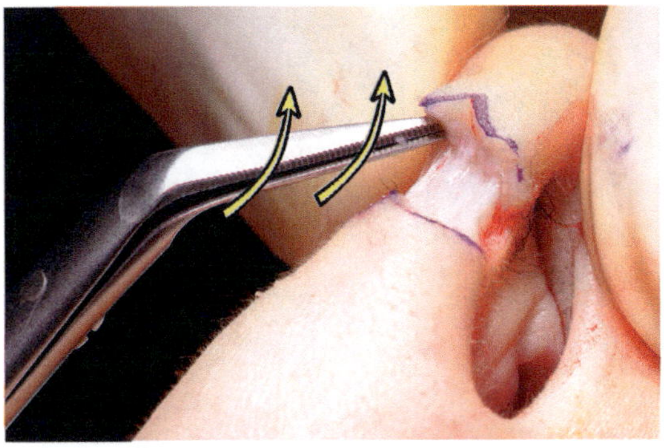

Fig. 13.14 Initial flap elevation. By holding the scissors with the tips closed and adhering to the cartilage, it is possible to lift the flap at full thickness

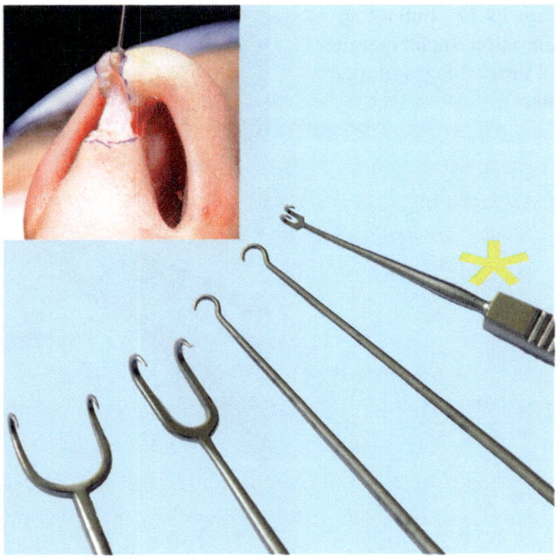

Fig. 13.15 Initial flap elevation. The columellar flap is supported by the surgeon's assistant with a delicate double hook applied centrally in the subcutaneous tissues

Fig. 13.16 The flap is elevated close to the medial crus of the left lower lateral cartilage with small spreading movements of the scissors tips

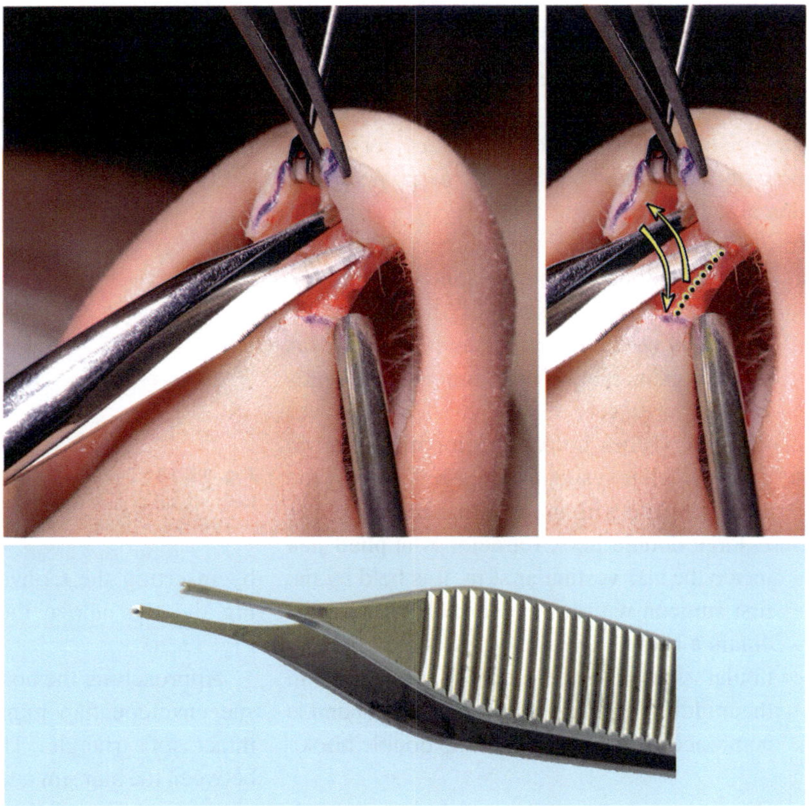

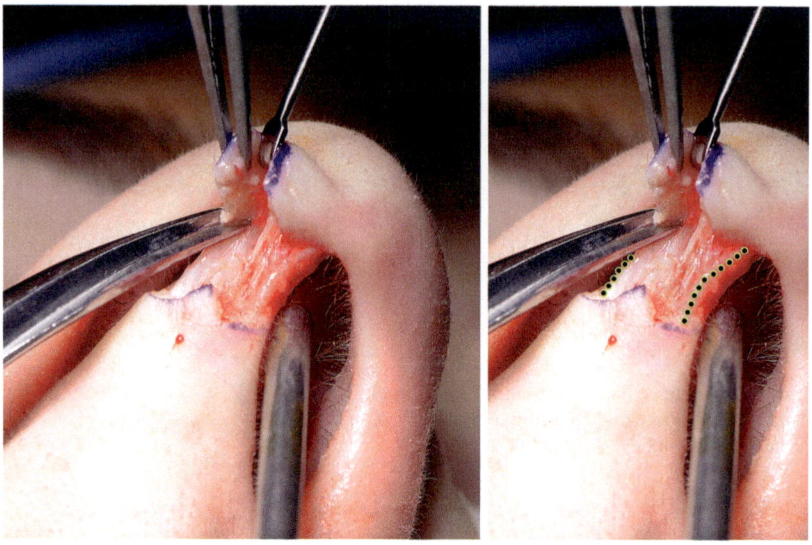

Fig. 13.17 Initial flap elevation. Intact margins of the cartilages (dotted lines)

13.4 Marginal Incision in the Domal Area

Before reaching the domal region it is necessary to tighten the lower lateral cartilage by adding two hooks. Figure 13.18 illustrates the so-called three-point countertraction technique for elevation of the skin/soft tissue envelope over the domal region:

1. A delicate double hook is applied centrally in the subcutaneous tissues of the columellar skin. It is held by the first assistant with his non-dominant hand. The dominant hand holds the suction tube.
2. A single Gillies hook retractor is applied in the columellar vestibular skin. It is held by the surgical nurse with the dominant hand.
3. A large double hook retractor is applied just inside the alar vestibular skin. It is held by the first surgeon with his non-dominant hand. To obtain a better exposure of the endonasal vestibular skin, a gentle external pressure with the middle finger of the non-dominant hand is combined with a rotation of the double hook.

Once again, before cutting the skin, the soft tissue attached to the intermediate crus is elevated close to the perichondrium (Fig. 13.19). To advance, it is necessary to create a small tunnel by inserting the Converse scissors and spreading the tips above the cartilage, as shown in Fig. 13.20.

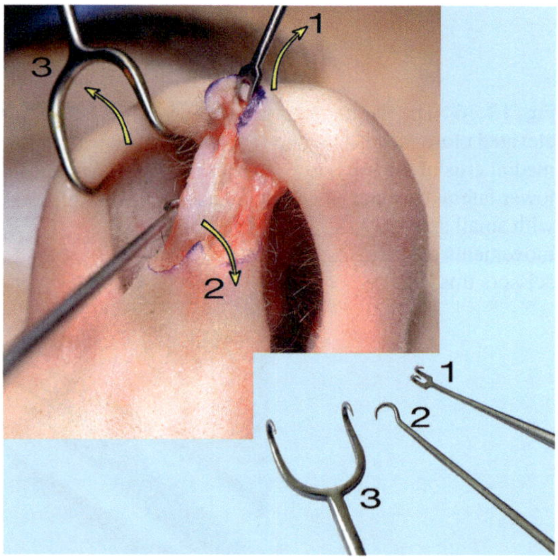

Fig. 13.18 The three-point countertraction technique to help visibility and dissection during flap elevation

Approaching the nostril apex, the skin/soft tissue envelope flap must include the whole and intact soft triangle. This is the thin skin fold between the alar rim and the curved caudal border of the junction of the medial and lateral crus. When this is well defined, it is referred to as a facet. No cartilage supports this extremely thin skin (Fig. 13.21).

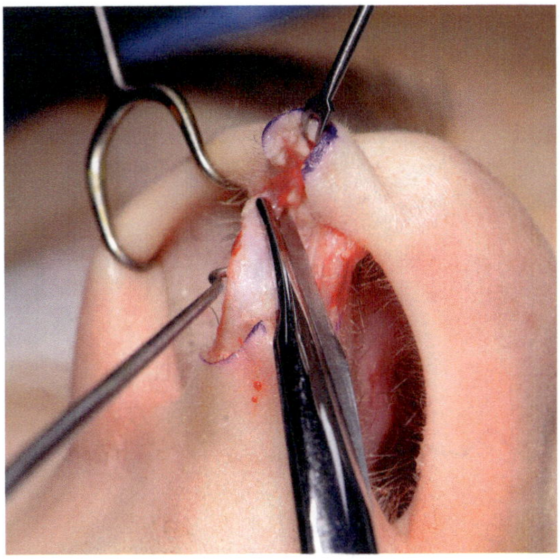

Fig. 13.19 Marginal incision in the domal area. Soft tissue elevation maintaining the scissors tips close to the perichondrium

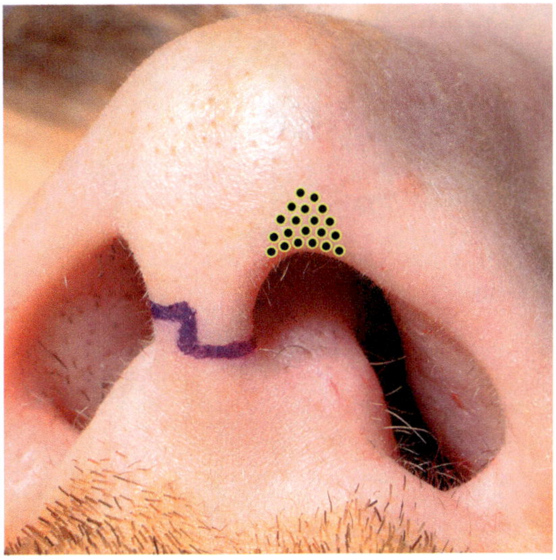

Fig. 13.21 Soft triangle (dotted area)

Fig. 13.20 Marginal incision in the domal area. To further elevate the flap it is necessary to create small tunnels by inserting the Converse scissors and spreading the tips above the cartilage

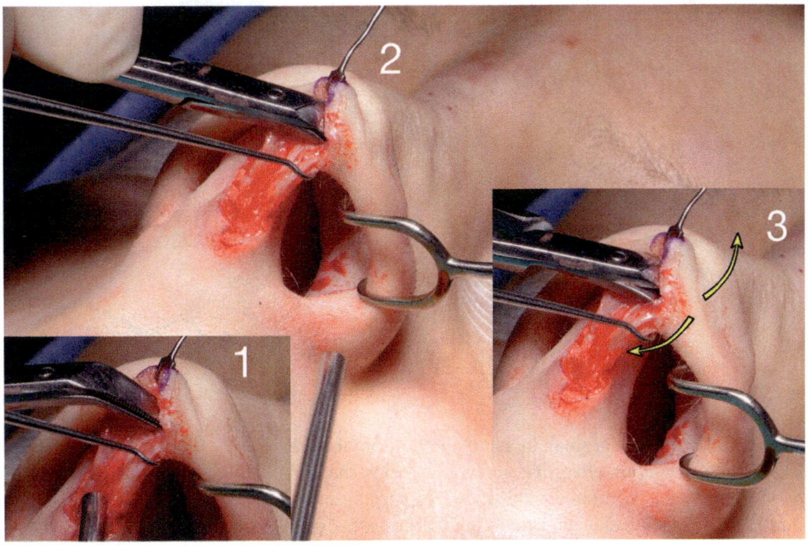

The three-point countertraction technique helps the surgeon to identify the vestibular skin of the soft triangle and direct the elevation only over the cartilage (Fig. 13.22a, b). The incision is then performed safely between the cartilage margin and the soft triangle maintaining the scissor blades perpendicular to the skin (Fig. 13.22c, d).

13.5 Finishing the Marginal Incision and Lower Lateral Dissection

To obtain the best aid from the three-point countertraction technique, the single Gillies hook retractor can be frequently changed in position

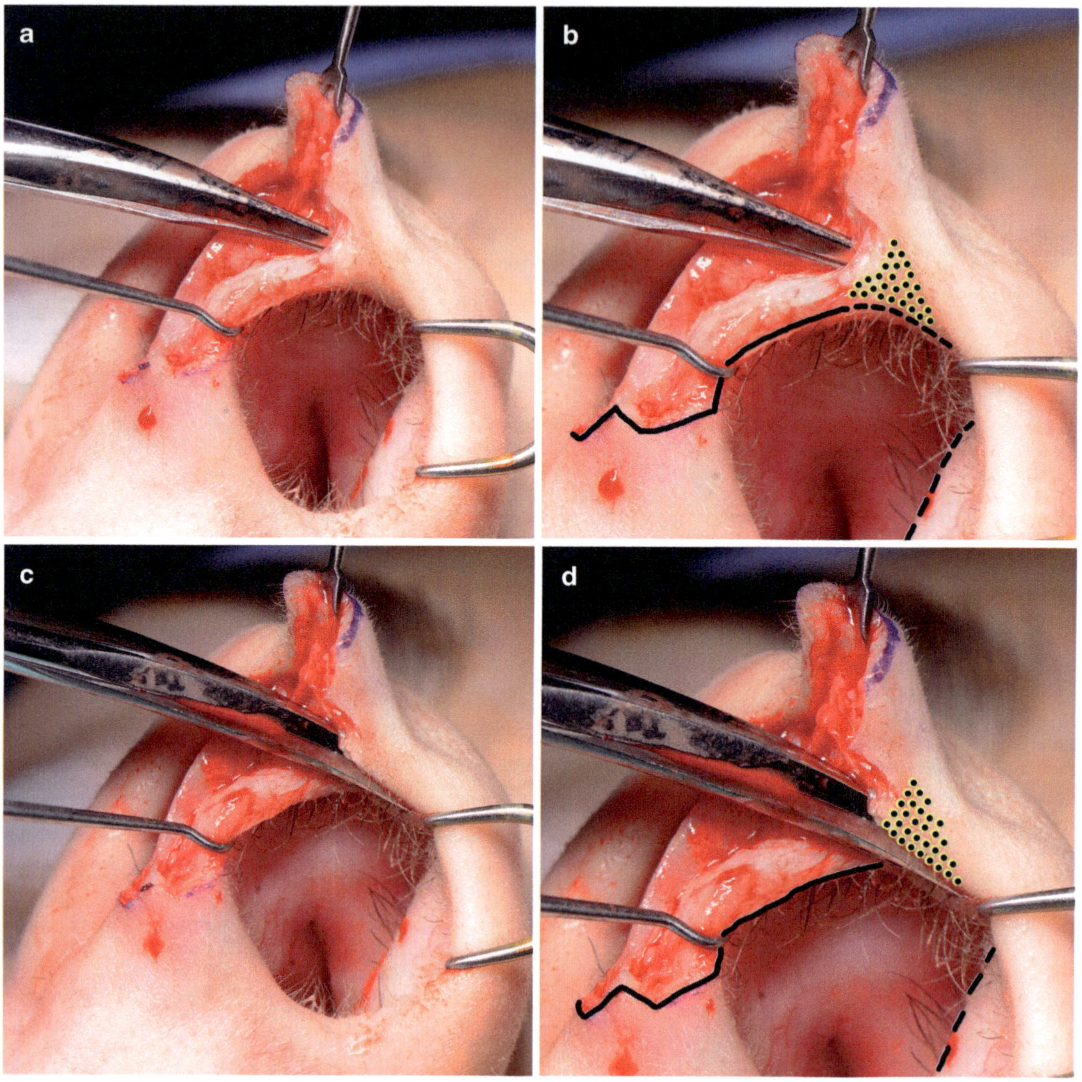

Fig. 13.22 (**a**–**d**) Marginal incision in the domal area. The three-point countertraction technique helps the surgeon identify the vestibular skin of the soft triangle and direct the soft tissue elevation maintaining the tunnel only over the cartilage (**a**, **b**). The incision is then performed safely between the cartilage margin and the soft triangle maintaining the scissor blades perpendicular to the skin (**c**, **d**)

and vector of traction. The other two hooks instead remain in their initial positions.

Approaching the lateral portion of marginal incision, the single Gillies hook retractor is placed in the vestibular skin just under the dome and, with the aid of gentle traction, the margin of the lateral crus becomes evident under the skin as shown by the dotted line of Fig. 13.23.

With some individual variation, the inferior margin of the lateral crus becomes divergent from the lateral margin of the nostril. The lateral skin incision line must follow the cartilage profile and not the nostril. It is performed with the 15c blade or, better, with pointed scissors such as the Converse scissors.

As a general rule, during nasal surgery we elevate the skin and mucosa flaps over three cartilages: the lower lateral, the upper lateral, and the septal cartilage. In every case the difficult and time demanding phase is the starting one.

A pointed instrument should be used initially to find the correct avascular anatomical plane with delicate scratching movements. This instrument should be inclined at 20–30° relative to the cartilage surface (Fig. 13.24a–c).

Complete exposure of the lateral crus may be obtained with a small double-ended elevator, such as a Freer or a Tebbetts elevator (Fig. 13.25) or a sterile cotton-tip applicator pushed in the deep areolar plane below the muscle and over the perichondrium (Fig. 13.26). The selection of the

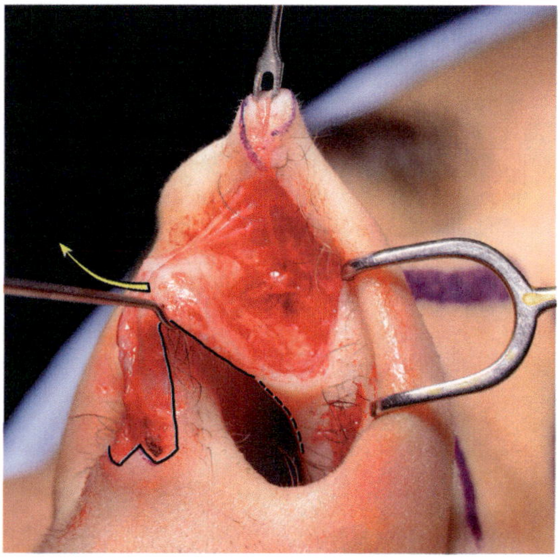

Fig. 13.23 Lateral portion of marginal incision. The Gillies single hook is positioned just under the dome and, with the aid of gentle traction, the margin of the lateral crus becomes evident under the skin (dotted line)

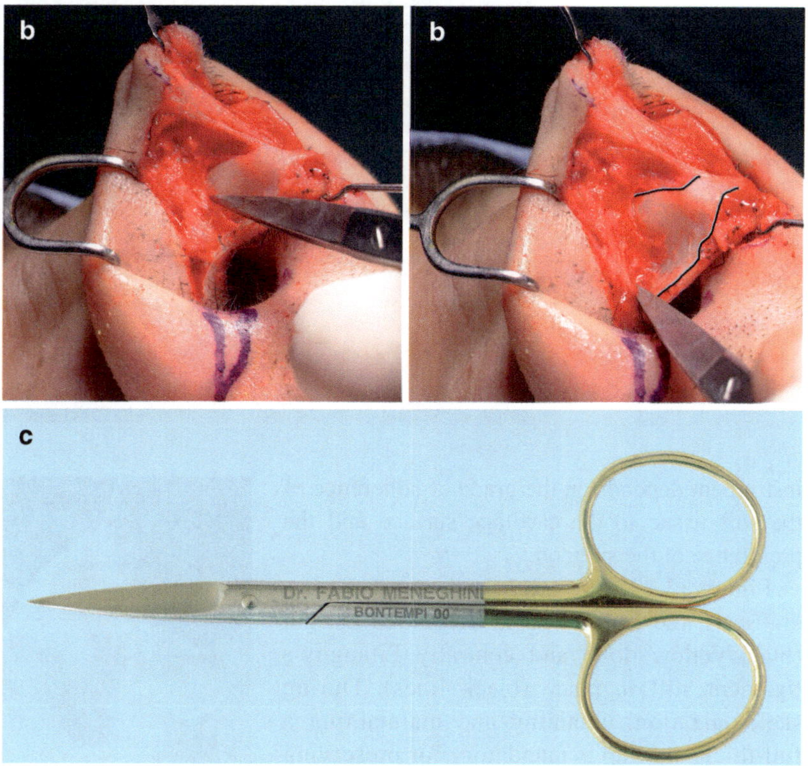

Fig. 13.24 (**a–c**) Pointed scissors (**c**) can be used initially to find the correct avascular anatomical plane and to elevate the flap over the lateral crura

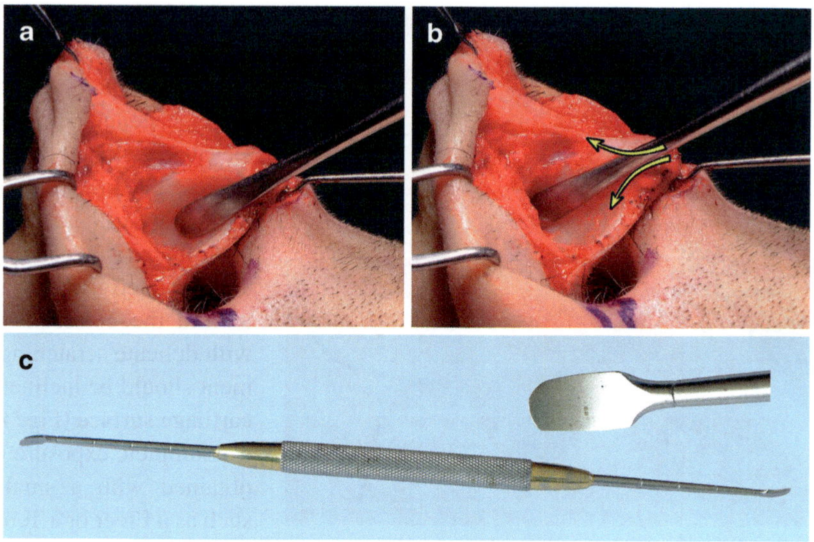

Fig. 13.25 (**a**–**c**) Complete exposure of the lateral crus may be obtained with a small double-ended elevator such as a Freer or Tebbetts elevator (**c**)

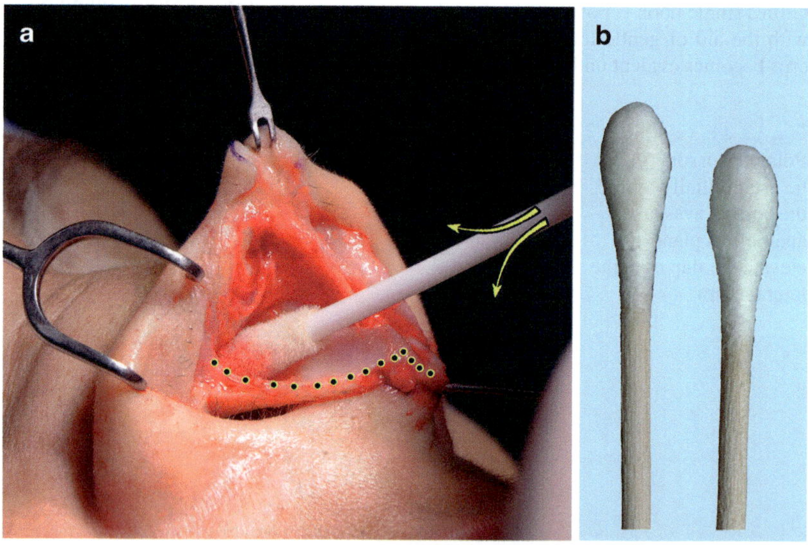

Fig. 13.26 (**a**, **b**) Complete exposure of the lateral crus over the correct avascular plane may also be obtained with a sterile cotton-tip applicator (**b**)

instrument depends on the grade of adherence of the soft tissue to the cartilage surface and the preference of the surgeon.

Figure 13.27 shows the exposure of the lateral crus, the free lower cartilaginous margin (black/yellow dots) and centrally Pitanguy's ligament still in place (black lines). During skeletonization, obtaining and maintaining a full-thickness flap is mandatory for preserving intact the vascular and muscular structures of the nasal tip.

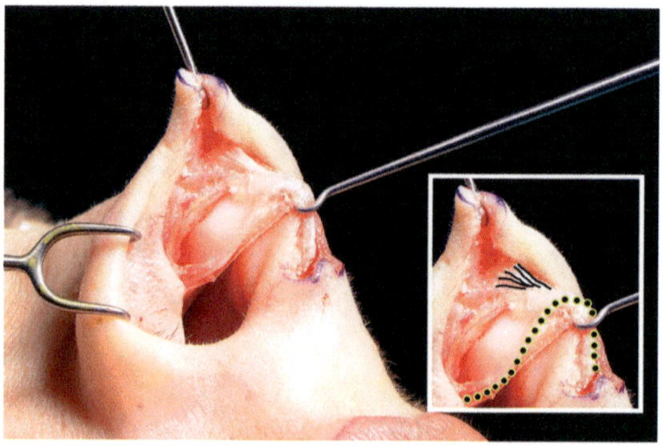

Fig. 13.27 Complete exposure of the lateral crus. Centrally Pitanguy's ligament is still in place (black lines)

13.6 Dealing with the Ligaments of the Nasal Tip

The previous steps of lateral flap elevation permit a clear preservation of the ligaments comprised between the medial crus and domes of the lower lateral cartilage. Clinically, at this stage, they appear as whitish fibers as shown in Fig. 13.28.

The surgical logic of BOR suggests maintaining all these tissues attached to the nasal tip skin by elevating the skin envelope flap towards the anterior septal angle at the deepest plane (Fig. 13.29). Once the tissue is well isolated from the cartilage, it is cut in its deepest part (Fig. 13.30). Later, during surgery, the posterior part of these ligaments can be removed or sutured to the cartilaginous dorsum to reduce the supratip dead space.

13.7 Midline and Lateral Dorsal Dissection

Approaching the dorsum, the surgeon's assistant holds the flap with a small retractor such as the double-ended Kasdan hand retractor and, if necessary, pushes inferiorly the two lower lateral cartilages with a large double hook (Fig. 13.31). Again, it is necessary to immediately reach the deep plane just above the perichondrium. To do this, Converse scissors should be used, pushing the closed pointed ends towards the dorsal cartilage and then opening them a little. These maneuvers should be done until a shiny and blue surface is seen that indicates that the right plan of dissection has been achieved (Fig. 13.32a).

The enlargement of the midline tunnel is continued with the Converse scissors, over the cartilaginous dorsum (Fig. 13.32b), and with the Obwegeser Periosteal elevator over the nasal bones. This instrument should be inclined 20–30°

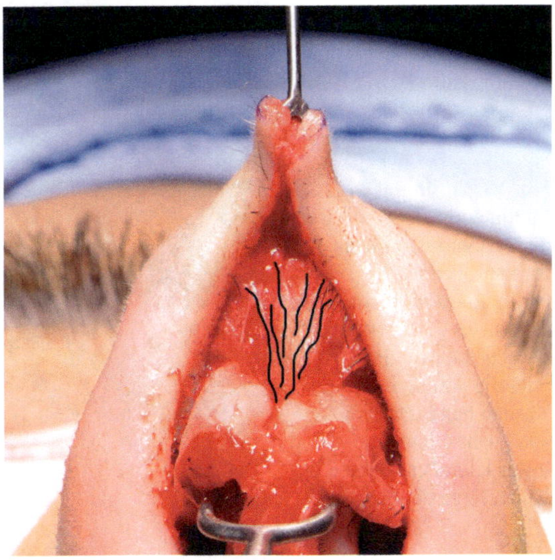

Fig. 13.29 Pitanguy's ligament

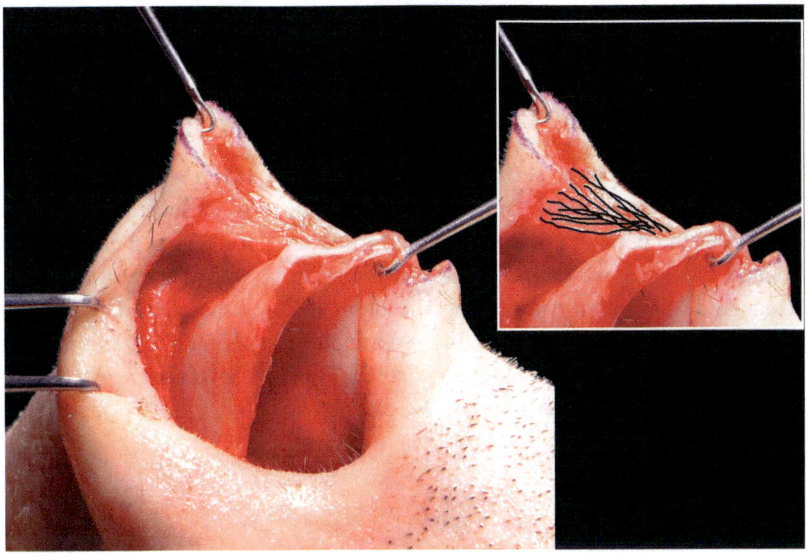

Fig. 13.28 Pitanguy's ligament

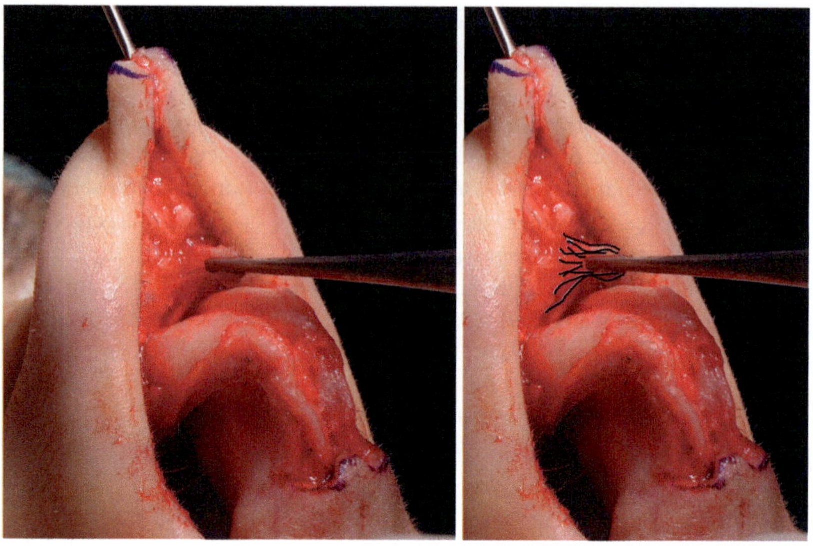

Fig. 13.30 Pitanguy's ligament after releasing its deepest part. Later, during surgery, the ligament can be removed or sutured to the cartilaginous dorsum to reduce the supratip dead space

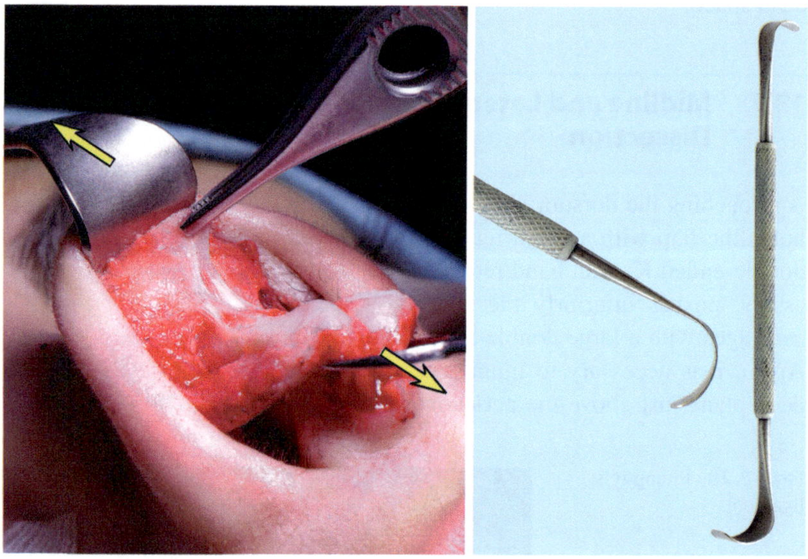

Fig. 13.31 Initial midline dorsal dissection: instruments for approaching the cartilaginous dorsum. The surgeon's assistant retracts the skin flap with the double-ended Kasdan hand retractor and pushes down the lower lateral cartilage with a large double hook

with respect to the bone surface (Fig. 13.33) and, with upward and lateral small movements the flap under the periosteum is dissected. For better control, the index and thumb of the non-dominant hand guide the instrument during the blunt dissection over the dorsum (Fig. 13.34). Approaching the junction between the triangular cartilages and the nasal bones (K-area) special care should be taken with the elevator. The junction normally is solid and resistant to penetration with the elevator between cartilage and bone.

The superior and lateral extents of the dorsal dissection depend on the treatment plan and should be monitored precisely by slowing the movements with the Obwegeser Periosteal elevator (Fig. 13.35a, b). If reduction of the nasal radix

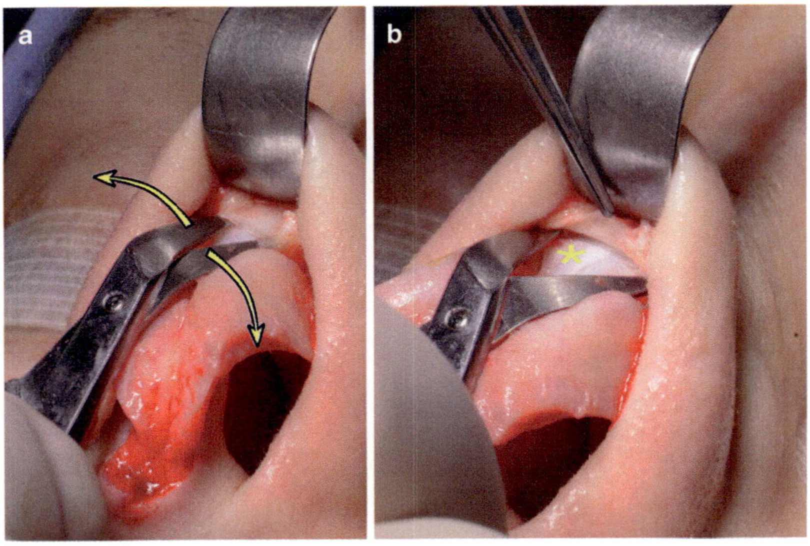

Fig. 13.32 (**a**, **b**) Initial midline dorsal dissection: pushing the closed pointed ends of the Converse scissors towards the dorsal cartilage and then opening them a little, spreading the tissue until the deep plane is reached (**a**). The enlargement of the midline tunnel is continued with the Converse scissors, over the cartilaginous dorsum (asterisk in **b**)

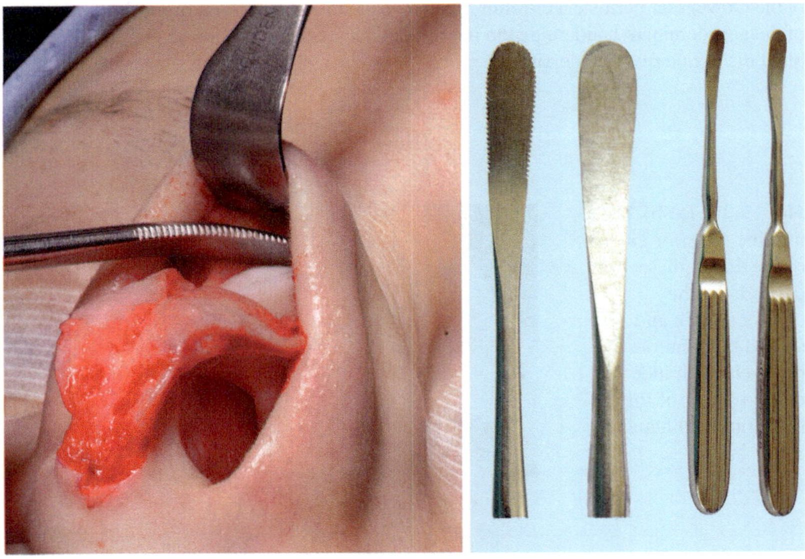

Fig. 13.33 The midline dorsal dissection is continued over the nasal bones with the Obwegeser periosteal elevator

is necessary, a large subperiosteal dissection must be performed superiorly and bilaterally to allow perfect exposure of the bony area to be modeled (Fig. 13.36a). In the opposite case, when a radix graft is planned, a small, precise, central subperiosteal pocket should be created in order to minimize the risk of graft displacement (Fig. 13.36b).

Frequently, at this step, the extent of dissection over the upper lateral cartilage is assessed under direct vision and limited laterally on the basis of the planned dorsal reduction. Figure 13.37a shows the extended flap elevation needed if a large nasal hump is to be removed, whereas Fig. 13.37b shows the limited flap elevation necessary if a minor reduction or augmentation of dorsal profile is required.

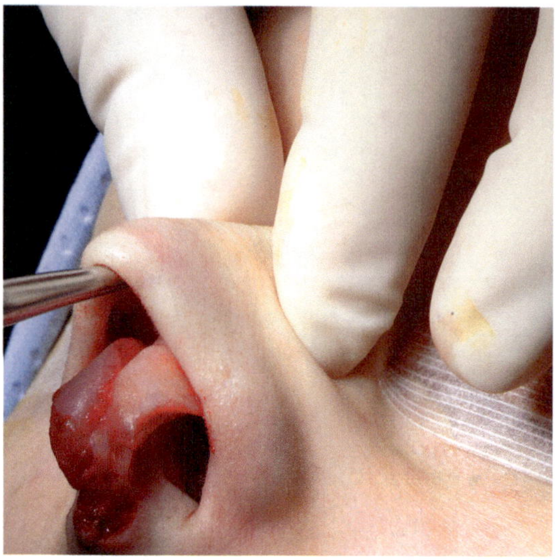

Fig. 13.34 Midline dorsal dissection. For better control of the Obwegeser periosteal elevator, the index and thumb of the non-dominant hand guide the instrument during the blunt dissection over the dorsum

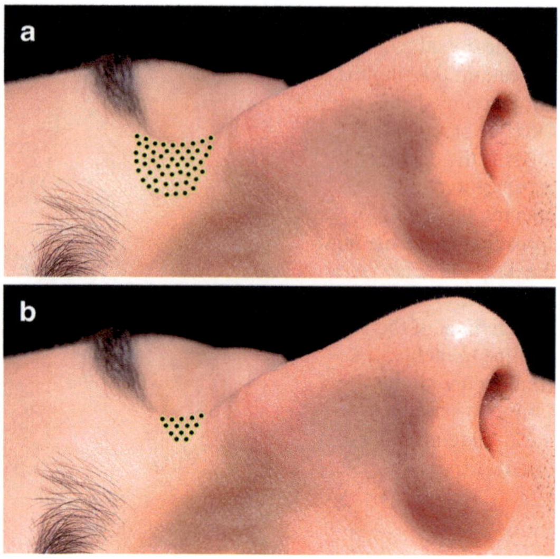

Fig. 13.36 (**a**, **b**) Radix area dissection. If dimensional reduction of the nasal radix is planned, a large subperiosteal dissection must be performed superiorly and bilaterally to allow perfect exposure of the bony area to be modeled (**a**). If a radix graft is planned, a small, precise, central subperiosteal pocket should be created in order to minimize the risk of graft displacement (**b**)

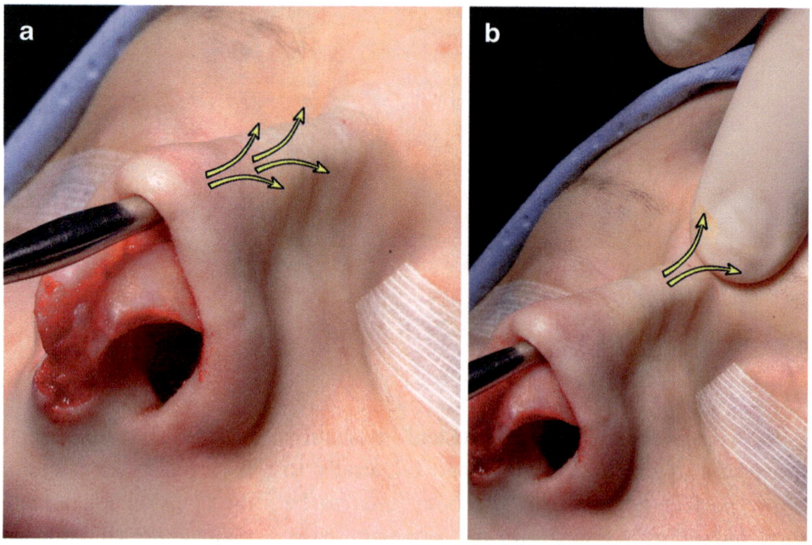

Fig. 13.35 (**a**, **b**) The midline superior extent of the dorsal dissection depends on the treatment plan and should be monitored precisely with index or middle finger of the non-dominant hand (**b**)

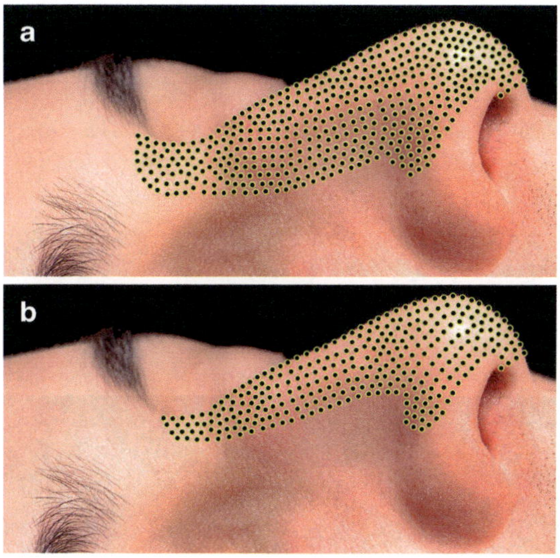

Fig. 13.37 (**a**, **b**) Lateral dorsal dissection planning. Extended flap elevation in the case of a large nasal hump (**a**) and limited flap elevation in the case of minor reduction or augmentation of dorsal profile (**b**)

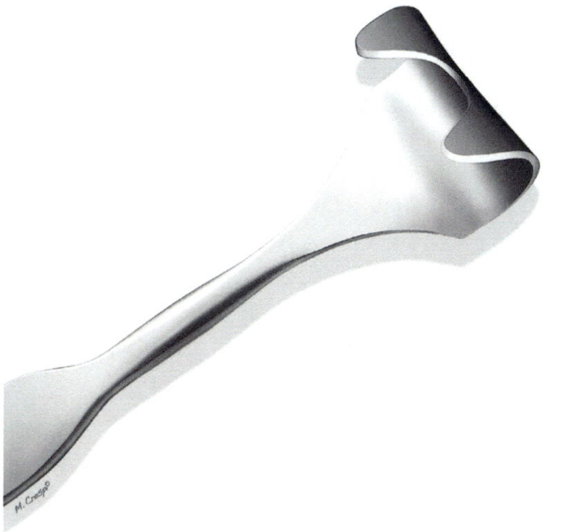

Fig. 13.38 Meneghini nasal skin retractor (MNSR). The instrument has two rounded, tapered edges with a grooved, concave tip for stabilization against the nasal dorsum; it is specifically designed to expose completely the nasal tip and partially the cartilaginous dorsum

13.8 Approaching the Septum with the "Tip Split" Technique

Skeletonization of the cartilaginous and bony nasal septum represents the next surgical phase.

The first step is the retraction and protection of the nasal skin flap. For this purpose a specially designed instrument, such as the Meneghini nasal skin retractor (MNSR), can be used.

The creation of my nasal skin retractor for the "open approach" followed the experience I had with pre-existent instruments proposed by three worldwide renowned rhinoplasty surgeons: Ronald P. Gruber, Gilbert Aiach, and John B. Tebbetts. Subsequently, I spent 5 years developing and clinically testing three consecutive series of prototypes with the aim of obtaining a safer, self-retaining, easy-to-use, time-saving, stable, light, small, durable, and cheap instrument.

The MNSR has two rounded, tapered edges with a grooved concave tip for stabilization against the nasal dorsum; it is specifically designed to minimize nasal flap trauma embracing the skin and exposing completely the nasal tip and partially the cartilaginous dorsum (Fig. 13.38). The flat and smooth handle easily adapts to the patient's forehead avoiding rotation of the instrument (Fig. 13.39). When the

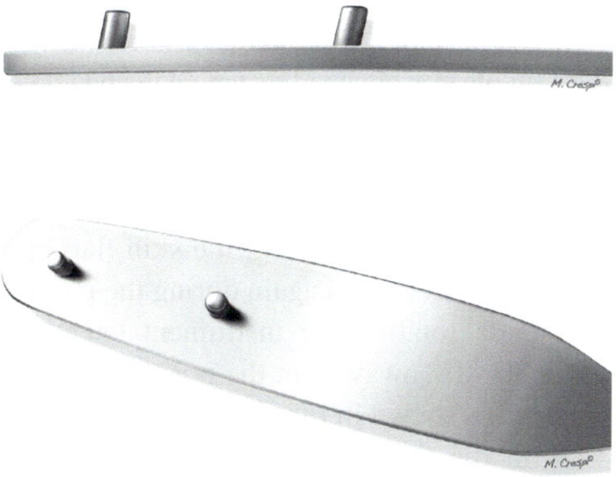

Fig. 13.39 Meneghini nasal skin retractor (MNSR). The flat and smooth handle easily adapts to the patient's forehead avoiding rotation of the instrument

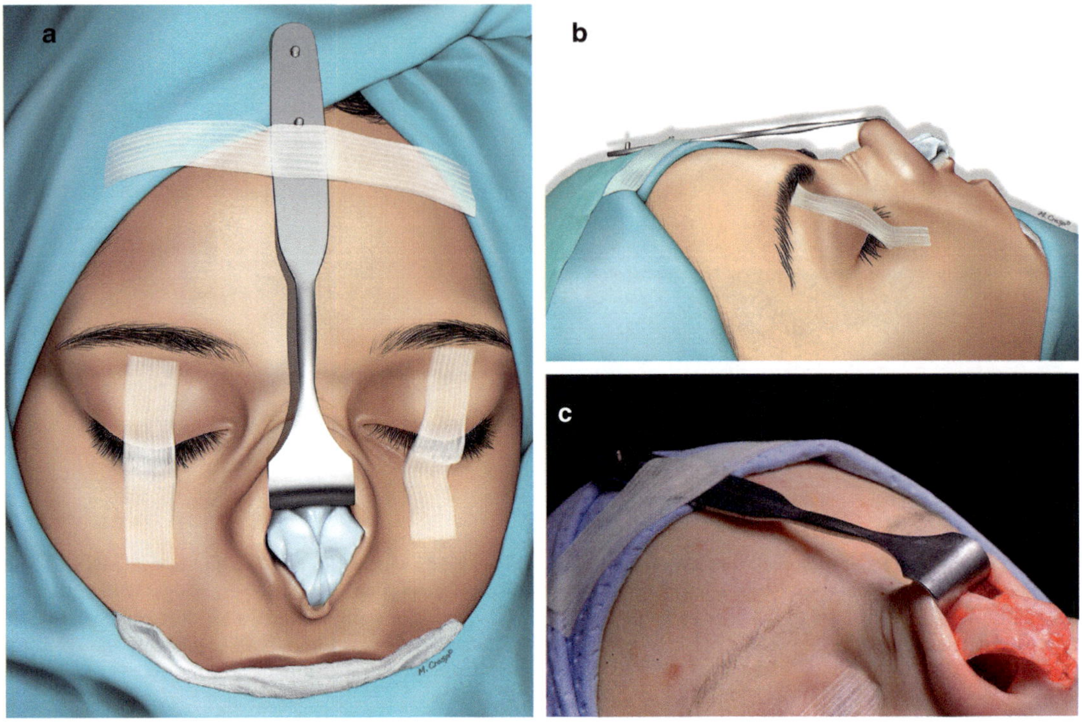

Fig. 13.40 (**a**–**c**) Meneghini nasal skin retractor (MNSR). Fixation into place is obtained by taping the handle inferiorly to one of the small hooks with one or two Steri-Strips, thus freeing the surgeon assistant's right hand

preferred position of the retractor is reached, fixation into place is obtained by taping the handle inferior to one of the small hooks (Fig. 13.40) with one or two Steri-Strips[2] thus freeing the surgeon assistant's right hand.

After initial positioning, the skin flap can be released and retracted again during the procedure by merely rotating the instrument laterally, by about 30–40°, away from the position of the first surgeon, as shown in Fig. 13.41.

With the flap retracted, the two lower lateral cartilages are grasped and separated from each other utilizing delicate pliers such as the Adson Brown or the DeBakey curved dissecting forceps (Fig. 13.42). In particular, the right ala is supported with the non-dominant hand of the first operator while the left ala is sup-

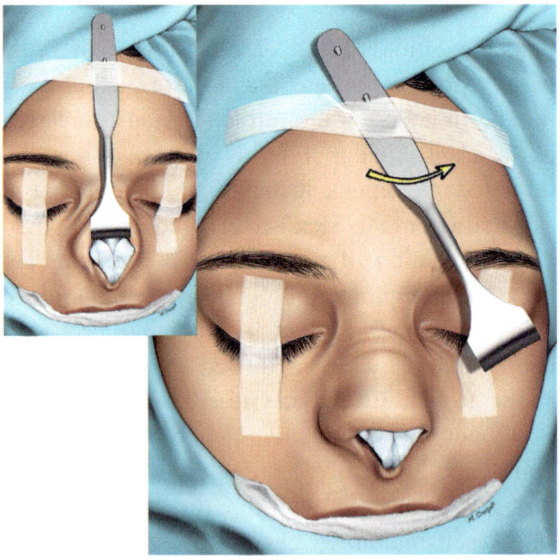

Fig. 13.41 Meneghini nasal skin retractor (MNSR). After initial positioning, the skin flap can be easily released and retracted again during the procedure by merely rotating the instrument laterally

[2]Steri-Strip, type R1547, ½ in X 4 in—12 mm X 100 mm (3 M Health Care).

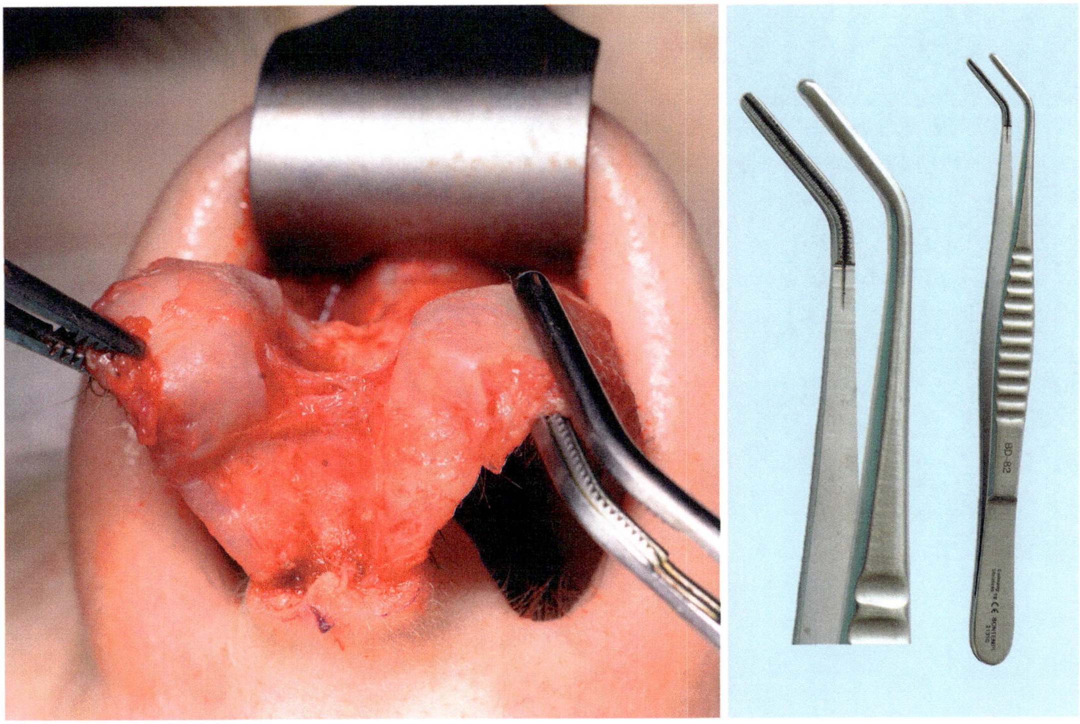

Fig. 13.42 "Tip Split" technique. The two lower lateral cartilages are grasped and separated utilizing two DeBakey curved dissecting forceps. The right ala is supported with the non-dominant hand of the first operator while the left ala is supported by the dominant hand of the assistant

ported by the dominant hand of the assistant. Once the cartilages have been stabilized, with the Converse scissors, a delicate dissection is performed between the medial crus and then into the membranous septum (Fig. 13.43). Maintaining the midline, in the case of a straight caudal septum, dissection can be performed more quickly using the Colorado microdissection needle (Fig. 13.44), setting the electrosurgery unit to low power (usually at 15 on a scale of 100).

This anterior-inferior approach to the septum, which involves the separation of the two domes and the two medial crura of the lower lateral cartilage, is named the "Tip Split" technique.

During dissection of the membranous septum, to avoid the risk of perforating the skin, the surgeon must respect these rules:

- Start dissection only when the surgical field is perfectly illuminated.
- Repeatedly clean the field from blood and serum with moistened gauzes.
- Maintain, with the aid of the assistant, a continued, delicate and balanced tension at both medial crura cartilages.
- Palpate several times, with the forefinger, the caudal margin of the septum to establish its exact spatial position and the thickness of the tissue still to be incised.
- Progress only with small dissections directly towards the caudal margin of the septum.

Next, with the aid of a small Killian nasal speculum, the connective fibers can be spread apart for a clear demonstration of the position of the inferior free margin of the septum (Fig. 13.45).

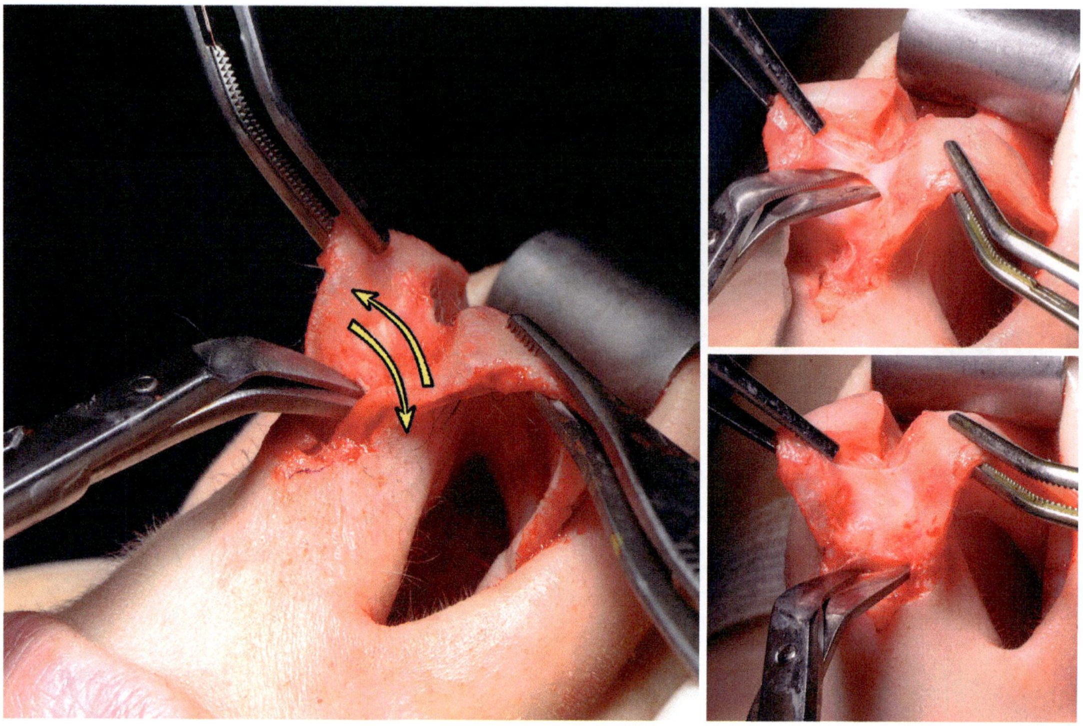

Fig. 13.43 "Tip Split" technique. A delicate dissection is performed between the medial crus and then into the membranous septum with Converse scissors

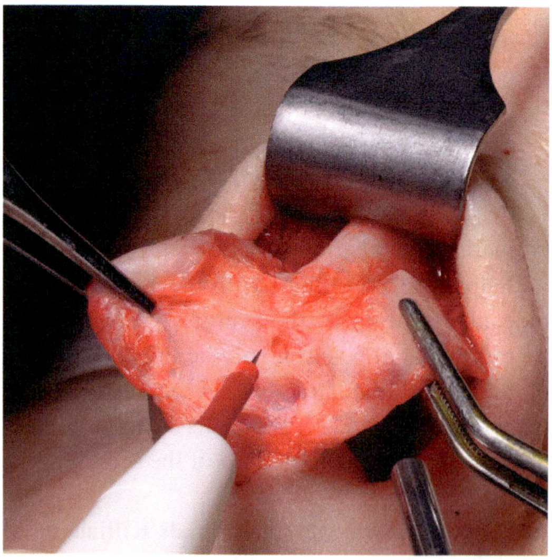

Fig. 13.44 "Tip Split" technique. In the case of a straight caudal septum, the dissection can be performed more quickly using a Colorado microdissection needle

13.9 Initial Nasal Septum Skeletonization

Once the inferior margin and the anterior septal angle are clearly identified, more time is spent in finding the subperichondrial plane. To do this, the author's preferred instruments are the 15c blade and the Iris sharp scissors. With the 15c blade some small incisions are performed to the tissue covering the septum close to the anterior nasal spine. For safety, to avoid inadvertently cutting the skin, the incisions are directed upwards as shown in Fig. 13.46; the asterisk indicates a small whitish area in which the subperichondrial space is just reached. The small upward incisions are then repeated following the edge of the cartilage until the anterior septal angle is exposed (Fig. 13.47).

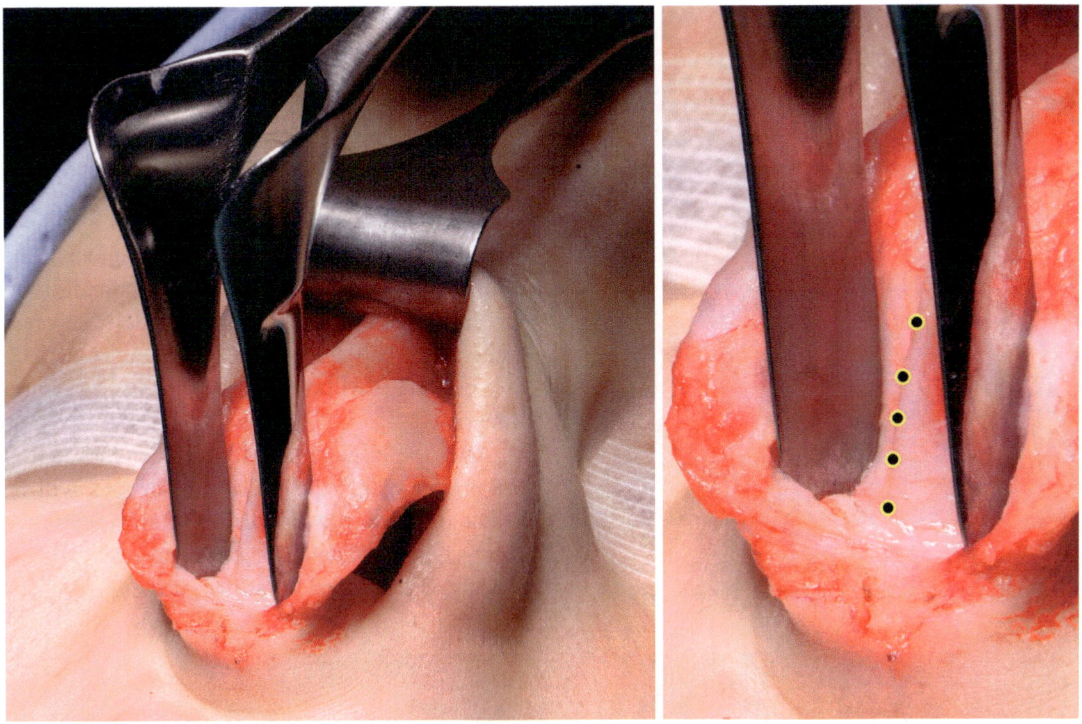

Fig. 13.45 "Tip Split" technique. With the aid of a small Killian nasal speculum, the connective fibers can be spread apart for a clear demonstration of the position of the inferior free margin of the septum

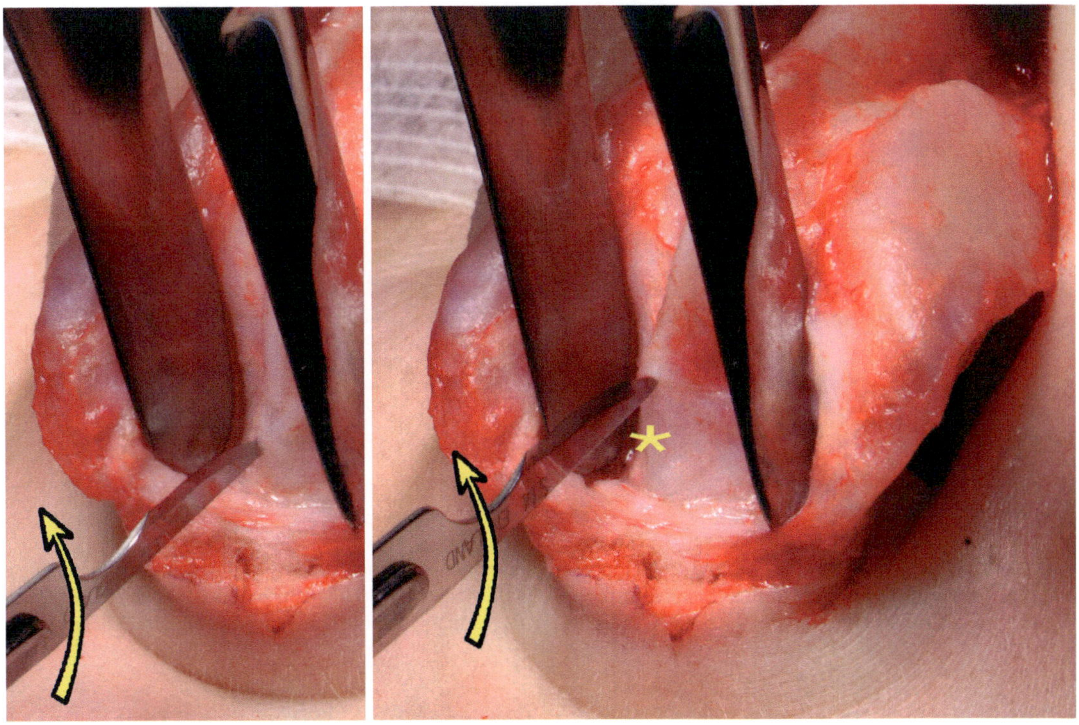

Fig. 13.46 Small incisions are performed to the tissue covering the septum close to the anterior nasal spine. The asterisk indicates a small whitish area in which the subperichondrial space is just reached

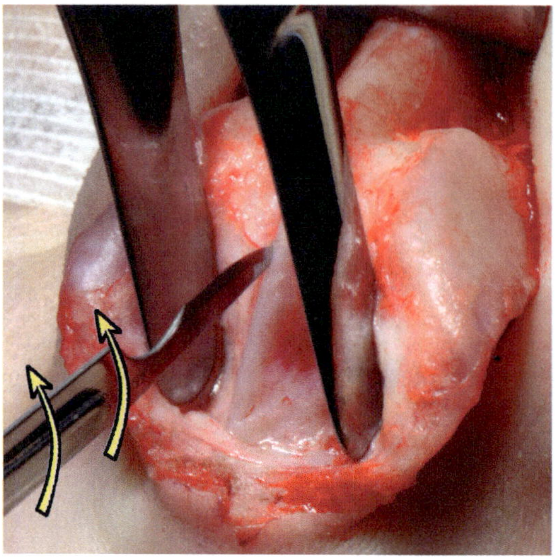

Fig. 13.47 The small upward incisions are then repeated along the caudal margin of the septal cartilage

The strong adherence of the perichondrium around the septal margin makes it necessary to proceed carefully. Every surgeon has his favorite instrument for cutting the perichondrium and preserving the cartilage intact. The author, for the initial bilateral elevation of the mucosa utilizes sharp pointed scissors as illustrated in Fig. 13.48; during the initial oscillating movements, the pointed tip is oriented almost perpendicularly to the cartilage while maintaining a delicate pressure. The main goal is to superficially scratch the cartilage without damaging its structural integrity.

After the bilateral flaps have been elevated in the proper plane, the tip of the scissors will be oriented more parallel to the septal cartilage (Fig. 13.49). The dissection then continues towards the anterior one-third of the quadrangu-

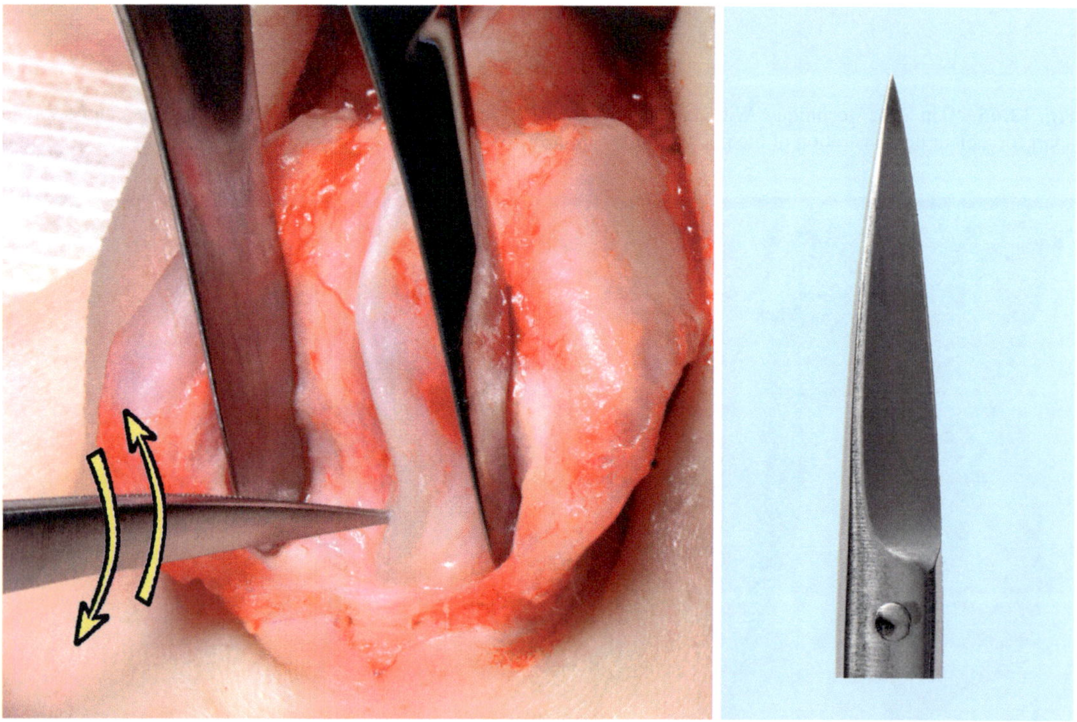

Fig. 13.48 Initial bilateral elevation of the septal mucosa. Sharp pointed scissors can be helpful in finding the proper deepest plane of dissection. Initially the pointed tip is oriented almost perpendicularly to the cartilage maintaining a delicate pressure. The main goal is to superficially scratch the cartilage without damaging its structural integrity

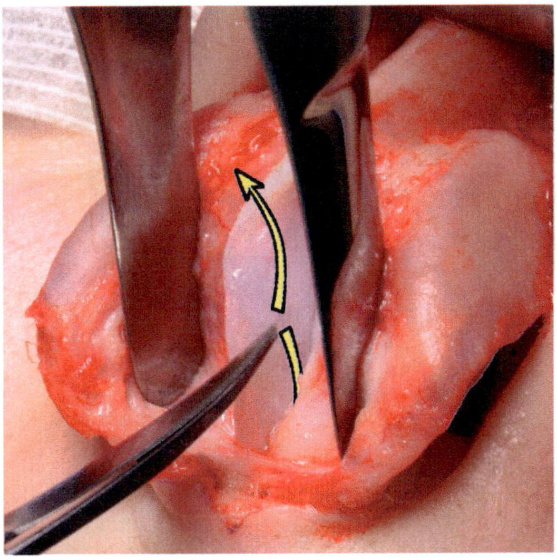

Fig. 13.49 Initial bilateral elevation of the septal mucosa. After the bilateral flaps have been elevated in the proper plane, the tip of the scissors will be oriented more parallel to the septal cartilage

lar cartilage. Now the resistance to elevation opposed by the perichondrium is decreased.

13.10 Variations in the Extent of Septum Skeletonization

The extent of septum skeletonization depends on both the planned esthetic correction and the functional problem related to septal deviation or spurs, and should be known in advance.

Also in the case of a straight osteocartilaginous septum, the need for large straight solid fragments or fine-diced pieces of cartilage for grafting can require a wide skeletonization of the quadrangular cartilage.

So, this is one of the several moments in the BOR sequence in which the operator takes a "surgical time out"[3] before proceeding with the subsequent steps.

[3]This interesting way of thinking, "take a surgical time out," comes from Daniel RK. Mastering Rhinoplasty. Berlin, Heidelberg: Springer Verlag; 2010. p. 24.

For safety and ergonomics during the work of the septum, the operating table must be lowered and the scialytic lamp vertically oriented over the surgical field. The nasal skin flap is still retracted upward and the mucoperiosteal flaps are bilaterally elevated with a Freer or Tebbetts double-ended elevator (Fig. 13.50b) or, in the case of moderate bleeding, with a Gorney suction elevator or similar instruments (Fig. 13.50c, d). For handling the most posterior portion of the quadrangular cartilage or the osseous septum, a long-blade nasal speculum is necessary (Fig. 13.50a).

The elevator must advance along the cartilaginous surface with lateral movements without ever using force when resistance is encountered. Any obstacle or firm adherence of the mucoperichondrium must be dealt with after the flap has been elevated all around. The most difficult anatomical areas to handle are:

- The caudal margin of the septum, from which the surgical flap elevation begins.
- The osteochondral junction at the level of the maxillary crest of the septum.
- The osteochondral junction at the level of the anterior nasal spine.
- Septal spurs.
- Any highly deformed and angled area as a result of previous nasal trauma.
- Any deformed and angled area as a result of previous septal surgery.

The goal is to keep intact the continuity of the full-thickness mucosal flaps as well as the integrity and stability of the quadrangular cartilage.

13.11 Splitting the Upper Lateral Cartilage from the Septum

The last step of nasal skeletonization is the separation of the upper lateral cartilages from the dorsal margin of the septal cartilage preserving the nasal mucosa intact. For this reason, the

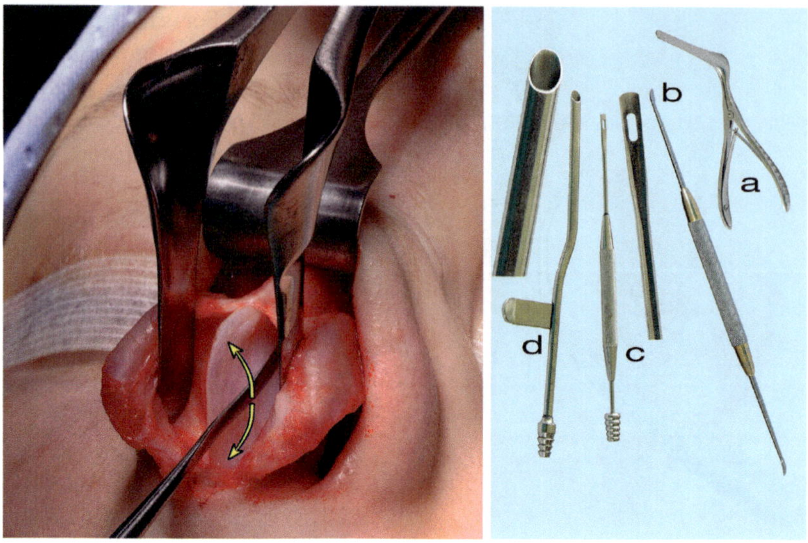

Fig. 13.50 (**a–d**) The bilateral mucoperiosteal flap elevation can be done with a double-ended elevator (**b**) or a suction elevator (**c, d**). For handling the most posterior portion of the quadrangular cartilage and the osseous septum, a long-blade nasal speculum is necessary (**a**)

splitting maneuver is performed only after verifying that the mucoperichondrium has been elevated perfectly along the dorsal margin of the septum.

In preparation, the surgical nurse holds the Maliniac or Tebbetts nasal retractor in place while the first surgeon and assistant spread laterally the alar cartilages with their respective nondominant hands. This action opens a small space for the insertion of the 15c blade (Fig. 13.51) which, oriented upwards, will allow the incision of the junction between the upper lateral cartilage and septum (Fig. 13.52). Alternatively, a pair of straight scissors can be used instead of the 15c blade.

The wide exposure obtained with this maneuver allows perfect analysis and treatment of the septal deformities (Fig. 13.53).

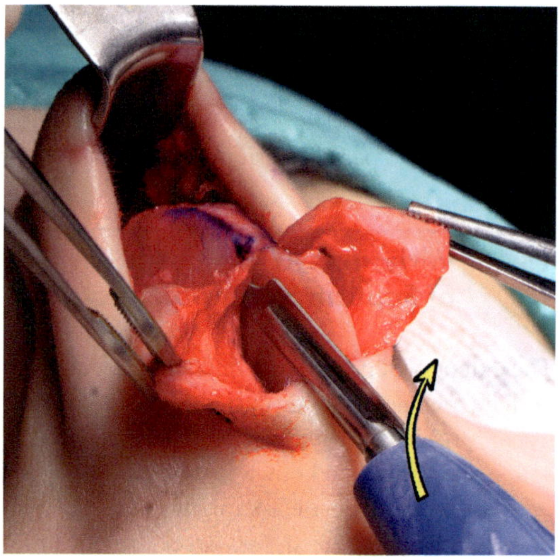

Fig. 13.51 Splitting the upper lateral cartilage from the septum. The action of spreading laterally the alar cartilages (straight arrows) opens a small space between the septum and the upper lateral cartilage for the insertion of the 15c blade (curved arrow)

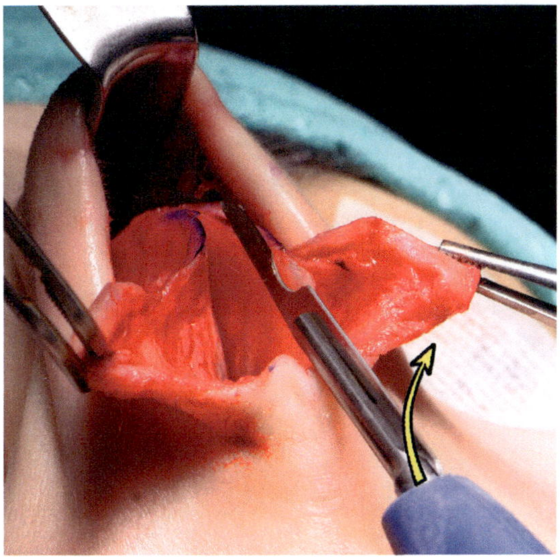

Fig. 13.52 Splitting the upper lateral cartilage from the septum. Incision of the junction between the upper lateral cartilage and septum with a 15c blade oriented upwards

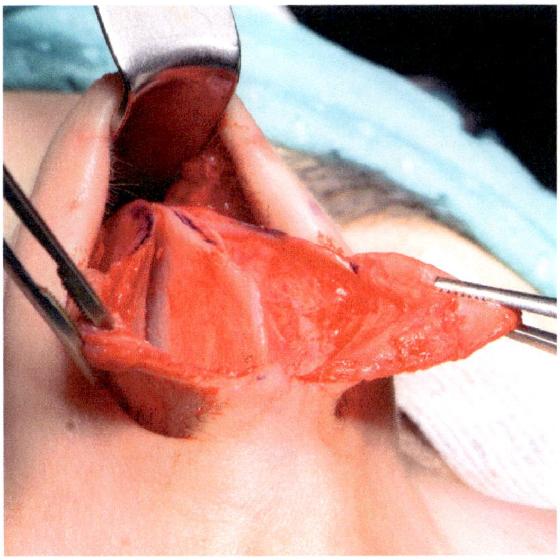

Fig. 13.53 Splitting the upper lateral cartilage from the septum. The wide exposure obtained with this maneuver allows perfect analysis and treatment of the septal deformities

Further Reading

A book full of anatomical and clinical images as well as of descriptions of many surgical techniques is: Daniel RK, Pálházi P. Rhinoplasty. Springer International Publishing AG; 2018.

14 Basic Open Rhinoplasty: Intraoperative Analysis

During surgery it is often necessary to stop for a moment to take stock of the situation. This is the main "surgical time out" before proceeding with the core part of BOR rhinoplasty.[1]

The skin of the face and nose is completely cleaned with moist gauze and a precise visual and tactile nasal inspection begins. The nasal flap is elevated, with a Maliniac or Tebbetts nasal retractor, irrigated with saline solution and cleaned. All bleeding points are checked and gently cauterized, except for the bleeding that occurs in the lower surface of the flap, although this is very rare if the correct plane of dissection has been followed.

The cartilaginous and bony components of the nasal framework are re-evaluated for shape, size, and strength. With a nasal speculum also the septum and both the inferior turbinates are inspected.

The main goals of the intraoperative analysis are:

- Re-evaluate the basic preoperative findings such as skin thickness, osteocartilaginous deformities and symmetry, any septal deviations and hypertrophy of the inferior turbinates.
- Study the peculiarities and fine details of the nasal deformities revealed during the early surgical phases.
- Confirm the treatment plan objectives.
- Confirm or change the next surgical steps.
- Check the quantity and quality of septal cartilage available for any structural or camouflage grafts.

This intraoperative analytical exercise is of great value for the next more operative steps of rhinoplasty.

14.1 Intraoperative Nasal Tip Analysis

For a better analysis of the nasal tip, special care should be taken not to stretch up or deform the alar cartilages with the instrument used to retract the skin flap. A description of a dedicated, light, self-retainer instrument for holding and protecting the skin flap was given in Chap. 13. Also the upper lip and the cheeks must be free and not constrained by the sheets or tapes used to isolate the surgical field and fix the endotracheal tube. Any traction to the nasal soft tissues should be carefully avoided.

During the intraoperative analysis, it is necessary to observe the nasal tip from several points of view such as:

[1]Previously cited: "take a surgical time out," Daniel RK. Mastering Rhinoplasty. Berlin, Heidelberg: Springer-Verlag; 2010. p. 24.

F. Meneghini, *Basic Open Rhinoplasty*, https://doi.org/10.1007/978-3-030-61827-8_14

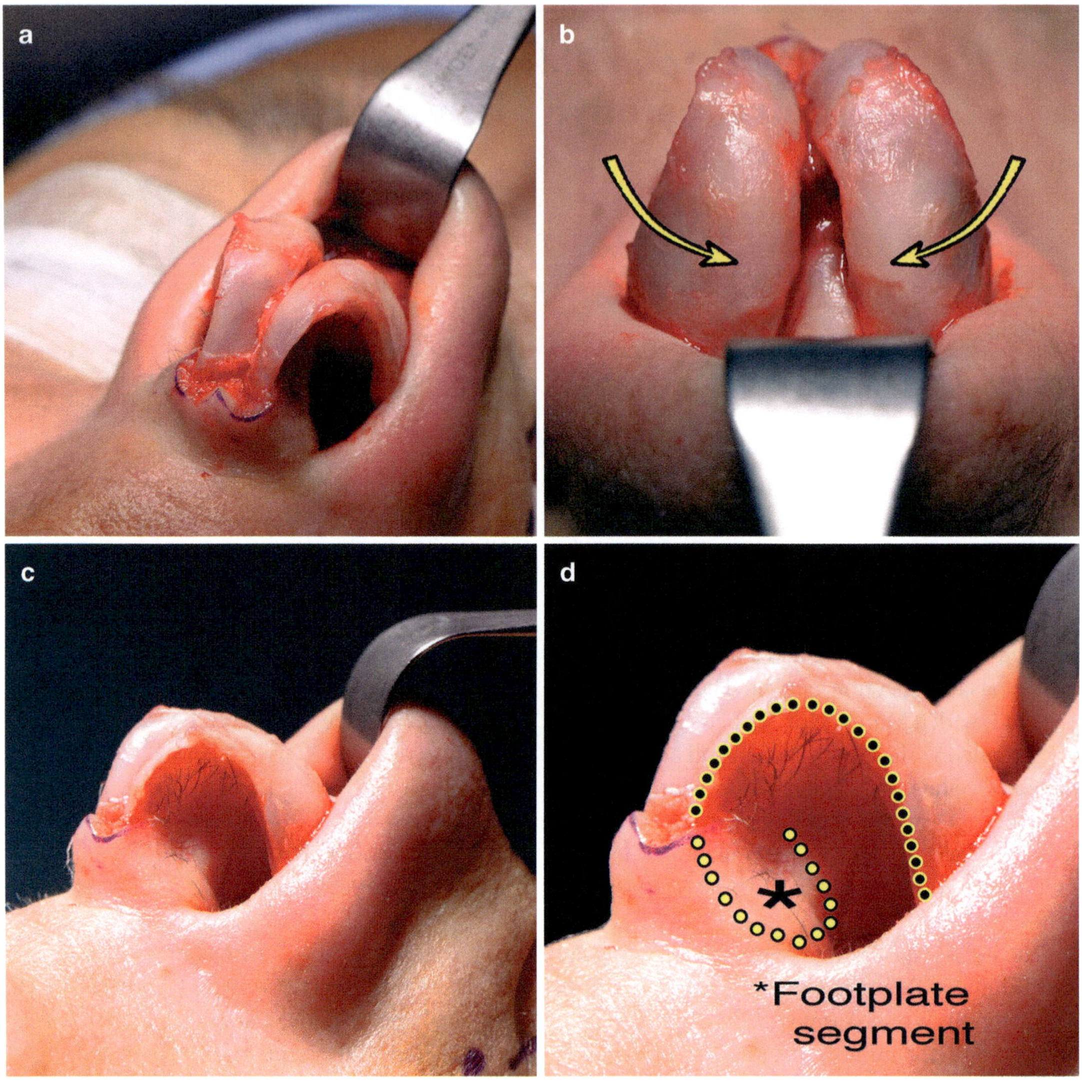

Fig. 14.1 (**a–d**) Intraoperative nasal tip analysis. The lower lateral cartilage should be analyzed from below (**a**), above (**b**) and in profile view (**c, d**)

- From below (Fig. 14.1a).
- From above (Fig. 14.1b).
- Profile view (Fig. 14.1c, d).

The lower lateral cartilages were divided by Rollin Daniel in his 1992 publication,[2] from medial to lateral, into three portions:

- Medial crus, subdivided into footplate (Fig. 14.2a) and columellar segments (Fig. 14.2b).
- Middle crus, subdivided into lobular (Fig. 14.2c) and domal segments (Fig. 14.2d).
- Lateral crus (Fig. 14.2e).

With daily practice, every young surgeon will discover how the anatomy of the alar cartilages found at surgery is quite different from Rollin Daniel's description as well as from the illustrations of the main rhinoplasty books and articles. There are many variables and it is always interesting to study every single clinical case as if it were a unique experience.

[2]Daniel RK. The nasal tip: Anatomy and aesthetics. Plastic Reconstr Surg. 1992;89(2):216–224.

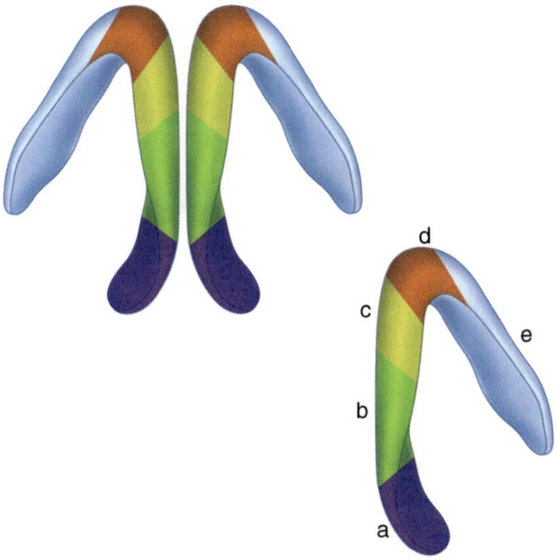

Fig. 14.2 The lower lateral cartilages have been divided by Rollin K Daniel from medial to lateral, into three portions: medial crus, subdivided into footplate (**a**) and columellar segments (**b**), middle crus, subdivided into lobular (**c**) and domal segments (**d**), and lateral crus (**e**)

Figure 14.1a–d shows a frequent intraoperative finding: a single strip of cartilage, without clear angulations and characters, shapes the nasal tip framework; none of the three crura is clearly distinguishable from the others. The only obvious feature, indicated by the two curved arrows, is represented by the position of the lateral crus parallel to the nasal dorsum. The corresponding visible external deformity is called "parenthesis tip" because it creates a "parenthesis" appearance on frontal view in thin skin patients.

A somewhat similar extreme anatomical variability of the alar cartilages can be found in dental occlusion. Lawrence F. Andrews, one of the fathers of modern orthodontics, in his cornerstone article "The six keys to normal occlusion" described his difficulty finding 120 dental casts of non-orthodontic patients with normal occlusion. His search took a period of 4 years (1960 to 1964) and cooperation with local dentists, orthodontists, and a major university. The models selected were of teeth which:

- Had never had orthodontic treatment.
- Were straight and pleasing in appearance.
- Had a bite which looked generally correct.
- Would not, according to Dr. Andrews, benefit from orthodontic treatment.

Subsequently Dr. Andrews himself admitted that the normal occlusion he described was not at all normal but statistically exceptional in the population. For this reason he changed the terminology from "normal" to "optimal," and today this rare and particular type of dental occlusion is considered the main objective of every orthodontic treatment.

Lawrence Andrews' experience on dental occlusion can be transferred to the field of rhinoplasty, in particular to when the surgeon is dealing with the intraoperative study of the anatomy of alar cartilages. In this way, Rollin Daniels' description of the alar cartilages is a fundamental template in the mental process of analysis and an aid for imagining the three-dimensional modifications necessary to give an "optimal" shape to the nasal tip even if it is rarely seen in non-operated noses.

To confirm the great variability of the shape of the alar cartilages, Fig. 14.3 presents one exceptional case documented by the author where the various segments are clearly recognizable after flap elevation:

(a) Footplate segment of medial crus.
(b) Columellar segment of medial crus.
(c) Lobular segment of middle crus.
(d) Domal segment of middle crus.
(e) Lateral crus.

Figure 14.4 illustrates a reverse nasal tip anatomy if compared to the amorphous one depicted in Fig. 14.1. In this clinical case:

- The alar cartilages display tight curves.
- Some areas of accentuated concavity-convexity are close together.
- The two domal regions have different width.
- On tactile analysis, these cartilages appeared hard and resistant to handling.

All these findings are causes of visible clinical skin bossae.

Figure 14.5 shows some preoperative close-up images of this nose. The main findings are:

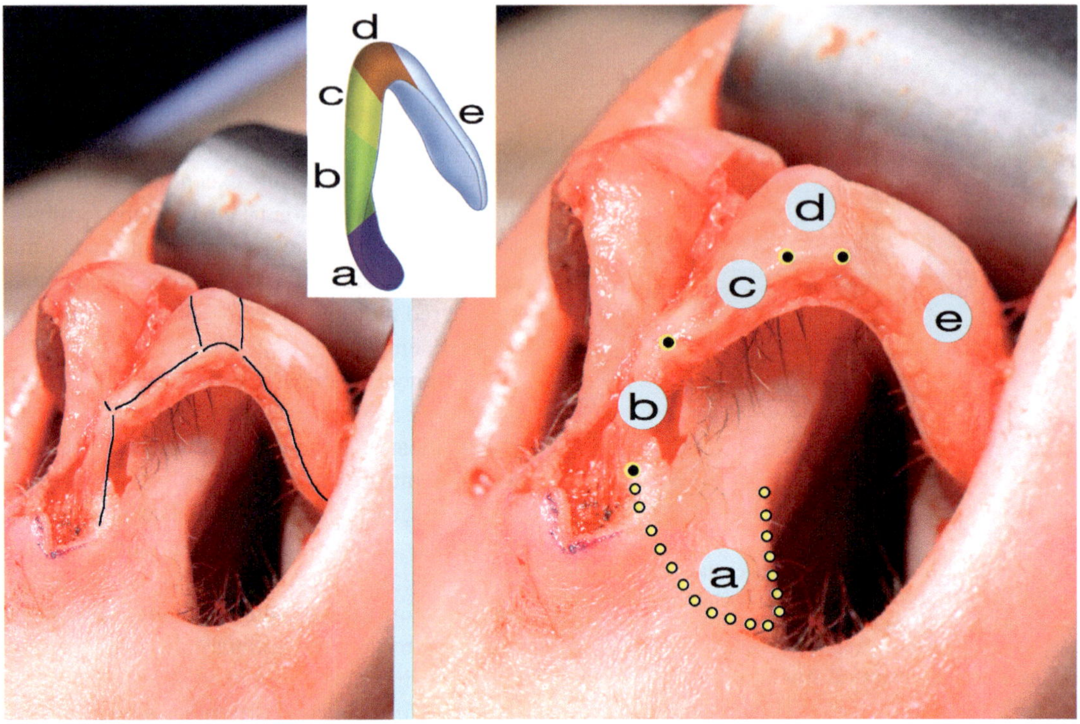

Fig. 14.3 Intraoperative nasal tip analysis. In this case all lower lateral cartilage segments are clearly recognizable: footplate (**a**) and columellar (**b**) segments of the medial crus, lobular (**c**) and domal (**d**) segments of the middle crus and lateral crus (**e**)

- The nasal root (nasion) is positioned inferiorly to the superior palpebral fold (lateral view).
- A small osteocartilaginous hump is present (lateral and oblique views).
- The domes diverge from each other creating a bifid lobule with bossae. Their underlying shapes are evident and asymmetric (frontal, oblique, basal, and face-down views). They are covered by whitish thin skin.
- The caudal septum is deviated to the left with respect to the anterior nasal spine. In basal view, the columella is also rotated counterclockwise producing an asymmetric nasal tip.
- The nasolabial angle is reduced due to the clockwise rotated columella (lateral view).
- The columellar/lobular angle is sharply evident (lateral view).
- The nose is deviated to the right (frontal and face-down views).

The association in the same nose of a very thin skin with "intractable," rigid, asymmetrical and deformed lower lateral cartilages, suspected from the preoperative analysis and confirmed during surgery, greatly reduces the surgeon's margin of error in shaping the tip. At the end of surgery the insertion of an autologous temporal fascia graft between the reconstituted cartilaginous nasal tip framework and the skin flap is an option to keep in mind to minimize late postoperative irregularities.

This condition, in which thin skin is associated with strong and deformed alar cartilage, must bring to mind the words of M. Eugene Tardy: "With the possible exception of the nasolabial angle, no abrupt sharp angles, edges, or offsets exist in the ideal nose."[3]

[3]Tardy ME. Rhinoplasty. The Art and the Science. Philadelphia: WB Saunders Company; 1997. p. 14.

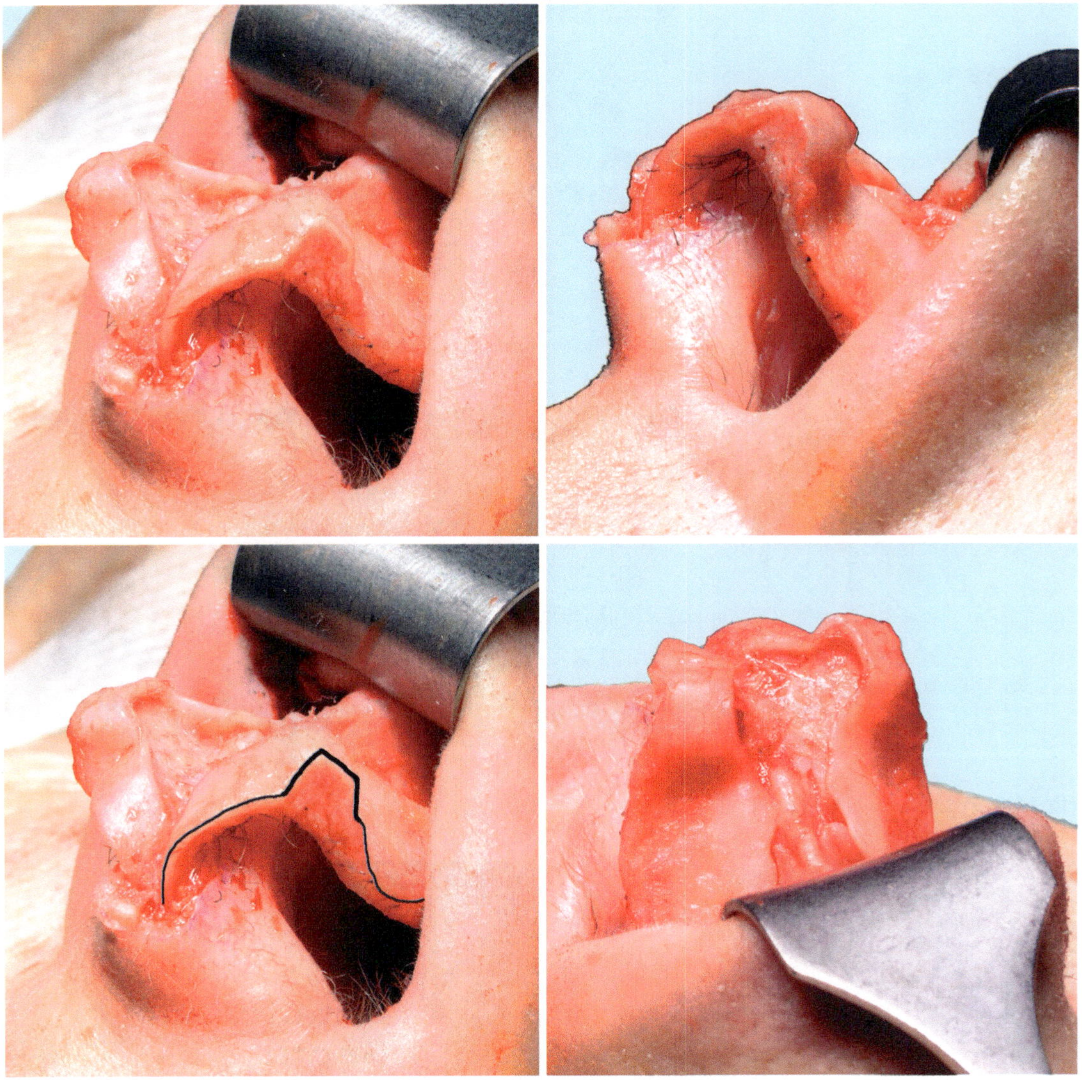

Fig. 14.4 Intraoperative nasal tip analysis. A case characterized by highly deformed strong lower lateral cartilages with tight curves and asymmetries. The accentuated concavities-convexities are too close to each other producing visible clinical nasal tip bossae

14.2 Intraoperative Dorsum Analysis

The morphology of the nasal dorsum is then studied looking also at the preoperative photographs.

Figure 14.6 shows some interesting intraoperative findings: the osteocartilaginous junction (K area) is broad and deformed by the presence of lateral asymmetric spurs while the anterior portion of the cartilaginous dorsum rapidly changes into a thin configuration (Tardy's words immediately come back to mind!). It seems that the upper lateral cartilages fail to support to the airway, with a bilateral collapse of the internal nasal valve. Preoperative photographs and tactile inspection of the nasal dorsum had already highlighted these problems (Fig. 14.7). In this particular case, nasal hump removal must be followed by a narrowing of the bony dorsum and reconstruction of the cartilaginous dorsum with autolo-

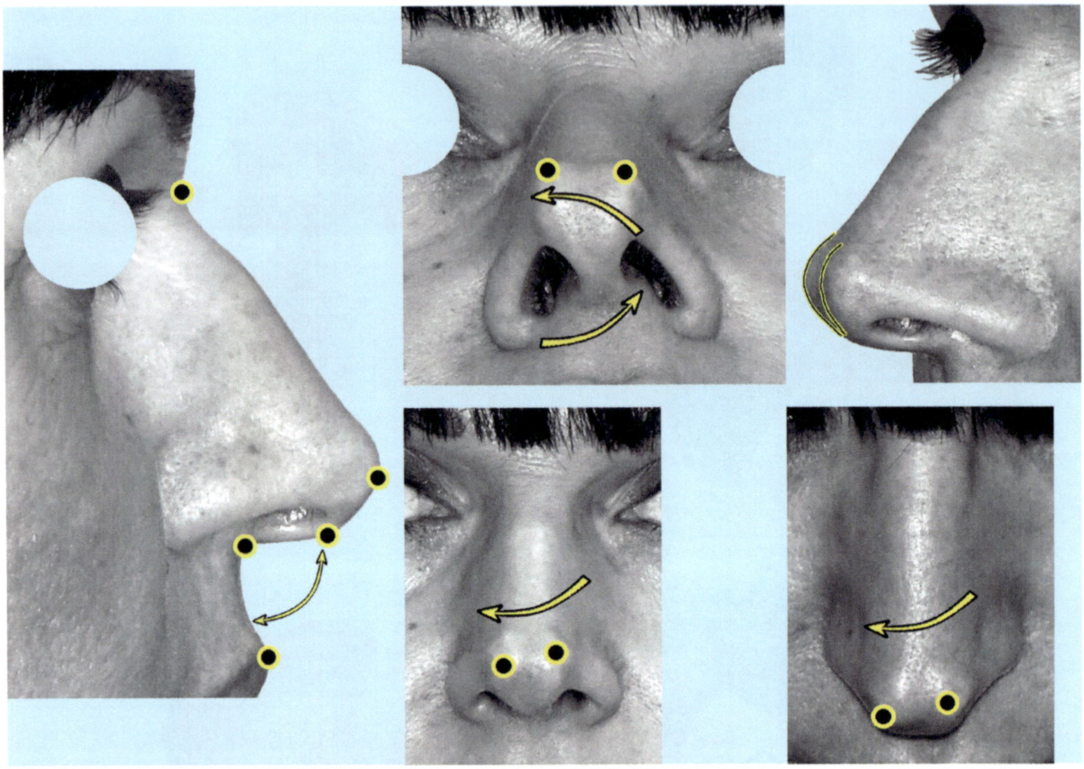

Fig. 14.5 Preoperative close-up images of the nose depicted in Fig. 14.4

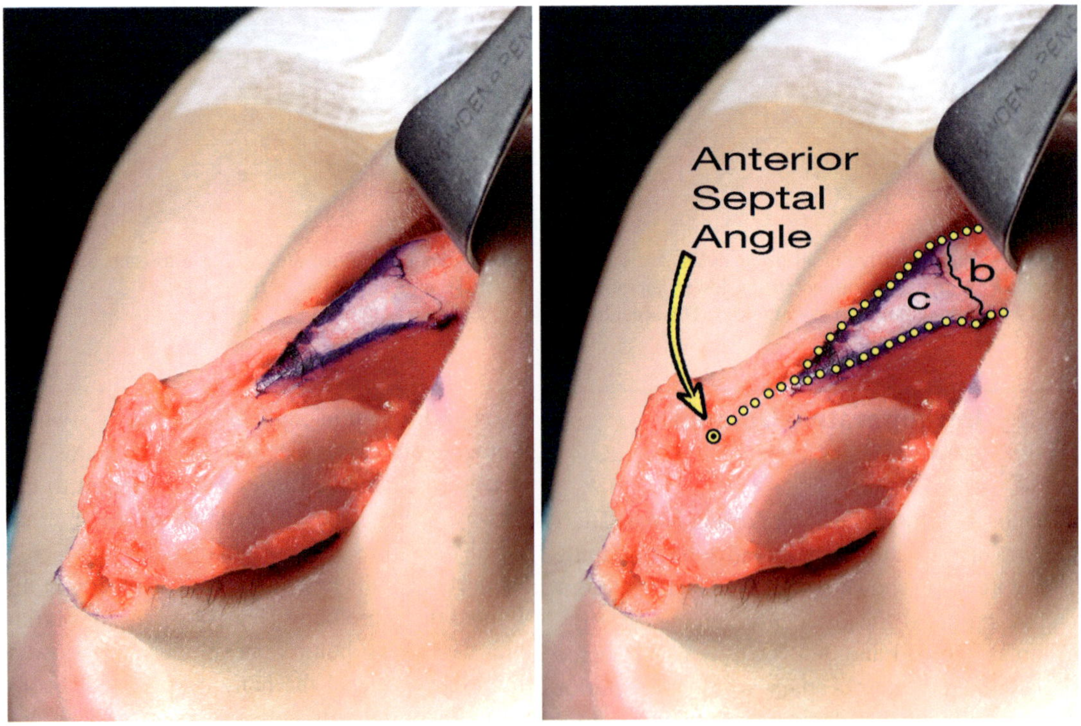

Fig. 14.6 Intraoperative dorsum analysis. Broad and deformed osteocartilaginous junction and thin configuration of the cartilaginous dorsum

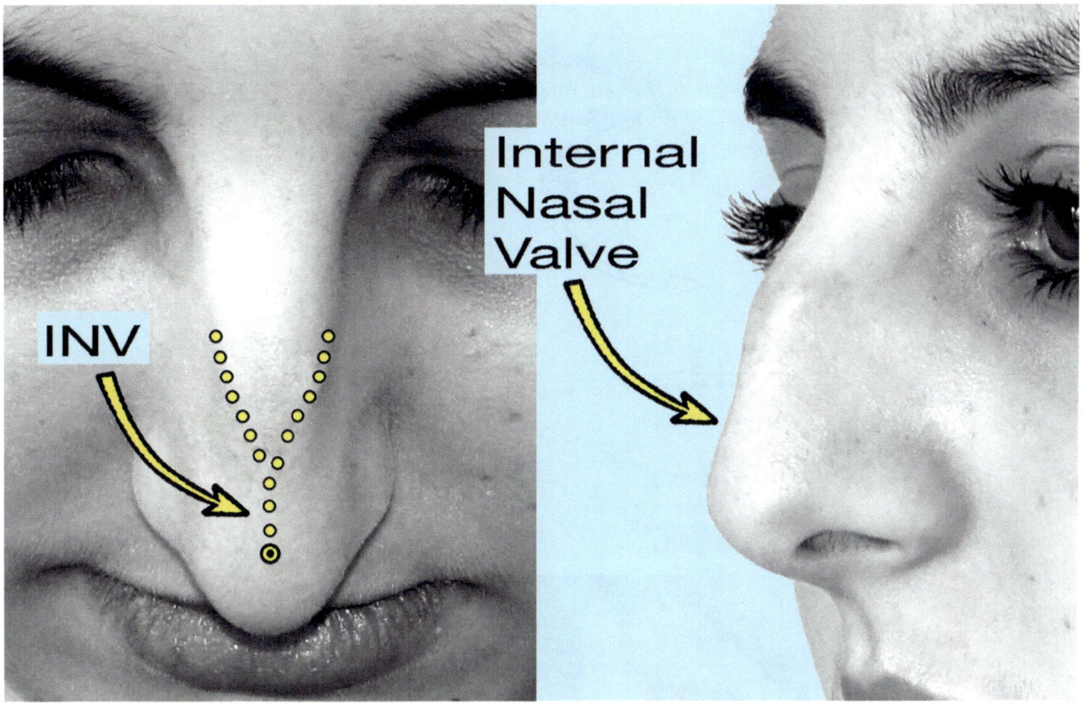

Fig. 14.7 Preoperative face-down and left oblique view of the patient depicted in Fig. 14.6. Broad and deformed osteo-cartilaginous hump and restricted nasal valve

gous spreader grafts both for aesthetic and functional reasons (Fig. 14.8a–c).

14.3 Intraoperative Tip/Dorsal Profile Assessment

Starting from this phase of rhinoplasty onwards it is necessary to frequently assess the projection of the nasal tip with respect to the dorsal profile and from time to time perform a nasal tip positioning exercise.

Figure 14.9a–d shows the significant difference in height between the two nasal domes and the more anterior profile of the cartilaginous septum is marked with the lines and the black dot (c, d). The situation is the opposite of the desired skeletal profile at the end of the surgery, in which the domes must be some millimeters more projected with respect to the anterior septal profile.

The cause of this temporary imbalance is due to various factors:

- The septal cartilage is rigid and therefore its spatial position is not affected by the elevation of flaps.
- In most primary cases the projection of the septum, at the level of the anterior septal angle, must be reduced during the intervention. So at this stage it should be considered a temporary condition.
- The original projection and shape of the lower lateral cartilages is largely lost after the initial flap elevation due to their deformability and pliability (curved arrows in Fig. 14.9c). In particular, the removal or cutting of the ligaments between the cartilages themselves and the surrounding structures cause this loss of support to the nasal tip.

With the endonasal approach the same and well-known condition is only partially hidden to

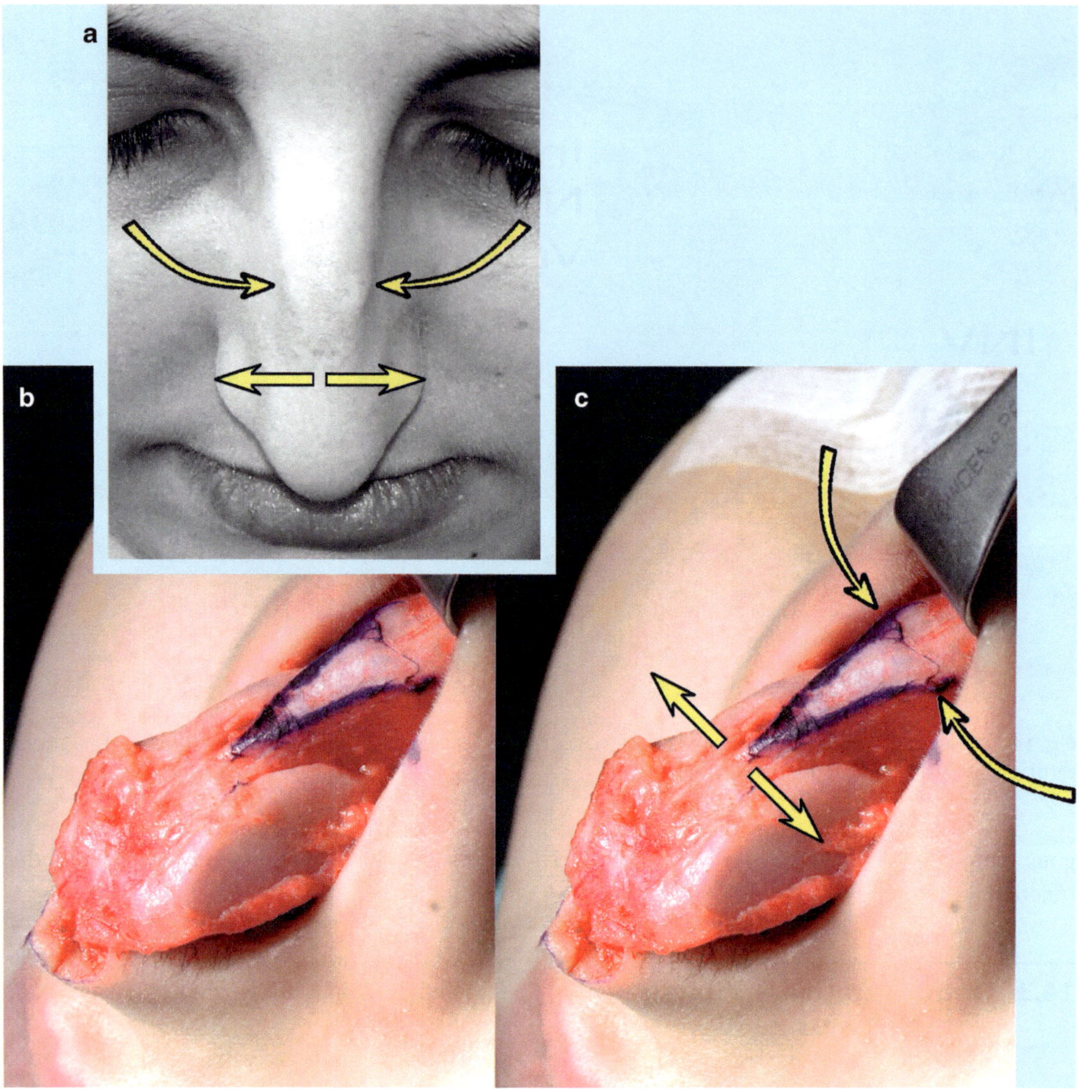

Fig. 14.8 (**a–c**) The preoperative treatment plan, made on clinical photography (**a**), is confirmed after the intraoperative analysis (**b**, **c**). It consists of narrowing and symmetrizing the bony nasal dorsum as well as widening the cartilaginous dorsum with a spreader graft both for aesthetic and functional purposes

the surgeon's view by the presence of the skin over the nasal tip.

By changing the perspective from which we look at surgical facts, rhinoplasty scholars tend to divide and think in one of these two ways:

- Those who hope to preserve more the ligamentous apparatus of the nose, especially of the nasal tip, hiding the action of the instruments from sight by keeping them under the skin.
- Those who decide to always and directly see the actions and effects of the instruments on the nasal structures, check all the surgical cuts and take responsibility for a difficult and precise process of reconstruction of the nasal structures, ligaments included.

With all the innumerable intermediate possibilities, it is often preferable to follow the second approach and operate directly previewing the framework reconstruction through some useful exercises. The most interesting, the nasal tip

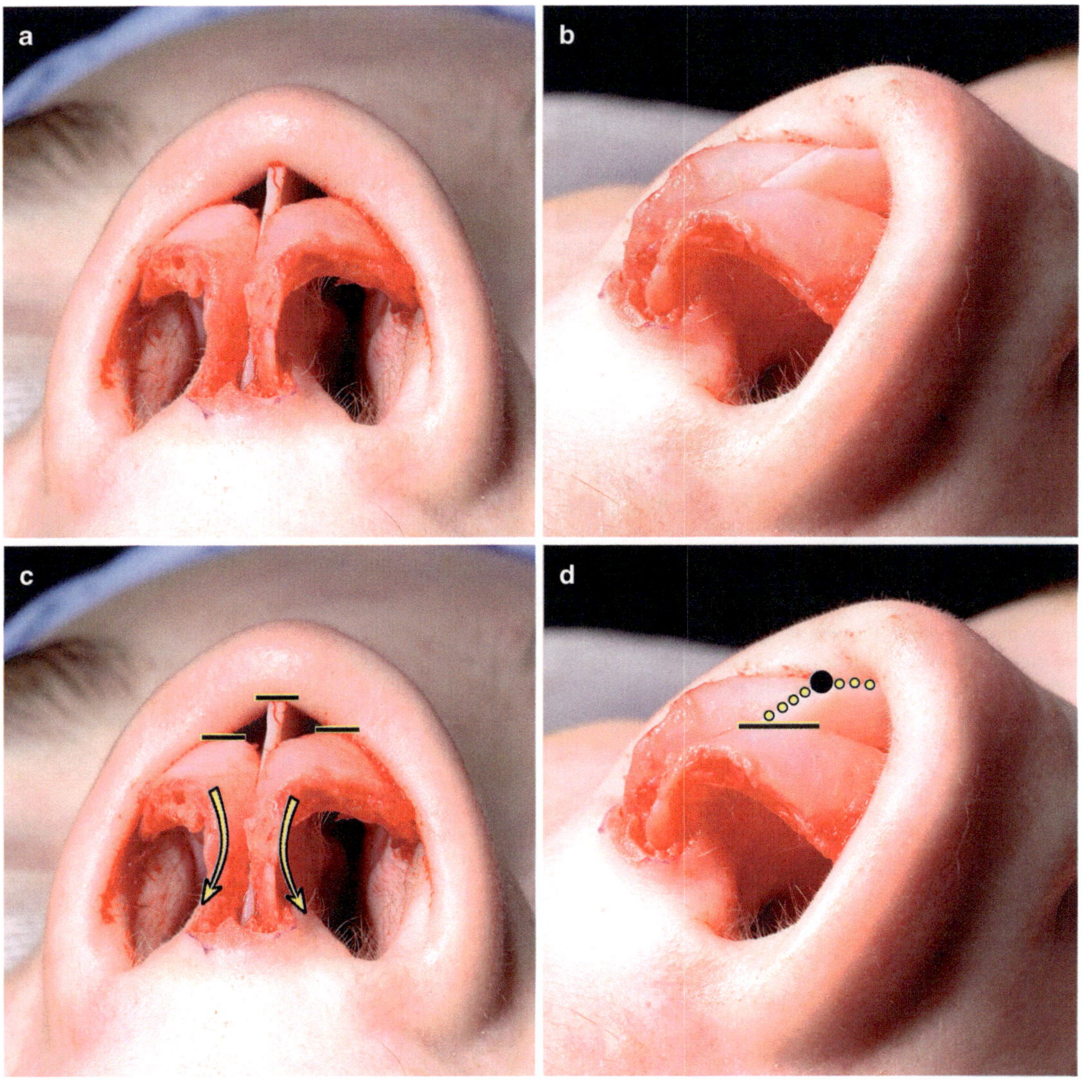

Fig. 14.9 (**a–d**) Intraoperative tip/dorsal profile assessment. The significant difference in height between the two nasal domes and the more anterior profile of the cartilaginous septum is marked with the lines and the black dot (**c**, **d**)

positioning exercise, is explained in Fig. 14.10a, b. Holding together the two middle crura just under the domes with a curved DeBakey dissecting forceps, the nasal tip can be freely moved both in the anterior-posterior and superior-inferior directions.

14.4 Intraoperative Septal and Inferior Turbinate Analysis

The intraoperative study of the septum and lower turbinates has several objectives:

- Confirm the deformities already seen on the CT scans.
- Identify the surgical strategy to obtain the straightening of the dorsocaudal L-strut of cartilage that should be maintained.
- Identify the extent of central cartilage harvesting to be used for grafts.
- Recognize absolute or compensatory hypertrophy of the inferior turbinates.
- Make sure there are no tears of the septal mucosa and, if present, perform their suture.

The endonasal steps of rhinoplasty aim to redistribute spaces and model anatomical

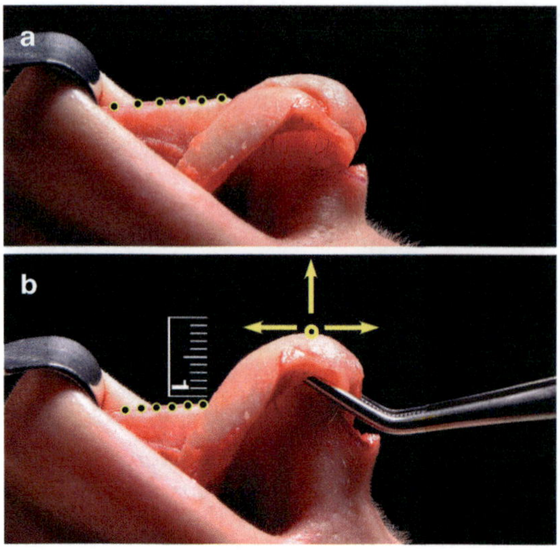

Fig. 14.10 (**a**, **b**) Nasal tip positioning exercise. Holding together the two middle crura just under the domes with a curve DeBakey dissecting forceps, the nasal tip can be freely moved both in the anterior-posterior and superior-inferior directions. In this way, it is possible to study the ideal position to be achieved with the reconstruction of the lower third of the nose

structures and, as happens with tip or dorsal cartilages, the surgeon must have in mind an ideal reference conformation suitable for his patient.

Further Reading

For further information on the segmentation and three-dimensional spatial arrangement of the lower lateral cartilage, you can read the article by Daniel RK. The nasal tip: anatomy and aesthetics. Plast Reconstr Surg. 1992;89(2):216–24. The terminology and content of this article, from publication to date, can be considered the standard reference for any rhinoplasty scholar.

15 Open Rhinoplasty: Initial Surgical Steps

All the operational steps of the basic open rhinoplasty method alternate details of great esthetic value, such as lowering the nasal dorsum, with details of great functional value, such as reducing the anterior volume of the inferior turbinate. So, a particular intraoperative skill of the surgeon is to continue to question himself about the functional and esthetic effects of each surgical maneuver.

After a complete surgical exploration of the nasal structure, the next steps will be directed to achieve the first objectives of the treatment plan.

15.1 Releasing the Depressor Septi Nasalis Muscle

Studying the nasal tip dynamics on lateral view images helps the surgeon to evaluate the activity of depressor septi nasalis muscle (Fig. 15.1a). The action of rotating the tip down of the depressor septi nasalis muscle must be separated from the contemporary action of the levator labii superioris alaeque nasi and other nasal muscles, as in the central and right clinical cases depicted in Fig. 15.1b, c. When the levator labii superioris alaeque nasi and other nasal muscles are also hyperactive, the clockwise rotation of the tip appears more evident and the patient must be advised of his particular condition which can only be partially improved.

The reduction of the activity of the depressor septi nasal muscle, with the BOR method, can be divided into three isolated steps:

- **T1**—During the approach to the caudal margin to the nasal septum and to the region of the anterior nasal spine, the simple tissue dissection releases part of the fibers of the depressor septi nasalis muscle. This step is practically mandatory in the BOR technique, being a part of the routine access to the nasal septum. It is described in Chap. 13, Sect. 13.8.
- **T2**—This step is optional and performed after the intraoperative analysis described in Chap. 14.

If the preoperative facial analysis showed a hyperactive depressor septi nasalis muscle, a further dissection of the soft tissues around the anterior nasal spine and the anterior maxilla is added. The intraoral access, used in the past, has been replaced by a direct access through the separation of the middle crura. Elevation of the skin of the base of the columella and central upper lip, with a delicate retractor, exposes the anterior nasal spine region and the underlying muscles fibers (Fig. 15.2a).

To avoid bleeding, the dissection from the orbicularis oris muscle can be initially accomplished with a Colorado microdissection needle until the periosteum of the anterior maxilla is reached (Fig. 15.2b), then a further muscu-

F. Meneghini, *Basic Open Rhinoplasty*, https://doi.org/10.1007/978-3-030-61827-8_15

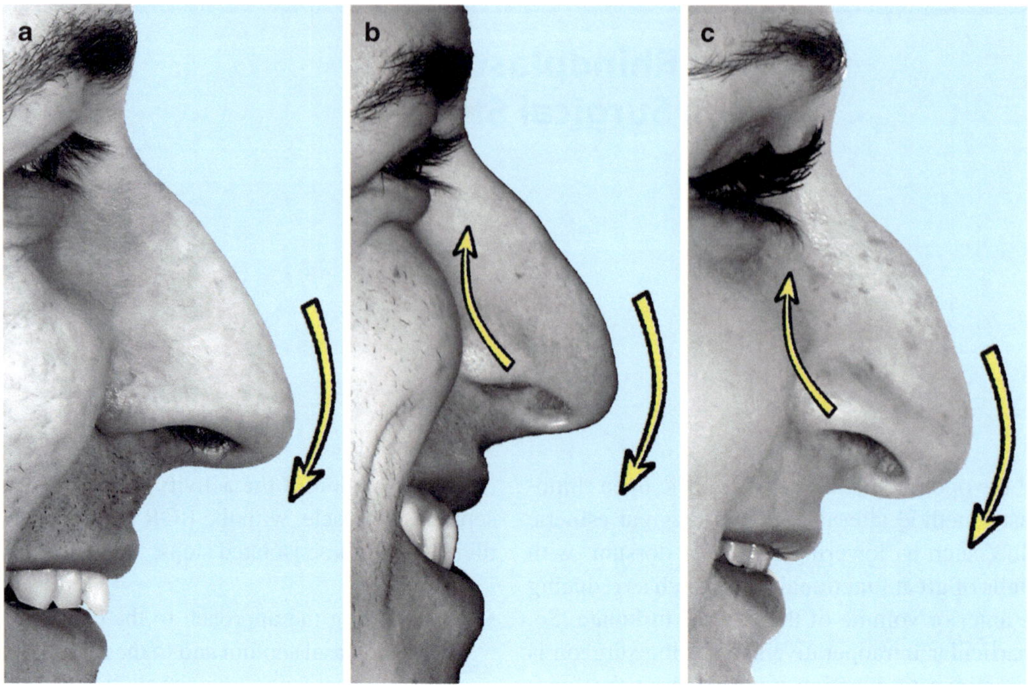

Fig. 15.1 (**a**–**c**) Depressor septi nasalis muscle activity in lateral view (**a**). The action of rotating the tip down of depressor septi nasalis muscle must be separated from the contemporary action of the levator labii superioris alaeque nasi and other nasal muscles (**b**, **c**)

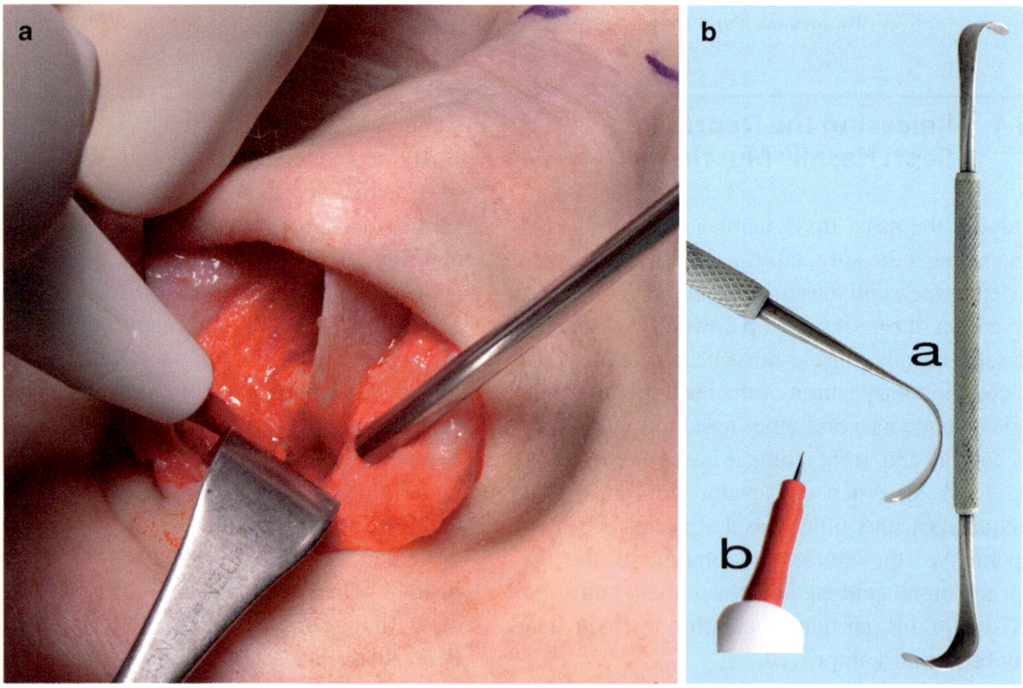

Fig. 15.2 (**a**, **b**) Release of the transnasal depressor septi nasalis muscle. Elevation of the skin of the base of the columella and central upper lip with a delicate retractor (**a**) exposes the anterior nasal spine region and the underlying muscles fibers. To avoid bleeding, muscle release can be accomplished with a Colorado microdissection needle (**b**) and a small or medium Obwegeser elevator

lar detachment from the bone can be obtained with a small or medium Obwegeser elevator.

- The extent of muscle release also depends on:
  - The patient's age. In adults and the elderly, a conservative approach is preferable so as not to worsen the tendency of the lip to drop with age.
  - The height of the upper lip. The larger the height of the lips, the more contraindicated it is to act on the septum depressor muscle.
  - The degree of exposure of the upper incisors and the gingiva at rest and during the smile.
- Figure 15.3 depicts the preoperative close-up views of a young female patient with short and incompetent upper lip, excessive exposure of the upper incisors at rest and wide exposure of the gingiva during smiling. In such cases, a more aggressive dissection of muscle fibers is indicated.

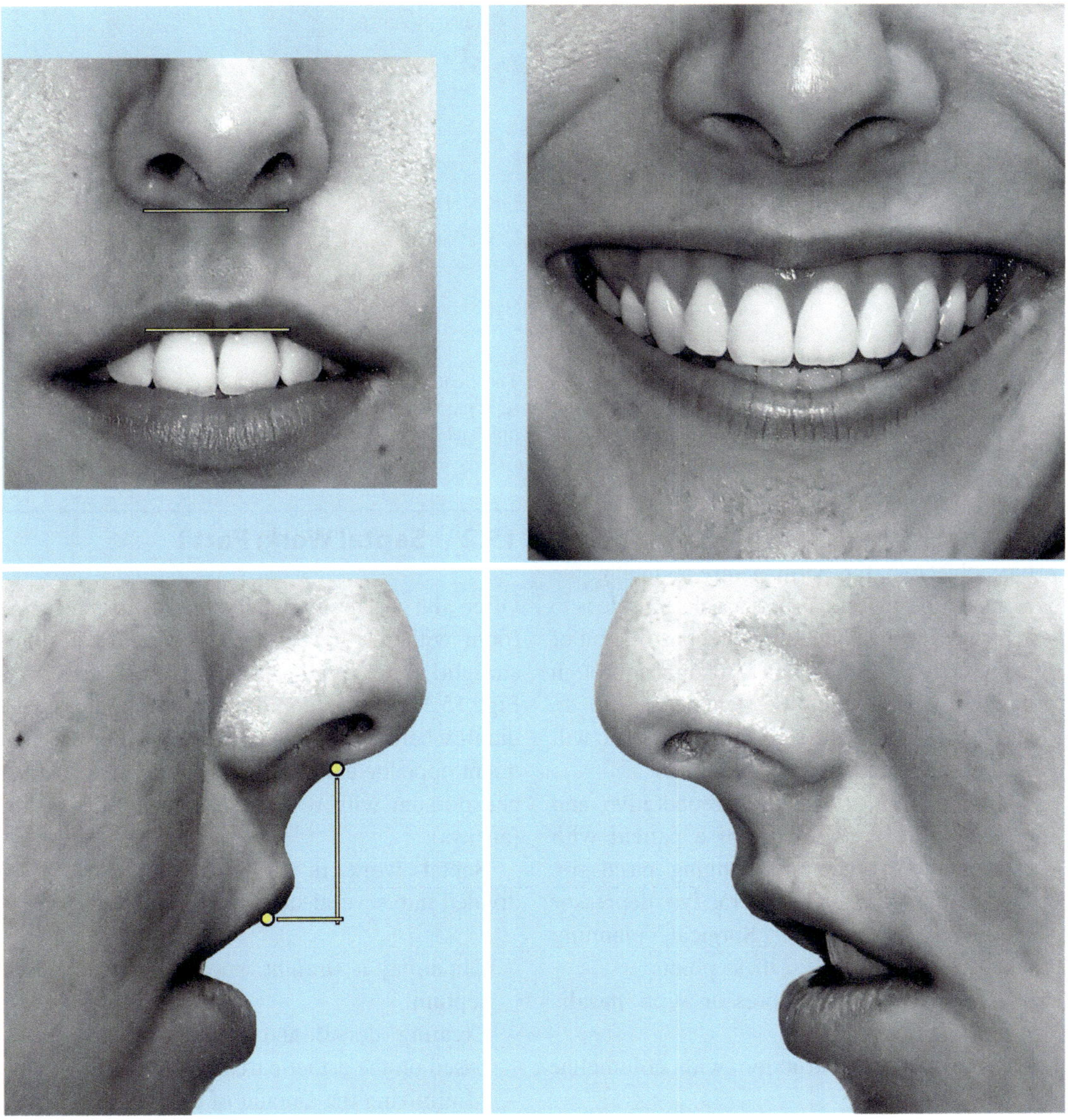

Fig. 15.3 Preoperative views of a clinical case with short and incompetent upper lip, excessive exposure of the upper incisors at rest, and wide exposure of the gingiva during smiling. In these cases a more aggressive dissection of muscle fibers is indicated

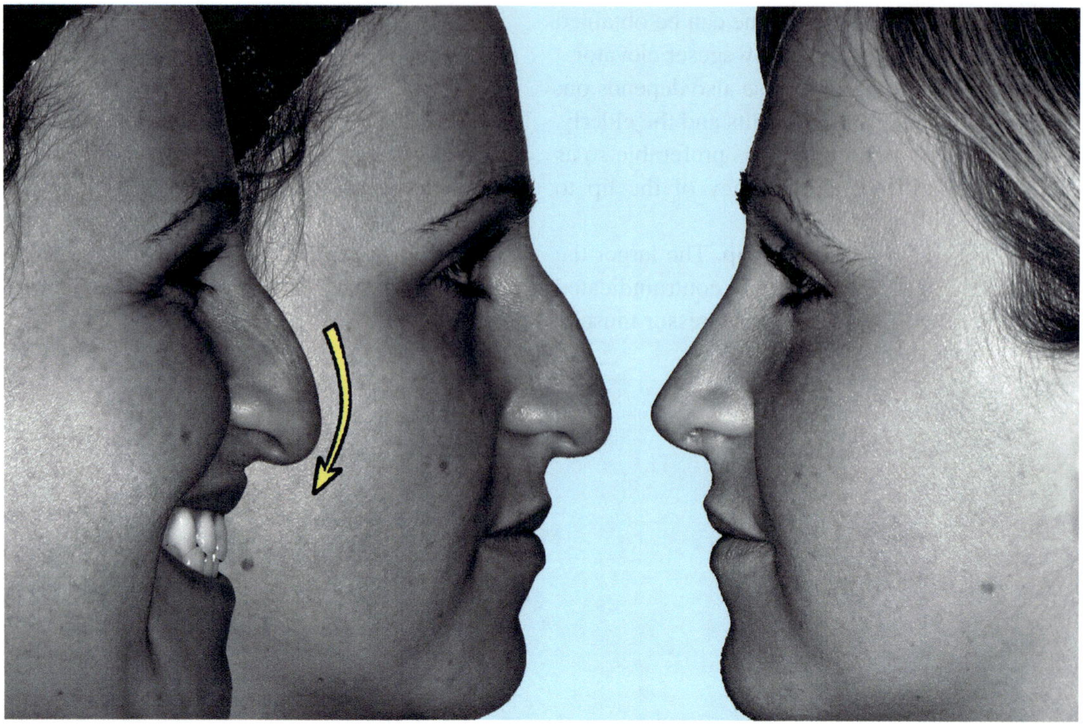

Fig. 15.4 Preoperative and postoperative profile view of a patient with moderate dorsal hump, plunging nasal tip, short columella, and hyperactive depressor septi nasalis muscle. The treatment plan included the release of the depressor septi nasalis muscle fibers, a columellar strut graft, and multiple stabilizing polydioxanone sutures to the alar cartilages

- **T3**—Probably the most important and mandatory objective for permanently reducing the action of the depressor septi nasalis muscle is to achieve a strong and resilient reconstruction of the nasal tip. This goal can be obtained through the reconstruction of the columella with an autologous septal cartilage graft. This topic will be described in the next two chapters.

  Figure 15.4 shows the preoperative and postoperative profile view of a patient with moderate dorsal hump, plunging nasal tip, short columella, and hyperactive depressor septi nasalis muscle. Surgical planning included, among others, these points:
  - Releasing of the depressor septi nasalis muscle fibers.
  - Nasal tip reconstruction with columellar strut.
  - Alar cartilage structural preservation and shaping with multiple polydioxanone sutures.

15.2 Septal Work: Part I

Often the nasal septum looks like a giant in a room with too low a ceiling. He cannot stand straight! The four preoperative CT scans in Fig. 15.5 visually confirm the metaphor of the giant, whereas the two axial views show the frequent opposite external deviation of the nasal tip and dorsum with respect to that of the septum (arrows).

Septal work in BOR septorhinoplasty is divided into several steps with four final goals:

- Obtaining a straight, supporting and stable septum.
- Creating dorsal and caudal septal profiles based on the esthetic treatment plan.
- Minimizing the amount of cartilage harvested for grafting.
- Preserving the integrity of the bilateral mucosal flaps.

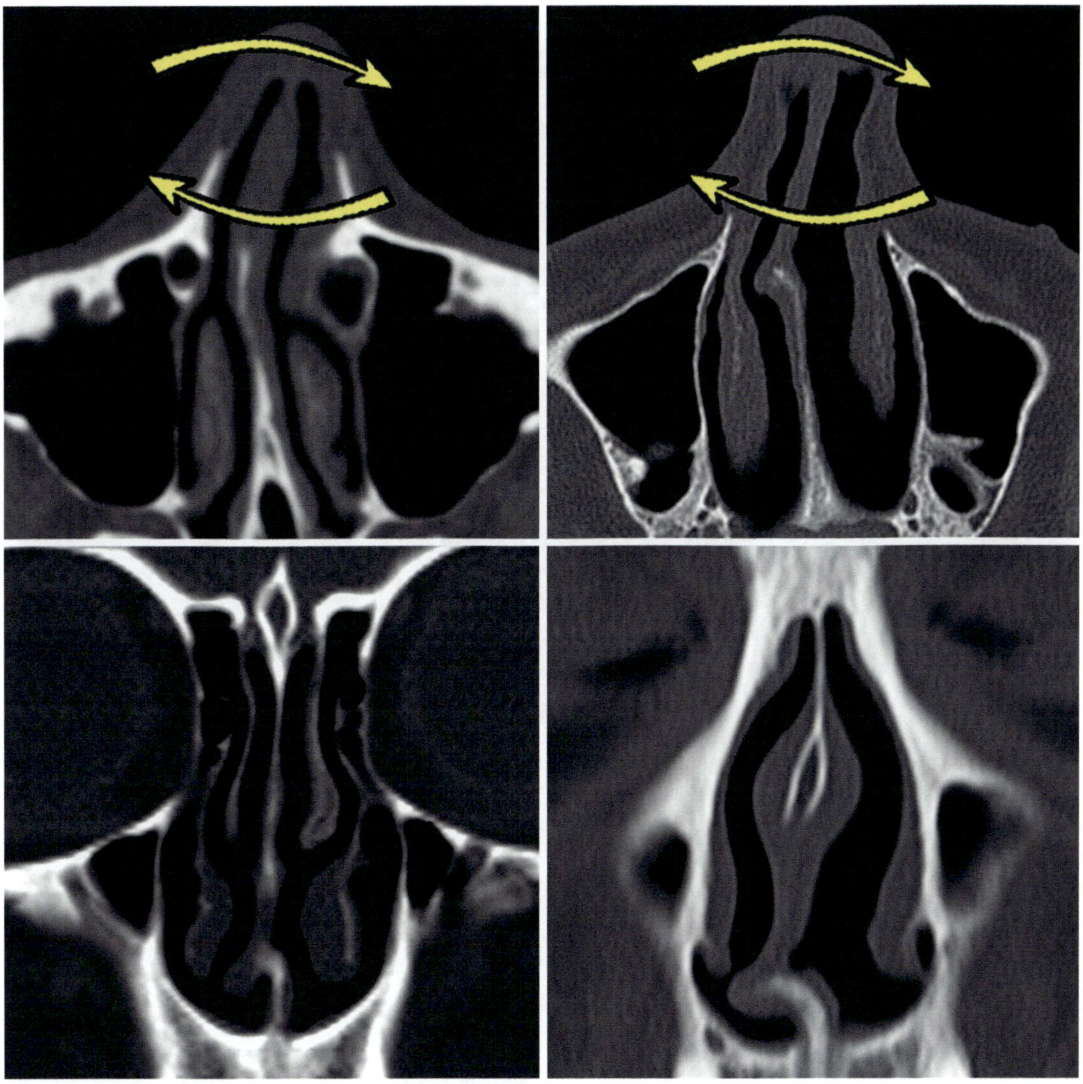

Fig. 15.5 The four preoperative CT scans show the excessive size of the septum with respect to the space in which it is contained, resulting in its inability to stand straight. Also evident is the frequent opposite external deviation of the nasal tip and dorsum with respect to that of the septum (arrows)

The first part of the septal work is, in the majority of cases, removal of a small strip of quadrangular cartilage along the maxillary crest in order to reduce the midline interference between the bone and the cartilage. Any overlapping between bone and cartilage should be eliminated.

Figure 15.6 shows the logic and quantity of this small resection that is extended as posterior as possible. At least initially, it is advisable not to remove the point of contact between the posterior septal angle and the anterior nasal spine (asterisk in Fig. 15.7).

To reduce the risk of tearing the mucosa, the incision of the cartilage is carried out with two small scalpels used in otologic surgery (Fig. 15.8a). Instead, if a 15c blade is used, to protect the opposite mucosa, it is useful to insert a small strip of plastic cut from the ruler that is usually supplied together with the skin marker.

Much attention must be paid to incise and harvest an intact long strip of cartilage, as depicted

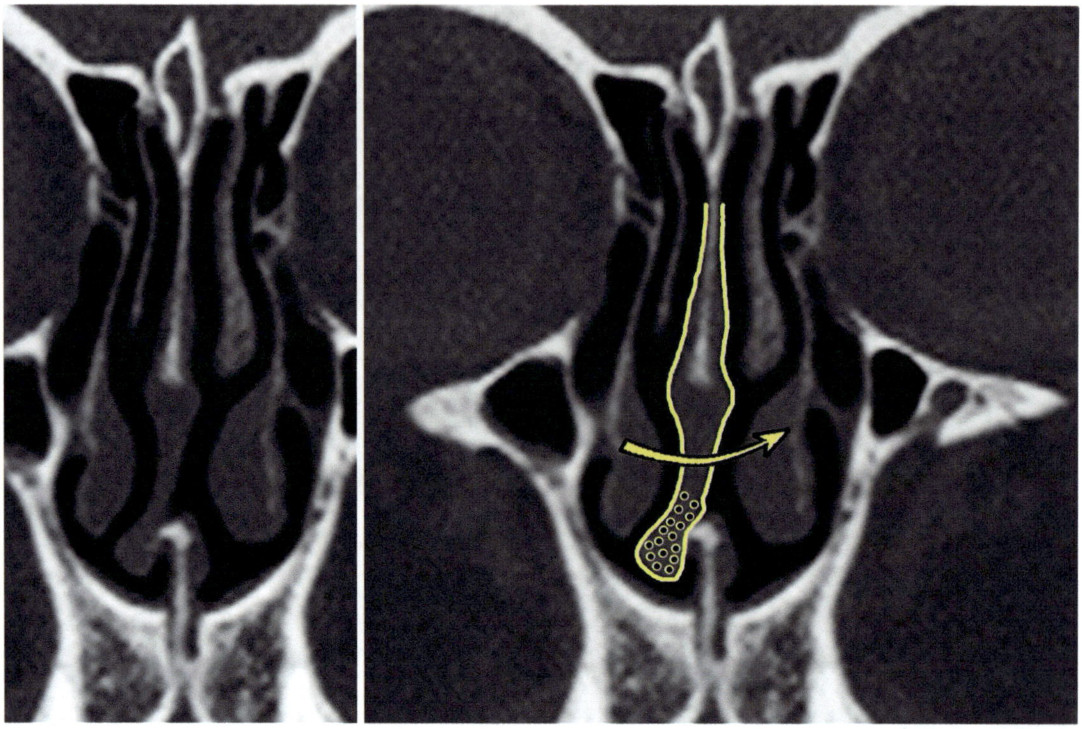

Fig. 15.6 The preoperative CT scan highlights the overlap of the quadrangular cartilage on the maxillary crest of the septum. To straighten the septum, any overlapping between bone and cartilage should be eliminated

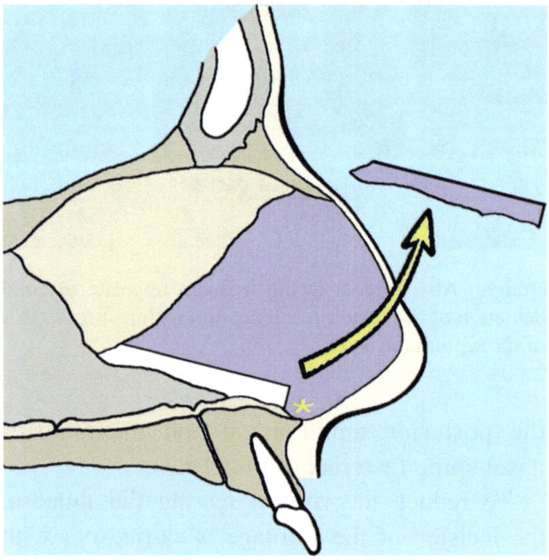

Fig. 15.7 The small initial resection is extended as posterior as possible and harvested in one piece. At least initially, it is advisable not to remove the point of contact between the posterior septal angle and the anterior nasal spine (asterisk)

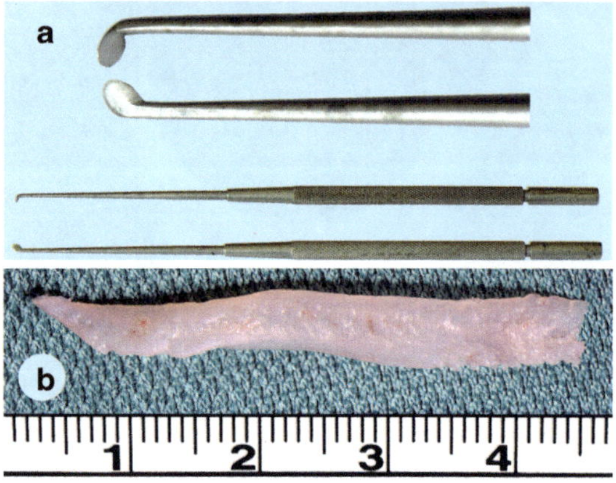

Fig. 15.8 (**a**, **b**) To reduce the risk of tearing the mucosa, the incision of the cartilage is carried out with small scalpels used in otologic surgery (**a**). The cartilage harvested should be intact and in one piece (**b**)

in Fig. 15.8b. In the general economy of rhinoplasty, a long and strong strip can have many useful uses while small and irregular pieces of cartilage can only serve for a subsequent diced graft. Like every piece of cartilage removed during surgery, also this fragment is gently cleaned with wet gauze by the surgical nurse and stored in saline solution.

Next, the portion of septal cartilage in direct contact with the anterior nasal spine is progressively trimmed to relieve any interference but maintain contact between them.

In this way, the so-called "swinging door" of the lower margin of the quadrangular cartilage is realized (see Fig. 12.4 in Chap. 12). Its effect on the septum is then evaluated; in many cases, a variable grade of improvement on anterior and dorsal deviation is obtained.

Finally, the deviated bone parts of the septum are addressed. The more frequent conditions are the removal of a central osteocartilaginous spur (Fig. 15.9) and/or a deviated maxillary crest.

A particular type of bone deviation can involve the perpendicular plate of the ethmoid close to the ipsilateral nasal bone. This anterior deviation should be recognized at preoperative CT scan analysis (Fig. 15.10). Sometimes, failure to treat the ethmoid deviation can be a cause of a clear postoperative high dorsal deviation due to incomplete unilateral mobilization of nasal bone after osteotomies. The surgeon must be careful resecting any ethmoid deviation due to the risk of damaging the cribriform plate and producing a cerebrospinal fluid leak.

The nasal skin flap is retracted with the Meneghini nasal skin retractor (MNSR) or a similar delicate retractor held in position with one or two Steri-Strips. The surgeon's non-dominant hand holds a Killian nasal speculum with thin long blades. The removal of the deviated bone can

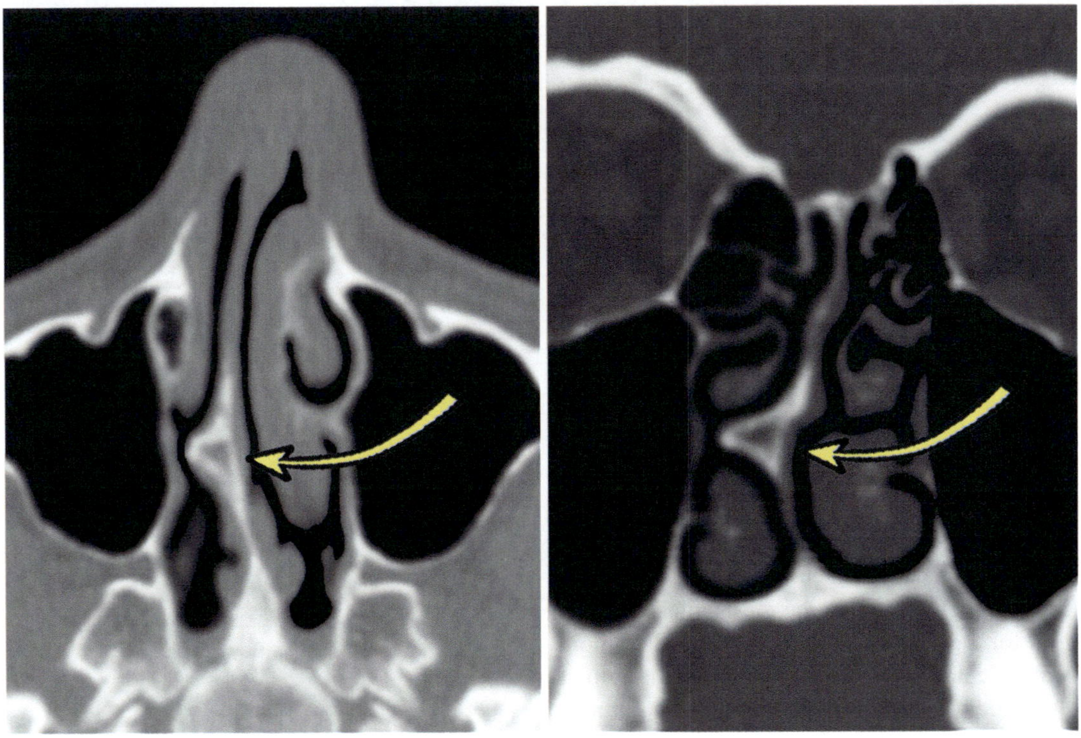

Fig. 15.9 Preoperative CT axial and coronal scans. Central osteocartilaginous spur (curved arrows) and contralateral hypertrophied inferior turbinate

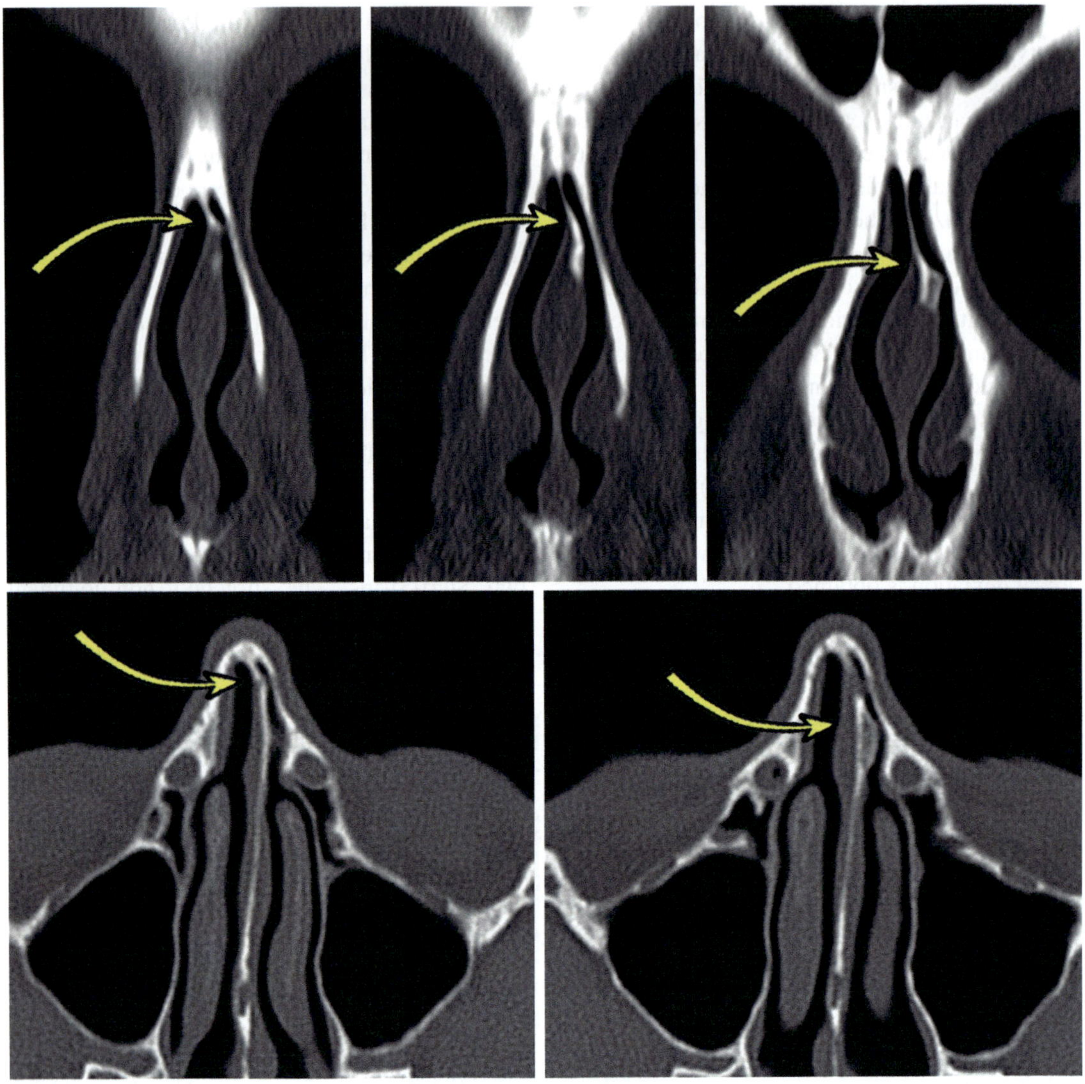

Fig. 15.10 Preoperative CT axial and coronal scans. High and anterior bony septal deviation of the perpendicular plate of the ethmoid close to the ipsilateral nasal bone (curved arrows)

be done gently in small bites and without any twisting movements utilizing a Beyer delicate double-action bone rongeur or Takahashi scissors (Fig. 15.11) but actually the most suitable instrument for a gentle resection of a deviated ethmoid perpendicular plate or an ethmoidal spur is a small ultrasonic bone saw (Fig. 15.12). This work must be performed slowly under direct vision and copious irrigation with sterile saline. Ultrasonic bone surgery technology (also named piezosurgery) will become the gold standard for safe reshaping and resection of small bones in the near future.

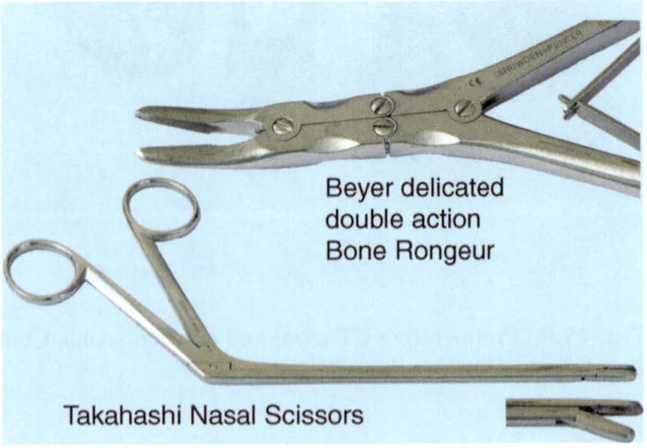

Fig. 15.11 Beyer delicate double-action bone rongeur and Takahashi scissors

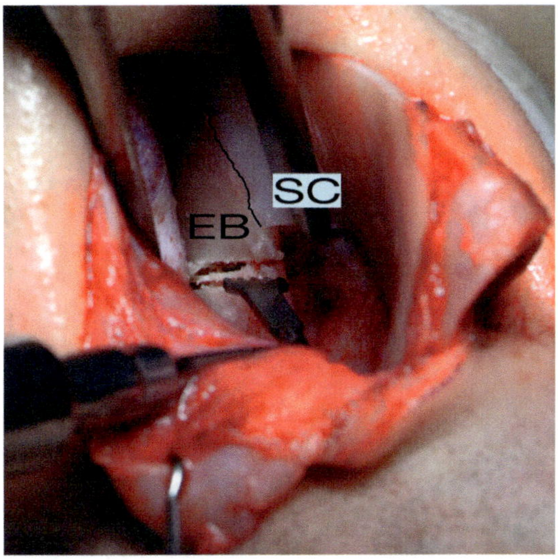

Fig. 15.12 Intraoperative view of a resection of a deviated ethmoid perpendicular plate using a small ultrasonic bone saw. This work must be performed slowly under direct vision and copious irrigation with sterile saline

All the described septal work can be done with a scialytic lamp after lowering the operating bed a little.

15.3 Shaping the Anterior Nasal Spine

Sometimes the anterior nasal spine is so prominent as to alter the esthetic columellar-upper lip contour (Fig. 15.13). In this case, the reduction can be performed under direct vision with a small osteotome (Fig. 15.14), a bone rongeur (Fig. 15.15), or a Piezosurgery saw. During these maneuvers, it is necessary to protect the lower margin of the columellar incision with a small retractor (Fig. 15.16). The use of a power burr is not recommended due to the risk of inadvertently damaging the soft tissues.

More rarely the anterior nasal spine is deviated on one side. The corrective choices in this case are between reshaping with reduction of the most deviated portion or performing an incomplete osteotomy followed by manual repositioning of the most protruding portion. The first method is preferred when a reduction of volume and projection of the anterior nasal spine is

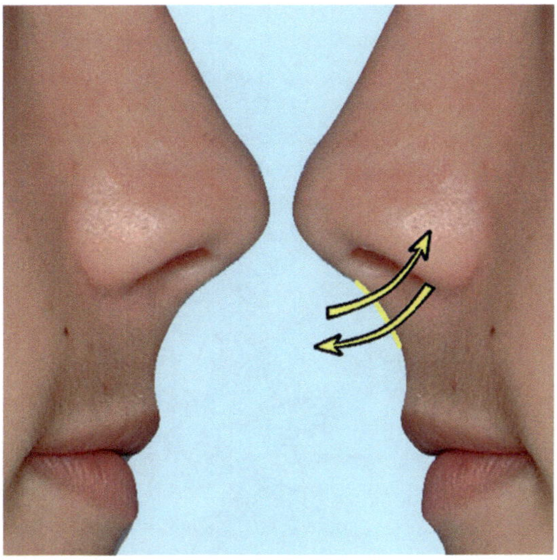

Fig. 15.13 Prominent columellar-upper lip contour

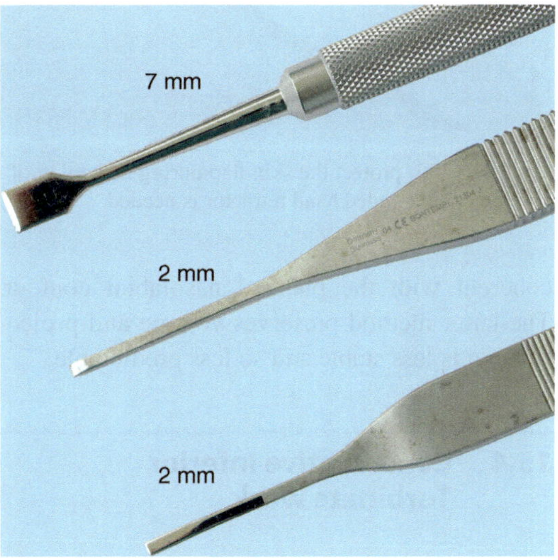

Fig. 15.14 Series of small osteotomes

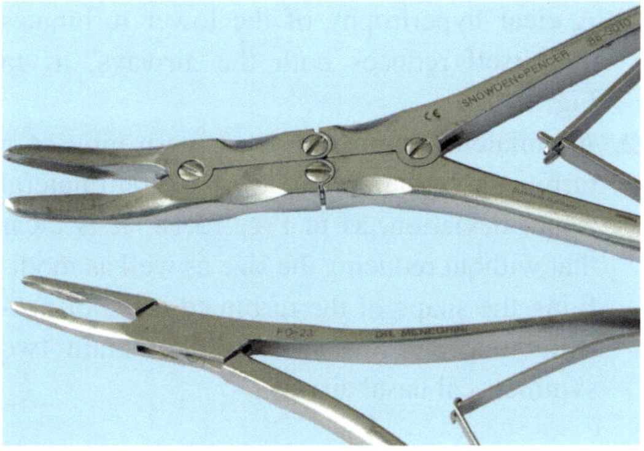

Fig. 15.15 Bone rongeurs

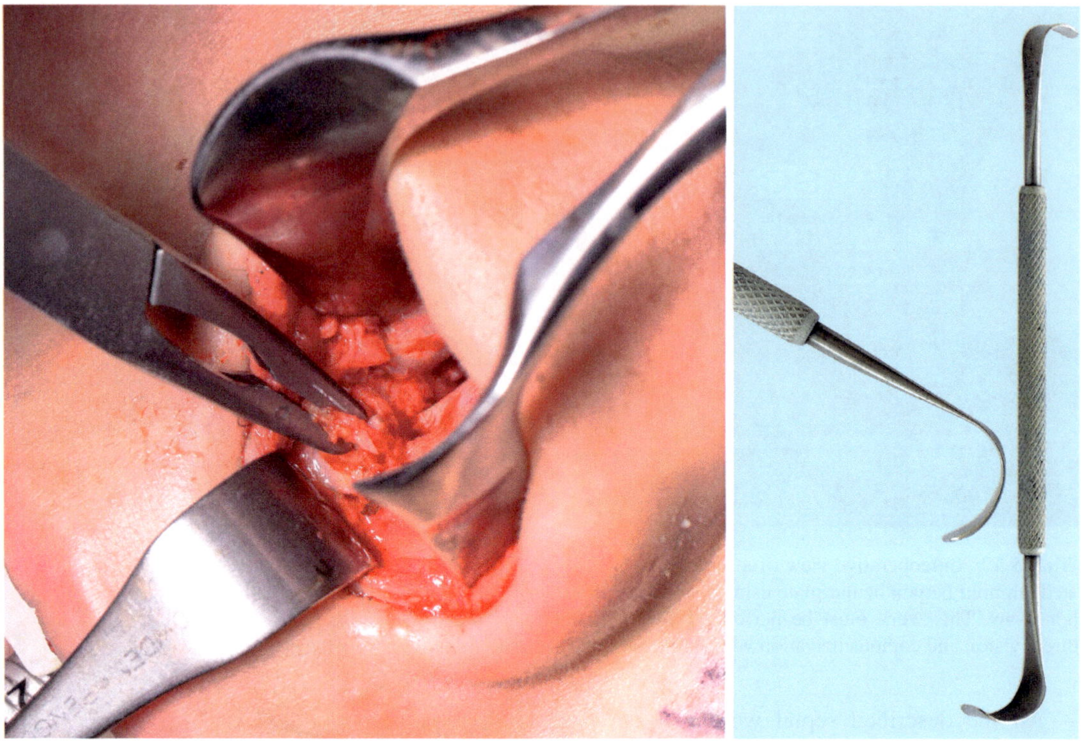

Fig. 15.16 To protect the skin flap during reshaping of the anterior nasal spine, a small delicate retractor such as the Kasdan double-ended hand retractor is needed

coherent with the planned nasolabial contour. The latter method preserves volume and projection but is less stable and so less predictable.

15.4 Conservative Inferior Turbinate Work

In rhinoplasty there are three main conditions related to the lower turbinates to consider:

1. A clear hypertrophy of the lower turbinates that itself reduces both the airways, as in Fig. 15.17.
2. A unilateral compensatory hypertrophy of a turbinate in the presence of a contralateral septal deviation, as in Fig. 15.18. It is clear that without reducing the size as well as modifying the shape of the turbinate it is not possible to center the septum and obtain two symmetrical nasal airways.
3. A relative hypertrophy in patients candidate to a reductive rhinoplasty. The head of the inferior turbinates, one of the elements of the internal nasal valve, potentially puts the airway patency at risk after surgery, as in Fig. 15.19.

If only one of these conditions is present, a conservative surgical treatment of the inferior turbinate should be considered mandatory.

In the author's clinical experience, in over 90% of BOR rhinoplasty cases, a simple and standard surgical treatment of the inferior turbinate was performed.

At this point of the surgical sequence, when soft tissue nasal and septal flaps are elevated and the "swinging door" of the quadrangular cartilage offers extra space, with a simple Killian speculum and scialytic lamp the operator can perfectly visualize and check his actions on the inferior turbinate.

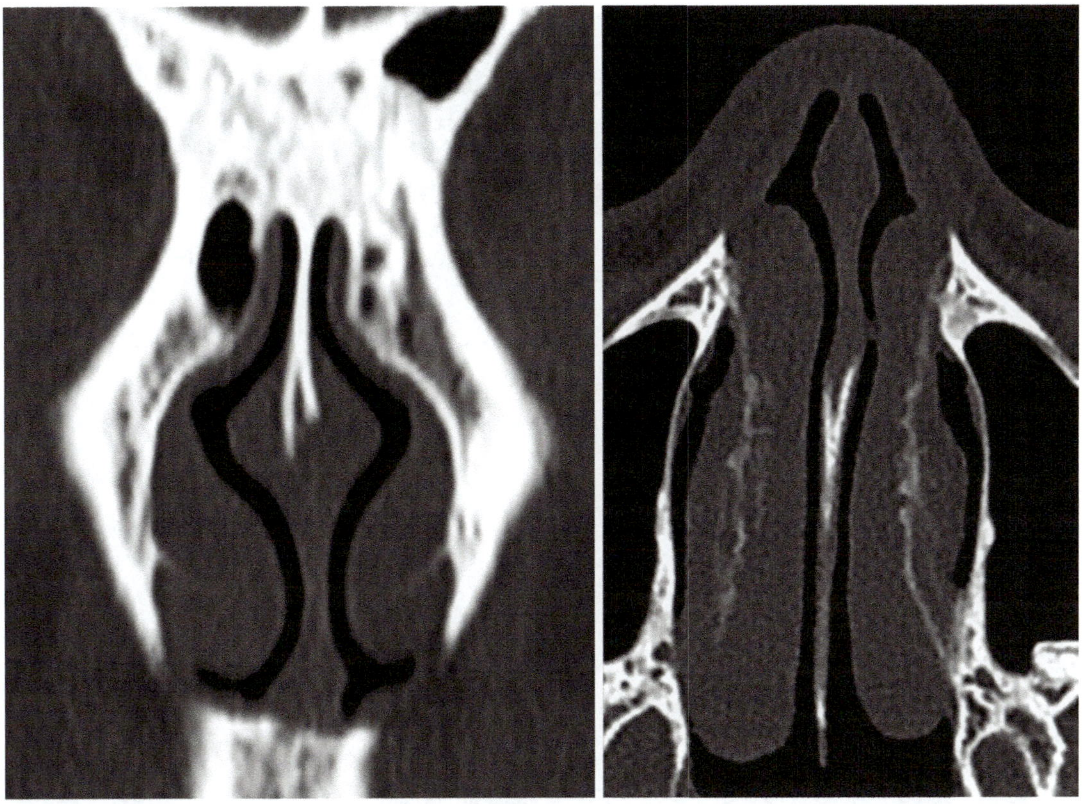

Fig. 15.17 Preoperative CT coronal and axial scans. Bilateral hypertrophy of the inferior turbinates with reduction of the nasal airways

The author has used the surgical technique presented here for more than 10 years with little modification. The inspiring principles are:

- Avoid heat injury to the mucosa and underlying soft tissue as well as to the bone.
- Avoid any mucosal resection.
- Remove the bone of the anterior one-third of the inferior turbinate and fracture in small pieces the remaining conchal bone of the posterior two-thirds.
- Effectively reduce postoperative swelling of the anterior portion of the inferior turbinate through medium- to long-term direct physical containment.
- Promote postoperative fibrosis of the anterior portion of the inferior turbinate in order to reduce the risk of late hypertrophy relapse close to the internal nasal valve.
- Reduce the risk of postoperative synechiae by avoiding mucosal raw surfaces.

The main steps of BOR turbinoplasty are:

- **T1**—A slow injection of local anesthetic at the level of the head of turbinate. A half dental carpule vial (0.9 mL) for each turbinate is the usual quantity.
- **T2**—A small longitudinal incision of the head of the turbinate is performed with the Colorado microdissection needle until the periosteum of the bone is reached. The total length of the incision is comprised between 1 and 1.5 cm (Fig. 15.20a, b).
- **T3**—With a small double-ended nasal elevator, such as a Freer or Tebbetts elevator, a delicate dissection of the soft tissue from the conchal bone is performed on the anterior third of the turbinate. The thin bone is then fractured and removed with a straight atraumatic Halsted Mosquito forceps (Fig. 15.21a). The quantity and thickness of bone removed will vary according to the anatomy encoun-

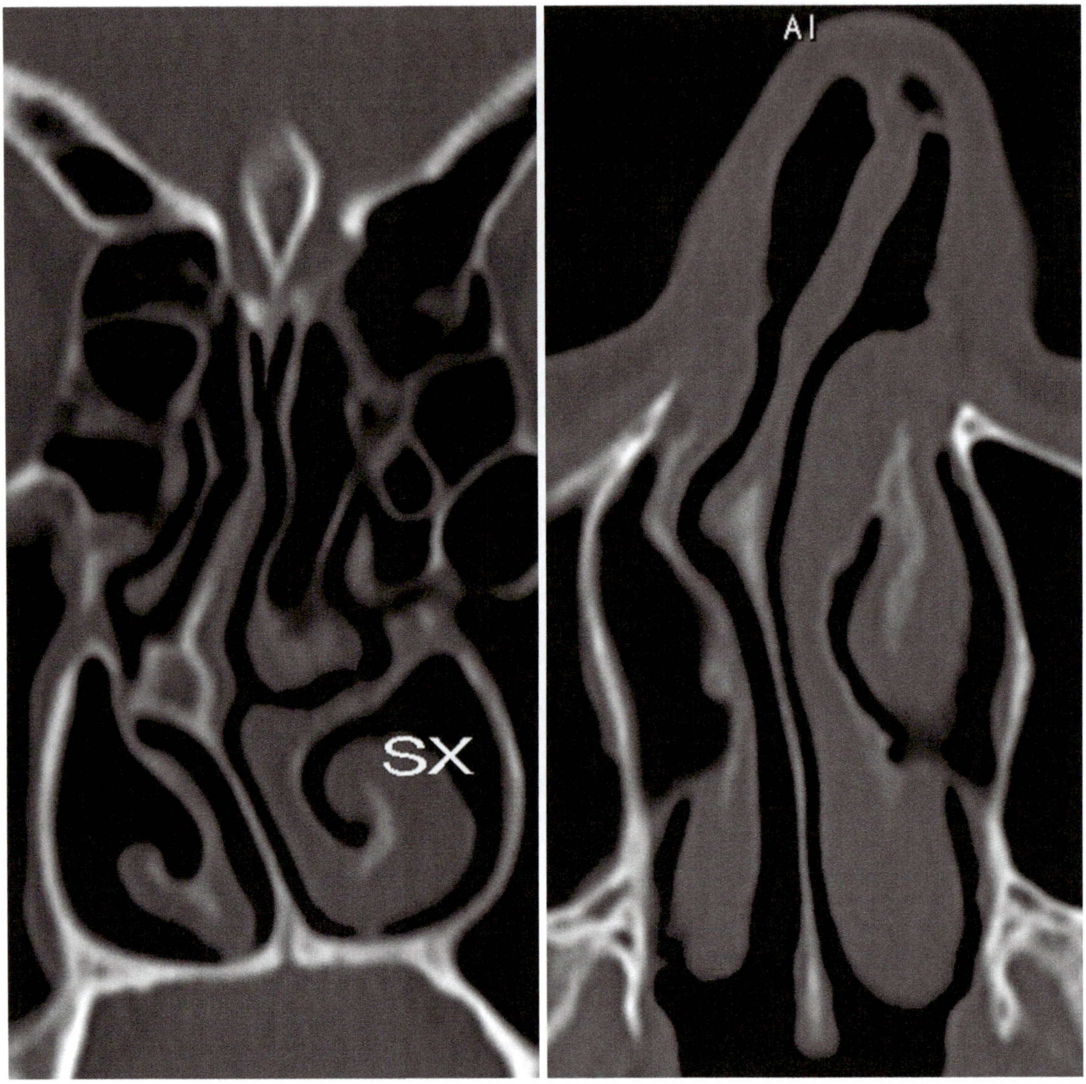

Fig. 15.18 Preoperative CT coronal and axial scans. Unilateral compensatory hypertrophy of the left inferior turbinate, ipsilateral enlarged middle turbinate (concha bullosa) in the presence of a contralateral septal deviation

tered; Figure 15.21b shows the bone removed in a single piece from a turbinate mainly composed of bone.

- **T4**—The remaining conchal bone is then microfractured in accordance with Rohrich et al.[1] With a Killian or Tebbetts long nasal speculum, the turbinate is gentle outfractured in a juddering motion proceeding from posterior to anterior while pushing the extremity of the speculum laterally on the turbinate. For a complete microfracture it is preferable to repeat the maneuver two or three times.

  The objective is to obtain a comminuted fracture inside an intact mucosal envelope instead of the classic simple outfracture of the entire conchal bone.

- **T5**—A double running suture, extending from the most anterior part to the central third of the turbinate, is done. To keep the knot completely

[1]Rohrich RJ, McKee D, Malafa M. Closed microfracture technique for surgical correction of inferior turbinate hypertrophy in rhinoplasty: Safety and technical considerations. Plast Reconstr Surg. 2015;136:607e.

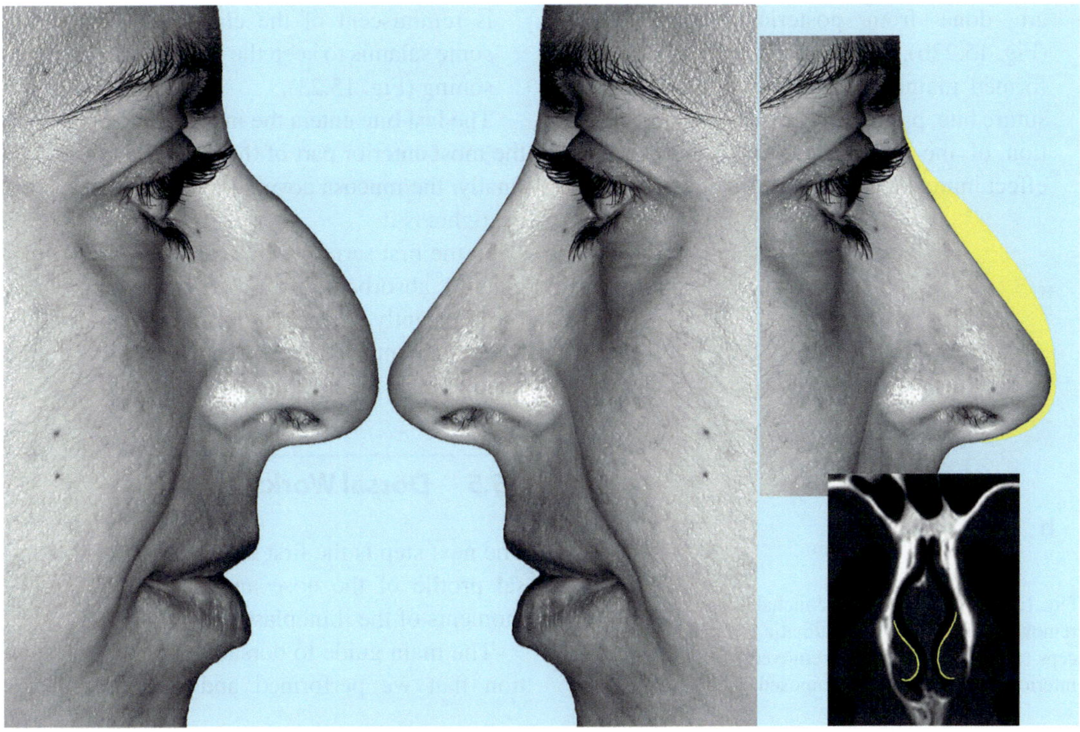

Fig. 15.19 "Mirror" and "Overlap" right profile simulations and preoperative CT coronal scan in a clinical case of reductive rhinoplasty. The relative hypertrophy of the head of the inferior turbinates potentially puts the airway patency at risk after surgery

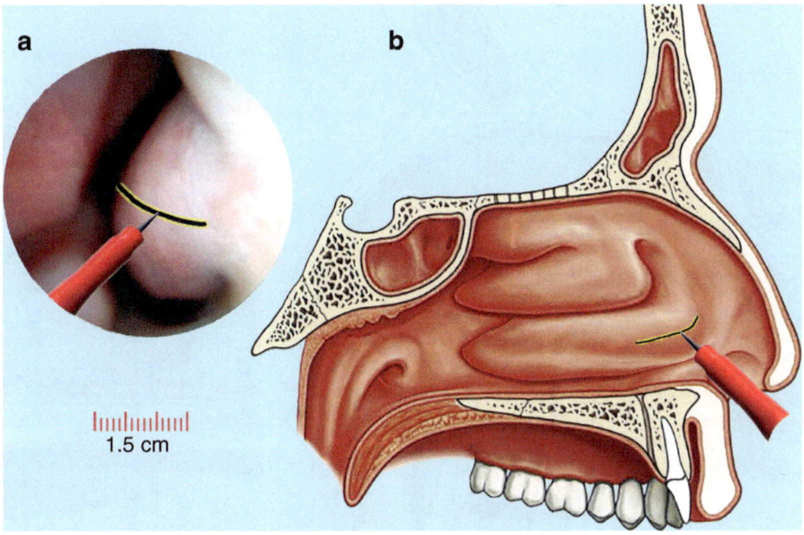

Fig. 15.20 (**a**, **b**) Endoscopic view (**a**) and anatomical drawing of the left nasal cavity (**b**). A small longitudinal incision of the head of the turbinate is performed with the Colorado microdissection needle until the periosteum of the bone is reached. The total length of the incision is comprised between 1 and 1.5 cm

under the mucosa at the end of the suture, the first bite enters directly into the mucosal incision. The next are large bites that continue well beyond the length of the mucosal incision and carry on to the middle of the turbinate. Eight or nine bites are performed from anteriorly to posteriorly (Fig. 15.22a) and then another series of similar large running bites are done from posteriorly to anteriorly (Fig. 15.22b). This double running suture, performed maintaining gentle tension on every suture bite, produces an evident volume reduction of the anterior turbinate. The shaping effect immediately appears to the operator and is reminiscent of the elastic net that wraps some salamis to keep the shape during the seasoning (Fig. 15.23).

The last bite enters the mucosa and exits from the most anterior part of the wound incision and, finally, the mucosa covers the knot as the operator tightens it.

In the first series of clinical cases, a 5/0 polyglactin, absorbable, braided suture was used. More recently, a 5/0 poliglecaprone, absorbable, monofilament has also been used with similar good clinical result.

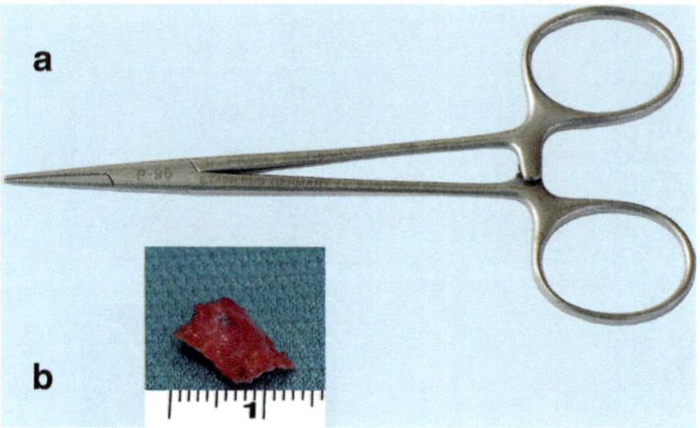

Fig. 15.21 (**a**, **b**) The thin conchal bone is fractured and removed with a straight atraumatic Halsted Mosquito forceps (**a**). A bone fragment removed from the head of an inferior turbinate mainly composed of bone (**b**)

15.5 Dorsal Work: Part I

The next step is the first modification of the dorsal profile of the nose and one of the crucial moments of the rhinoplasty.

The main guide to dorsal work is the simulation that we performed and shared with the

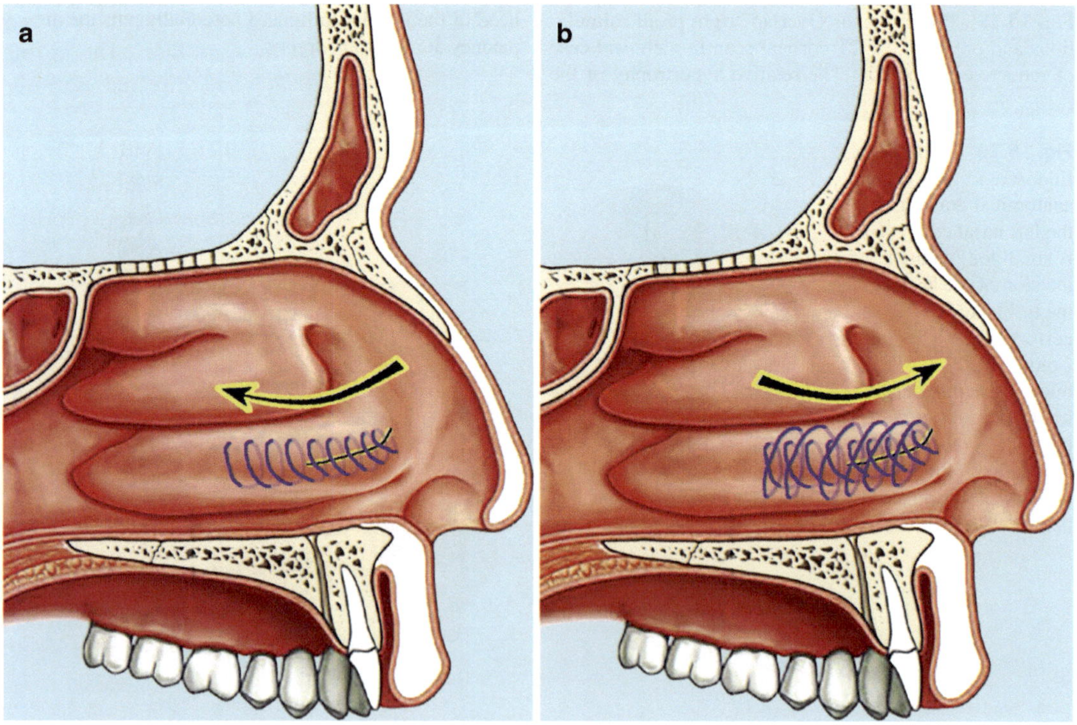

Fig. 15.22 (**a**, **b**) Modeling double running sutures of the inferior turbinate. Eight or nine bites are performed from anteriorly to posteriorly (**a**) and then another series of large running bites are done from posteriorly to anteriorly (**b**) maintaining gentle tension on every suture bite and so producing an evident volume reduction of the anterior turbinate

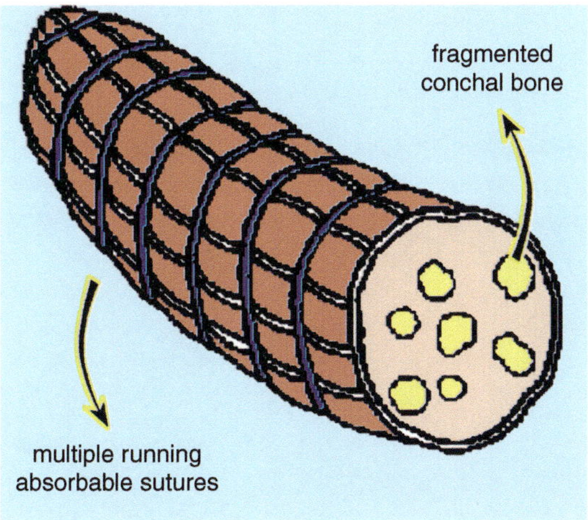

Fig. 15.23 The shaping effect of the two running suture series on turbinate volume and shape recall the elastic net that wraps some salamis to keep their shape during the seasoning. In a similar way, the running sutures can maintain the shape of the turbinate during the healing steps

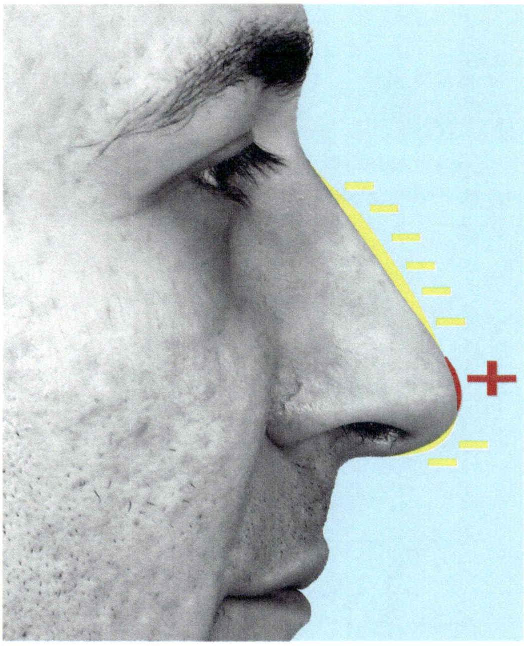

Fig. 15.24 "Overlap" right profile simulations. An enlarged printed simulation with the subtraction areas well marked, and sometimes also the more rare areas, where the profile should be increased, is the best guidance for profile alignment

patient, and is now hanging close to the first surgeon. An enlarged printed simulation with the subtraction areas well marked and also the more rare areas where the profile should be increased (Fig. 15.24) is more useful than the classic simulations printed on separate sheets of paper (Fig. 15.25).

Figure 15.26a, b helps to understand the enormous variations of the dorsal modification even in simulations where the common goal is to obtain a straight profile. It is therefore evident that without a good preoperative simulation it is difficult, also for an experienced surgeon, to appreciate exactly where and how much the nasal profile should change.

Then there is the variability of the adaptation ratio of the nasal soft tissue envelope to the changes in the shape of the osteocartilaginous nasal skeleton realized by surgery. In many classical rhinoplasty texts, as well as in Chap. 5 of this book, the difference of the thickness of the skin and underlying soft tissue is described, from cephalic to caudal, as a sequence of thick-thin-thick thicknesses. Figure 15.27a shows a diagram with the regional soft tissue envelope thickness in a case of evident osteocartilaginous hump. If the final goal is a straight dorsal profile, the new shape of the supporting framework should resemble a small and less accentuated hump such as that shown in Fig. 15.27b.

The potential risk of removing en bloc a dorsal hump with a large straight base (Fig. 15.27a–c) is the saddle nose deformity. It can be defined as a concave and over-reduced nasal dorsum (Fig. 15.27c).

This condition is not to be confused with soft tissue pollybeak deformity, the fullness of the supratip due to excess skin and scar tissue (Figs. 15.28 and 15.29).

The approaches recommended by BOR are therefore more conservative and gradual than in the past. For simplicity they are subdivided into two main techniques:

- Limited osteocartilaginous hump resection and progressive septal profile adjustment.
- Partial and conservative nasal bone resection and conservative adjustment of cartilaginous hump.

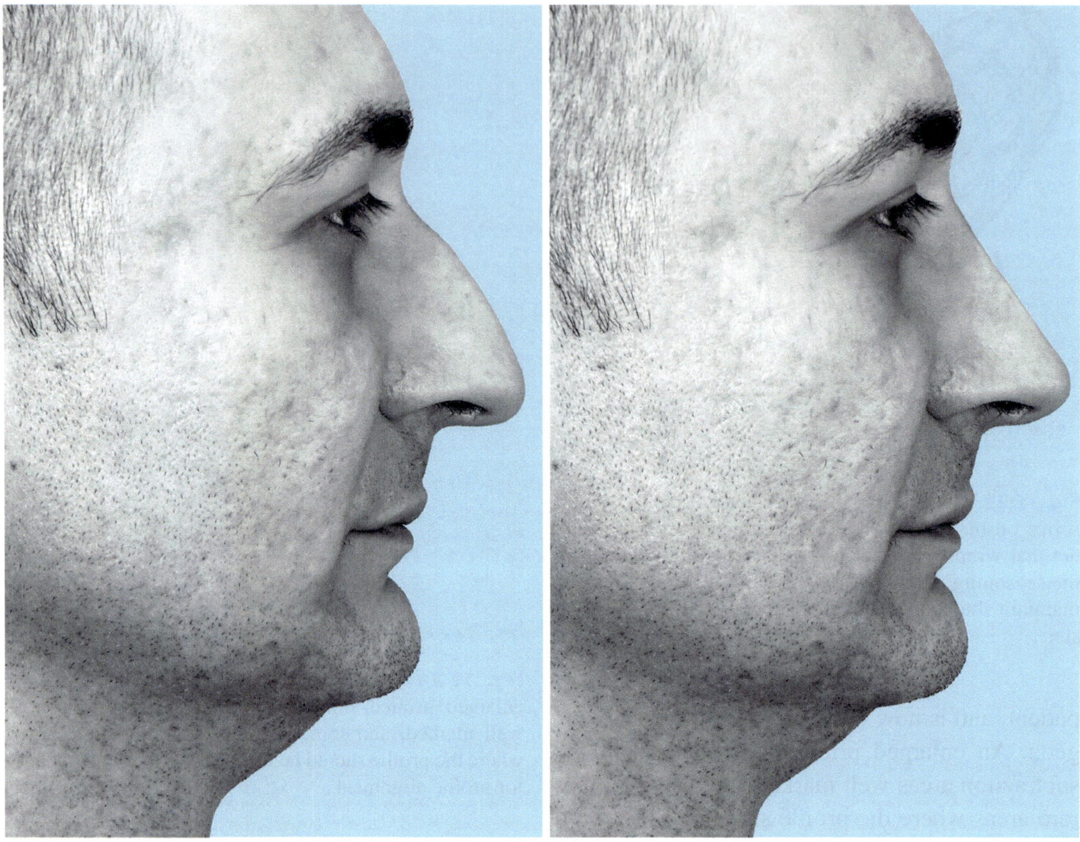

Fig. 15.25 The classic simulation and the initial profile view printed on separate sheets of paper is of less help for the surgeon in identifying the specific areas to be corrected

15.6 Limited Osteocartilaginous Hump Resection and Progressive Profile Adjustment

This technique is preferred in the case of a noticeable hump and its goal is to keep intact part of the excess of the upper lateral cartilage for a later dorsal reconstruction.

The most utilized method in the past was the complete en bloc removal of the nasal hump. It consists of a single piece composed of a strip of the anterior cartilaginous septum, part of the upper lateral cartilages, and part of the nasal bones (Fig. 15.30a, b). The cartilages are cut with a 15c or similar blade under direct vision, whereas the bone osteotomy is performed with a sharp Rubin (Fig. 15.31) or Tebbetts osteotome. Despite the accuracy of the operator and the direct vision offered by the open approach, frequently the hump removed appears on close observation asymmetric or excessive. Figure 15.32 shows a specimen in which the left upper lateral cartilage is over-resected compared to the opposite side and the bone is over-resected on the right side. These findings suggest that the surgeon will be

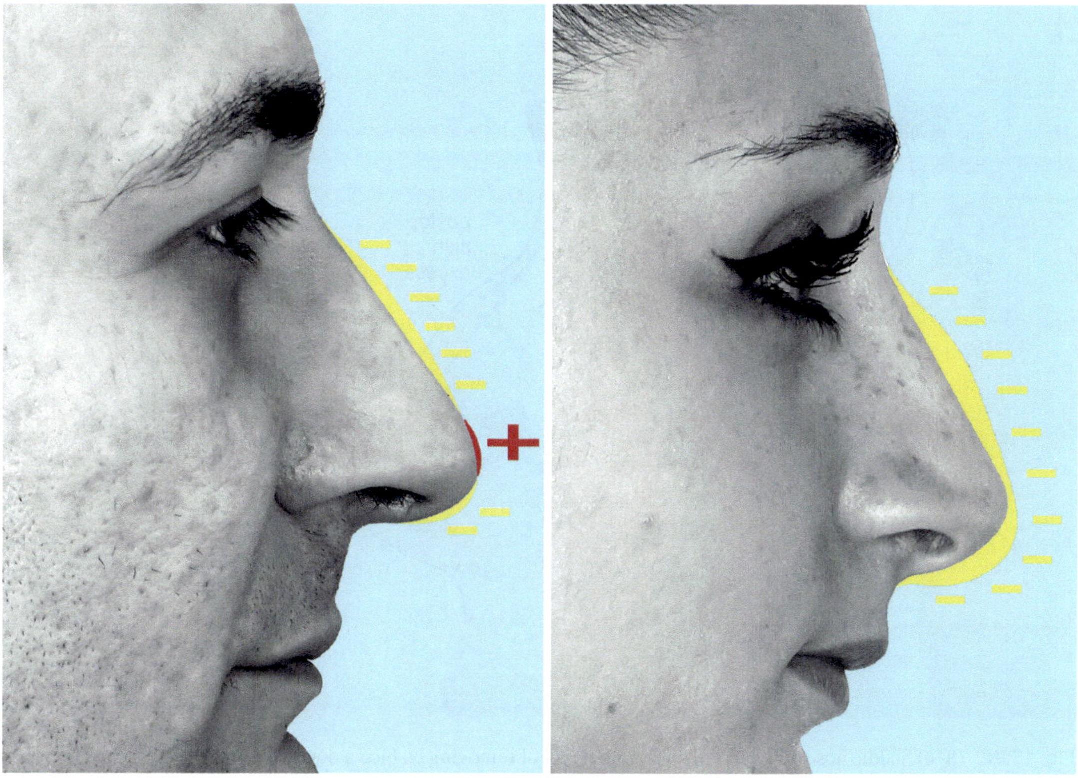

Fig. 15.26 (**a**, **b**) The enormous variations of the dorsal modification even in two "Overlap" simulations where the common goal is to obtain a straight profile

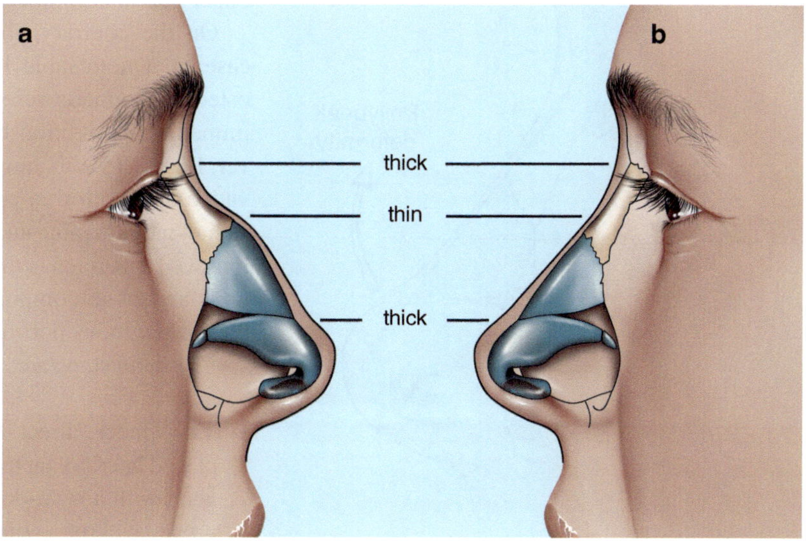

Fig. 15.27 (**a**, **b**) The regional soft tissue envelope midline thickness in a case of evident osteocartilaginous hump (**a**). If the final goal is a straight dorsal profile, the new shape of the supporting framework should resemble a small and less accentuated hump and not a straight line (**b**)

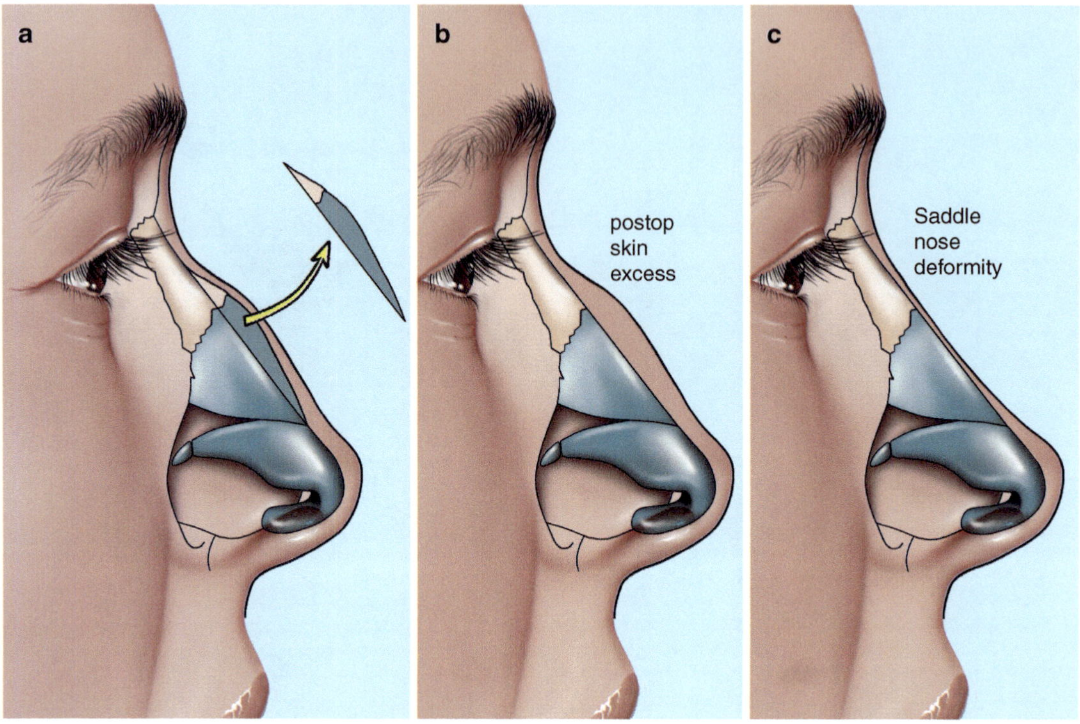

Fig. 15.28 (**a**–**c**) Saddle nose deformity. The potential risk of removing en bloc a dorsal hump with a large straight base (**a**) is the saddle nose deformity. It can be defined as a concave and over-reduced nasal dorsum (**c**)

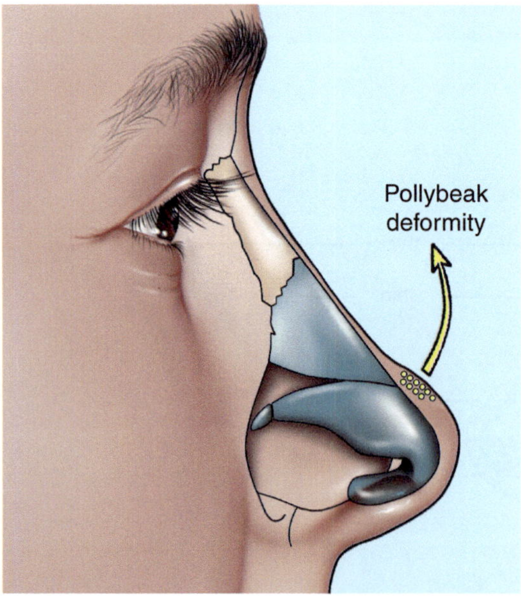

Fig. 15.29 Soft tissue pollybeak deformity. Secondary deformity marked by the fullness of the supratip area due to excess skin and scar tissue (dots). This condition is not to be confused with the cartilaginous pollybeak secondary to under-resection of the quadrangular cartilage close to the anterior septal angle

forced to balance these asymmetries by removing some nasal bone on the left and reducing the right upper lateral cartilage.

On the contrary, the BOR approach, in the case of a noticeable hump, suggests a limited osteocartilaginous resection without seeking an immediate correction based on a single maneuver. Figure 15.30b simply illustrates this conservative approach that can be performed with the same instruments and the same steps. The removed specimen is thinner both in the cartilaginous and bone components while the length of the cartilaginous portion is significantly shorter.

The main steps are:

- **T1**—Under direct vision, the 15c blade is placed laterally on the left nasal bone (for a surgeon with a right-dominant hand) at an appropriate level for a conservative hump removal.
- **T2**—The blade is then moved caudally from the nasal bone to the upper lateral cartilage to start the incision. The pressure of the instrument should be directed medially to incise

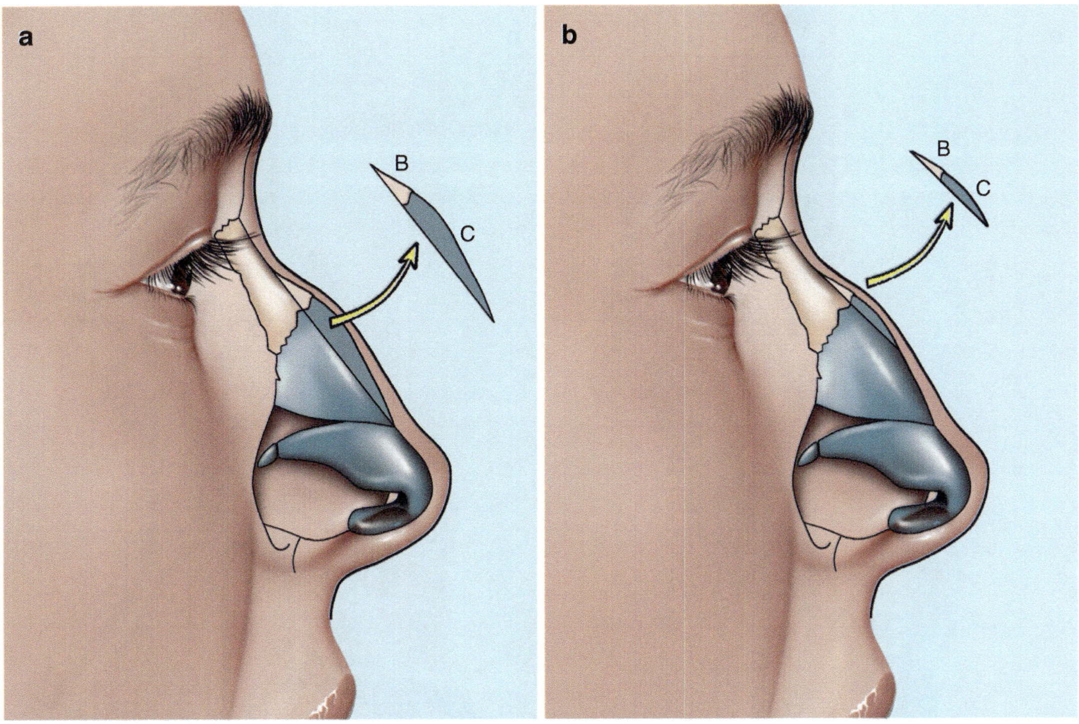

Fig. 15.30 (**a**, **b**) En bloc removal of the nasal hump. It consists of a single piece composed of a strip of the anterior cartilaginous septum, part of the upper lateral cartilages, and part of the nasal bones. A conservative approach (**b**) with under-resection is mandatory

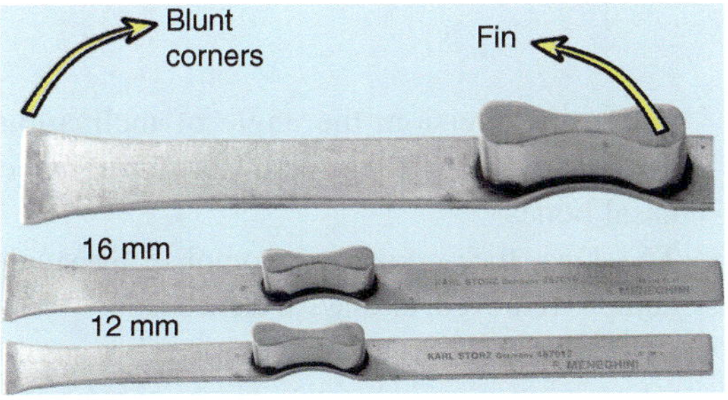

Fig. 15.31 Rubin osteotome. The fin helps the surgeon in orienting the instrument, whereas the blunt corners avoid accidental soft tissue injury during nasal osteotomy

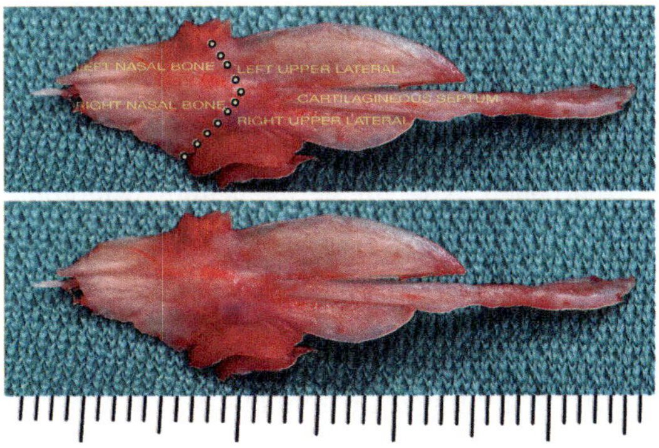

Fig. 15.32 En bloc removal of the nasal hump. The left upper lateral cartilage is over-resected compared to the opposite side and the bone is over-resected on the right side. These findings suggest that the surgeon will be forced to balance these asymmetries by removing some nasal bone on the left and reducing the right upper lateral cartilage

also the septum and the contralateral upper lateral cartilage in a single gesture as depicted in Fig. 15.33a. If a conservative resection is followed, the blade does not injure the underlying nasal mucosa.

- **T3**—To complete the cartilage incision, the blade is directed caudally (Fig. 15.33b) with the aim of keeping the resection limited and as symmetrical as possible.
- **T4**—Under direct vision the Rubin osteotome is positioned under the cartilaginous hump in contact with the bone (Fig. 15.34). It is essential to check the angle of inclination and the

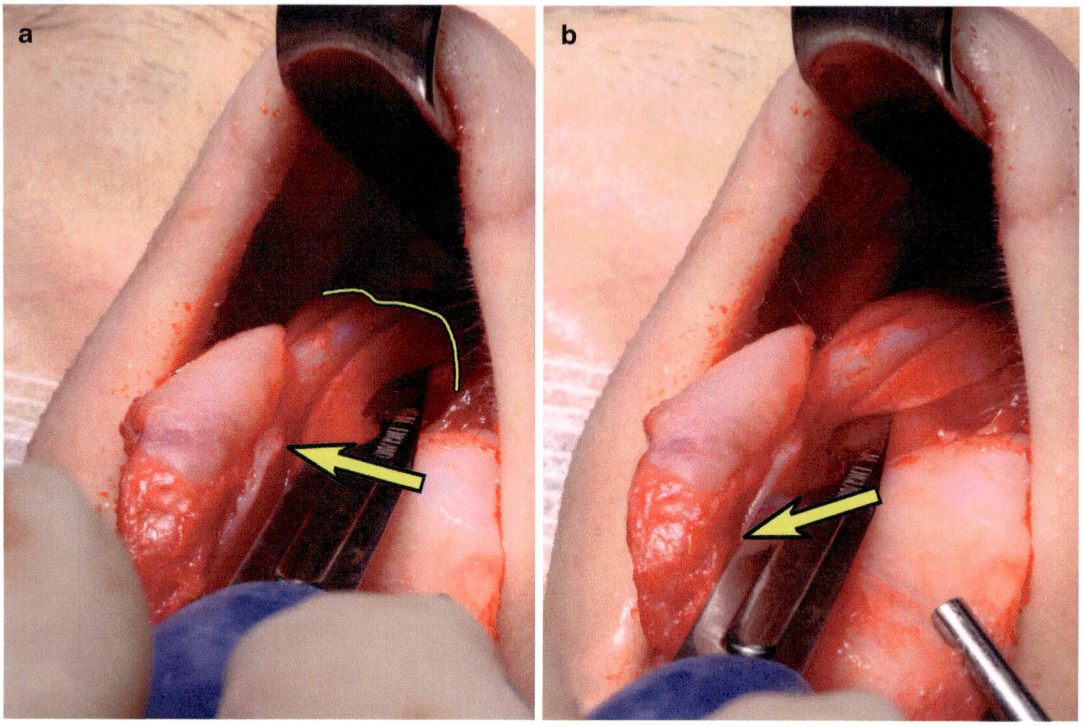

Fig. 15.33 (**a**, **b**) En bloc removal of the nasal hump. The cartilaginous portion is incised with the 15c blade. The blade is then moved caudally from the nasal bone to the upper lateral cartilage to start the incision. The pressure of the instrument should be directed medially to incise also the septum and the contralateral upper lateral cartilage in a single gesture (**a**). To complete the cartilage incision, the blade is directed caudally (**b**) keeping the resection limited and as symmetrical as possible

rotation along the axis of the instrument. It is equally important that the osteotome is well sharpened. The fin of the Rubin osteotome helps the surgeon to hold and properly orient the instrument before and during hammering.

- **T5**—Initially the nasal skin flap is maintained elevated by the operator's non-dominant hand with a Maliniac or Tebbetts nasal retractor while the assistant holds the mallet. The osteotome is then advanced under the power generated by the mallet blows. The surgeon directly controls, with his dominant hand and under direct vision, the angle of inclination and precise osteotome pathway through the nasal bones.
- **T6**—Once the osteotomy is complete, the small hump is removed, cleaned and checked for symmetry and thickness. It is then stored in sterile saline solution with the other pieces of bone and cartilage previously harvested. Also the surgical field is cleaned with sterile saline and visually inspected. A careful assessment by palpation of the intermediate nasal profile is done with the nasal flap repositioned (Fig. 15.35).

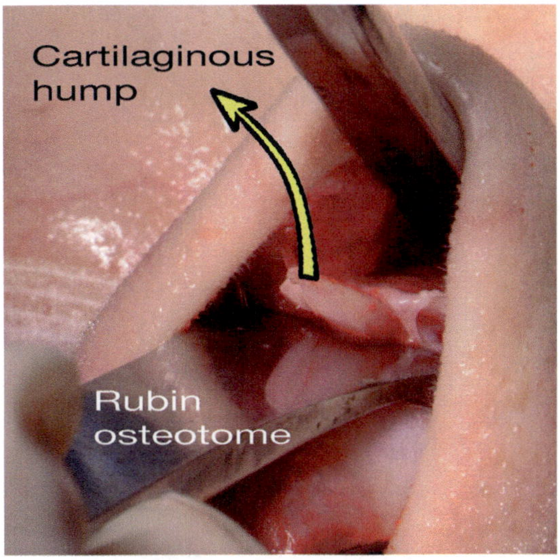

Fig. 15.34 En bloc removal of the nasal hump. Under direct vision the Rubin osteotome is positioned under the cartilaginous hump in direct contact with the bone. It is essential to continuously check the angle of inclination and the rotation along the axis of the instrument previewing the planned line of osteotomy. To avoid transmitting too much energy on the bone with the hammer and to guide the osteotomy with greater precision, a well-sharpened osteotome is also fundamental

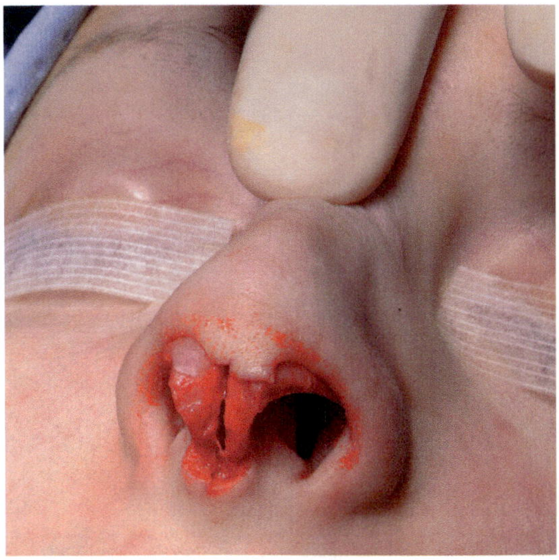

Fig. 15.35 Assessment by palpation of the intermediate nasal profile after en bloc removal of the nasal hump. A direct visual inspection with cleaning of the surgical field is also mandatory

In recent years, technological evolution has allowed the replacement of the classic osteotome and the hammer with piezoelectric saws for a more precise and controlled hump osteotomy, as shown in the next section.

15.7 Partial Conservative Nasal Bone Resection and Conservative Profile Adjustment

This technique is preferred in the case of minimal hump, a very frequent case. Its goal is to approach the dorsum maintaining the upper lateral cartilages completely intact and removing only the bony part of the deformity.

The main steps are:

- **T1**—With the aid of sharp scissors or the sharp end of a Tebbetts elevator, the most anterior portion of nasal bone is skeletonized from the underlying upper lateral cartilage (Fig. 15.36b). This area, named "nasal keystone region," consists of contributions from the paired nasal bones cephalically, paired upper lateral cartilages caudally, quadrangular cartilage anterior-inferiorly, and perpendicular plate of the ethmoid posterior-inferiorly (Fig. 15.36a). The dissection is difficult and must be limited only to the undersurface of the paired nasal bones to maintain the structural strong adherence between the bone and cartilage in both the lateral aspects (Fig. 15.37).
- **T2**—The recommended instrument for bone removal is the ultrasonic saw under copious sterile saline irrigation. Under direct vision, all the osteotomy lines can be drawn and completed slowly by passing several times the oscillating saw over the bone surface with gentle pressure (Fig. 15.38a–c). Usually the specimen consists of a thin triangular-shaped bone with the base oriented caudally and the apex cephalically (Fig. 15.39).

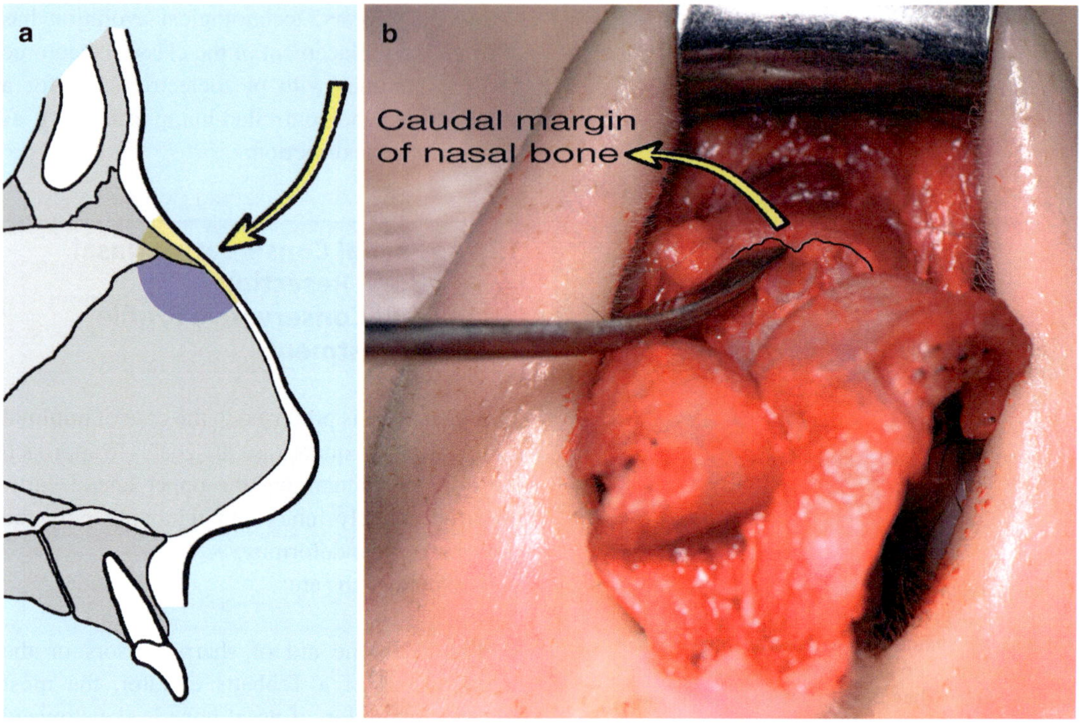

Fig. 15.36 (**a**, **b**) Nasal keystone region (**a**). With the aid of a sharp-end elevator, the most anterior portion of the nasal bones is skeletonized from the underlying upper lateral cartilage (**b**)

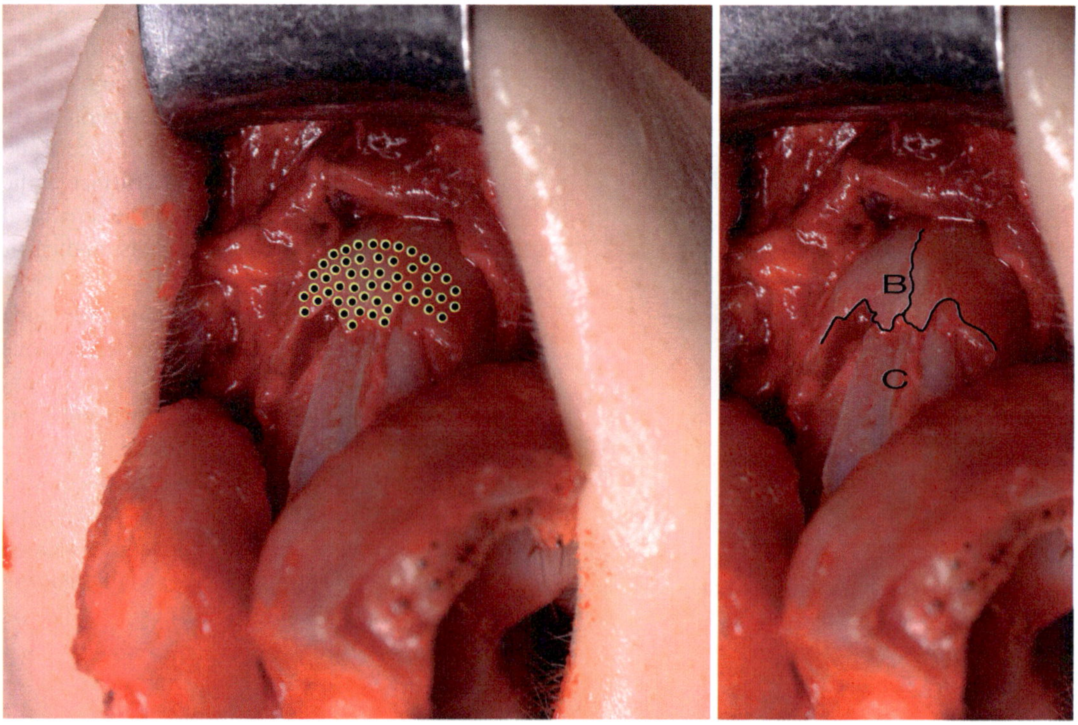

Fig. 15.37 The dissection is difficult and must be limited only to the undersurface of the paired nasal bone (dotted area) to maintain the structural strong adherence between the bone and cartilage in both the lateral aspects. *B* nasal bone, *C* cartilage

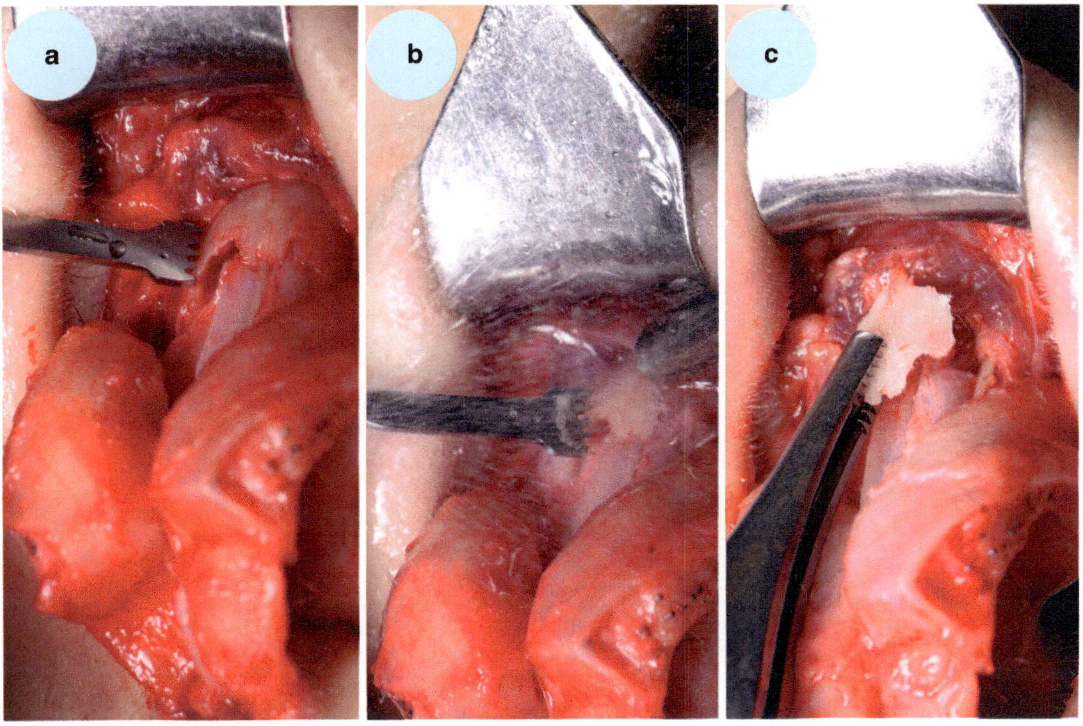

Fig. 15.38 (**a–c**) Ultrasonic removal of the bony hump. Under direct vision, all the osteotomy lines can be drawn and completed slowly by passing several times the ultrasonic oscillating saw over the bone surface with gentle pressure

Fig. 15.39 Ultrasonic removal of the bony hump. Usually the specimen consists of a thin triangular-shaped bone with the base oriented caudally and the apex cephalically

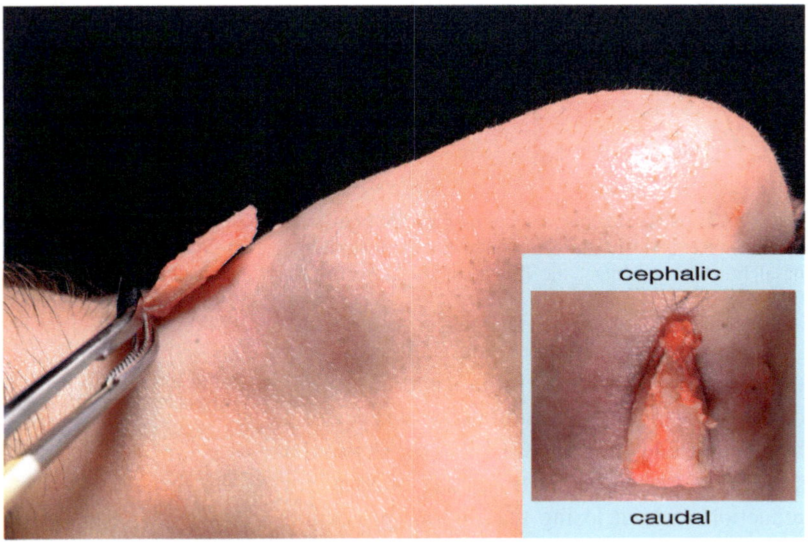

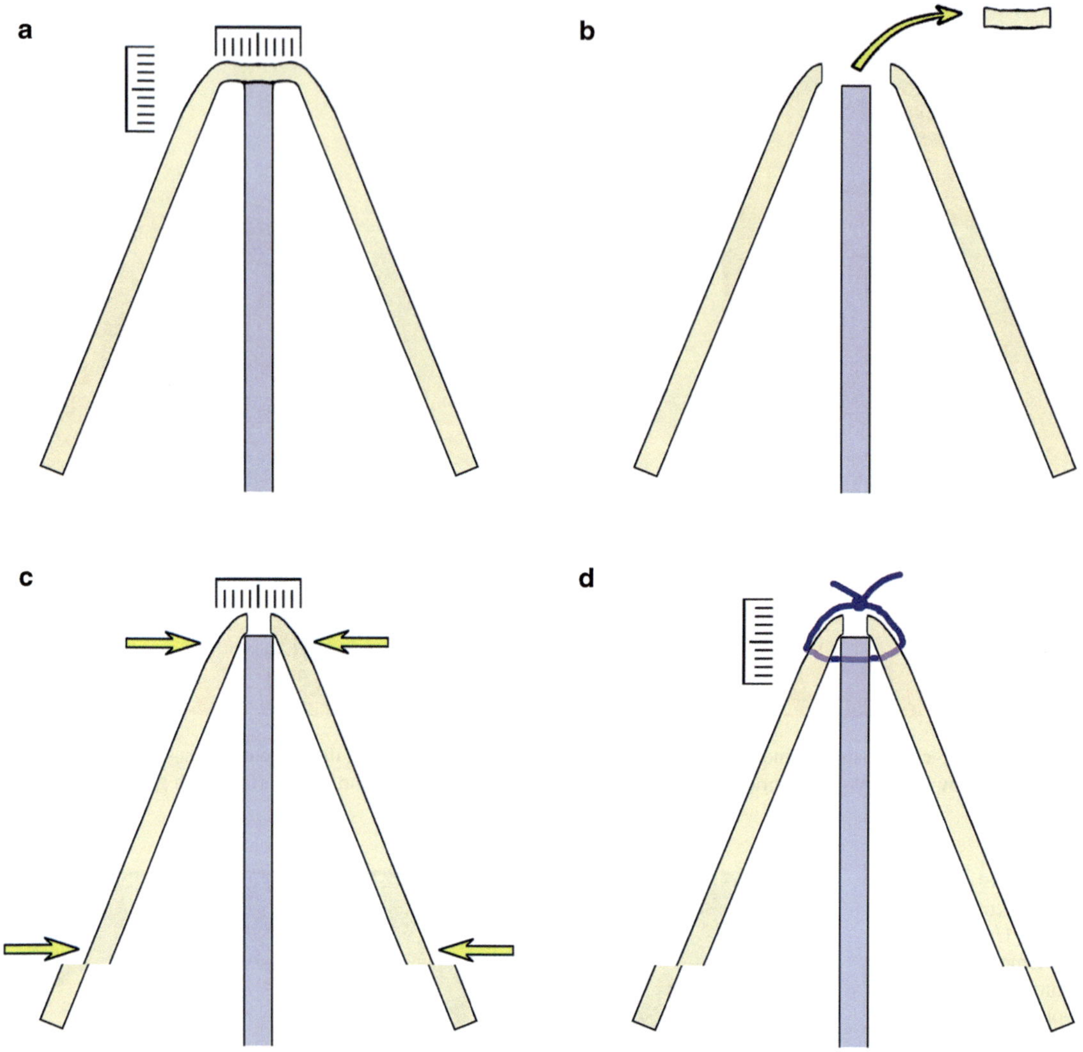

Fig. 15.40 (**a**–**d**) Schematic section of a wide bony dorsum (**a**). Removal of the transverse component of the nasal bone leaves intact the height of the dorsum (**b**). Closure of the residual open roof with basal osteotomies (**c**). Stabilization of the transverse width by suturing both the nasal bones to the cartilaginous septum (**d**)

This very conservative ultrasonic surgical technique can become useful in a particular condition: the wide bony dorsum in the absence of a hump in profile view. Figure 15.40a–d shows the surgical sequence of the transverse bony width reduction without losing the anterior projection of the dorsum.

In the case of a planned deepening of the nasal radix, it is also possible to remove a unique long piece of bone with the piezoelectric oscillating saw (Fig. 15.41).

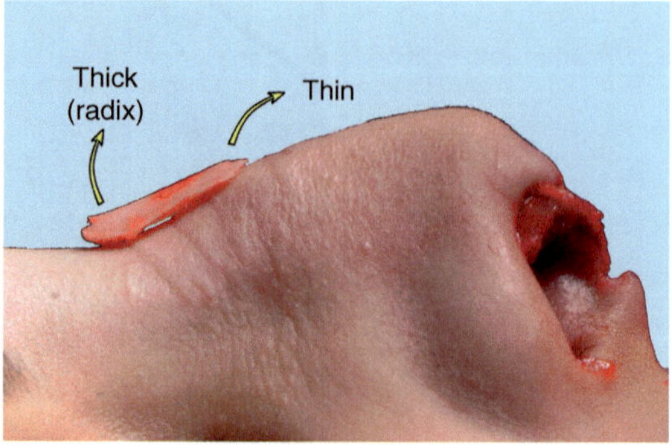

Fig. 15.41 Ultrasonic removal of the bony hump. In the case of a planned deepening of the nasal radix, it is also possible to remove a single long piece of bone

15.8 Deepening the Nasal Radix with an Electric Power Burr

Deepening the nasal root region poses some problems even though, in selected cases, it represents an important esthetic goal. From the anatomical point of view, there are two elements that prevent the achievement of the desired results:

1. The soft tissue envelope is thicker than in all other nasal regions (Fig. 15.42a). It responds little or very little to the reduction of the underlying bone.
2. The nasal radix bone almost always is thicker and denser than all the other nasal and maxillary regions (Fig. 15.42b). It responds little or not at all to manual rasping.

Before engaging in an attempt to deepen the root, it is advisable to review the median sagittal section of preoperative CT. Figure 15.43a illustrates a relatively favorable case with a thin skin for the radix and a thick underlying bone to work on. The opposite condition is a major contraindication to deepen the radix. It consists of a thick soft tissue envelope and a thin underlying bone (Fig. 15.43b).

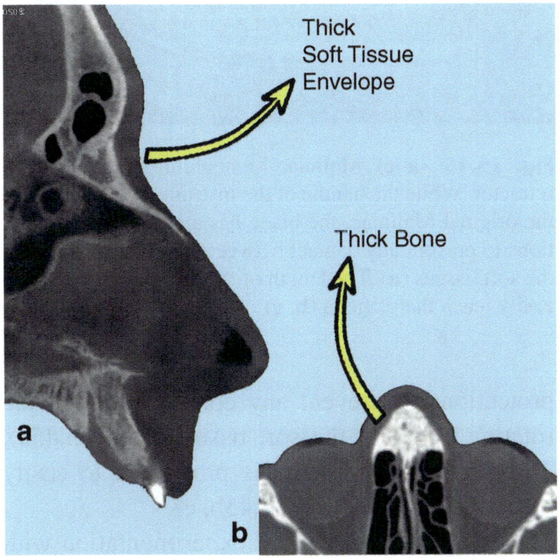

Fig. 15.42 (**a**, **b**) CT scans of the nasal radix. The soft tissue envelope is thicker than in all other nasal regions (**a**). The nasal radix bone almost always is thicker and denser than all the other nasal and maxillary regions (**b**)

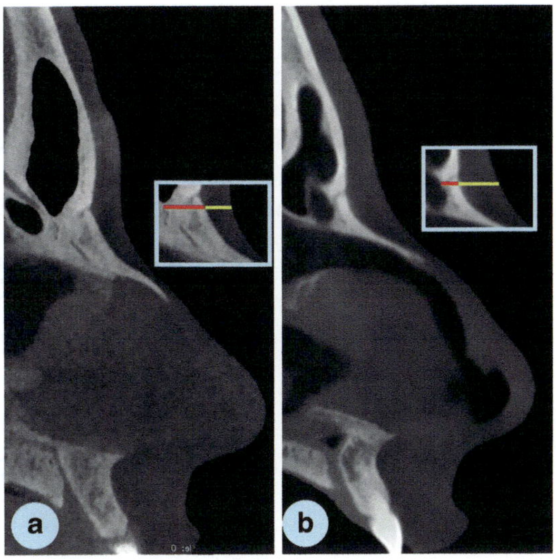

Fig. 15.43 (**a**, **b**) Deepening of the nasal root. CT midline sagittal scans show a favorable case due to a thick bony radix (**a**) and the opposite condition with a thin bone that represents an absolute contraindication to deepen the radix (**b**)

Figure 15.44 shows an example of an evident shallow and caudally positioned nasofrontal angle. The simulation of the profile preferred by the patient, highlighted in yellow, shows how only a marked variation of the nasal radix creates a balance between the nasal structures. Unfortunately, the CT study in the sagittal projection reveals the unfavorable relationship between bone and soft tissue thickness.

Whichever technique is chosen for lowering the nasal radix, it should leave a smooth bony surface and an intact anterior frontal sinus wall.

The use of a rasp is indicated only if small cephalic irregularities appear after removal of the hump but with these kinds of instruments a real radix deepening is not feasible. In other words, it is a matter of superficial polishing and not of real deepening. Furthermore, a prolonged rasping time is considered a major trauma for the overlying soft tissue and a cause of prolonged swelling and ecchymosis.

In the past, some authors suggested "marking" an upper horizontal osteotomy line utilizing a 2 mm sharp osteotome introduced directly over the radix with a transcutaneous approach and then removing part of the radix en bloc with the

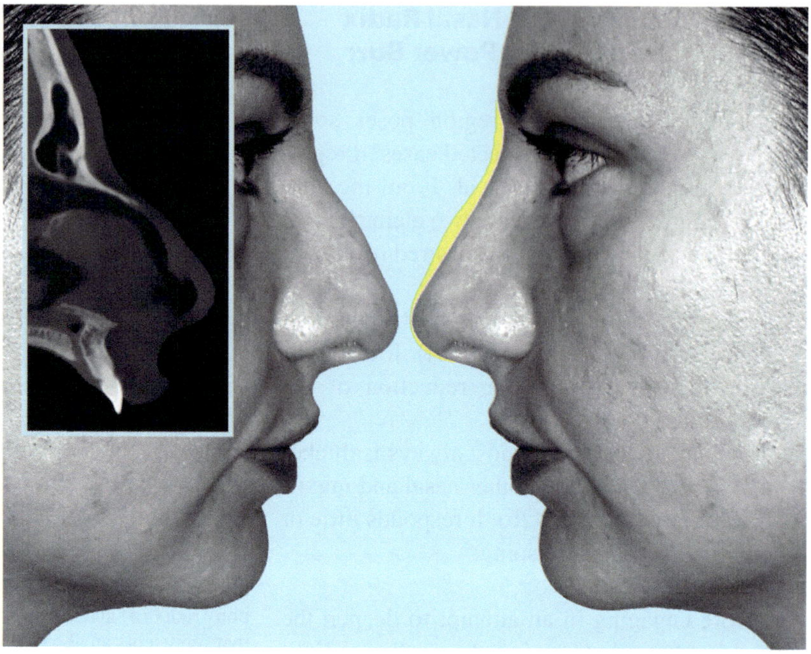

Fig. 15.44 Deepening of the nasal root. Right profile view, "Overlap" profile simulations, and CT midline sagittal scan of a patient with a shallow and caudally positioned nasofrontal angle. Even if a nasal radix reduction and its upward placement may be desirable, the CT study reveals the unfavorable relationship between bone and soft tissue thickness

nasal hump utilizing a Rubin or similar osteotome. This technique is not recommended as it is unpredictable and aggressive to the frontal sinus and bone even though it is the only viable route in the absence of dedicated electromedical equipment.

An effective and safe, though time-demanding, technique consists of tracing and deepening three or more vertical and horizontal sulci with the ultrasound saw and then fracturing the remaining weakened bone radix with the Rubin osteotome. The procedure can be better done in an incremental manner until the desired radix deepening is obtained. The role of ultrasound bone surgery is that of promoting a safe and limited bone resection.

The author's preferred technique for deepening the radix and also for smoothing the cranial nasal bone after hump resection is an evolution of that described by Rudolf Meyer in his 1967 book consisting of the use of a dental burr. Differently from Guyuron, who proposed a unique olive-shaped guarded burr, we designed and developed a modified Maliniac nasal retractor which completely protects the soft tissue during milling. While the handle of the instrument is identical to the original Maliniac, the blade has ample lateral protections to prevent any contact between the rotating burr and the soft tissues (Fig. 15.45a). The length of the blade is prolonged to easily reach the glabella (Fig. 15.45b, c).

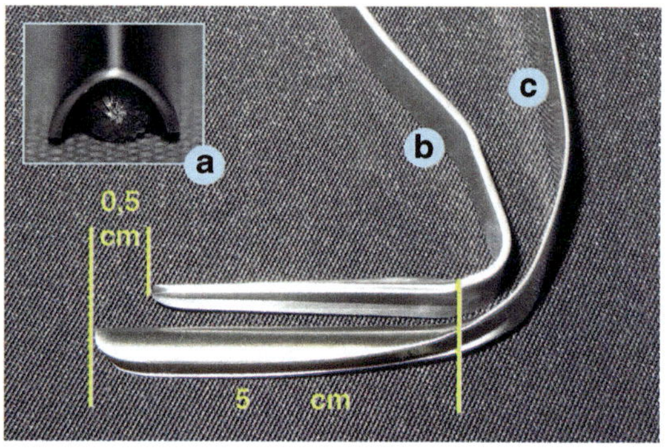

Fig. 15.45 (**a–c**) Maliniac-Meneghini modified nasal retractor. While the handle of the instrument is identical to the original Maliniac, the blade has ample lateral protections to prevent any contact between the rotating burr and the soft tissues (**a**). The length of the blade is prolonged to easily reach the glabella (**b**, **c**)

During the first year of experimentation with the retractor prototype, different types of rotating drills were compared (Fig. 15.46). The ideal one has the following characteristics:

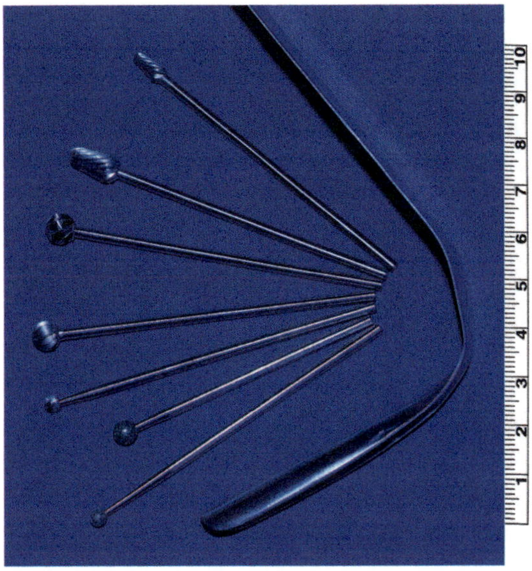

Fig. 15.46 Maliniac-Meneghini modified nasal retractor. During the first year of experimentation with the initial retractor prototype, different types of rotating burrs were compared

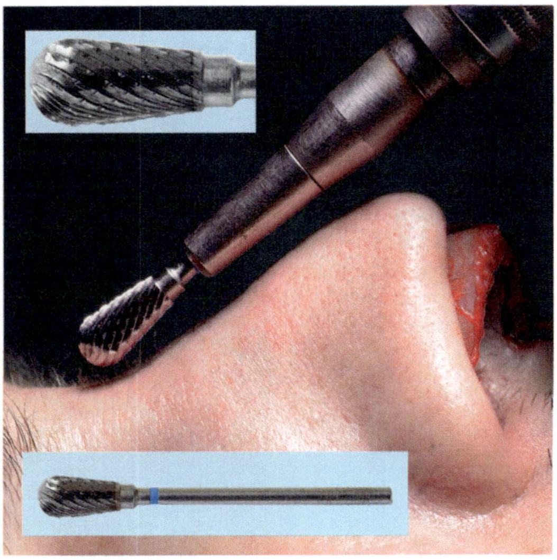

Fig. 15.47 Pear-shaped multiple-blade bur. This is the ideal instrument to uniformly deepen the nasal root. It also produces a smooth and continuous transition line with the profile of the nasal bones

- It fits the maximum diameter allowed by the sulcus of the Maliniac-Meneghini blade. The rule is that the small burs create new irregularities whereas the large burs smooth the preexisting irregularities.
- It must not create step deformities. The pear-shaped multiple-blade bur with larger distal diameter uniformly deepens the nasal root and produces a smooth and continuous transition line with the profile of the nasal bones (Fig. 15.47).[2] Olive-shaped burs, as those proposed by Guyuron, are not effective in the cranial portion of the radix where there is a greater need when deepening the nasal radix. Ball-shaped burs really deepen the nasal radix but can create a stairstep deformity.
- It is made of tungsten carbide with a multiblade X-cut surface.
- It can be used with a standard straight handpiece.

With his non-dominant hand, the surgeon positions the extremity of the retractor blade in direct contact with the glabella and examines the radix area to be treated. Maintaining firmly in place the Maliniac-Meneghini, the bur is positioned precisely over the nasal radix and a first short period of milling is done while the assistant irrigates the field with sterile saline (Fig. 15.48). As suggested by Guyuron, with gentle movement along the line connecting the canthi, the desired amount of bone can be removed from the nasofrontal junction with little time consumed. So, the goal is achieved with multiple incremental steps interrupted frequently to check the result (Fig. 15.49) and to wash again the bone surface with sterile saline. It is important to avoid heat production and thereby thermal injury to the soft tissue envelope and bone.

The electric power bur, utilized with the Maliniac-Meneghini nasal retractor, can also be useful for reducing the bony dorsum or refining the bony profile after hump removal with the osteotome or ultrasonic (piezoelectric) saw (Fig. 15.50). Compared to manual rasping, the procedure is faster, more effective, and less traumatic for the soft tissues.

[2] Meisinger Germany: code HM77 GX 060104 tungsten carbide bur or similar product.

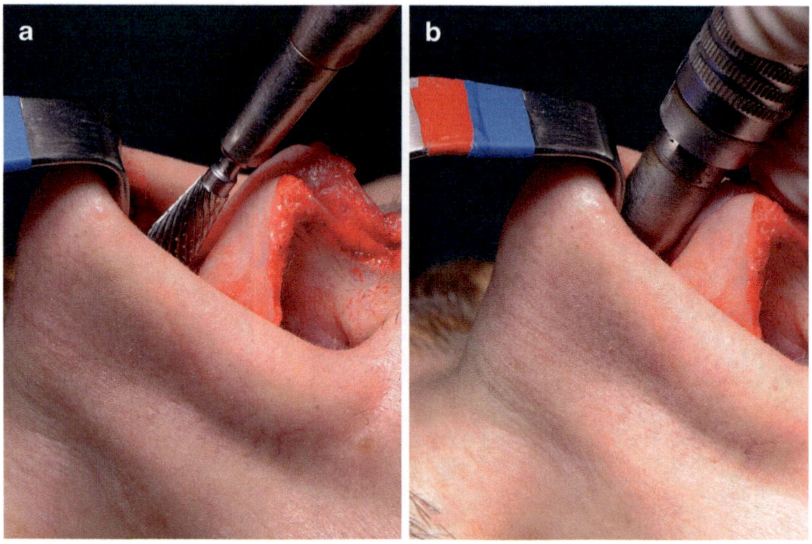

Fig. 15.48 (**a**, **b**) Deepening of the nasal root. Maintaining firmly in place the Maliniac-Meneghini nasal retractor, the bur is positioned precisely over the nasal radix and a first short period of milling is done while the assistant irrigates the field with sterile saline

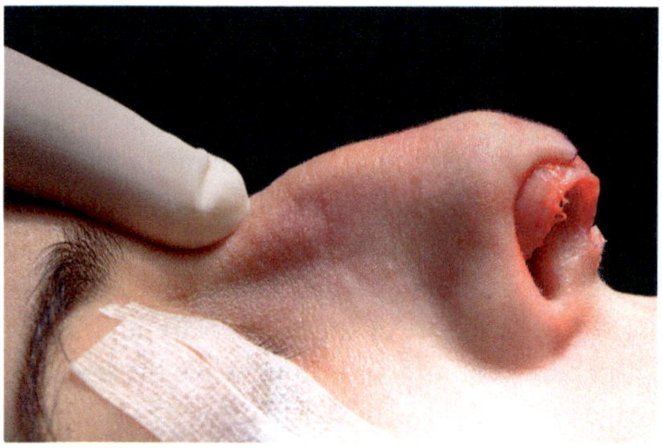

Fig. 15.49 Deepening of the nasal root. The goal is achieved with multiple incremental steps interrupted frequently to check the result by inspecting the radix area and palpating the skin

Figure 15.51 shows some detail of a glabella rasp. This is a useless and expensive surgical instrument and the two sharp angles of the working end of the instrument are traumatic for the skin flap, and increase swelling and bleeding. Rasping is no longer an acceptable method for reducing and smoothing the nasal radix.

15.9 Lowering the Dorsal Profile of the Quadrangular Cartilage

After shaping the bone component of the nasal profile, it is relatively easier to decide how much to reduce and the final inclination of the dorsal profile of the quadrangular cartilage.

For a precise adjustment, under direct vision the skin flap and the upper lateral cartilage should be retracted to expose the quadrangular cartilage. The angulated serrated Fomon scissors improve the view of the operative field and help the surgeon control both the amount and the inclination of the cartilage being cut (Fig. 15.52).

If a large reduction of the quadrangular cartilage is planned, instead of proceeding with progressive removal of small cartilage strips, it is preferable to start with an initial generous removal. For a secure and precise resection, the piece of cartilage can be measured and marked as shown in Fig. 15.53. Harvesting a long piece of intact cartilage, rather than many

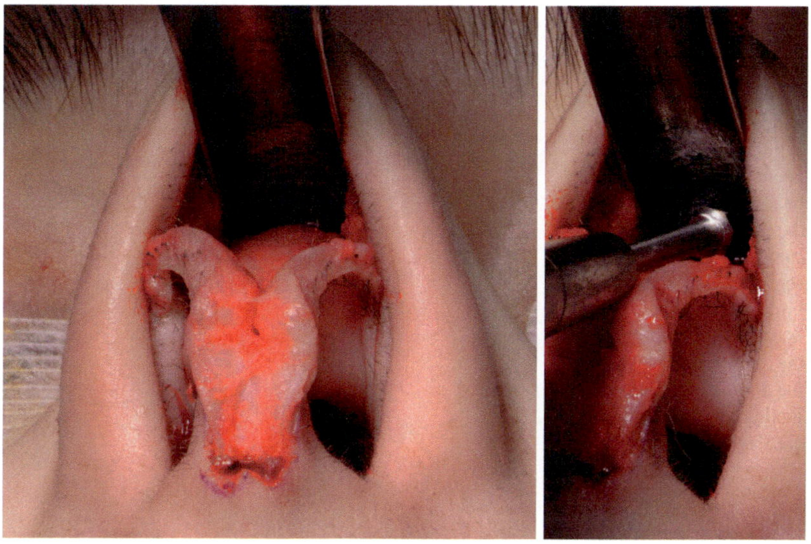

Fig. 15.50 The electric power bur, utilized with the Maliniac-Meneghini nasal retractor, can also be useful for reducing the bony dorsum or refining the bony profile after hump removal

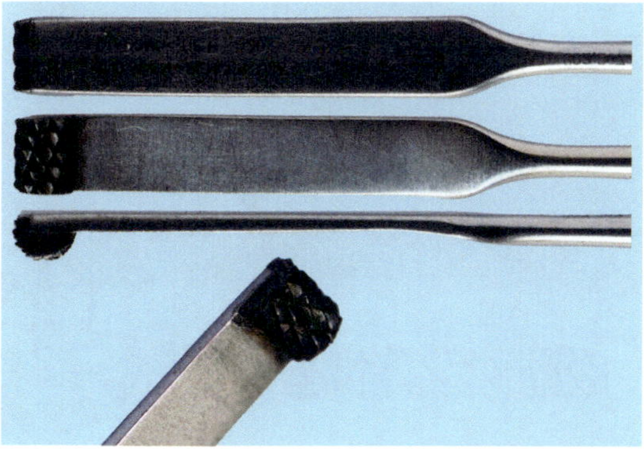

Fig. 15.51 Glabella rasp (working end details)

thin strips, at the beginning of the procedure can prove useful later, for example for structural grafting.

Until a few years ago, the next step after lowering of the quadrangular cartilage profile was to reduce the corresponding excess of the upper lateral cartilages. However, the introduction of a conservative option, the spreader flap, has modified the operative sequence.

15.10 Lowering and Refining the Nasal Bones

After a conservative reduction of the hump, further lowering and reshaping of the nasal bones is often required. In the past, the most utilized instruments were rasps. Figure 15.54a, b shows the shape and a working end of an aggressive rasp used to lower the bony hump and the dorsal margin of nasal bones in the first steps. Figure 15.54c, d instead shows two less aggressive nasal rasps used for the finishing steps. Rasping involves performing one or more series of back and forth movements until the desired result is obtained. It is often necessary to stop rasping to re-evaluate the nasal profile, wash the surgical field with sterile saline solution and clean the working end of the instrument. During the procedure the index finger of the dominant hand is kept over the rasp to modulate the pressure on the bone (Fig. 15.55) while the axis of the instrument with respect to the midline of the nose varies frequently (Fig. 15.56a, b). Special care is taken to maintain the rasp par-

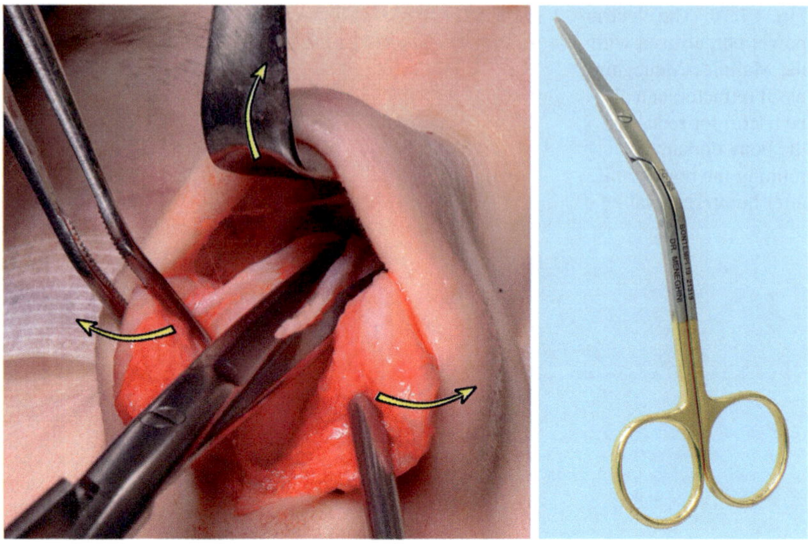

Fig. 15.52 Lowering of the dorsal profile of the quadrangular cartilage. For a precise adjustment, under direct vision the skin flap and the upper lateral cartilage should be retracted to expose the quadrangular cartilage. The angulated serrated Fomon scissors improve the view of the operative field and help the surgeon control both the amount and the inclination of the cartilage being cut

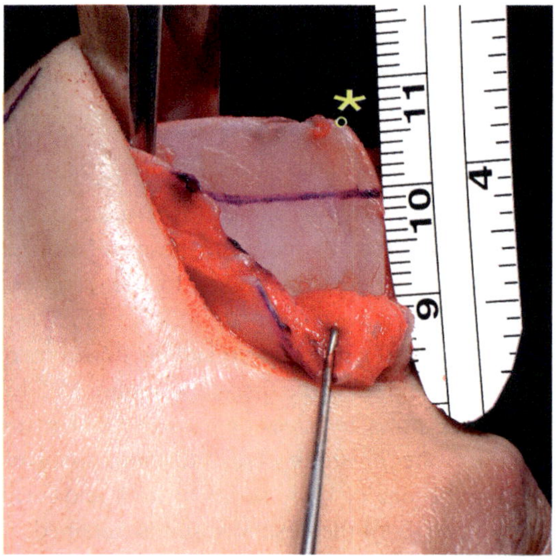

Fig. 15.53 Lowering of the dorsal profile of the quadrangular cartilage. If a large reduction of the quadrangular cartilage is planned, instead of proceeding with progressive removal of small cartilage strips, it is preferable to start with an initial generous removal. For a secure and precise resection, the piece of cartilage can be measured and marked (the dots on the septal margin marked with the asterisk highlight the anterior septal angle)

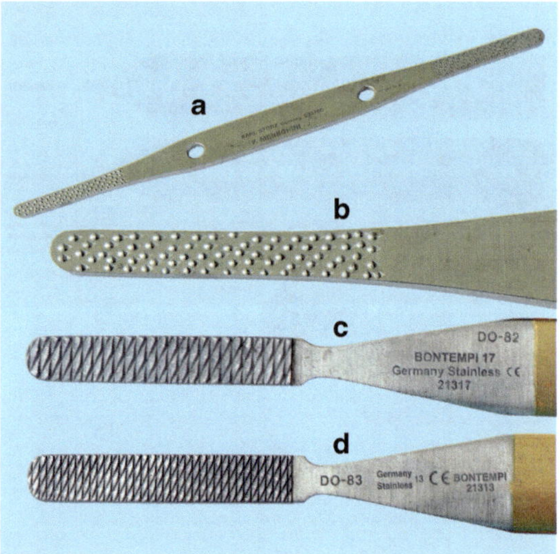

Fig. 15.54 (**a**–**d**) Aggressive rasp used to lower the bony hump and the dorsal margin of nasal bones in the first surgical steps (**a**, **b**). Less aggressive double-ended forward and reverse cutting nasal rasps with tungsten carbide inserts used for the finishing steps (**c**, **d**)

allel to the bone. At the same time, the thumb and the index finger of surgeon's non-dominant hand hold the nasal radix to stabilize the patient's head. For safety it is mandatory to avoid any pressure with the rasp over the cartilaginous septum and the upper lateral cartilages. The use of the rasps before osteotomies is an acceptable, though not ideal, method for shaping and refining the nasal bone. After osteotomies, their use should be avoided owing to the high risk of damaging both the septum and the lateral osteocartilaginous nasal wall (see Chap. 16).

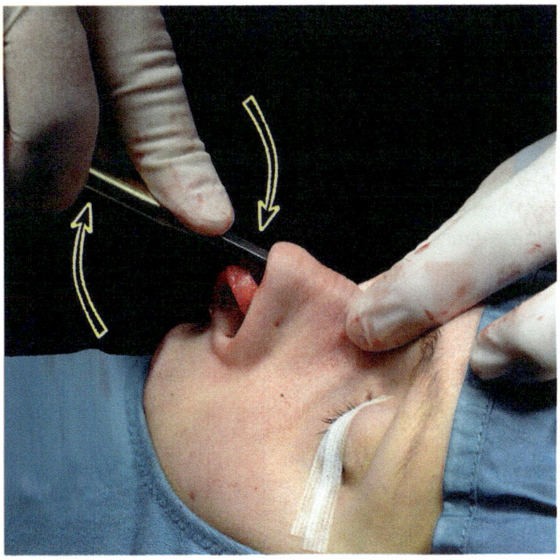

Fig. 15.55 The index finger of the dominant hand is kept over the rasp to modulate the pressure on the bone. Special care is taken to maintain the rasp parallel to the bone

15.11 Take Another "Surgical Time Out"

In BOR rhinoplasty, as in other surgical procedures or in some artistic practices, some passages guide the rest of the procedure. A sort of chain reaction that can no longer be stopped or a slope that drives the surgeon's actions in a well-defined direction. Part of the new nose has been shaped. The final result is not yet evident but, from now on, all the elements to be addressed will have to fit together perfectly as in a puzzle.

After setting the line and the slope of the osteocartilaginous dorsum, now the treatment plan has one less variant. A perfect time to clean the nose again with moistened gauze, recheck the written treatment plan and think about the details of the next steps.

Fig. 15.56 (**a**, **b**) During rasping the axis of the instrument with respect to the midline of the nose varies frequently

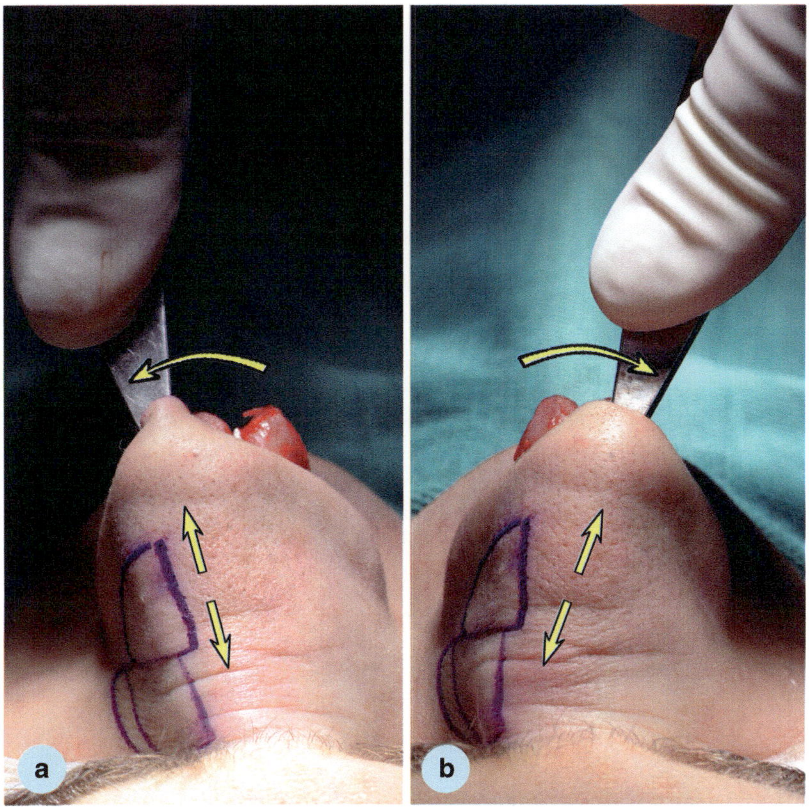

Further Reading

The description of surgical techniques can be further explored in these classic books on the open approach. They are presented here in order of publication. Even though this does not indicate the mandatory reading sequence, the historical evolution of the open approach represents an ideal way to study it. Daniel RK. Aesthetic plastic surgery: rhinoplasty. Boston: Little, Brown; 1993. p. 525–53; Jugo S. Surgical atlas of external rhinoplasty. Edinburgh: Churchill Livingstone; 1995; Tebbetts JB. Primary rhinoplasty. a new approach to the logic and the techniques. St. Louis: Mosby; 1998; Daniel RK. Rhinoplasty. An atlas of surgical techniques. Berlin, Heidelberg: Springer-Verlag; 2002; Daniel RK. Mastering rhinoplasty. a comprehensive atlas of surgical techniques. New York: Springer; 2010; Guyuron B. Rhinoplasty. Elsevier Saunders: Edinburgh; 2012; Daniel RK, Pálházi P. Rhinoplasty. Berlin: Springer International Publishing AG; 2018.

More data on ultrasound (piezoelectric) technology applied to rhinoplasty can be found in: Gerbault O, Daniel RK, Kosins AM. The role of piezoelectric instrumentation in rhinoplasty surgery. Aesthet Surg J. 2016;36(1):21–34. Epub 2015 November.

Basic Open Rhinoplasty: Intermediate Surgical Steps

16

The core of BOR surgery is full of fundamental decisions and the principles to be respected are many and demanding. The surgeon should work progressively from the depth of the nose towards the more superficial elements of the external framework. Any action should be done conservatively and preferably utilizing the instruments and techniques that maximize the preservation of bone and cartilage tissue. Each piece of cartilage removed must be stored in sterile saline solution in anticipation of its possible use during the final phases of the surgery; in the last few minutes even a small cartilage fragment can be decisive for the final result. Every modification of the nasal framework should be corresponded by a direct stabilizing and reconstructive maneuver; nasal packing and external splinting done at the end of surgery are ineffective if compared with multiple bone and cartilage direct sutures.

Due to the complexity of rhinoplasty, the surgeon should ask himself some basic questions during the central phases of the intervention:

- Have I harvested enough cartilage for the reconstructive needs of this nose? How are the quality and the sizes of these fragments?
- Is the residual septum sufficiently stable, straight, and strong?
- How to optimize and simplify the reconstruction of the new nasal framework according to the planned nasal shape and profile?
- Are the previewed projection, orientation, and shape of the nasal tip achievable?
- Am I following closely the priorities shared with the patient during the preoperative meetings?

Even in the simplest cases, the risk of forgetting a question and the related "operative surgical answer" is dangerous for the final achievable result. Only by following a basic frequently used operative sequence and consulting the treatment plan from time to time during surgery can the operator reduce this risk.

16.1 Septal Work: Caudal Reshaping

An overused step of rhinoplasty consists of a wide reduction of the caudal septum to rotate the tip and shorten the nose. With BOR rhinoplasty, the caudal septum shape and dimension is conserved or minimally reshaped in the majority of clinical cases.

In particular, the area close to the anterior nasal spine is considered for a reduction only in the case of an excessively wide nasolabial angle with an unpleasant fullness. The need for a reduction and its precise localization is previewed on the preoperative "Overlap" simulation. Figure 16.1a shows a case in which no changes are planned in the caudal profile of the nose. Figures 16.1b, c show two cases in which the area close to the anterior nasal spine is previewed as stable, whereas the upper tip rotation

F. Meneghini, *Basic Open Rhinoplasty*, https://doi.org/10.1007/978-3-030-61827-8_16

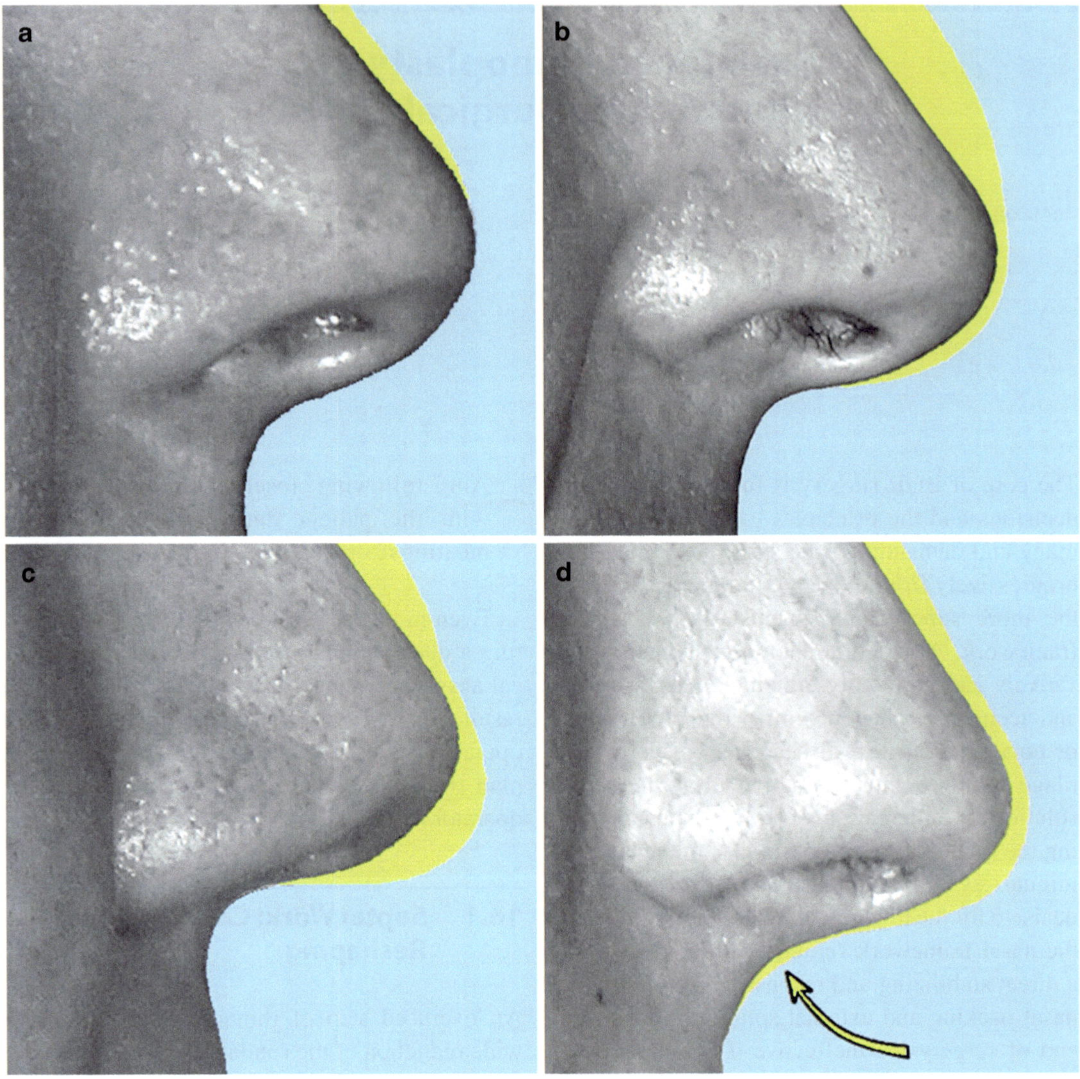

Fig. 16.1 (**a–d**) Caudal septum reshaping. Planned nasolabial contour in four different cases. A small variation of the nasolabial contour close to the anterior nasal spine is a fairly rare case (**d**)

and projection change. Finally, Fig. 16.1d shows a fairly rare case in which even a small variation of the nasolabial contour is wanted.

The thickness of the soft tissues around the anterior nasal spine and at the base of the columella is considerable and the relationship between surgical removal and bone and profile modification is low. This limiting aspect needs to be taken into account when performing the simulation of the planned result.

With the BOR approach the caudal septum is widely exposed (Fig. 16.2). Figure 16.3a–c shows the basic three types of caudal septum reshaping: **a**—anterior triangular, **b**—total caudal septum reduction, and **c**—posterior triangular (close to anterior nasal spine). If a straight reduction is planned, as depicted in Fig. 16.3b, the surgeon should remove the excess in one single piece to gain the maximum advantage later, when it can be used as a structural graft.

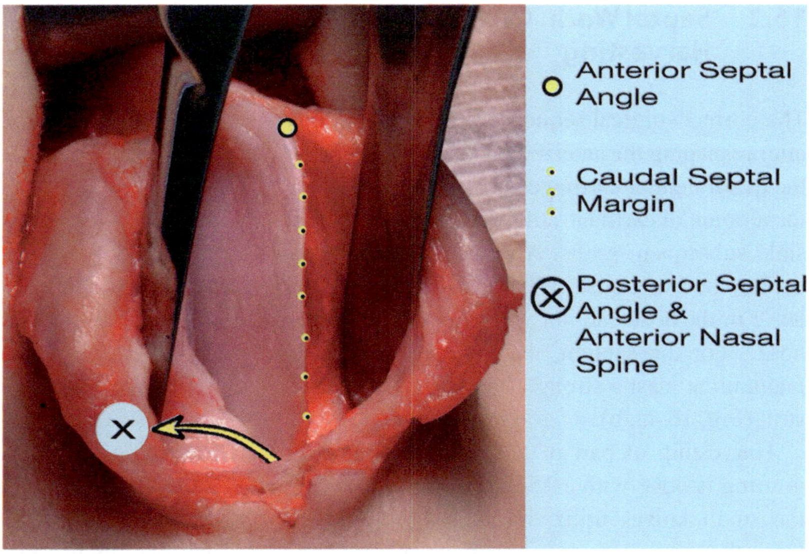

Fig. 16.2 Caudal septum reshaping. With the BOR approach the caudal septum is widely exposed

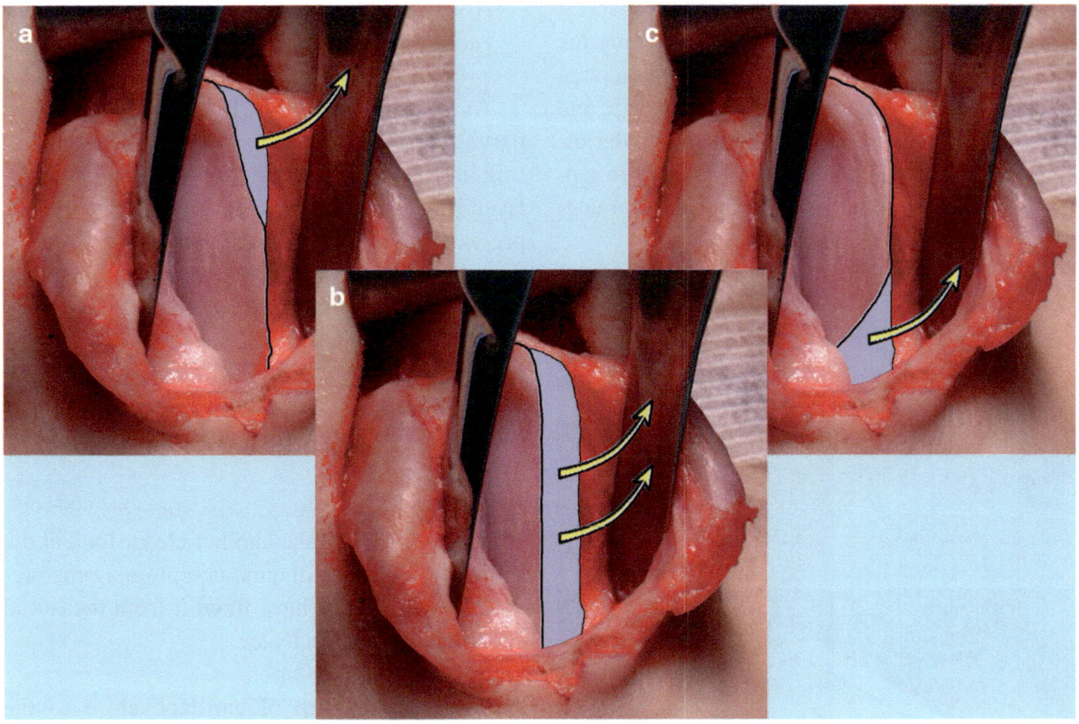

Fig. 16.3 (**a**–**c**) Caudal septum reshaping. The basic three types of caudal septum reshaping: (**a**) anterior triangular, (**b**) total caudal septum reduction, and (**c**) posterior triangular (close to the anterior nasal spine)

16.2 Septal Work: Cartilage Harvesting

The correct surgical sequence provides that only after reshaping the anterior and caudal margins of the quadrangular cartilage is it possible to decide the amount of cartilage still available for any possible subsequent grafts. A phrase that circulates among the experts is: "What matters is what you leave in the nose and not what you take from the nose." For the septum, the first objective is to maintain at least a strong 10 mm wide L-shaped strut (Fig. 16.4a, b).

Harvesting of part of the central septum for grafting is done with a 15c blade scalpel or with the small knives utilized for otologic surgery. Once the cartilage is cut in its main margins, the complete release of the piece is carried out with a Freer elevator. Care should be taken to harvest a single piece of cartilage without damaging the residual L-shaped strut. Figure 16.5 shows a large and intact piece of harvested central cartilage and describes its anatomical and surgical boundaries.

During harvesting, to protect the opposite septal mucosa, a small strip of sterile plastic material obtained from the disposable ruler is inserted between the quadrangular cartilage and the opposite side of the septal mucosa (Fig. 16.6). In this way, even if the blade passes through the cartilage, it cannot reach the contralateral mucosal flap.

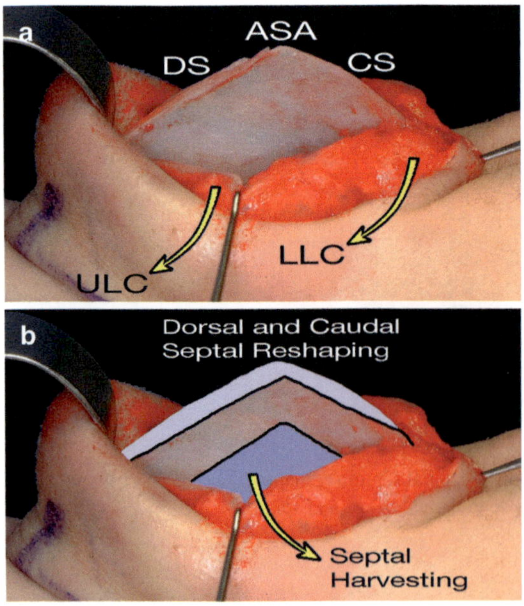

Fig. 16.4 (**a**, **b**) Septal cartilage harvesting. The objective is to maintain in place at least a strong 10 mm wide L-shaped strut

The extension of the septal harvesting is based on the need for the subsequent reconstructive phases and on the amount of cartilage already removed and stored at the moment. The main guidelines are:

- Be conservative and consider any other option for grafting.
- Re-evaluate several times during the procedure the cartilage stored in sterile saline solution to optimize its use in the next steps in the ideal attempt to avoid further septal harvesting.
- Always think in terms of final practical utilization when harvesting any piece of cartilage.

As shown in Fig. 16.7, from a single piece of harvested septal cartilage, by optimizing the cutting lines, more structural grafts can be obtained. Even if the septal area being harvested may have pre-existing folds, fractures, and other deformities, the surgeon's ability to remove the cartilage in one piece without further damaging it will lead to more reconstructive options later.

16.3 Straightening the Dorsal Septum

This is the time to take another closer look at the symmetry of the cartilaginous septum. Some previous specific steps have freed it from the initial deformed shaped such as:

- Removing a strip of cartilage close to the maxillary crest.
- Removing any osteocartilaginous septal spur and any midline bony deviation.
- Obtaining an anterior and caudal "swinging door"-type free movement without interference with the anterior nasal spine.
- Harvesting a central piece of cartilage (if needed).

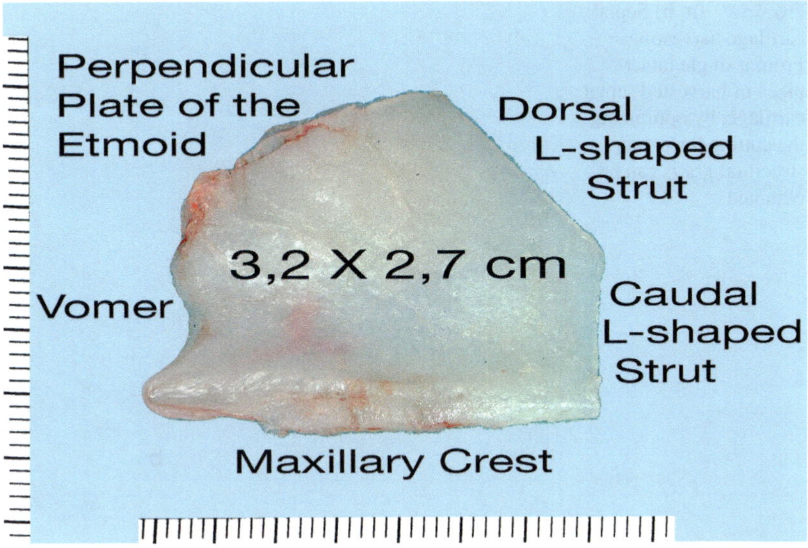

Fig. 16.5 Septal cartilage harvesting. Large and intact piece of harvested central cartilage. Its anatomical and surgical boundaries are described

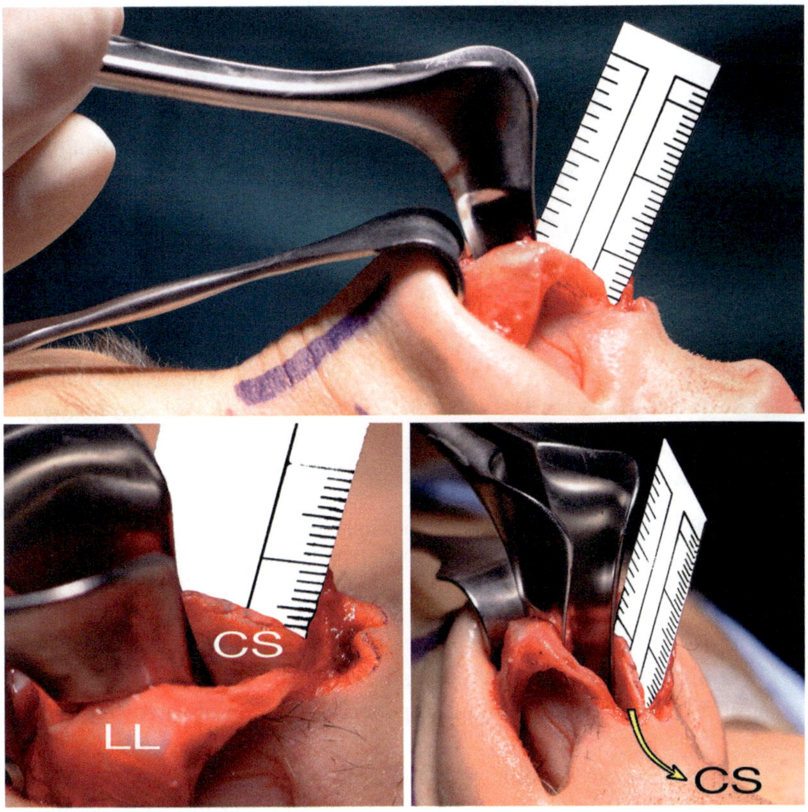

Fig. 16.6 Septal cartilage harvesting. During harvesting, to protect the opposite septal mucosa, a small strip of sterile plastic material obtained from the disposable ruler is inserted between the quadrangular cartilage and the opposite side of the septal mucosa. In this way, when the blade passes through the cartilage, it cannot reach the contralateral mucosal flap (*CS* caudal septum, *LL* right lower lateral cartilage)

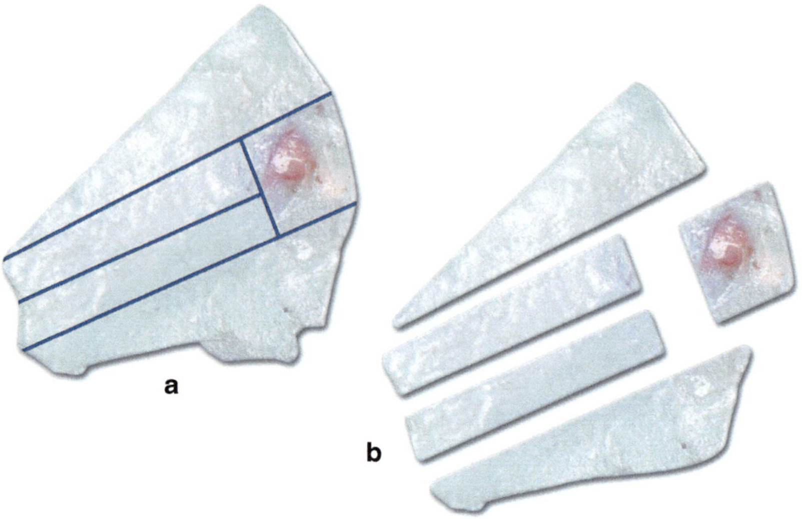

Fig. 16.7 (**a**, **b**) Septal cartilage harvesting. From a single intact piece of harvested septal cartilage, by optimizing the cutting lines, more structural grafts can be obtained

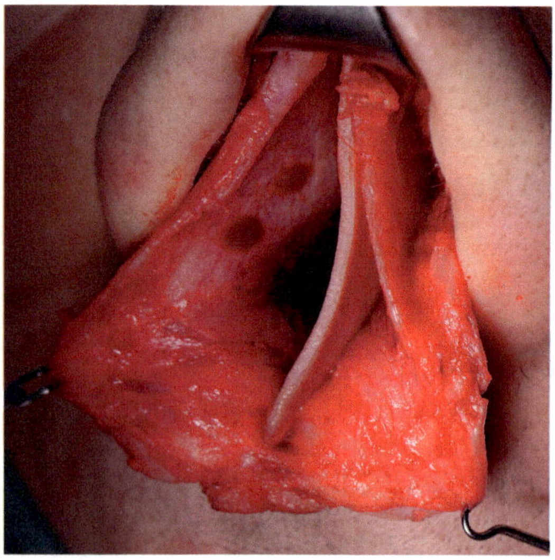

Fig. 16.8 Residual septal deformity after bilateral mucosal flap elevation and caudal "swinging door"-type free movement

To straighten a residual curved L-shaped septal strut (Fig. 16.8), the next main steps are:

- Release cartilage tension with multiple and very superficial scoring, in an anteroposterior direction, of the perichondrium on the concave side (Fig. 16.9).
- Carve and fix in position, with multiple 5/0 polydioxanone mattress sutures, a paired bilateral spreader graft or, rarely, a unilateral spreader graft (see below).
- Lower the anterior edge of the superior lateral cartilage bringing it to the level of the new anterior septal margin and reconstruct the integrity of the nasal dorsum with multiple 5/0 polydioxanone mattress sutures. The stitch of every suture passes through the septum, both spreader grafts and both margins of the upper lateral cartilages (see below).
- Suture the caudal septum to the anterior nasal spine (see below).

16.4 Spreader Grafts

Spreader grafts do not only serve the purpose of straightening the dorsal margin of the nose. In 1984, Sheen first described the use of spreader grafts as a method of reconstructing the internal nasal valve and the nasal dorsum in both primary and secondary rhinoplasty. Ideally, a spreader graft consists of a long straight and strong strip of cartilage placed and usually fixed parallel to the dorsal margin of the septum. It can be unilateral or bilateral depending upon the needs.

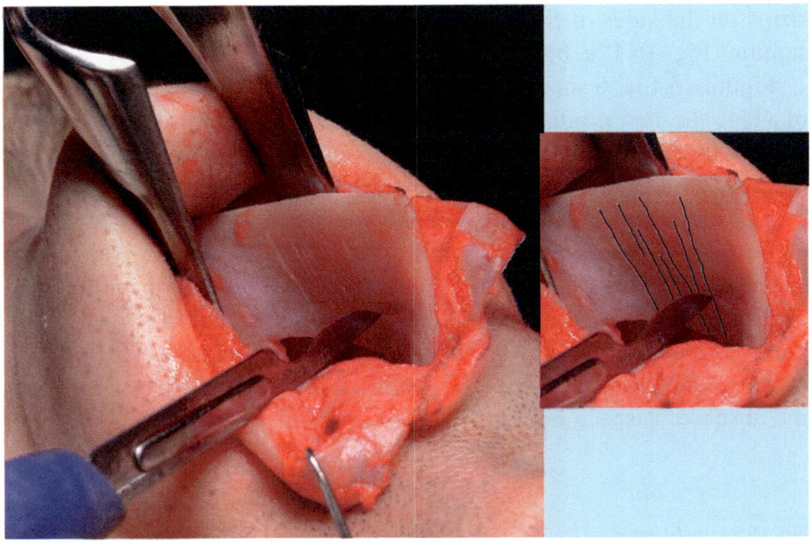

Fig. 16.9 Straightening of the dorsal septum. Release of cartilage tension with multiple and very superficial scoring, in an anteroposterior direction, of the perichondrium on the concave side

Following the removal of the nasal hump, the purposes of a spreader graft are to:

- Maintain or create an adequate width of the nasal dorsum.
- Displace the upper lateral cartilages from the septum to increase the nasal airways (internal nasal valve reconstruction).
- Due also to long-lasting meticulous sutures, stabilize the new shape of the osteocartilaginous nasal dorsum to avoid deformities such as inverted-V deformity, asymmetries, and palpable or visible irregularities.

The larger and higher the hump being removed, the greater the need to reconstruct the dorsum with a spreader graft.

The ideal spreader graft can be carved from a long, straight piece of septal cartilage. Figure 16.10 shows the original piece and the drawing of the final dimension of the graft prior its placement. Most often it is necessary to obtain two spreader grafts for a bilateral reconstruction from a large piece of cartilage. As always happens in rhinoplasty, it is necessary to optimize the resource by splitting it in a logical way so as not to preclude the subsequent creation of other grafts (Fig. 16.11).

Two fine needles can be used to position and facilitate suturing of the two cartilage

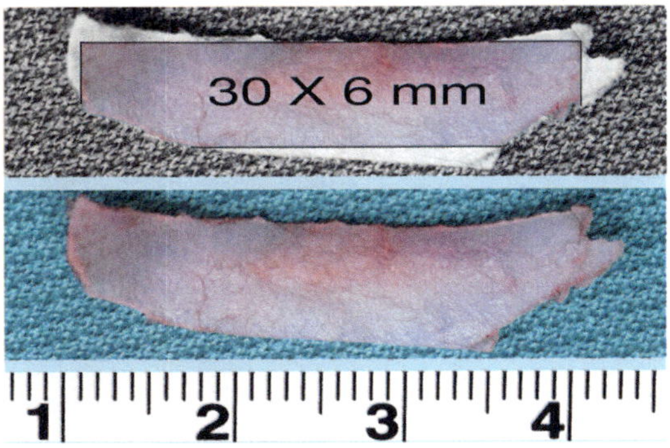

Fig. 16.10 The ideal spreader graft can be carved from a long, straight piece of septal cartilage. The figure shows the original piece and the drawing of the final dimension of the graft prior to its placement

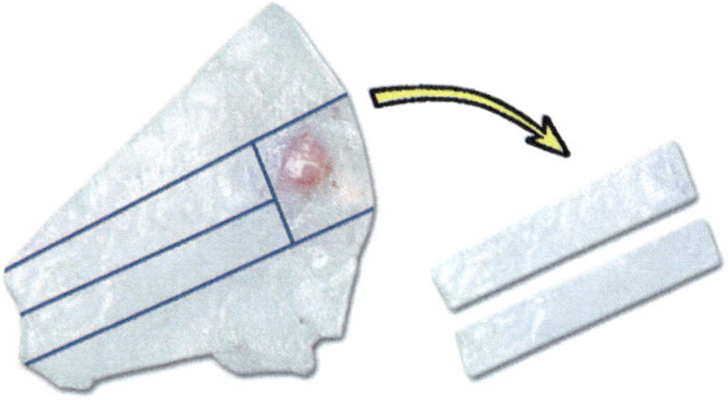

Fig. 16.11 Most often, for a bilateral reconstruction it is necessary to obtain two spreader grafts from a large piece of cartilage. As always happens in rhinoplasty, it is necessary to optimize the resource by splitting it in a logical way so as not to preclude the subsequent creation of other grafts

strips on the sides of the dorsal profile of the septum (Fig. 16.12a, b).

Figure 16.13a, b shows, from a lateral point of view, the two grafts, which must be stabilized with at least three 5/0 polydioxanone mattress sutures. The grafts should follow the dorsal margin of the septum without protruding externally to avoid a palpable or visible ridge. The thicker end of the graft is placed cephalic, between the septum and the nasal bone, to reconstruct the widest portion of the dorsum, the keystone area. The stability and the absence of space between the septum and the grafts should always be checked and often improved by adding one or two additional sutures. Once the grafts are fixed, their anterior ends must be beveled to guarantee a smooth transition towards the nasal tip and avoid visible irregularities.

In some cases, in order not to enlarge the dorsum too much, the spreader grafts should lie half a millimeter below the septal margin. Figure 16.14a, b shows an example of bilateral spreader graft in which the right one was correctly beveled in its anterior end (a), whereas the left one is still raw (b).

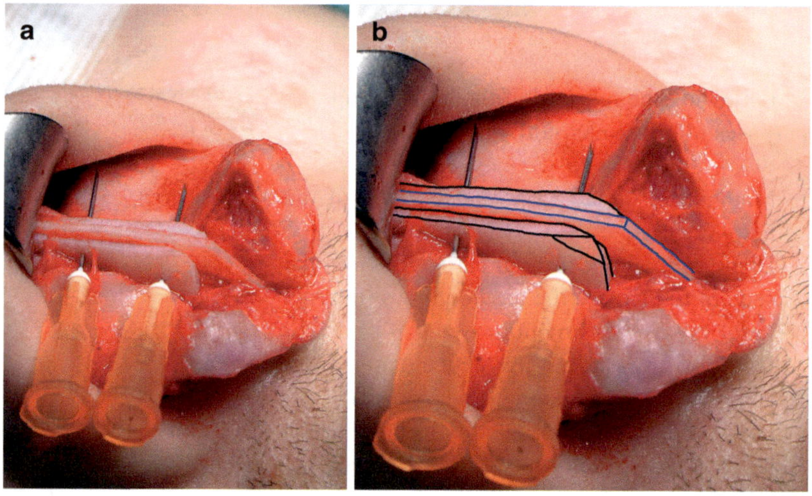

Fig. 16.12 (**a**, **b**) Spreader grafts. Two fine needles can be used to position and facilitate suturing of the two cartilage strips on the sides of the dorsal profile of the septum

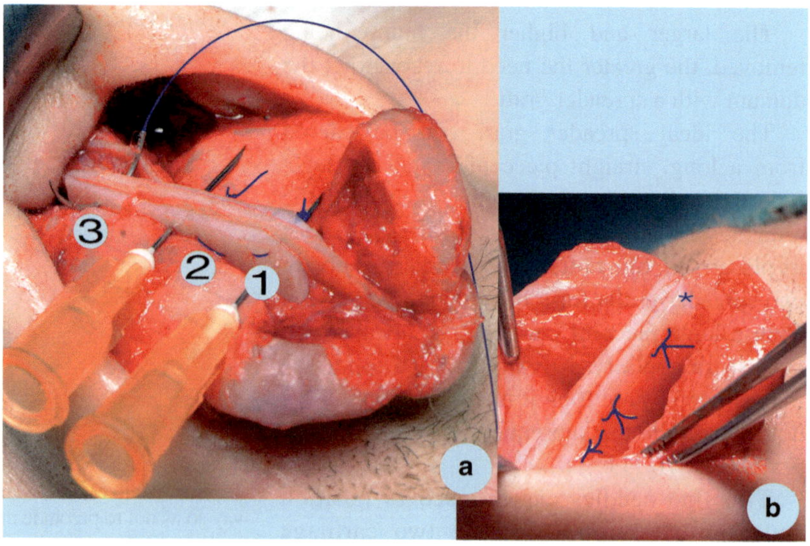

Fig. 16.13 (**a**, **b**) Spreader grafts. The two grafts must be stabilized with at least three 5/0 polydioxanone mattress sutures

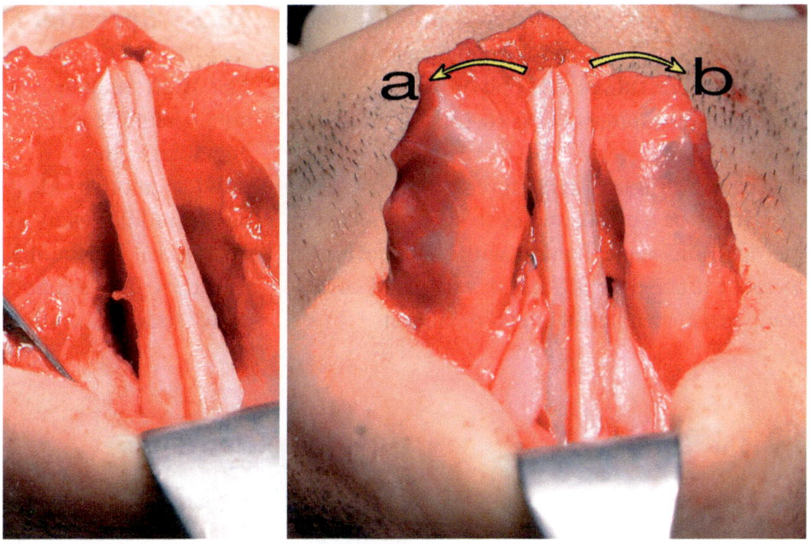

Fig. 16.14 (**a**, **b**) An example of bilateral spreader graft in which the right one was correctly beveled in its anterior end (**a**), whereas the left one is still raw (**b**)

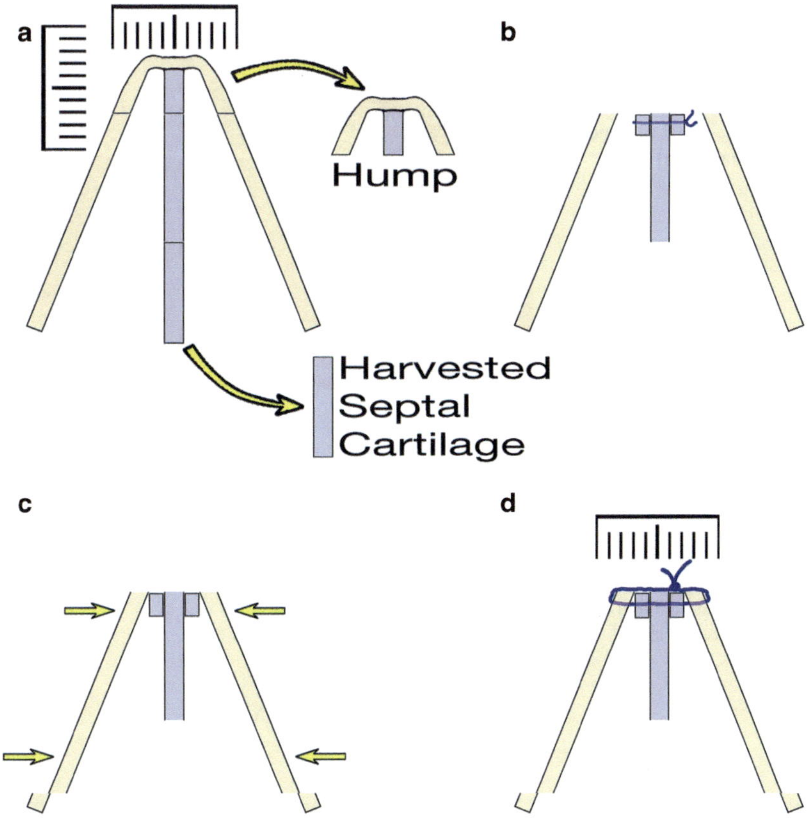

Fig. 16.15 (**a**–**d**) Most utilized steps of dorsal reconstruction with spreader graft after hump removal

Figure 16.15a–d schematically summarizes the principal and most utilized steps of dorsal reconstruction with spreader graft after hump removal:

- Hump removal and then septal cartilage harvesting from the central portion of the quadrangular cartilage (Fig. 16.15a).
- Spreader graft carving and fixation with at least three 5/0 polydioxanone mattress sutures to the dorsal septal margin (Fig. 16.15b).
- Basal osteotomies and controlled closure of the open roof maintain an adequate width of the dorsal profile (Fig. 16.15c).

– Suture of the upper lateral cartilages to the septal margin incorporating the spreader graft with at least three 5/0 polydioxanone simple or mattress sutures (Fig. 16.15d).

The use of a unilateral spreader graft is quite rare. It can be a useful choice to support an asymmetrical mid-vault dorsum with a concave side, to reconstruct a single nasal valve and also to compensate an anterior septal deviation.

16.5 Spreader Flaps

The BOR sequence defers the trimming of the upper lateral cartilage after the trimming of the dorsal margin of the quadrangular cartilage to provide another ideal option for restoring the nasal middle vault structure (Figs. 16.16 and 16.17a, b). If a hump is 1.5 mm or more above the ideal dorsal line and the dorsal septum is quite straight, clinically a frequent condition,

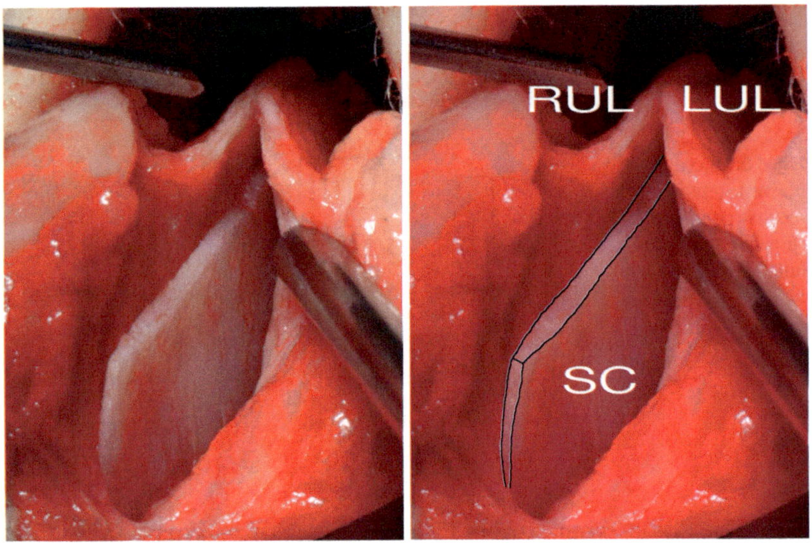

Fig. 16.16 Spreader flaps. To reconstruct the vault of the nasal dorsum after hump removal with spreader flaps, it is necessary to maintain intact the upper lateral cartilages (*SC* septal cartilage, *RUL* right upper lateral cartilage, *LUL* left upper lateral cartilage)

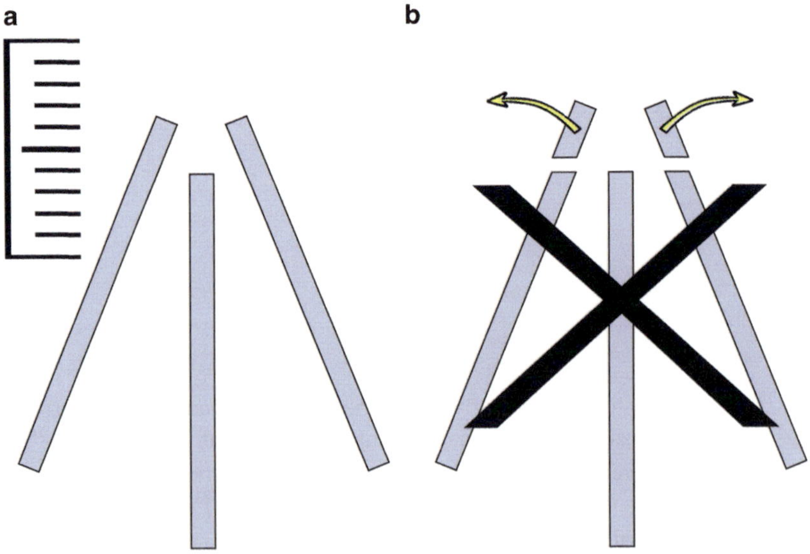

Fig. 16.17 (**a**, **b**) Spreader flaps. To reconstruct the vault of nasal dorsum after hump removal with spreader flaps, it is necessary to maintain intact the upper lateral cartilages

the dorsal reconstruction can be done better with spreader flaps than with spreader grafts.

The main steps of spreader flaps are:

- The perichondrium is meticulously dissected from the excess of the upper lateral cartilages. As the perichondrium is elevated, more pliability is obtained for the flap.
- Instead of trimming it at the new dorsal level, the excess of the upper lateral cartilages is marked (Fig. 16.18a, b) and folded on itself doubling its thickness and creating a new margin parallel to the septal dorsal margin (Fig. 16.19a, b). To favor a more angulated and easy-to-fold flap as well as a narrow dorsum, some small and superficial incisions can be made with 15c blades exactly along the expected new dorsal lines (Figs. 16.20a, b and 16.21).
- With three 5/0 polydioxanone horizontal mattresses or simple sutures to the septum, the bilateral spreader flaps are secured in position reconstructing anatomically the nasal dorsum

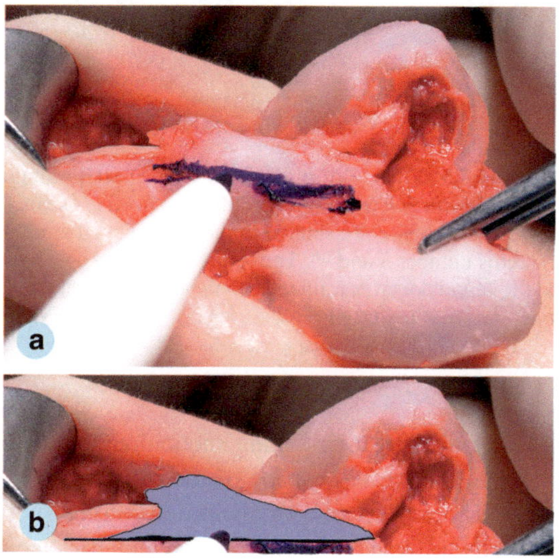

Fig. 16.18 (**a**, **b**) Spreader flaps. The excess of the upper lateral cartilages is marked with a sterile fine-tip skin marker

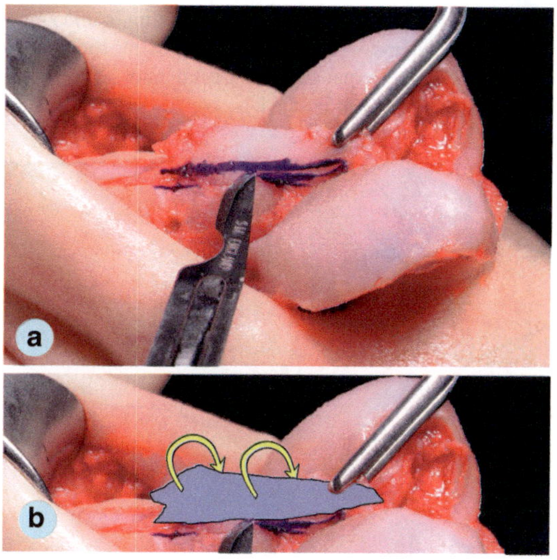

Fig. 16.20 (**a**, **b**) Spreader flaps. To favor a more angulated and easy-to-fold flap as well as a narrow dorsum, some small and superficial incisions can be made with 15c blades exactly along the expected new dorsal lines

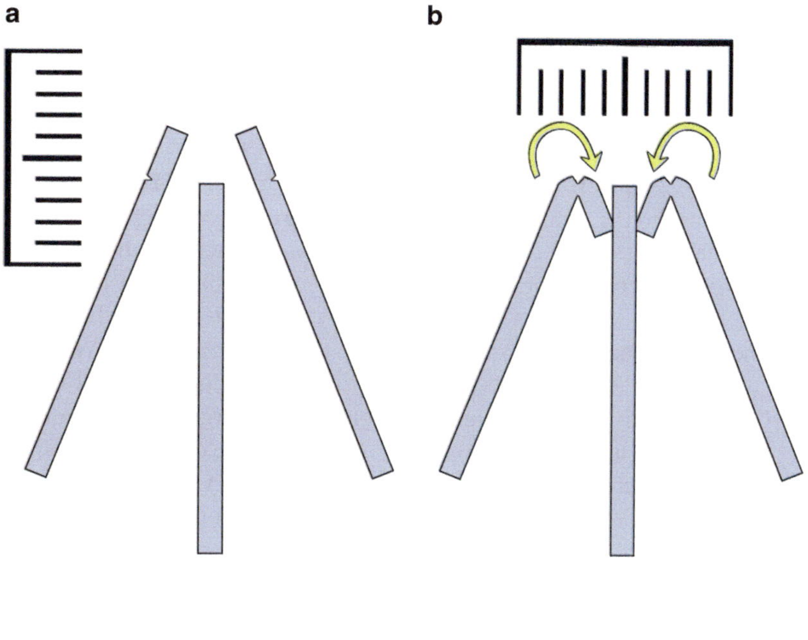

Fig. 16.19 (**a**, **b**) Spreader flaps. The excess of the upper lateral cartilages is folded on itself doubling its thickness and creating a new margin parallel to the septal dorsal margin

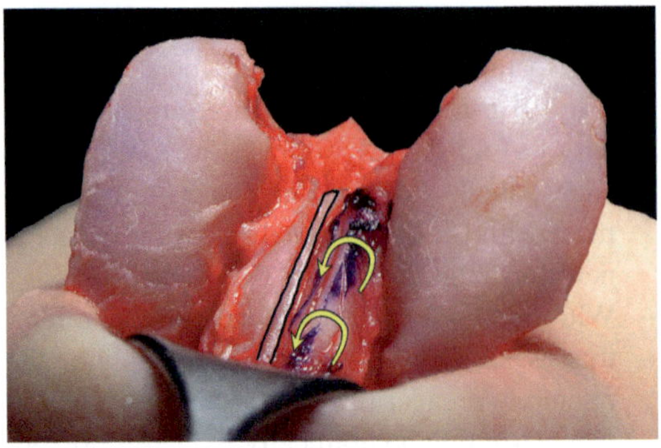

Fig. 16.21 Spreader flaps. To favor a more angulated and easy-to-fold flap as well as a narrow dorsum, some small and superficial incisions can be made with 15c blades exactly along the expected new dorsal lines. The septal dorsal margin is drawn in black

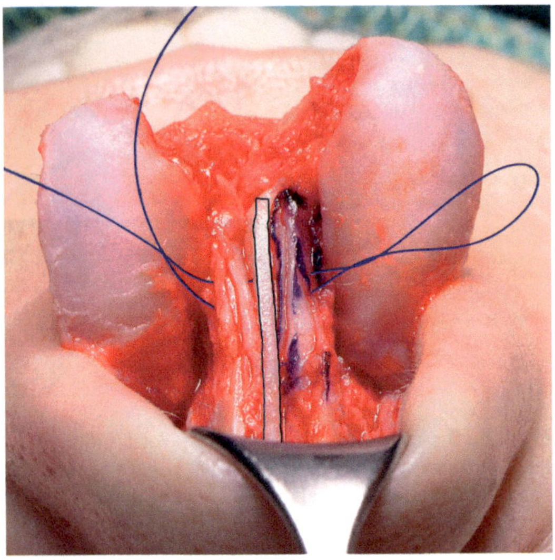

Fig. 16.22 Spreader flaps. The bilateral spreader flaps are secured in position with three 5/0 polydioxanone horizontal mattresses or simple sutures to the septum. The septal dorsal margin is drawn in black

(Figs. 16.22 and 16.23). The sutures must be kept close to the septal dorsal margin to keep the internal nasal valve open and the underlying nasal mucosa intact.

The main objectives of spreader flaps are to:

- Close perfectly the cartilaginous open roof of the nasal dorsum.
- Maintain or create an adequate width of the nasal dorsum.

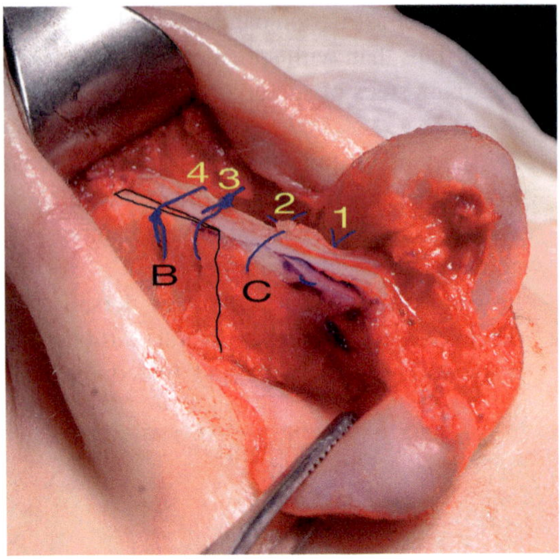

Fig. 16.23 Final dorsal reconstruction after hump removal with bilateral spreader flaps. Also the osteotomized nasal bones are sutured to the septal dorsal margin (sutures number 3 and 4). The sutures must be kept close to the septal dorsal margin to keep the internal nasal valve open and the underlying nasal mucosa intact. The right nasal bone is drawn in black

- Due also to long-lasting meticulous sutures, stabilize the new shape of the osteocartilaginous nasal dorsum to avoid deformities such as the inverted-V deformity, asymmetries, and palpable or visible irregularities.
- Reduce the amount of cartilage to be harvested from the central portion of the quadrangular cartilage, compared to a pair of spreader grafts.
- Reduce operative time compared with spreader graft carving, positioning, and suturing.

16.6 Trimming and Reattaching the Upper Lateral Cartilage

Trimming the dorsal excess of the upper lateral cartilage can be performed at this stage after the first surgeon has decided not to carry out the spreader flap. With Fomon dorsal nasal scissors the upper lateral cartilage exceeding the septum margin is easily reduced with two or three progressive conservative adjustments (Fig. 16.24a, b).

A mandatory step in the BOR sequence is the reconstruction of the cartilaginous nasal roof.

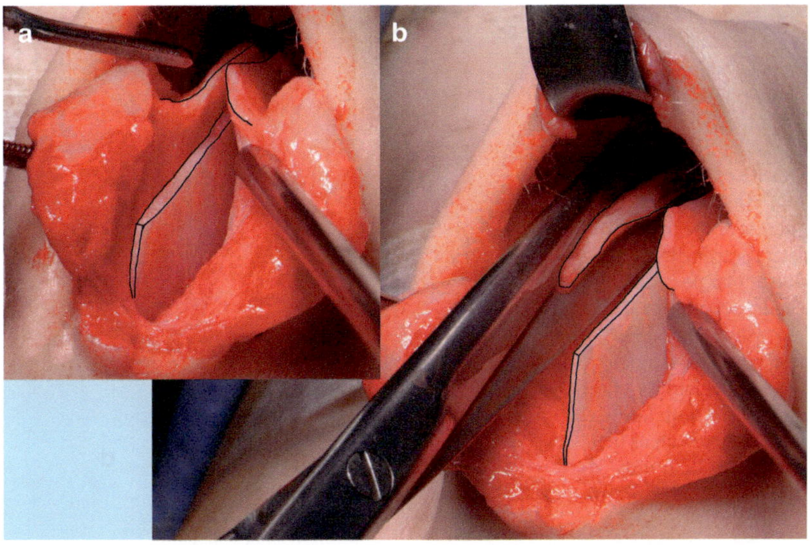

Fig. 16.24 (**a**, **b**) Trimming of the upper lateral cartilage. With Fomon dorsal nasal scissors the upper lateral cartilage exceeding the septum margin is easily reduced with two or three progressive conservative adjustments (**b**)

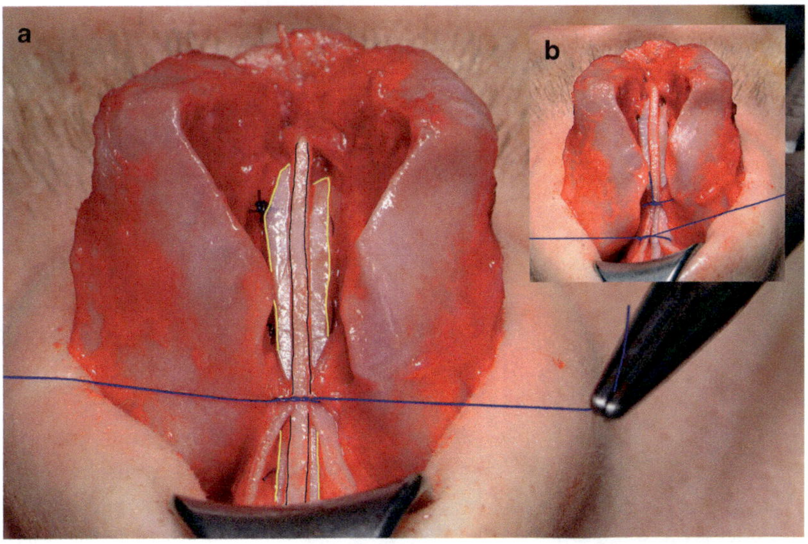

Fig. 16.25 (**a**, **b**) Direct suture of the upper lateral cartilages to the dorsal margin of the caudal septum. In this case the septum was previously straightened with bilateral spreader grafts (yellows lines)

Also in the simplest cases, where the hump reduction is less than 1.5 mm and the dorsum does not show deviations, three or more 5/0 polydioxanone horizontal mattress sutures between the septum and the two upper lateral cartilages are done. The same suture must also be done in the case of dorsal reconstruction with spreader grafts (Fig. 16.25a, b).

This search for the stability of the dorsum may seem excessive but it must be clear that in this surgical sequence osteotomies have not yet been made. The logic of these last steps is to define and stabilize the upper and middle part of the profile in order to achieve a fixed reference for the next shaping and projecting of the lower third as well as for setting the width of the nasal pyramid. A visual recall of the main steps of osteocartilaginous dorsum reconstruction is shown in Fig. 16.26a-d.

Before continuing, it is a good time to wash internally (Fig. 16.27) and externally the nose with sterile saline once again and to re-evaluate the goals achieved so far. Palpating the dorsum with the moistened index finger of the dominant hand carries out a further evaluation of the result.

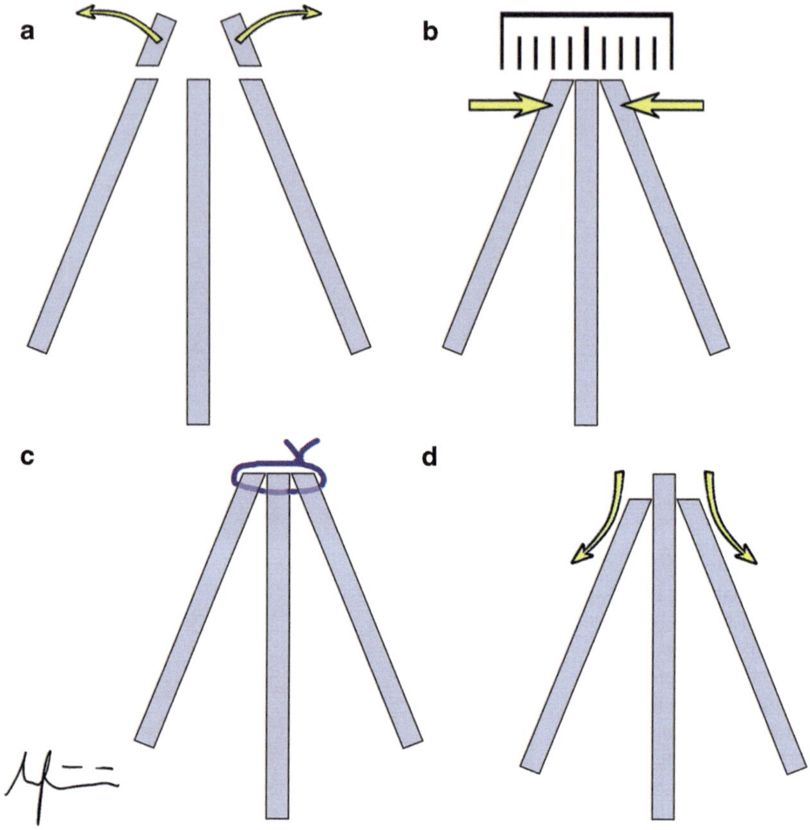

Fig. 16.26 (**a**–**d**) Basic steps in nasal dorsum reconstruction after hump removal. Trimming of the upper lateral cartilage (**a**), closure of the "open roof" (**b**), stabilizing sutures of the upper lateral cartilages to the dorsal margin of the caudal septum (**c**). The reconstruction of the framework is mandatory to avoid instability of the nasal walls with late deformities such as the inverted-V deformity (**d**)

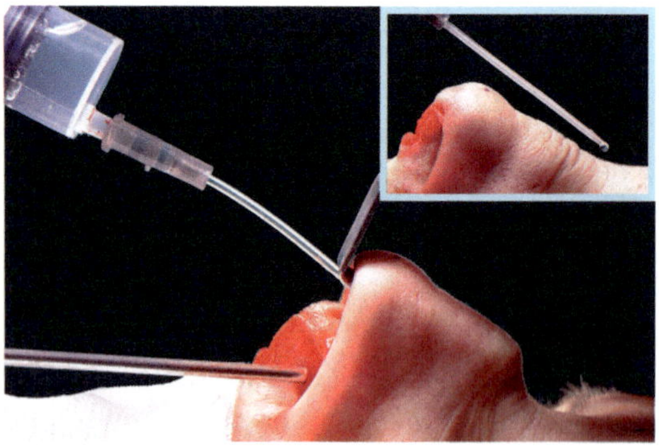

Fig. 16.27 For an evaluation of the result obtained so far, it is essential to wash the nose internally and externally with sterile saline solution. Frequent cleaning of the operating field is one of the most important aspects of rhinoplasty

16.7 Septal Fixation to the Anterior Nasal Spine

The essential goal of obtaining a straight and stable septum frequently requires a suture of the posterior septal angle to the anterior nasal spine. A stitch of a 5/0 polydioxanone or 4/0 polyglactin suture can be anchored to the dense fibrous tissue surrounding the anterior nasal spine or, better, passed through a hole drilled into the bone (Fig. 16.28).

The stitch is then passed through the posterior septal angle and then the knot is gently tightened until the cartilaginous septum reaches the mid-

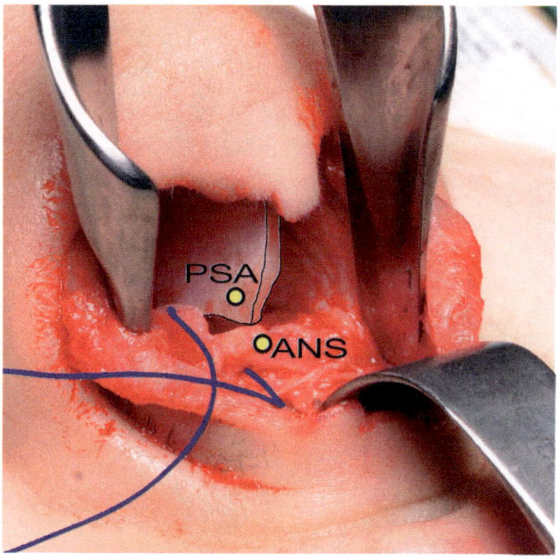

Fig. 16.28 Septal fixation to the anterior nasal spine. A stitch of a 5/0 polydioxanone or 4/0 polyglactin suture can be anchored to the dense fibrous tissue surrounding the anterior nasal spine or, better, passed through a hole drilled into the bone. The stitch is then passed through the posterior septal angle and then the knot is gently tightened until the cartilaginous septum reaches the midline (*PSA* posterior septal angle, *ANS* anterior nasal spine)

line. Any further tension risks deforming or tearing the cartilage and should be strictly avoided.

Figure 16.29a, b shows the cheap manual handpiece realized by the author for a safe manual drilling of small facial bones. It avoids the specific risks of high-speed electric drills of heating the bone and tearing the soft tissue. A more expensive but equally safe way to drill the anterior nasal spine is with an ultrasound tip under copious irrigation.

16.8 Septal Extension Graft

The preceding section illustrated the most common clinical situations in which the dimension of the cartilaginous septum is reduced or maintained. More rarely, as in the short nose, there is a need to elongate the septum.

Figure 16.30 shows a secondary rhinoplasty case in which the surgical exploration discovered an iatrogenic amputation of the anterior and caudal cartilaginous septum. The central and poste-

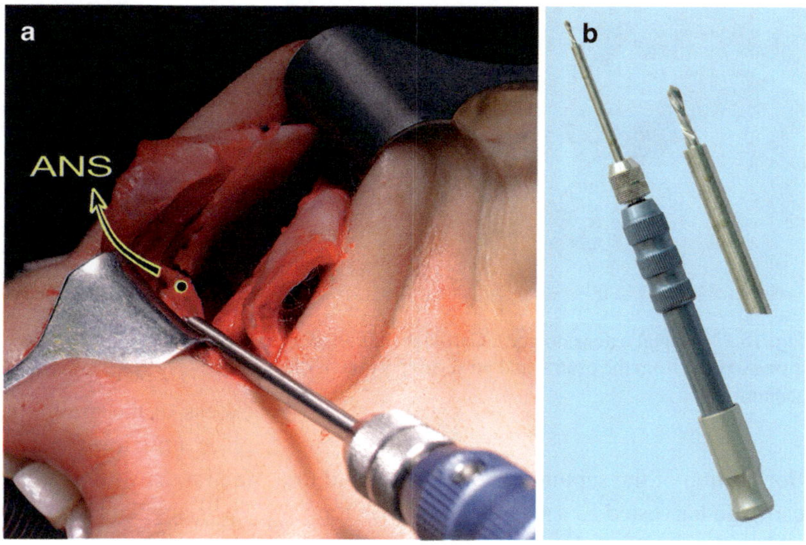

Fig. 16.29 (**a**, **b**) Septal fixation to the anterior nasal spine. Manual drilling of a hole just under the anterior nasal spine (**a**). The cheap manual handpiece realized by the author for a safe manual drilling of small facial bones (**b**). It avoids the specific risks of high-speed electric drills of heating the bone and tearing the soft tissue (*ANS* anterior nasal spine)

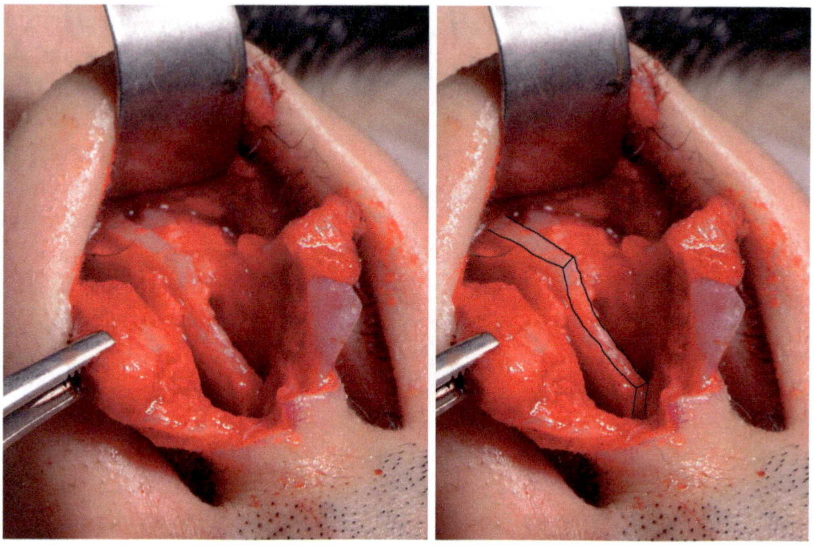

Fig. 16.30 Septal extension graft. Iatrogenic amputation of the anterior and caudal cartilaginous septum in a secondary rhinoplasty case

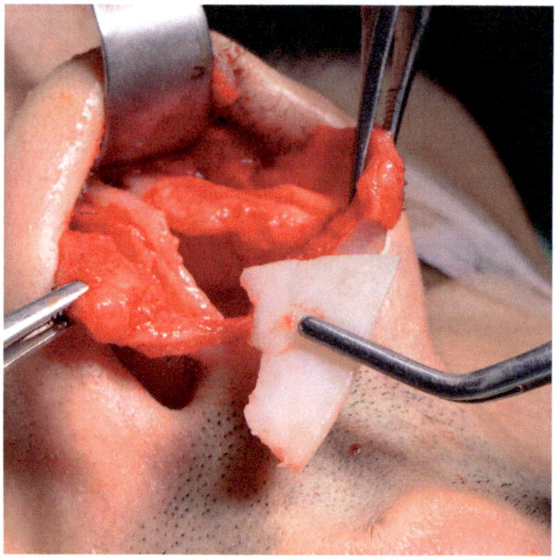

Fig. 16.31 Septal extension graft. Cartilage harvested as a single piece from the central and posterior portion of the septum

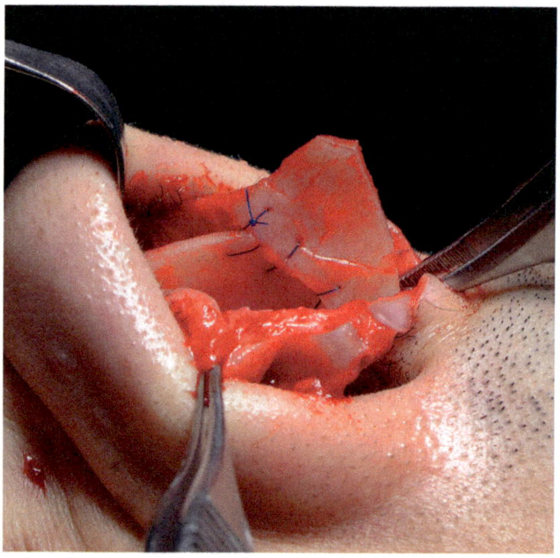

Fig. 16.32 Septal extension graft sutured in place

rior portion of the septum was still intact and the cartilage harvested as a single piece made it possible to have appropriate material for reconstruction with a septal extension graft (Fig. 16.31). The residual septum as well as the graft were carved in order to fit one in the other and fixed between them with four figure-of-eight 5/0 polydioxanone sutures (Fig. 16.32). A further stabilization was obtained with a heavy 3/0 polyglactin suture to the anterior nasal spine. The caudal and anterior excess of the graft was then precisely shaped in place utilizing the 15c blade (Fig. 16.33). The final reconstruction involved multiple suturing of the triangular cartilages to the new dorsal margin of the septum and quilting sutures of the septal mucosa (see below). The main steps of caudal septal reconstruction are also schematically presented in Fig. 16.34a, b.

If an adequate fragment of septal cartilage had not been available, the septal extension graft would have been performed with autologous rib cartilage.

16.9 Quilting Suture of Septal Mucosa

Quilting suture of the septal mucosa is a fixed step in the BOR method after completing surgery on the septum and inferior turbinate. The most frequent septal surgery associated with rhinoplasty is summarized in Fig. 16.35.

The many intended objectives of a quilting suture are to:

- Further stabilize the cartilaginous septum components.
- Avoid septal hematoma.
- Promote serum and blood drainage.
- Close and stabilize small tears of the septal mucosa. Large mucosal tears require specific meticulous single sutures.
- Eliminate the need for postoperative internal splinting and postoperative packing in over 50% of the patients and reduce to a minimum of 24 h nasal packing in the remaining patient population. The main requirement for reducing the need for nasal splinting only to few cases is to pursue the perfect integrity of the mucosal surface at the end of septal and turbinate surgery.
- Reposition the two septal mucosal layers in order to produce a light cephalic traction to the nasal tip and columella. Only in the case of a short nose, large nasolabial angle and retracted columella is it logical to follow the opposite repositioning vector.
- Avoid any redundancy of mucosa in the area of the membranous septum as well as any tendency to postoperative secondary local deformities such as a hanging columella. In BOR practice, the excess of mucosal lining is not trimmed and sutured but is spread posteriorly and cephalically over a large area preserving its surface and vascular integrity.

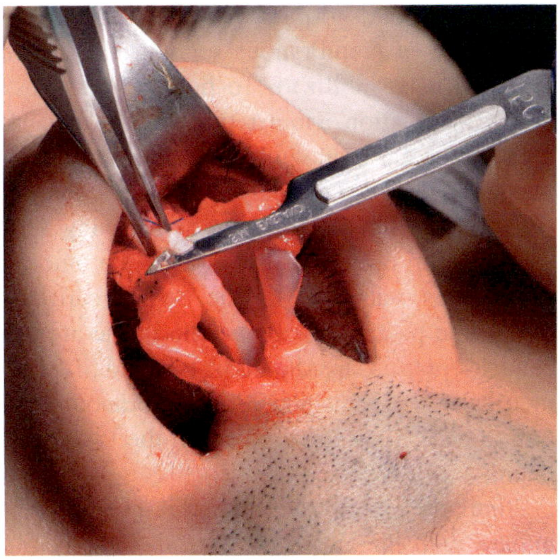

Fig. 16.33 Septal extension graft. The caudal and anterior excess of the graft was precisely shaped in place utilizing the 15c blade

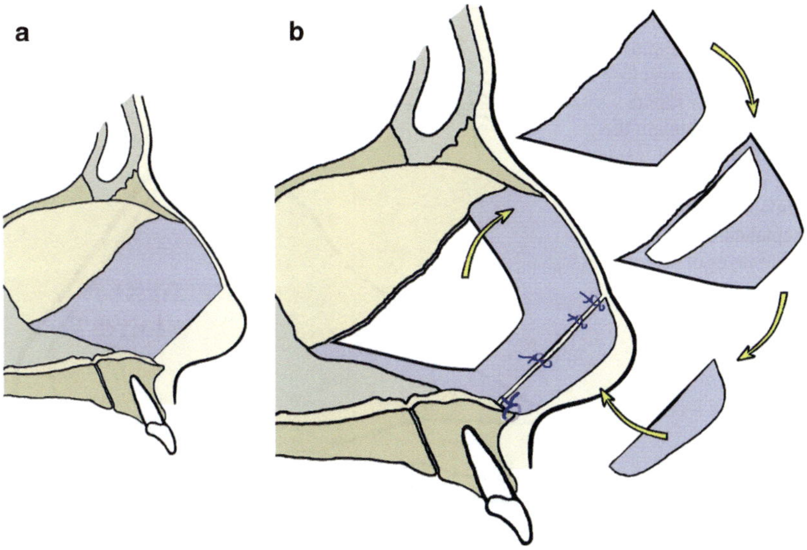

Fig. 16.34 (a, b) Main steps of caudal septal reconstruction: cartilage harvesting from the central portion of septal cartilage, carving of the septal extension graft and its stabilization in place with multiple suture fixation

Before starting the quilting suture, it is important to be sure that there is no longer a need to harvest septal cartilage and that the septal reconstruction can be considered complete. Instead of multiple single sutures, it is better and quicker to do a continue mattress suture with a 5/0 poliglecaprone or polydioxanone absorbable monofilament. The suture starts close to the posterior septal angle (Fig. 16.36). To maintain the final suture knot inside the mucosa, the first bite should pass through the septal cartilage and the right layer of septal mucosa (for right-dominant hand surgeons).

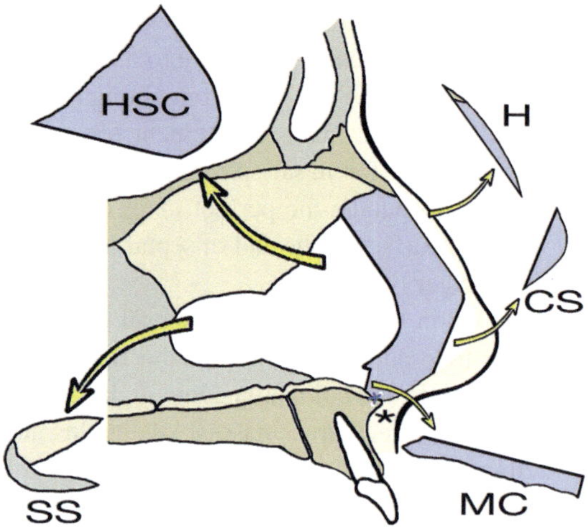

Fig. 16.35 Before starting quilting suture of the septal mucosa, it is necessary to check the completion of all septal work, namely: removal of septal spurs (*SS*) and of any interferences with the maxillary crest (*MC*), harvesting a central portion of cartilage for grafting (*HSC*), removing the dorsal hump (*H*), and reshaping the caudal margin of the septum (*CS*). Also the suture of the caudal septum to the anterior nasal spine comes before the quilting suture (asterisk)

The subsequent suture bites pass through the full thickness of the septum and should be taken maintaining the mucosa layers in a very light and cephalic-oriented tension. An average of ten come-and-go passages are done starting in the area of membranous septum that should be lifted and stabilized. To hold both mucosa layers in position against the septal cartilage, the surgeon can use, with his left non-dominant hand, a curved DeBakey dissecting forceps (Fig. 16.37). This instrument, by applying delicate but firm pressure, should keep the mucous membranes adherent to the septal cartilage during the passage of the needle in the area of caudal septum. Care should be taken to lift symmetrically the right and left membranous septum in order to maintain parallel the two lower lateral cartilages.

Similarly to Fred and tongue-in-groove techniques, with the aid of the DeBakey dissecting forceps, an additional anterior or posterior vector of the membranous septum mucosa can contribute to adding or reducing the final tip projection.

Fig. 16.36 Quilting suture of septal mucosa. The suture starts close to the posterior septal angle. To maintain the final suture knot inside the mucosa, the first bite should pass through the septal cartilage and the right layer of septal mucosa (for right-dominant hand surgeons)

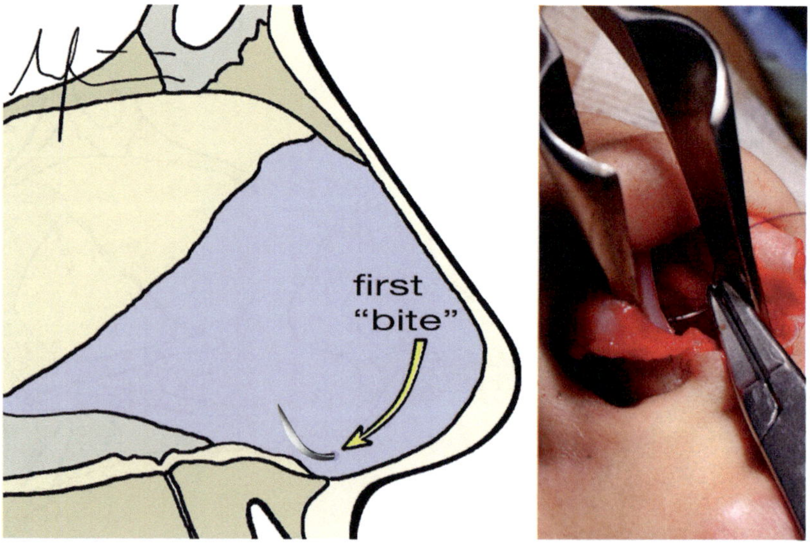

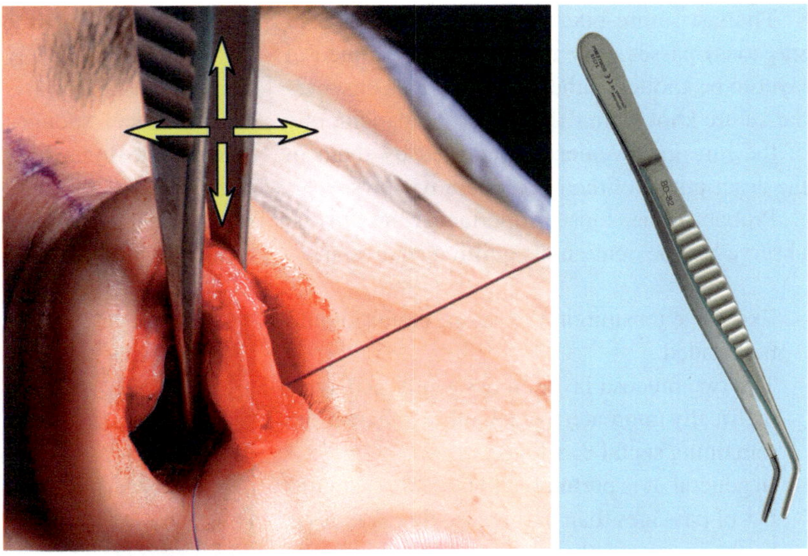

Fig. 16.37 Quilting suture of septal mucosa. To hold in position both mucosa layers against septal cartilage, the surgeon can use, with his left non-dominant hand, a curved DeBakey dissecting forceps. This instrument, by applying delicate but firm pressure, should keep the mucous membranes adherent to the septal cartilage during the passage of the needle in the area of the caudal septum

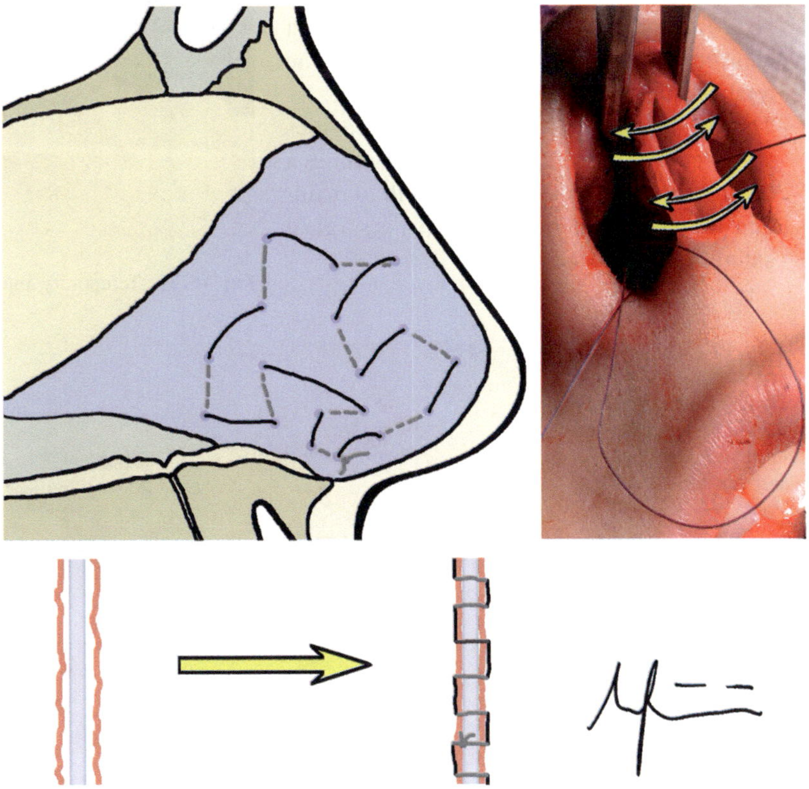

Fig. 16.38 Quilting suture of septal mucosa. An average of ten come-and-go passages are done starting in the area of membranous septum that should be lifted and stabilized with the curved DeBakey dissecting forceps. They are carried out progressively in a posterior and cephalic direction always maintaining a light tension in this direction of the mucosal layers

To better obliterate dead space and further stabilize the septal segments, the passes are at intervals of about 0.5 to 1.0 cm. They are carried out progressively in a posterior and cephalic direction always maintaining a light tension in this direction of the mucosal layers with the DeBakey dissecting forceps (Fig. 16.38). They also are closer to each other in the area of the membranous septum and then wider in the central portion of the quadrangular cartilage.

The last suture bite (for right-dominant hand surgeons) passes only through the left mucosal layer to be knotted at the other end. This obscures the suture knot from the sight of the patient, one of the rare inconveniences reported by them in the descriptions of their postoperative days.

Probably the most important rules to be observed in the continuous quilting sutures are:

- Excessive tension on the suture thread should be avoided.
- The two mucosa layers must gently and symmetrically approach to each other and over the remaining septal cartilage.
- In general, it is preferable to increase the number of passages than to increase thread tension to obtain a perfectly splinted and centered septal mucosa.
- A 5/0 absorbable monofilament is the first choice suture for its slight rigidity and the relative splinting effect on the septum.
- The patient should wash the nasal cavities with sterile seawater spray four or five times a day for the first postoperative month to maintain the endonasal mucosa with its surgical sutures clean and moist.

16.10 Temporary Nasal Packing

To improve hemostasis, a bilateral nasal packing with Merocel sponges soaked with tranexamic acid can be done (Figs. 16.39 and 16.40a, b). In over 50% of patients, the sponges can be removed at the end of the procedure a few minutes before awakening the patient.

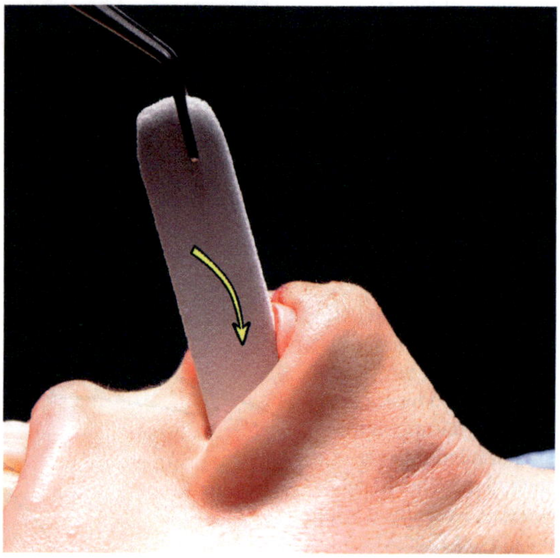

Fig. 16.39 Temporary anterior nasal packing

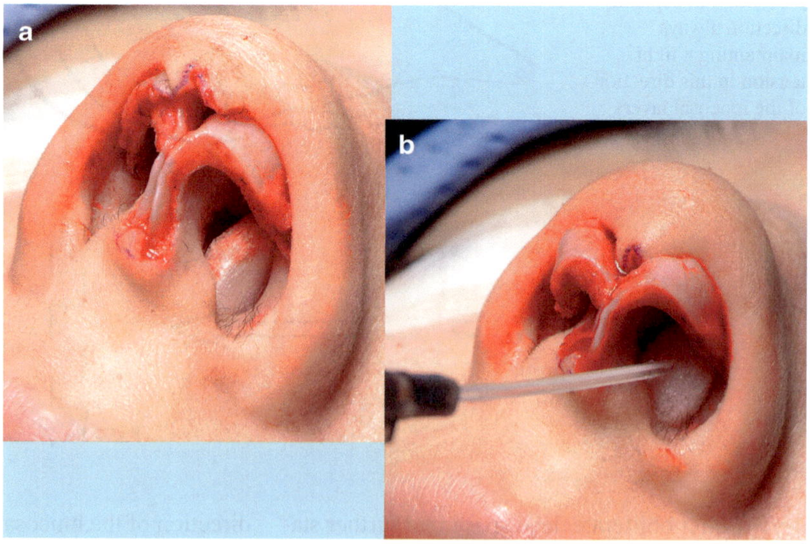

Fig. 16.40 (**a**, **b**) Temporary anterior nasal packing. The sponges are soaked with tranexamic acid immediately after their placement into the nasal fossa

Precise and deep positioning of the sponges parallel to the floor of the nasal cavities is mandatory to avoid unwanted interference during the mobilization of the nasal bones after the osteotomies as well as during tip shaping (Fig. 16.41).

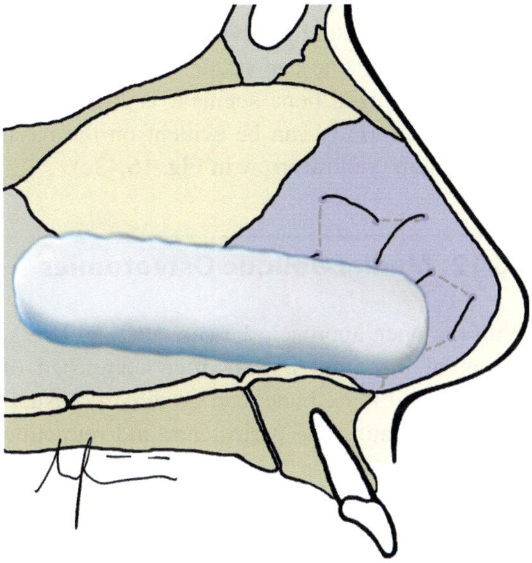

Fig. 16.41 Temporary anterior nasal packing. Precise and deep positioning of the sponges parallel to the floor of the nasal cavities is mandatory to avoid unwanted interference with the mobilization of the nasal bones after the osteotomies and during tip shaping

16.11 Nasal Osteotomies

Osteotomies involve the nasal bones as well as the frontal process of the maxilla and represent one of the fundamental steps of primary rhinoplasty. Mobilization of bones, by osteotomies and finger pressure, directly influences also the position of the upper lateral cartilages, which are strongly attached to the nasal bones.

The basic objectives of osteotomies are to:

- Close the open roof after hump removal with a reciprocal and symmetrical movement of approximation of the anterior osteocartilaginous margins.
- Reduce the width of the base of the nasal pyramid with a reciprocal and symmetrical movement of approximation of the posterior osteocartilaginous margins.
- In a crooked nose, center the nasal dorsum with a reciprocal but asymmetrical movement of the anterior osteocartilaginous margins.

Figure 16.42 shows:

- The open roof (dotted area) created with hump removal.
- The osteocartilaginous unit composed of nasal bones, frontal process of the maxilla

Fig. 16.42 Nasal osteotomies. Open roof (dotted area), osteocartilaginous unit composed by nasal bone plus part of the frontal process of the maxilla (*B*) and the upper lateral cartilage (*UL*), medial oblique osteotomy (continuous line), and basal osteotomy (dashed line). The small bone area in which the osteotomy lines converge is marked with an *X*

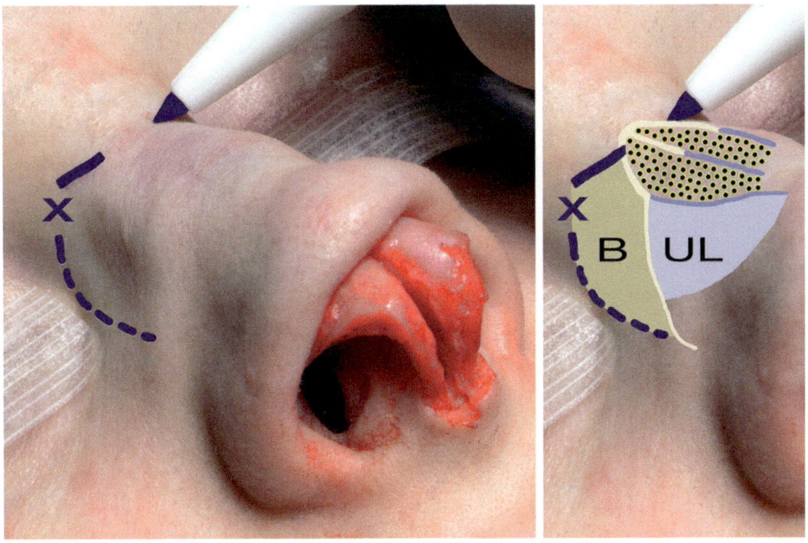

and upper lateral cartilage. The bone portion is marked with a B and the cartilaginous portion with a UL.

- The medial oblique osteotomy line (continuous line).
- The basal osteotomy line (dashed line).
- The small bone area, in which the osteotomy lines converge (marked with an X).

In cases of thin bone and elderly patients, area X is gently fractured with finger pressure to reduce the possibilities of excessive mobility with an unstable bony segment. If the resistance opposed by the bone is excessive, it is not advisable to press harder to obtain the fracture of the nasal wall but it is preferable to lengthen the basal osteotomy towards the medial one, reducing the X area by bringing the two osteotomy lines closer together.

In thick bone and young patients, the X area is reduced to a minimum by elongating the basal osteotomy towards the medial one until a completely mobilized osteocartilaginous segment is obtained.

Ideally, the entire portion of the nasal wall within the osteotomy lines should be comprised in one piece, as depicted in Fig. 16.43a, b. Sometimes, due to a large area of intact bone between the osteotomy lines, excessive pressure is needed to fracture the bone and an unwanted caudal fracture line can occur (Fig. 16.43c, d). The osteotomized bone segment is smaller and a visible deformity can be evident on the nasal dorsum skin (yellow arrow in Fig. 16.43c).

16.12 Medial Oblique Osteotomies

With the open approach the cephalic and lateral region of the nasal bones, often composed of compact and thick bone, can be directly visualized by elevating the periosteum and retracting

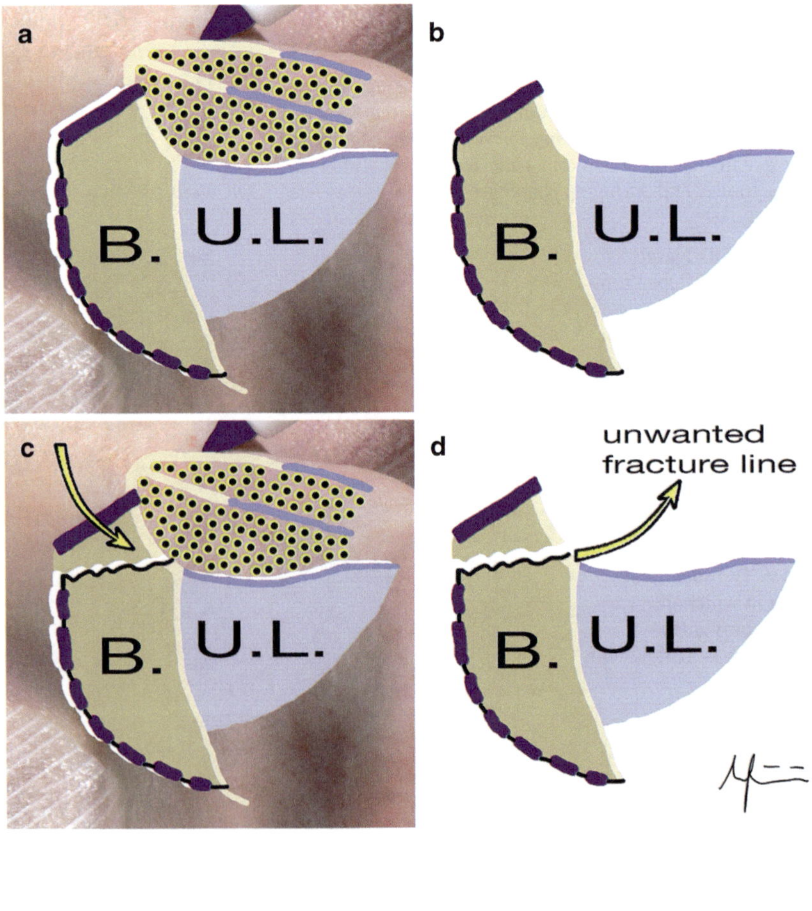

Fig. 16.43 (**a**–**d**) Nasal osteotomies. Correct pattern of fracture that follows the osteotomy lines (**a**, **b**). Unwanted fracture line (**d**) with production of stairstep deformity indicated with a curved arrow in **c**

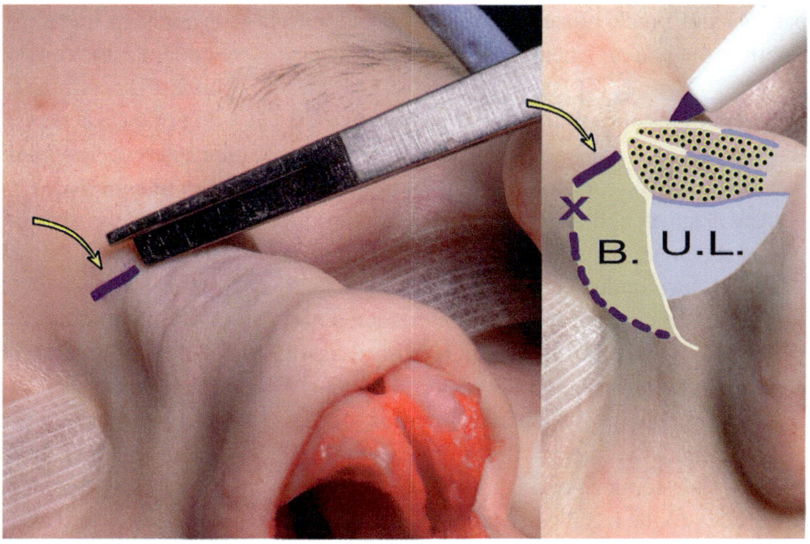

Fig. 16.44 The right medial oblique osteotomy line is traced for demonstration over the corresponding skin. A 3 mm guarded osteotome shows the correct orientation of the instrument to be maintained under the skin flap to perform the medial oblique osteotomy

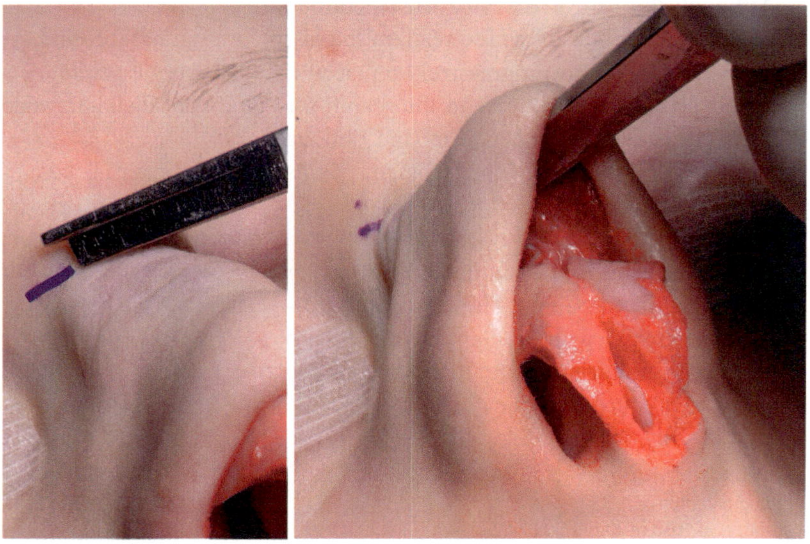

Fig. 16.45 Medial oblique osteotomy. With the open approach the correct positioning of the 3 mm guarded osteotome can be done under direct vision

the skin. In this region a bilateral medial oblique osteotomy can be carried out with a 2 or 3 mm guarded osteotome starting precisely at the level of the upper extremity of the open roof and inclining properly the osteotomy line towards the medial canthus (Figs. 16.44 and 16.45).

Small tilt differences of the osteotomy line depend on the level of the cephalic end of the open roof. The bone thickness encountered during the medial osteotomies is generally greater than during the basal ones. This anatomical condition dictates the rationale to perform the medial osteotomies first and then the basal ones.

Under direct vision, the guarded osteotome is placed in direct contact with the nasal bone and properly inclined towards the medial canthus. The skin flap is released over the instrument and the surgeon, with the index finger of his non-dominant hand, palpates the tip of the guarded osteotome through the skin to be sure of its positioning. During the entire procedure, the thumb and the index finger of the non-dominant hand palpate and pinch bilaterally the nasal radix to stabilize the patient's head and check:

- The progression of the osteotome through the bone.
- The correct direction of the osteotomy line.
- Any loss of contact between the osteotome and the bone, with the risk of traumatizing the soft tissues under the mallet blows. If this is the case, the skin flap should be retracted and the osteotome repositioned under direct vision to its initial position on the bone.
- The rare but possible fragmentation of the bone into small pieces. In this case the procedure is stopped and the operator passes directly to the basal osteotomies.

Although the use of the guarded osteotome for medial osteotomies is widespread, in the last 10 years the author has progressively replaced it with a small piezoelectric saw in the search for precise, clean, limited and safe medial oblique osteotomies (Fig. 16.46). The advantages of this method are that it:

- Avoids the risks of a comminuted fracture or unwanted fracture lines. These risks progressively increase with a not perfectly sharp osteotome requiring more force and mallet blows to produce the bone cut.
- Produces a linear groove of about 1 mm with a moderate and regular full-thickness removal of bone that permits easy mobilization and rotation of the osteocartilaginous segment with less interference compared with the irregular fracture line produced by an osteotome.
- Reduces the risk of visible irregularities and step deformities.

16.13 Basal Osteotomies

With the term "basal osteotomies" we refer to a broad range of osteotomy lines. Also the technique and the relative instruments proposed to do them are different. Basically, we can divide the basal nasal osteotomies into three main groups:

- Endonasal (blinded procedure).
- External percutaneous (blinded procedure).
- With small ultrasonic saw (under direct vision).

The external percutaneous and the endonasal osteotomies are the most commonly performed procedures. As other procedure requiring an osteotome and some mallet blows, they sometimes cause a wide range of well-known problems:

- Imprecise or irregular osteotomy lines.
- Bone fragmentation (unwanted fracture lines).

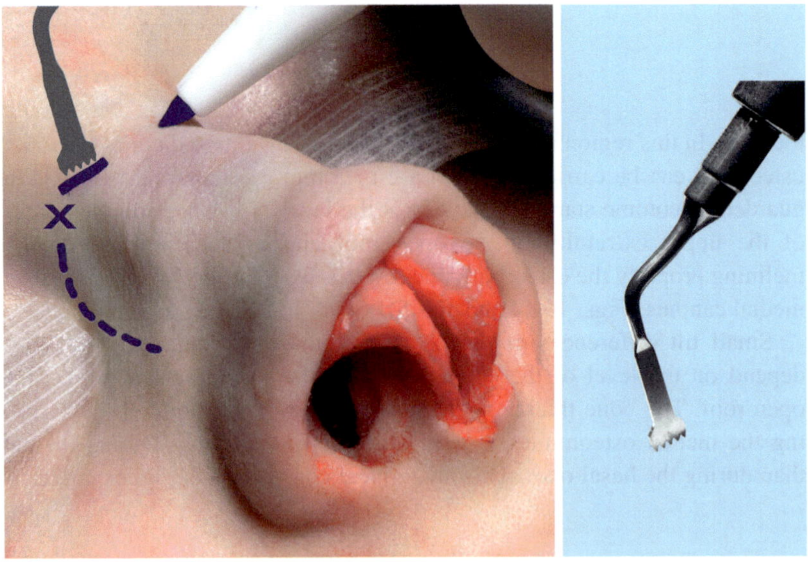

Fig. 16.46 Medial oblique osteotomy. Although the use of the guarded osteotome for medial osteotomies is widespread, in the last 10 years the author has progressively replaced it with a small piezoelectric saw in the search for precise, clean, limited and safe medial oblique osteotomies

- Asymmetries between the two bony fragments.
- Excessive mobility of one or both bony fragments.
- Excessive resistance to the planned movement of one or both bony fragments due to greenstick bone fracture or increased thickness of the nasal bone and septum.

A useful exercise is to thoroughly study as many axial CT scans of secondary cases as possible. Initially it will seem strange but in the long run we should admit that obtaining ideal osteotomies, with symmetrical movements of proper and intact bone fragments, is the exception rather than the rule. Fortunately, the bony irregularities produced with osteotomies do not always cause significant visible deformities due to the smoothing effect produced by the soft tissue envelope.

Utilizing a small ultrasonic saw (piezosurgery) under direct vision as well as suturing together the anterior edges of the two bone fragments, also under direct vision, can be a major advance in reducing postoperative deformities in the upper third of the nose. With the aid of piezosurgery oscillating instruments is also possible to reduce the thickness of the bony septum as well as model the points of interference that restrain a complete medial movement of the two osteotomized fragments.

16.14 Endonasal Basal Osteotomies

The endonasal technique requires a small vertical full-thickness skin incision in the lateral nasal vestibule. With the small 15c blade the bone surface of the piriform aperture is easily reached.

The most utilized instruments for endonasal osteotomies are the curved (one left and one right) or straight guarded osteotome. The dimension and thickness of the cutting extremity has been reduced over the years in an attempt to perform osteotomies preserving the endonasal periosteum and reducing the trauma to the external soft tissue envelope.

A small area of periosteum is elevated over the piriform aperture to favor the correct placement of the osteotome as well as to reduce the direct trauma by the instrument to the soft tissue. Some authors favor the creation of a complete subperiosteal tunnel over the entire planned osteotomy lines, whereas others prefer to avoid this step considering this an additional soft tissue trauma as well as a cause of bone instability.

Once the guarded osteotome is positioned on the larger portion of the piriform aperture, the classic low-to-high basal osteotomy can be divided into three steps. Figure 16.47 illustrates these three steps from the lateral point of view and Fig. 16.48 from above; the osteotome is placed over the skin for didactic purposes to better show the lines followed.

As for the medial oblique osteotomies, initially the surgeon with his index finger of his non-dominant hand palpates the tip of the guarded osteotome through the skin to be sure of its positioning. During the entire procedure, the thumb and the index finger of the non-dominant hand palpate and pinch bilaterally the nose to stabilize the patient's head and control the progression and the direction of the osteotome.

16.15 External Percutaneous Basal Osteotomies

Percutaneous basal osteotomies, performed with a 2 mm sharp osteotome, are an effective and less traumatic technique compared with the endonasal one. This is the procedure of first choice in adults or elderly patients, owing to their lower tendency to develop a greenstick fracture, as well as in the case of thin nasal bones.

The main steps of the percutaneous basal osteotomies are:

1. Identify and draw where to place the skin incision (Fig. 16.49a, b). For beginners it is helpful to draw the following visual references on the skin: the actual bony dorsal margin (after hump resection), the inferior margin of the nasal bone, the medial oblique osteotomy line, and the planned basal osteotomy line. The skin incision should lie anterior to the angular artery (depicted in red in

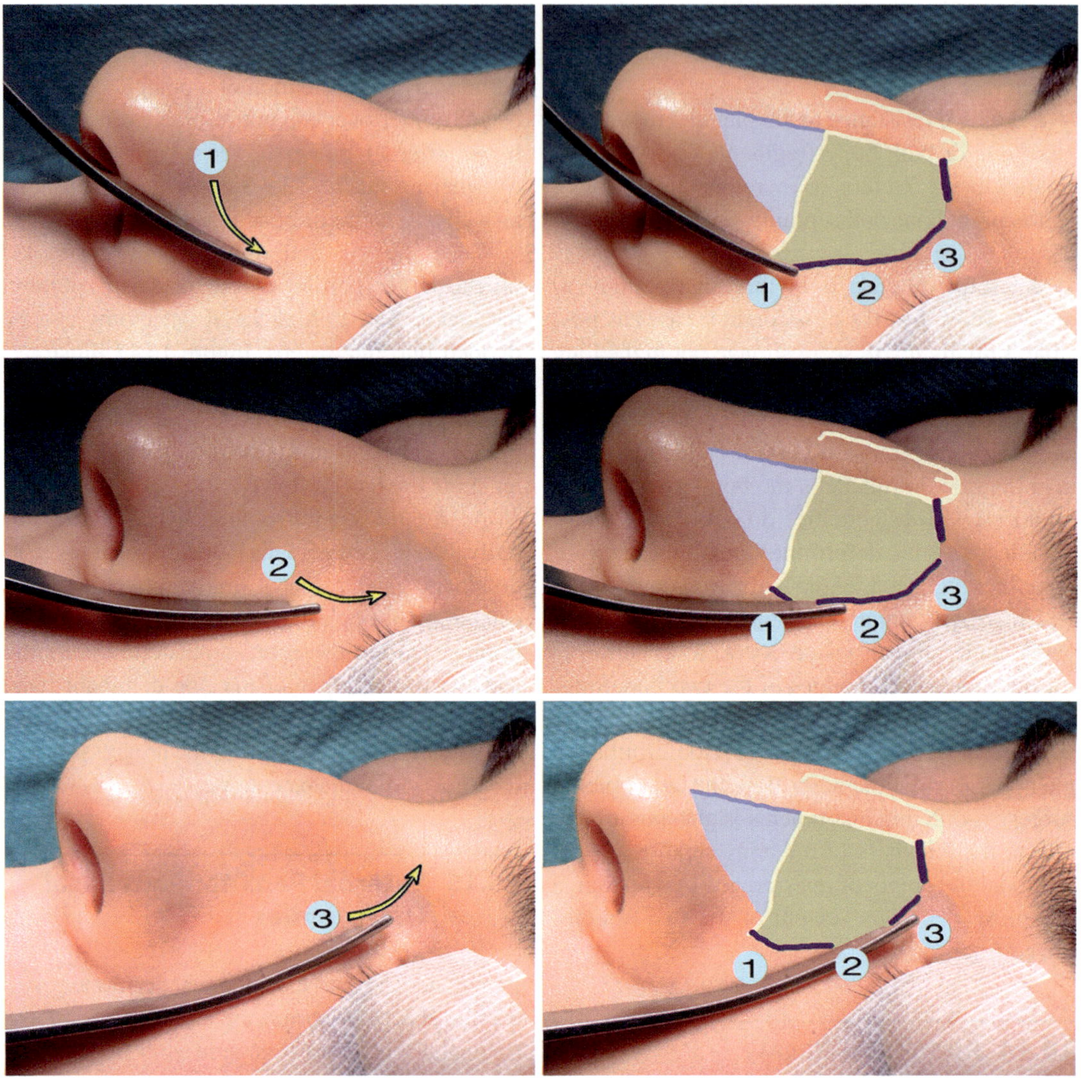

Fig. 16.47 Endonasal basal osteotomies. The three steps of the low-to-high basal osteotomies viewed from the lateral point of view

Fig. 16.49) to avoid its injury and equidistant from the ends of the osteotomy line.

2. Inject deeply (close to the periosteum) the soft tissue over the nasal pyramid with 0.8–1.0 cc of local anesthesia with epinephrine immediately before the osteotomies (Fig. 16.50).
3. Incise directly the nasal skin pushing the sharp 2 mm osteotome firmly against the bone. This is a single and quick action without uncertainty, to puncture precisely and without damaging the skin. It is mandatory to reach the subperiosteal plane. All the next steps should be done maintaining the tip of the 2 mm osteotome in contact with the bone surface in order to avoid any damage to the angular artery branches and generally to the nasal soft tissue envelope.
4. Move the tip of the osteotome posteriorly until it reaches the planned osteotomy line without losing contact with the bone surface. Figure 16.51 shows how the soft tissue follows the tip of the osteotome and the displacement effect on the angular artery.

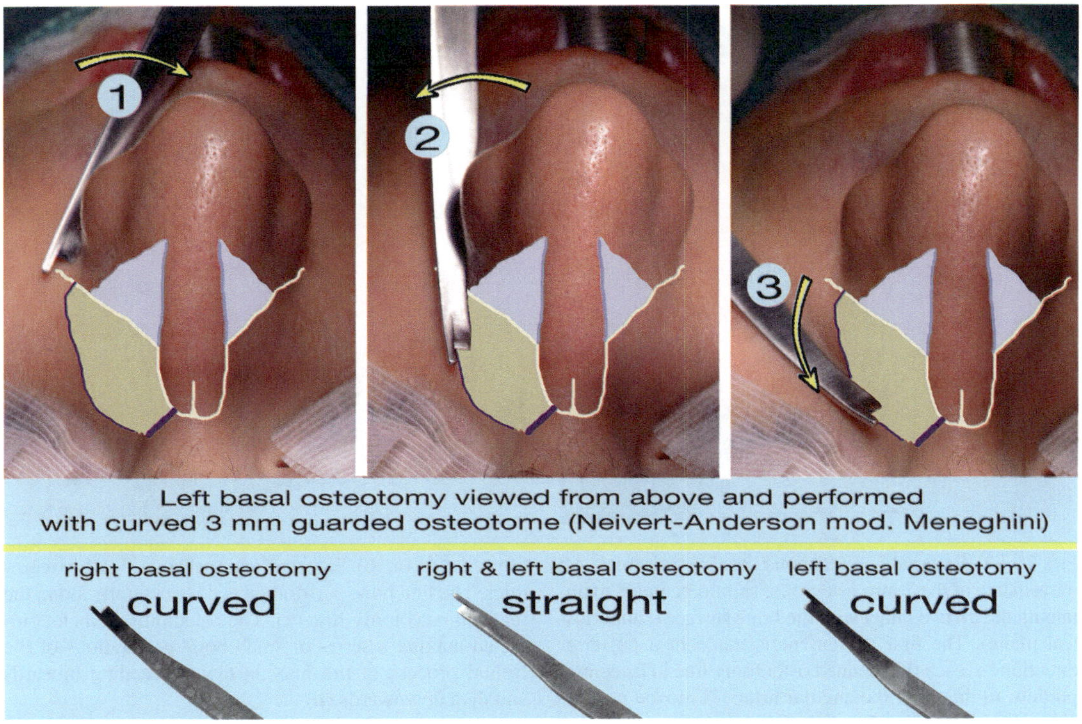

Fig. 16.48 Endonasal basal osteotomies. The three steps of the low-to-high basal osteotomies viewed from above

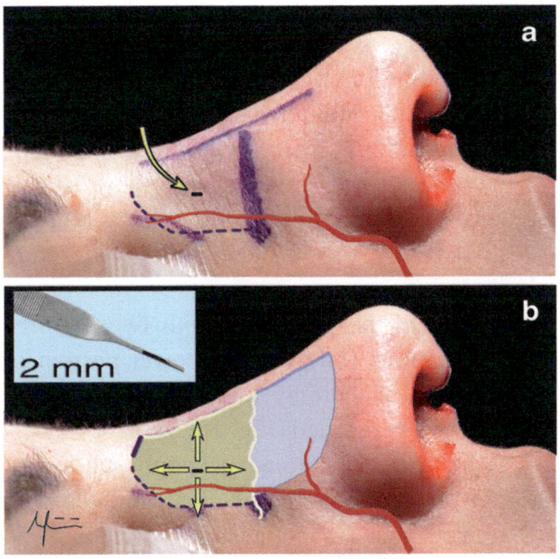

Fig. 16.49 (**a**, **b**) External percutaneous basal osteotomies. Identify and draw where to place the skin incision to avoid damaging the angular artery (depicted in red)

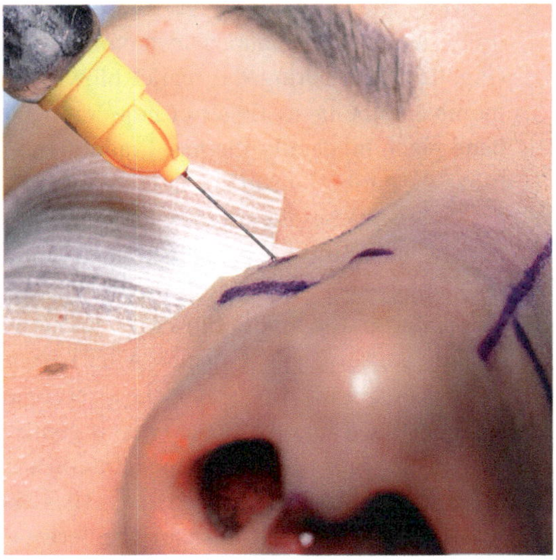

Fig. 16.50 External percutaneous basal osteotomies. A quantity of 0.8–1.0 cc of local anesthesia with epinephrine is injected over the nasal bone immediately before the osteotomies

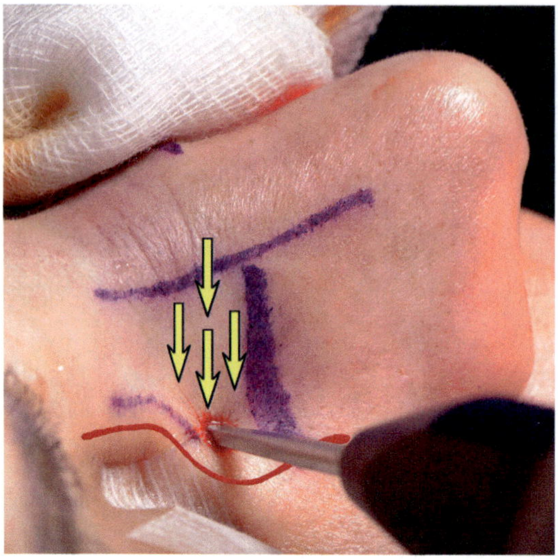

Fig. 16.51 External percutaneous basal osteotomies. All movements of the 2 mm osteotome should be made maintaining the tip in contact with the bone surface (subperiosteal plane). The first movement is made in a posterior direction to reach the planned osteotomy line in its central portion. In this way, the angular artery is moved posteriorly, thereby avoiding the risk of damaging it

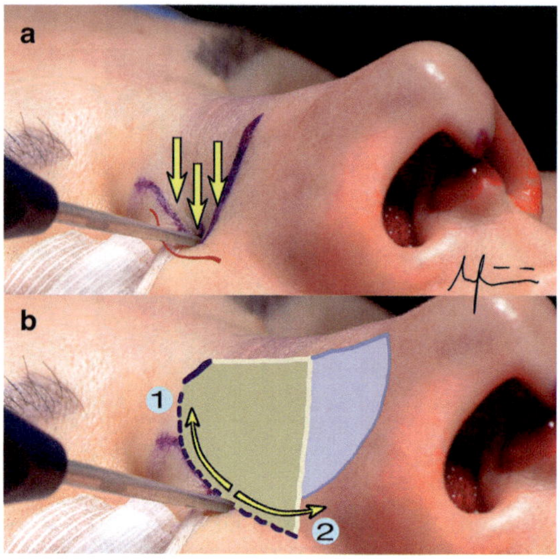

Fig. 16.52 (**a**, **b**) External percutaneous basal osteotomies. The first bone perforation is done centrally along the planned osteotomy line (**a**). The osteotomy is then completed making a series of small bony perforations of the frontal process of the maxilla first proceeding upwards and then downwards (**b**)

5. Perform the first bone perforation centrally along the planned osteotomy line (Fig. 16.52a). During the mallet blows, the thumb and the index finger of non-dominant hand pinch bilaterally the nasal radix to stabilize the patient's head and at the same time the thumb touches the osteotome giving support to maintain its exact position over the osteotomy line. Similarly to other procedures, during the mallet blows the mallet is held by the surgeon's assistant. After two or three mallet blows, to check if the osteotome has penetrated into the bone, twist it gently; also in the case of minimal penetration the osteotome is firmly positioned and resists the twisting movement. In this case the perforation should be stopped to avoid the risk of a deep penetration with injury to the internal periosteum and the nasal mucosa.
6. Retract the osteotome only from the bone without losing the subperiosteal plane (continue to maintain the bone contact) and move the tip of the osteotome upwards along the osteotomy line for the next bone perforation, about 2–3 mm away from the first one and following the same rules reported in point 5.
7. Continue the perforation following the upper portion of the osteotomy line until the medial oblique osteotomy is reached (Fig. 16.52b). The thickness of the bone increases progressively and the distance between the perforations should be reduced to decrease the risk of unwanted fracture lines or fragmentation.
8. Complete the procedure with two or three perforations following the lower portion of the basal osteotomy line until the piriform aperture is reached (Fig. 16.52b).
9. Remove the osteotome and apply gentle digital pressure for one or more minutes with soaked gauze over the small skin incision and the entire line of the basal osteotomy to favor hemostasis.
10. Perform the same procedure from point 1 to 8 on the opposite side of the nose taking care to avoid any trauma or pressure on the side that has just been done.
11. Maintain a thin moistened gauze over the nose and reposition the nasal bones by apply-

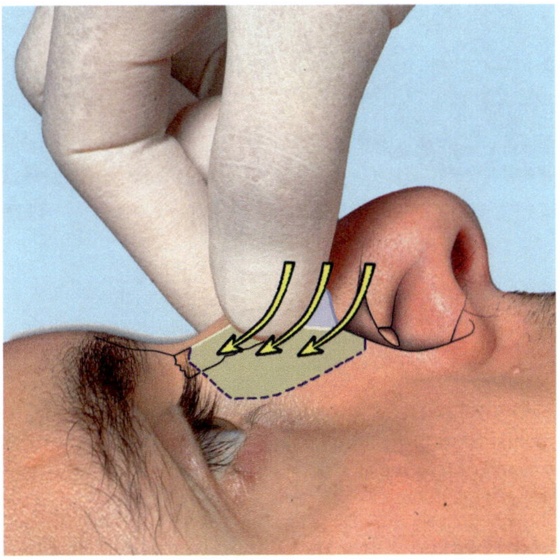

Fig. 16.53 External percutaneous basal osteotomies. The objective of the small perforations is to permit a controlled greenstick fracture along the planned osteotomy lines with very gentle external pressure. In the case of resistance, do not increase the pressure against the bone but reinsert the osteotome, displacing posteriorly the soft tissue and complete the osteotomy following the same rules as previously described

ing very gentle pressure with the thumb and forefinger taking care to distribute the force over the entire lateral surface of the osteotomized bone area (Fig. 16.53). The objective is to gently induce a greenstick fracture that permits accurate repositioning of the paired bones in the desired symmetrical location. In the case of incomplete osteotomy, do not force the repositioning of the nasal bone by increasing the pressure against the bone but reinsert the osteotome, displacing posteriorly the soft tissue and complete the osteotomy following the same rules as previously described.

16.16 Basal Osteotomies with Ultrasonic Instruments

The basal osteotomies can also be performed under direct vision with the aid of very small straight or dedicated saws vibrating at an ultrasonic frequency (also called piezosurgery). The dedicated saws are properly angled, one for right

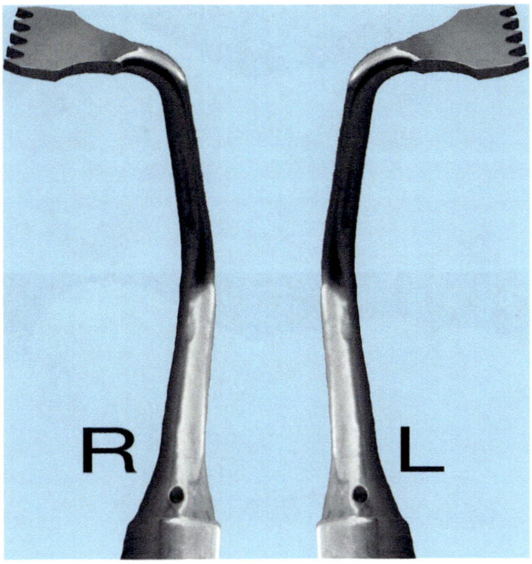

Fig. 16.54 Basal osteotomies with ultrasonic instruments. A couple of dedicated properly angled ultrasonic saws, one for right (*R*) and one for left (*L*) basal osteotomies

and one for left basal osteotomies, for a precise action in the limited space comprised between the frontal process of the maxillary bone and the elevated soft tissue flap (Fig. 16.54). However, from the author's direct experience, in some favorable cases all the nasal osteotomies can be done more quickly with a standard straight piezoelectric saw only.

If the surgeon decides to perform also the basal osteotomies with piezosurgery, the initial soft tissue elevation must be extended bilaterally over the upper lateral cartilage and the frontal process of the maxilla. Figure 16.55a, b shows the corresponding skin area of the usual soft tissue elevation (yellow dots) utilized in open rhinoplasty compared with the more extended area of elevation necessary for performing the basal osteotomies with piezosurgery (yellow-black dots). This adjunctive elevation should be done initially in the exploratory phase of the rhinoplasty and not later, as shown in Fig. 16.56. Figure 16.57 clearly depicts the skin projection of the osteotomy lines as well as the position of the saw during right basal osteotomy. The ideal posterior extent of subperiosteal flap elevation over the frontal process of the maxilla can be drawn over the skin

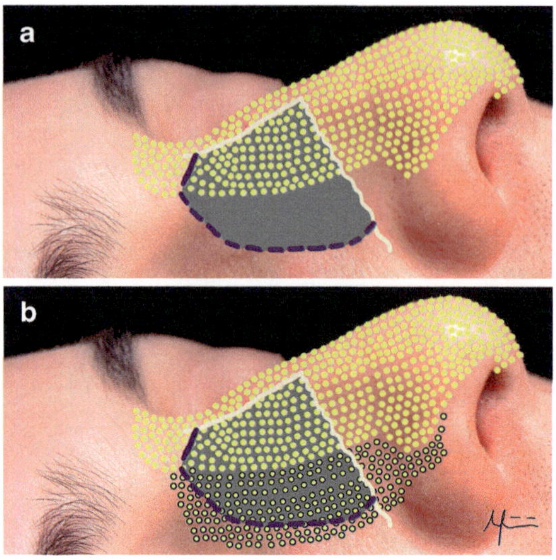

Fig. 16.55 (**a**, **b**) Comparison of the usual soft tissue elevation utilized in open rhinoplasty (yellow dots) with the more extended area of elevation necessary for performing the basal osteotomies with an ultrasonic saw (yellow-black dots). In particular, the soft tissue elevation must be extended bilaterally over the upper lateral cartilage and the frontal process of the maxilla (**b**)

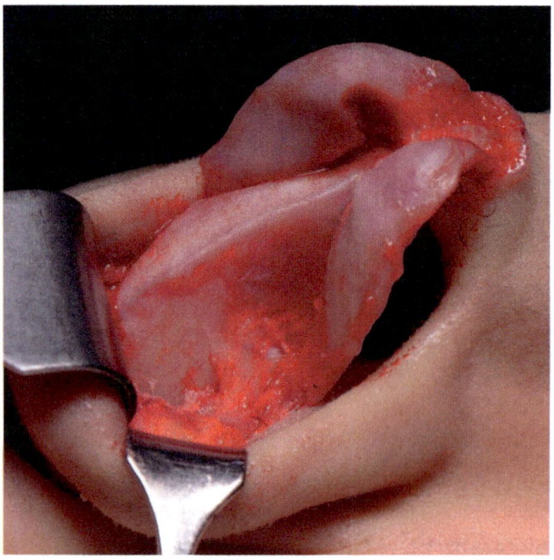

Fig. 16.56 Intraoperative view of the extended soft tissue elevation necessary for performing the basal osteotomies with an ultrasonic saw

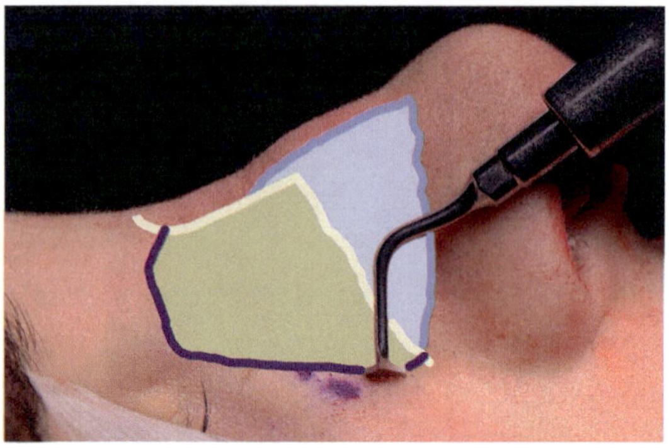

Fig. 16.57 Basal osteotomies with ultrasonic instruments. Skin projection of the osteotomy lines as well as the position of the saw during right basal osteotomy

and checked with an Obwegeser elevator positioned over the bone (Fig. 16.58).

The key objective is to widely expose all the site of the osteotomies to perform the entire bone job under direct vision and not merely create a tunnel under the periosteum to introduce the piezoelectric saw (Fig. 16.59). Protection of the skin soft tissue envelope as well as of the nasal mucosa under the osteotomy line are both obtained.

Execution of basal osteotomies with piezosurgery is a recent acquisition and can be considered the yet missing link in the intraoperative sequence of the BOR discipline. With the introduction of the piezosurgery technology in rhinoplasty, it is therefore possible to:

- Perform all the surgical steps under direct visualization.
- Visually check all the effects of any surgical maneuver.
- Work on the nasal septum, radix, pyramid and tip through a single skin incision approach.
- Avoid any incision of the nasal mucosa.
- Avoid the use of the mallet and osteotome as a probable cause of mucosal tears.
- Avoid the use of the mallet and osteotome as a probable cause of uncontrolled fractures and nasal wall bone fragmentation.

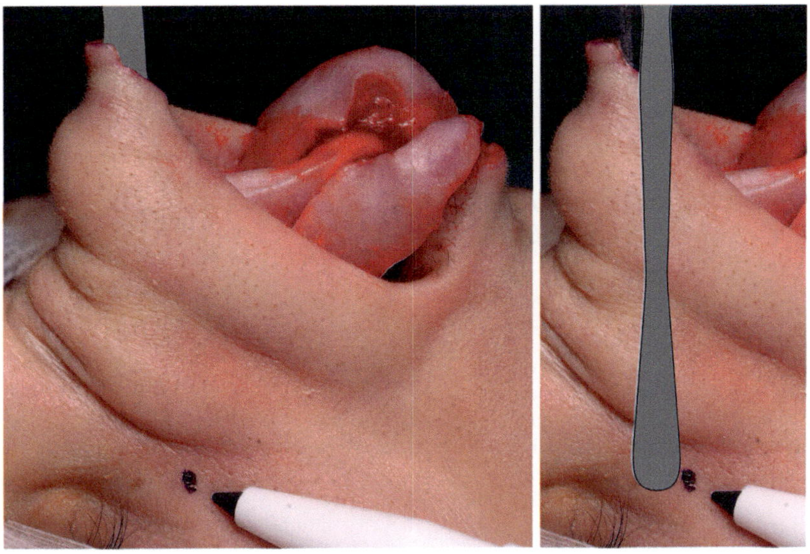

Fig. 16.58 Basal osteotomies with ultrasonic instruments. The ideal posterior extent of subperiosteal flap elevation over the frontal process of maxilla can be drawn externally with a skin marker and intraoperatively checked with an Obwegeser elevator positioned over the bone

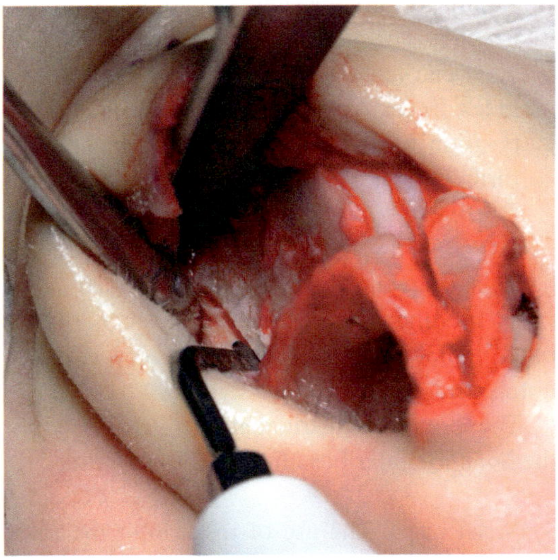

Fig. 16.59 Intraoperative view of nasal osteotomies with ultrasonic instruments

– Avoid or limit the use of rasps.
– Extend the use of internal fixation of nasal structures with long-lasting absorbable sutures to the bones reducing the postoperative instability of the nasal framework.

16.17 Nasal Osteotomies: Refinements and Stabilization

Whatever technique has been used, the final phase of the nasal osteotomies requires some free space around the patient's head. The surgeon must evaluate from all points of view the new position of the nasal bones obtained with his gentle finger pressure. The three main inspection tests are done in this sequence:

1. Palpatory inspection with the nasal skin flap repositioned over the nasal framework. The surgeon wears a pair of new clean gloves and wets the nose skin with sterile saline to better slide over the skin with the forefinger of his dominant hand. For a better appreciation of any small irregularities of the nasal framework, the surgeon can tense the skin with the thumb and index finger of the non-dominant hand. Palpating the dorsum is not only a static pressure over the nose but a dynamic come-and-go movement of the finger over the skin

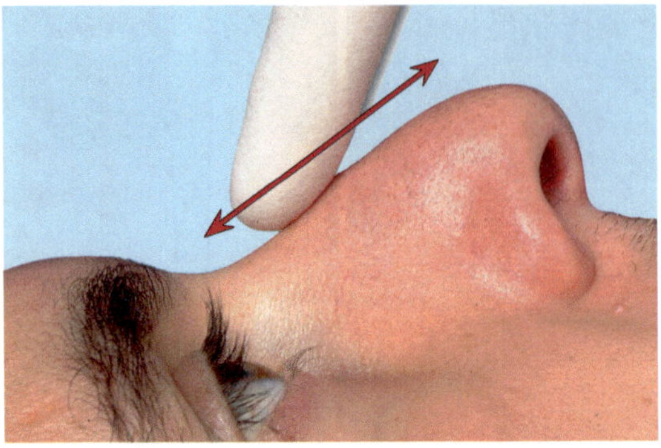

Fig. 16.60 Palpatory inspection after osteotomies. Palpating the dorsum is a dynamic come-and-go movement of the finger over the skin in the whole dorsal region from the radix to the tip

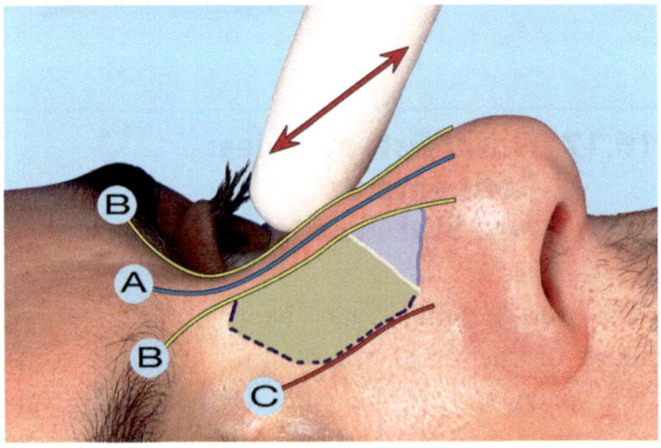

Fig. 16.61 Palpatory inspection after osteotomies. Ideally, the surgeon should imagine five lines running from cephalic to caudal: (**a**)—the median line, which follows the anterior margin of the septum after hump removal, (**b**)—the surgical margins of the nasal bones and upper lateral cartilages produced with hump removal (one left and one right), and (**c**)—the base of nasal pyramid ones corresponding to the basal osteotomy line (one left and one right). All these lines should be palpated and judged for symmetry and smoothness

in the whole dorsal region from the radix to the tip and side-to-side (Fig. 16.60). Ideally, after osteotomies the surgeon should imagine five lines running from cephalic to caudal (Fig. 16.61): **A**—the median line, which follows the anterior margin of the septum after hump removal; **B**—the surgical margins of the nasal bones and upper lateral cartilages produced with hump removal (one left and one right); and **C**—the base of the nasal pyramid ones corresponding to the basal osteotomy line (one left and one right). All these lines should be palpated and judged for symmetry and smoothness.

2. Endonasal visual inspection with the nasal skin flap superiorly retracted to completely expose the nasal framework. After copious irrigation with sterile saline to remove any small bone fragments and blood clots, the position of the two nasal bones with respect to the septum as well as the symmetry of the new dorsal framework is directly visualized. Any irregularities should be modeled conservatively with the less aggressive technique at the surgeon's disposal to avoid the risk of creating depressions or structural instability of the osteocartilaginous framework.
3. External visual inspection with the nasal skin flap repositioned over the nasal framework. Again, for a better appreciation of any small irregularities of the nasal framework, the surgeon can tense the skin with the thumb and index finger of the non-dominant hand. The position of the bones can be changed with further gentle pressure with the thumb and forefinger.

This sequence should be repeated after every modification of the dorsal osteocartilaginous components until a satisfactory result is obtained.

The principal instruments utilized to adjust the bone irregularities after osteotomies are:

- Nasal rasps. The use of rasps after the nasal osteotomies should be avoided for the risk of damaging both the septum and the lateral osteocartilaginous nasal wall. The unwanted increased mobility of these supporting structures can be a cause of visible deformities such as saddling, inverted-V deformity and asymmetries but also of nasal obstruction. Unfortunately, for modeling bony irregularities the basic surgical instrument kits are composed only of rasps, leaving the surgeon without any safe alternatives.
- Electric burr. The multiple-blade pear-shaped burr with a larger distal diameter presented in Chap. 15 can be used at a low speed under direct vision in the case of a

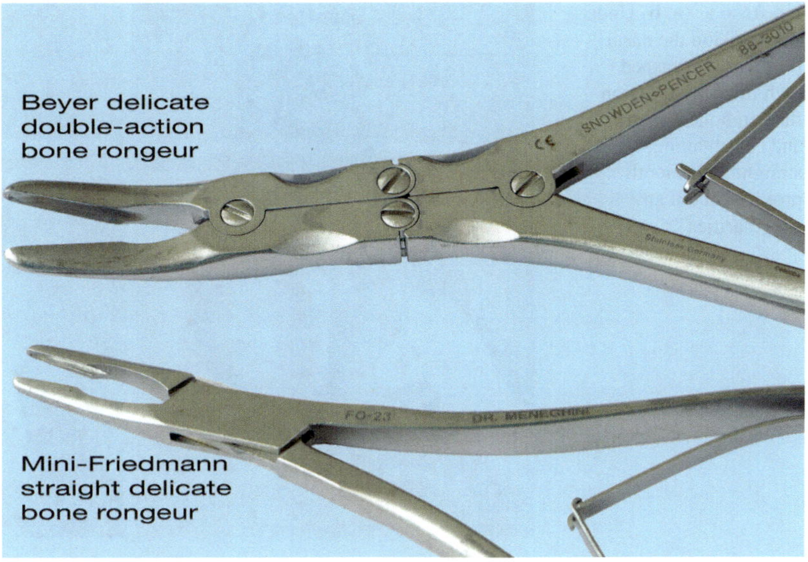

Fig. 16.62 Fine-tip bone rongeur and double-action fine-tip bone rongeur

bony spur emerging in the fixed upper margin of the medial oblique osteotomy. In this case the problem is an overly protruding step-shaped deformity produced by an effective medialization of the nasal bone; it should not be confused with the so-called Rocker deformity in which the bone portion that protrudes under the skin is represented by the cephalic anterior angle of the mobilized nasal bone. In general, when using the electric burr, care should be taken to avoid any contact of the burr with the soft tissue envelope as well as with any osteotomized bones. At first glance the multiple-blade pear-shaped burr's dimensions seem excessive but, as a general rule, it is important to remember that a large diameter burr removes irregularities while a small burr creates irregularities.

- Fine-tip bone rongeur and double-action fine-tip bone rongeur (Fig. 16.62). This cutting surgical instrument can be safely used to lower incrementally the dorsal profile of the nasal bones instead of the rasps even if the osteotomies have already been carried out. Under direct vision, the bone can be grasped and cut obtaining a new straight and smooth profile without any bone irregularities (Fig. 16.63a, b). The only recommendation is to check every time the condition of the cutting blades of the instrument; any irregularities of the instrument tips can produce a corresponding irregular bone cut.
- Piezosurgery rasps or saws. After years of experimentation there are no more doubts about the efficacy and safety of piezoelectric surgery in cutting and modeling small bones. So almost every nasal bone irregularity can be addressed before and after osteotomies under direct vision.

In BOR, the nasal osteotomies should be carried out after complete stabilization of the cartilaginous dorsum. The necessary sutures of the upper lateral cartilage to the septum, with or without spreader flaps or spreader grafts, indirectly stabilize also the mobilized nasal bone due to the strong connection between nasal bone and upper lateral cartilage.

To further stabilize the dorsum at the end of the osteotomies, an additional suture between the two nasal bones and the septum is indicated. With the aid of a manual or electric drill, or better with a small ultrasonic tip, a small hole can be drilled close to the inferior anterior angle of the nasal bone (Fig. 16.64). The interposing septum in this region is made of cartilage and therefore it must not be perforated. A 4/0 polyglactin absorbable suture is then gently tied to stabilize the nasal bones (Fig. 16.65). An excessively tightened suture disrupts the septal cartilage and has no favorable effects.

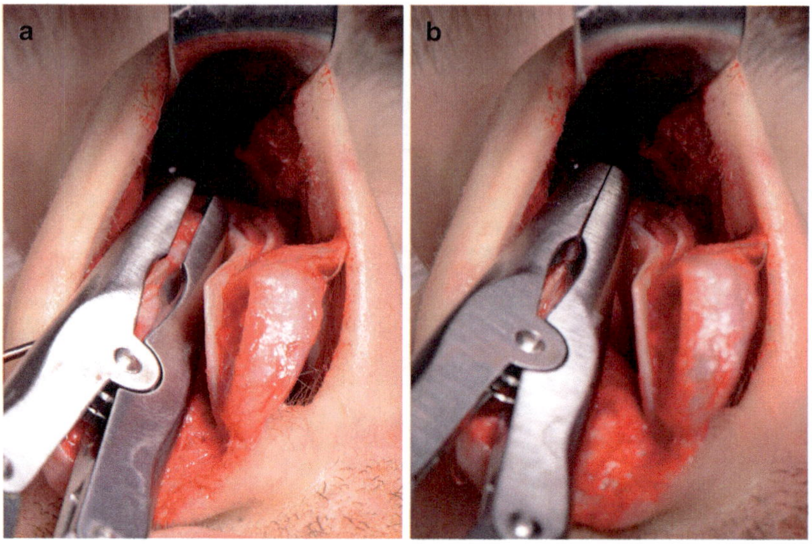

Fig. 16.63 (**a**, **b**) Under direct vision the nasal bone can be grasped with the double-action fine-tip bone rongeur and cut obtaining a new straight and smooth profile without any irregularities

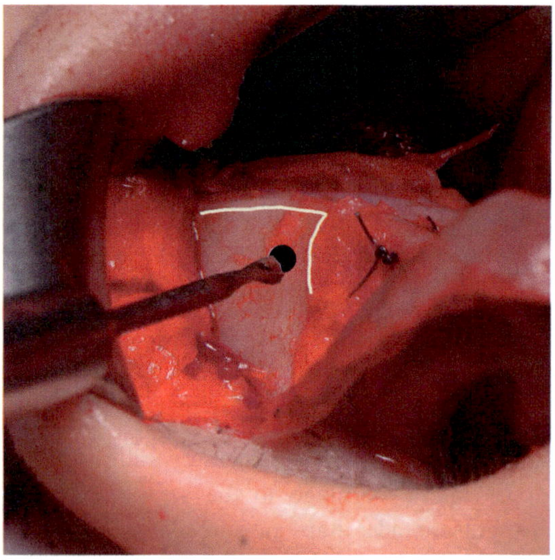

Fig. 16.64 Osteotomy internal stabilization. Drilling of a small hole close to the inferior anterior angle of the nasal bone. Drilling of a small hole close to the inferior anterior angle of the nasal bone

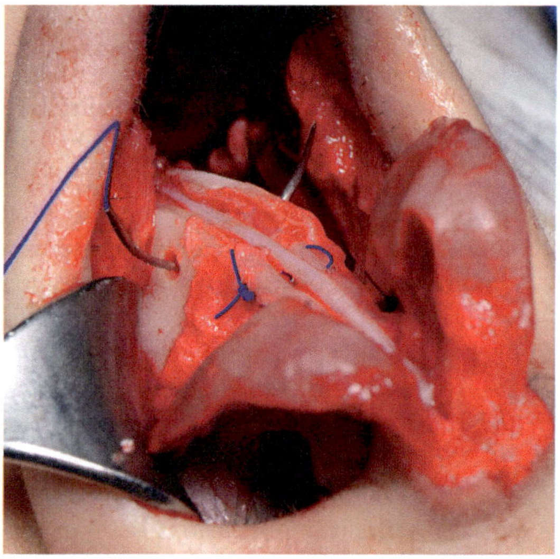

Fig. 16.65 The internal stabilization after osteotomies and the open roof closure are done with a simple suture of both nasal bones to the septum

The extra time spent to add this suture is about 3–4 min, not too much considering the purposes to be achieved:

- Avoiding the "open roof" deformity secondary to lateral back rebound of one or both nasal bones.
- Avoiding or reducing the extent of the inverted-V deformity secondary to instability and inferior posterior rotation of the lateral nasal walls.
- Stabilizing the cartilaginous septum. In the case of abnormal septal mobility, this suture is mandatory as are the sutures of the septum to the nasal spine and to the dorsal margin of the upper cartilages.
- Preventing the risk of inadvertently displacing the nasal bones during nasal cast removal or for early accidental trauma.

Sometimes the knot can be palpable under the skin but in some weeks the polyglactin suture gradually dissolves leaving a smooth area.

It must be clear that suturing the nasal bones is part of a more complex and articulated technique of reconstruction and stabilization of the osteo-cartilaginous dorsum. Used as a unique step to close the nasal roof it makes no sense.

16.18 Take Another "Surgical Time Out"

The next steps instead will surely be challenging and mostly focused on nasal tip reshaping and reconstruction. A "surgical time out" of 1 or 2 min is important for the surgeon to regain concentration and make decisions.

The skin flap should be repositioned and cleaned to check the result obtained so far at the level of upper and middle third of the nose. The previous steps, dedicated to the reconstruction of the nasal dorsum, are summarized schematically in Fig. 16.66a–d. Even if these local results will be often confirmed and maintained, some refinements can still be considered later in the surgery. The BOR sequence and techniques are not composed of a rigid and definitive scheme but form a highly flexible, reversible and customizable intraoperative approach.

The main objective of this "surgical time out" is to visualize the shape and projection of the best nasal tip for the actual dorsum. Dr. Ronald Gruber of San Francisco realized a plastic standard model to help the surgeon in his mental effort of visualizing the sculpted and repositioned alar cartilages. The greatest difficulty lies in the ability to obtain a given shape and position of the nasal tip framework starting from the initial deformity and utilizing the quality and quantity of cartilage available.

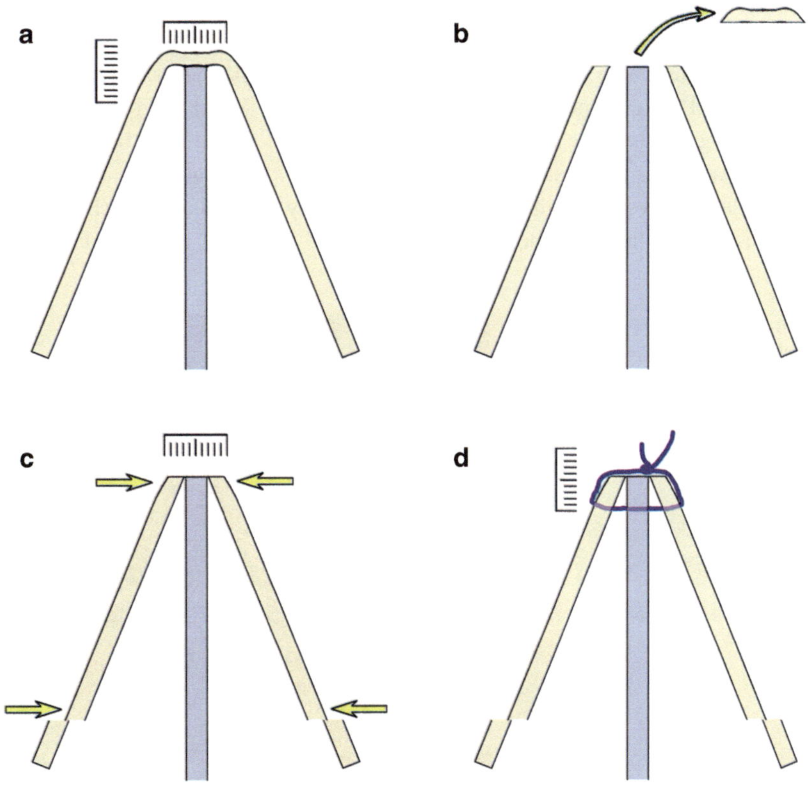

Fig. 16.66 (**a–d**) Schematic drawings of dorsal reconstruction. Removal of the bony hump (**b**). Closure of the residual open roof with basal osteotomies (**c**). Stabilization by suturing both the nasal bones to the cartilaginous septum (**d**). The anterior projection of the nasal dorsum is reduced, thereby maintaining the proportion of the framework

16.19 Columellar Reconstruction with Autologous Strut

The BOR discipline provides a fixed exploratory access to the caudal septum and, in many cases, the attenuation of the depressor septum muscle. This approach requires the splitting of the two medial crura of the lower lateral cartilages and partial removal of the interposed tissue between them. Also the membranous septum will be split (see Chap. 13).

The advantages of the "Tip Split" technique are:

- Obtaining unrestricted access to the whole septum without any mucosal incisions and reducing the incidence of mucosal tears.
- Performing a reconstructive septoplasty under direct vision.
- Mobilizing the medial crura of the lower lateral cartilages for their later spatial repositioning in a cephalic-caudal and anterior-posterior direction.

The method also involves a mandatory reconstruction of the columella through the insertion of an autologous cartilage strut fixed with polydioxanone absorbable sutures. In nearly every primary rhinoplasty as well as in the majority of secondary cases, a columellar strut should be utilized.

In summary, the objectives of the columellar strut are to:

- Provide stable support to the nasal tip.
- Help in creating and testing the "new surgical domes."
- Help in reducing or increasing tip projection.
- Help in maintaining or realizing a symmetric tip and columella structure.
- Correct the deformities of the medial crura (Fig. 16.67a, b) and repair them if injured.

The strut should be carved from an intact piece of solid septal cartilage. Figure 16.68a–d shows how a fragment of cartilage removed from the inferior margin of the septum close to the maxillary crest can be shaved to plane any irregularities and sculpted in two long and straight pieces that are ready to use. As previously mentioned, often it is necessary to obtain the strut from a large piece of cartilage harvested in the central portion of the cartilaginous septum (Fig. 16.69).

Before positioning the graft it is necessary to create a precise pocket between the footplates of the medial crura in order to stabilize and maintain separate from the anterior nasal spine the posterior end of the strut. In practice, with the aid of the assistant, the two domes are retracted anteriorly and laterally (Fig. 16.70) to separate the medial crura and facilitate the insertion of the Converse

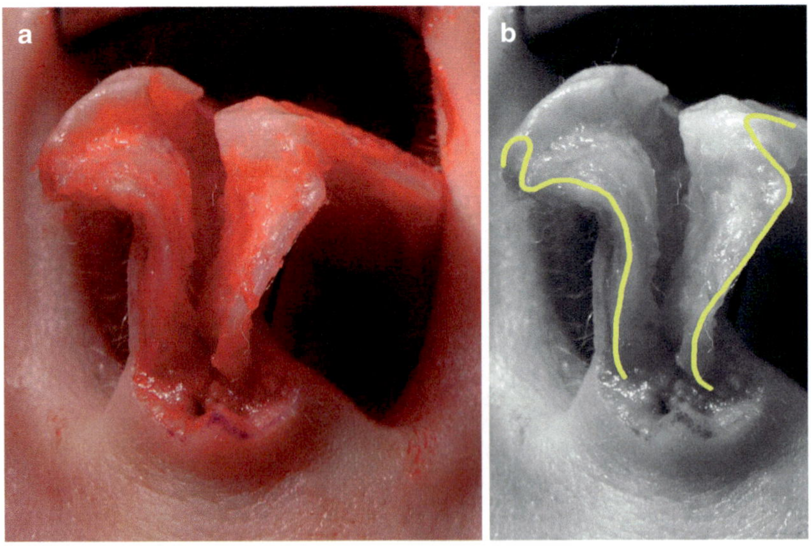

Fig. 16.67 (**a**, **b**) A columellar reconstruction with autologous strut is mandatory in case of deformed medial and middle crura

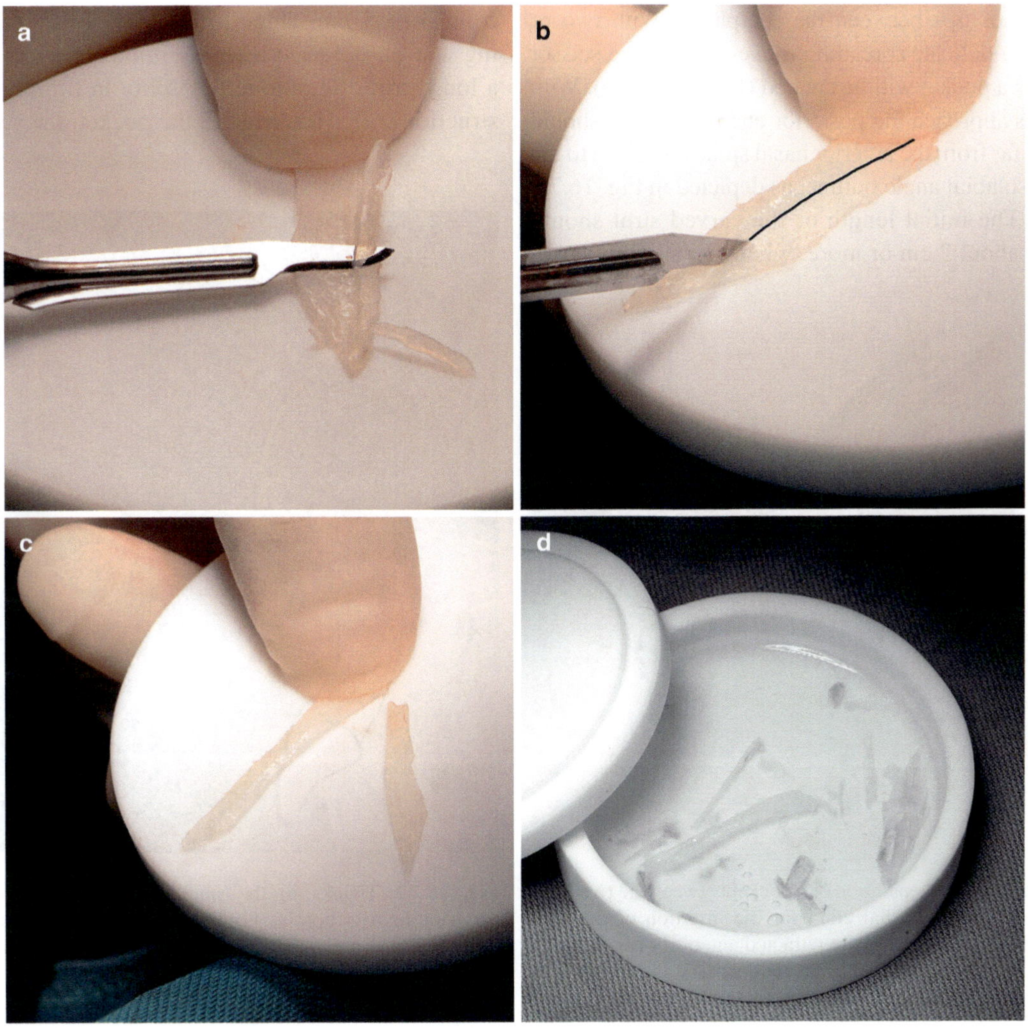

Fig. 16.68 (**a–d**) Columellar reconstruction with autologous strut. A fragment of cartilage removed from the inferior margin of the septum close to the maxillary crest can be shaved to plane any irregularities (**a**) and sculpted in two long and straight, ready-to-use pieces (**b**, **c**). Even the smallest discarded cartilage fragments should be stored again in the sterile solution (**d**)

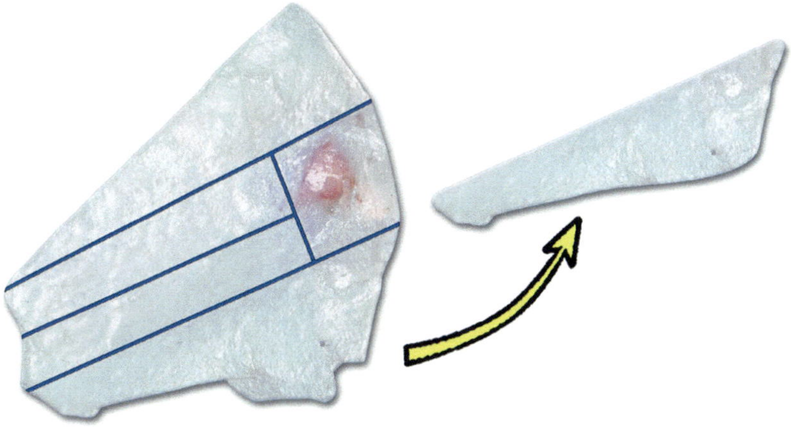

Fig. 16.69 Columellar reconstruction with autologous strut. More often it is necessary to obtain the strut from a large piece of cartilage harvested in the central portion of the cartilaginous septum

scissor tips between the footplates. With two or three delicate spreading movements of the scissor tips a pocket will be created (Fig. 16.71a, b). With this approach the posterior end of the strut should lie far from the anterior nasal spine and close to the nasolabial angle outline, as depicted in Fig. 16.72.

The initial length of the carved strut should be about 2 cm or more, whereas its width varies from 3 to 5 mm (Fig. 16.73). The final shaping can be deferred after its initial fixation so a long strut offers more flexibility in tip reconstruction. After insertion in the pocket, the strut

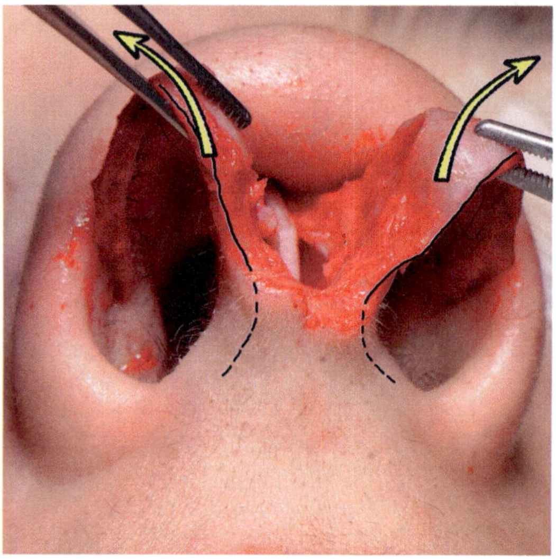

Fig. 16.70 Preparation of a pocket between the two footplates of the medial crura for the insertion of the strut graft: the two domes are retracted anteriorly and laterally to separate the medial crura and facilitate the insertion of the Converse scissor tips between the footplates

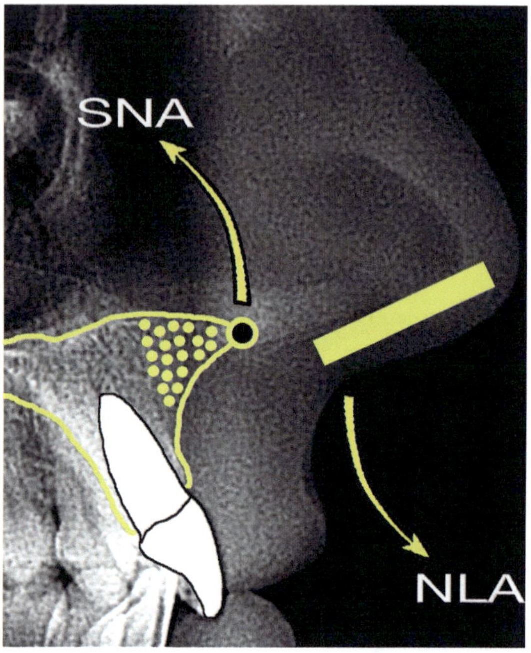

Fig. 16.72 Thanks to the small and precise pocket between the two footplates of the medial crura the posterior end of the strut should lie far from the anterior nasal spine (*ANS*) and close to the nasolabial angle outline (*NLA*)

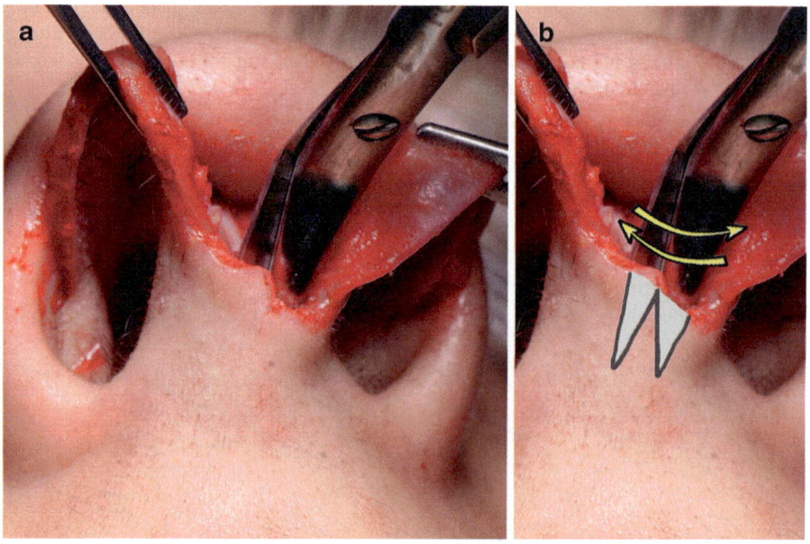

Fig. 16.71 (**a**, **b**) Preparation of a pocket between the two footplates of the medial crura for the insertion of the strut graft: with two or three delicate spread movements of the scissor tips a pocket will be created

must be oriented parallel to the medial crura (Fig. 16.74a, b).

In these moments the surgeon must resist the temptation to start suturing the medial crus of the lower lateral cartilage to the strut. First, it is better to stabilize the anterior end of the strut with a fine needle passing also through the lower lateral cartilages (Fig. 16.75a, b). Care should be taken to:

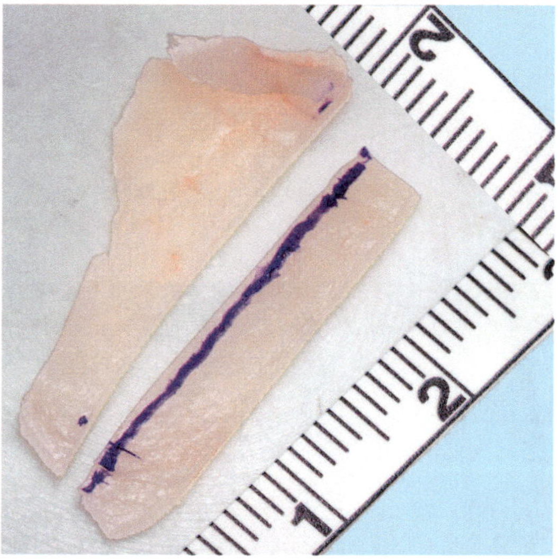

Fig. 16.73 Columellar reconstruction with autologous strut. The initial length of the carved strut should be about 2 cm or more, whereas its width varies from 3 to 5 mm. The final shaping can be deferred after its initial fixation so a long strut offers more flexibility in tip reconstruction

- Maintain or create a symmetric columella.
- Maintain the strut orientation parallel to the medial crura.
- Avoid any protrusion of the strut off the inferior margins of the medial crura.

For correct positioning of the strut, the surgeon with his non-dominant hand pushes the strut gently down in its pocket between the footplates and, with his dominant hand, lifts up the medial crura (Fig. 16.76a, b). This maneuver straightens any small folds of the medial crura and produces a favourable support effect on the nasal tip. It should be done putting a little tension in the cartilages taking care to avoid an excessive distorting force.

To stabilize the graft in position, a first single 5/0 polydioxanone simple suture should be placed close to the columellar skin incision margin (Fig. 16.77a, b). The objective of this suture is to cross over the inferior margins of the medial crura to prevent any accidental inferior dislocation of the strut subsequently producing tension and bulging on the skin columellar suture. The subsequent one or two stabilizing sutures are placed centrally in a horizontal mattress fashion. For the moment, the anterior third of the graft is instead left free between the domes, and the small stabilizing needle is removed to check the efficacy and symmetry of the strut.

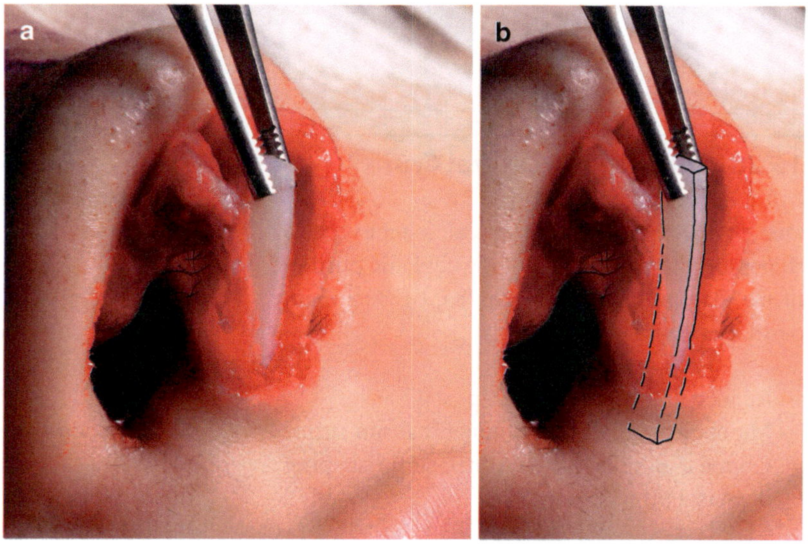

Fig. 16.74 (**a**, **b**) Columellar reconstruction with autologous strut. The strut after its insertion in the pocket must be oriented parallel to the medial crura

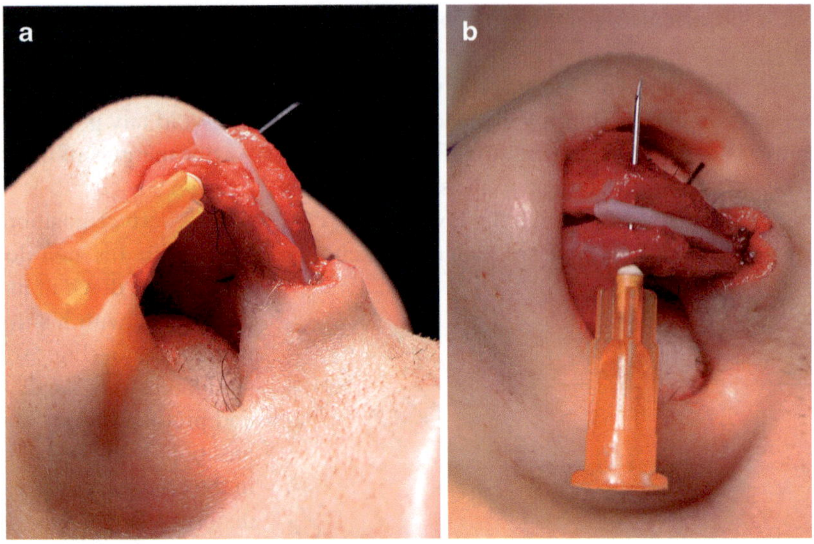

Fig. 16.75 (**a**, **b**) Columellar reconstruction with autologous strut. The anterior end of the strut is temporarily stabilized with a fine needle passing also through the lower lateral cartilages

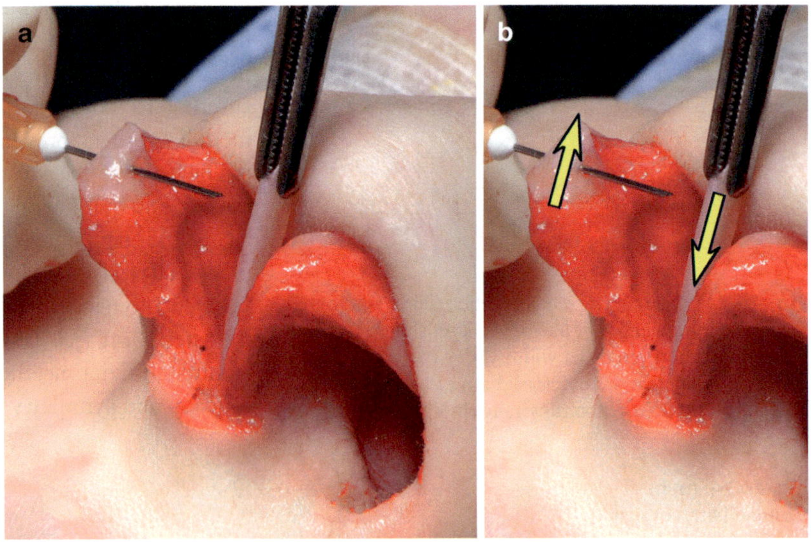

Fig. 16.76 (**a**, **b**) Columellar reconstruction with autologous strut. For correct positioning of the strut, the surgeon with his non-dominant hand pushes the strut gently down in its pocket between the footplates and, with his dominant hand, lifts up the medial crura

16.20 Shaping the Lateral Crura

One of the over-abused surgical maneuvers in rhinoplasty is the excision of the cephalic portion of the alar cartilages (Fig. 16.78a, b). The main desired effects are to:

- Reduce the volume of the tip.
- Maintain or create two symmetrical rim strips.
- Obtain a more malleable cartilage for shaping the nasal tip with sutures.

Usually a continuous strip of lateral crus with a regular width comprised between 6 and 8 mm is preserved to avoid secondary problems such as:

- Excessive weakening of the cartilage with compromise of the airway.
- The so-called "pinched nasal tip" deformity due to an anomalous concavity of the lateral crura.
- A superior alar retraction deformity.

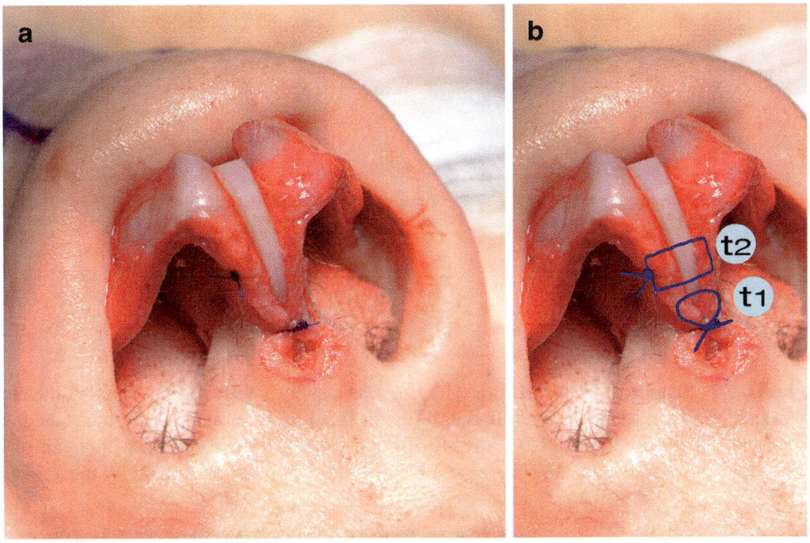

Fig. 16.77 (**a**, **b**) Columellar reconstruction with autologous strut. To stabilize the graft in position a first single 5/0 polydioxanone simple suture should be placed close to the columellar skin incision margin. The subsequent one or two stabilizing sutures are placed centrally in a horizontal mattress fashion

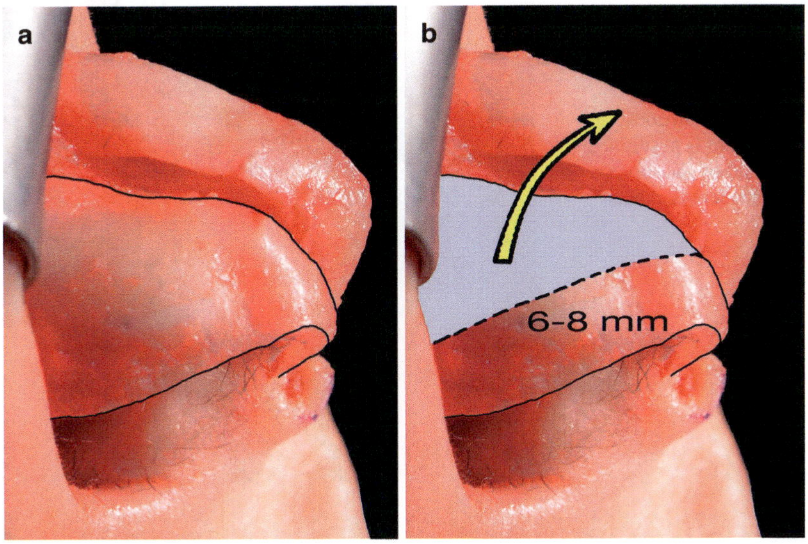

Fig. 16.78 (**a**, **b**) Shaping the lateral crura. Excision of the cephalic portion of the alar cartilages leaving at least a 6–8 mm wide intact strip

The preferred operative sequence is:

- Draw and measure the incision line.
- Inject the underlying mucosa of the lateral crura with 0.5 cc of local anesthetic to facilitate dissection.
- Retract the skin flap with the Meneghini nasal skin retractor fixed to the forehead with a pair of R1547 Steri-Strips[1] or a similar retractor held by the assistant (Figs. 16.79 and 16.80).
- Support and stabilize the lateral crura with the Meneghini delicate alar clamp or similar instruments. This instrument is positioned and held by the surgeon with his non-dominant hand (Figs. 16.81a, b and 16.82a, b). The definitive version of the Meneghini delicate alar clamp[2] is a forceps with a rectangular steel plate soldered on each arm of the instrument. These two plates are slightly convex and the inferior one is larger than the other. The

[1] 3M, R1547 Steri-Strip, 12 mm × 100 mm. The author has no conflict of interest with this or other 3M products.

[2] Bd-350, Meneghini Delicate Alar Clamp—Bontempi Chirurgische Instruments.

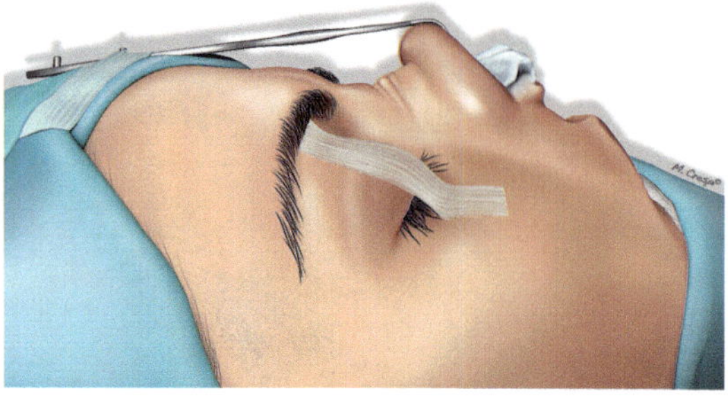

Fig. 16.79 Shaping the lateral crura. The skin flap can be retracted with the Meneghini nasal skin retractor fixed to the forehead with a pair of R1547 Steri-Strips or a similar retractor held by the assistant (lateral view)

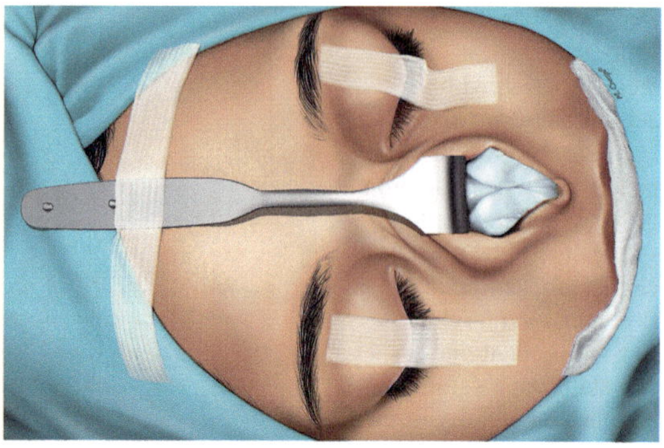

Fig. 16.80 Shaping the lateral crura. The skin flap can be retracted with the Meneghini nasal skin retractor fixed to the forehead with a pair of R1547 Steri-Strips or a similar retractor held by the assistant (frontal view)

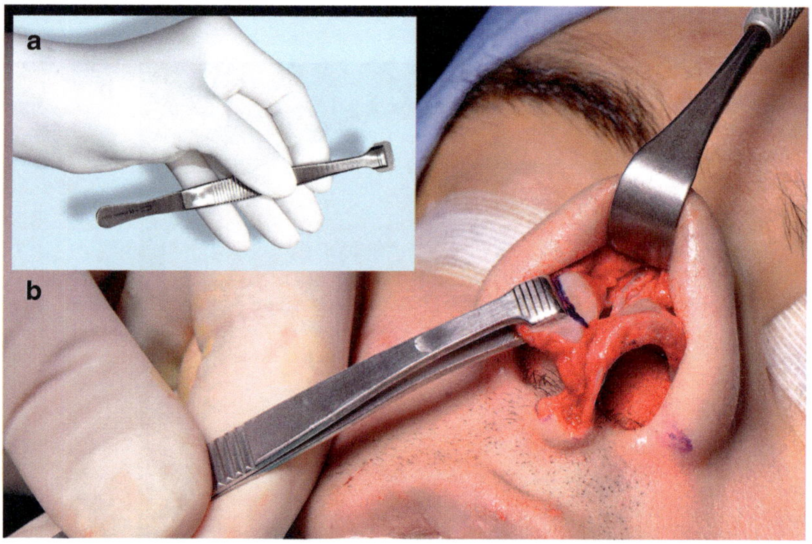

Fig. 16.81 (**a**, **b**) Shaping the lateral crura. Support and stabilize the lateral crura with the Meneghini delicate alar clamp or similar instruments. The instrument is positioned and held by the surgeon with his non-dominant hand

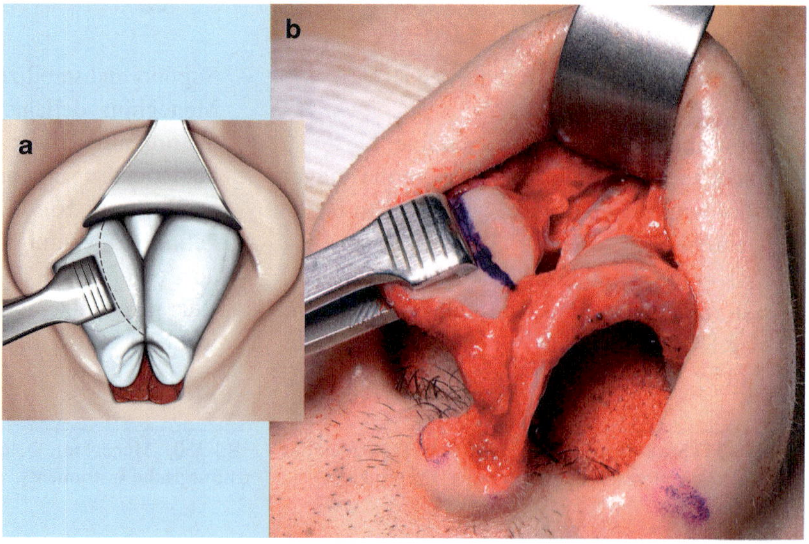

Fig. 16.82 (**a**, **b**) Shaping the lateral crura. Support and stabilize the lateral crura with the Meneghini delicate alar clamp or similar instruments. The instrument is positioned and held by the surgeon with his non-dominant hand (close-up view)

large lower plate has a crosshatched internal surface for a better grasping effect on tissue. When the forceps are tightened, a free space remains between the two arms and only the serrated distal edge of the small upper plate is in contact with the large lower one. During measurement and sculpturing of the lateral crus, the surgeon inserts the large plate into the nostril and gently grasps the lateral crura of the cartilage. The millimetric marking displayed on the external surface of the small plate helps in measuring the planned width of the cartilaginous strip, which remains covered and thereby protected by the same small plate.

- Precisely incise the lower lateral cartilages with a 15c scalpel blade (Figs. 16.83a, b and 16.84a, b). The gentle pressure of the sharp blade over the cartilage must avoid damaging the underlying nasal mucosa.
- Excise the cephalic portion of the alar cartilage with pointed scissors inserted between the margins of the incision and under the perichondrium taking care to avoid any mucosal tears (Fig. 16.85).

Even if a small resection of the cephalic portion of the alar cartilage is planned, every effort is made to remove it as a single and structurally intact piece, as this can be a useful graft source for the next nasal tip reconstruction steps (Fig. 16.86a, b).

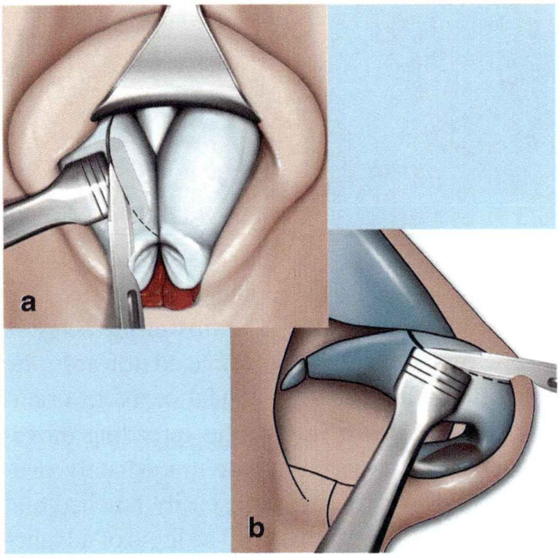

Fig. 16.83 (**a**, **b**) Shaping the lateral crura. Precisely incise the lower lateral cartilages with a 15c scalpel blade (schematic drawings)

16.21 Shaping and Reinforcing the Lateral Crura

The reduction in nasal tip volume is synonymous of cartilage removal and sometimes of interruption of the continuity of the lower lateral cartilage. Fortunately, the principles of conservative reshaping and reinforcing of the supporting tissues of the nose are becoming the rule and not the exception.

A useful way to reduce the width of the lateral crura and, at the same time, maintain the entire cartilage structure is to fold the cephalic strip over or under the main caudal strip instead of removing it. The author's preferred and most utilized technique is the lateral crura turn-in flap. Its main objectives are to:

- Reduce the excess of concavity or convexity of the lateral crus. It can be considered an equalizer of the pre-existing deformities.
- Maintain or enhance the rigidity and resilience of the cartilage with a little increase in thickness. Septal autologous onlay grafts usually further increase the thickness of the lateral crus and sometimes produce evident skin deformities.
- Balance the upward rotation effect of the columellar strut on the nasal tip.
- The main steps of the lateral crura turn-in flap are:
- Draw with a skin marker the cephalic excess of lateral crura that can be elevated and folded under the intact and continuous caudal strip. The latter should maintain a width comprised between 6 and 8 mm (Fig. 16.87).
- Calculate all the area of lateral crura elevation from the underlying skin to permit a complete rotation of the cephalic flap under the caudal strip. This area is exactly double the cephalic excess area (Fig. 16.88).

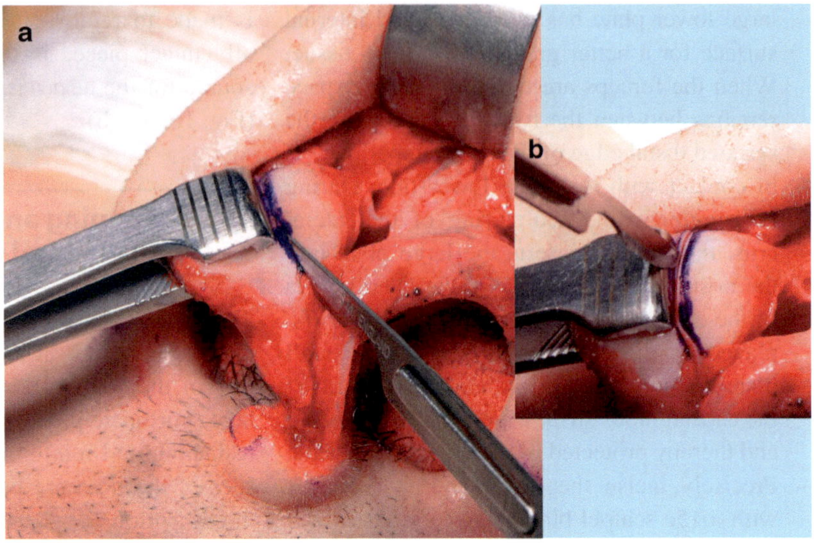

Fig. 16.84 (**a**, **b**) Shaping the lateral crura. With a 15c scalpel blade the lower lateral cartilages are incised precisely (intraoperative views)

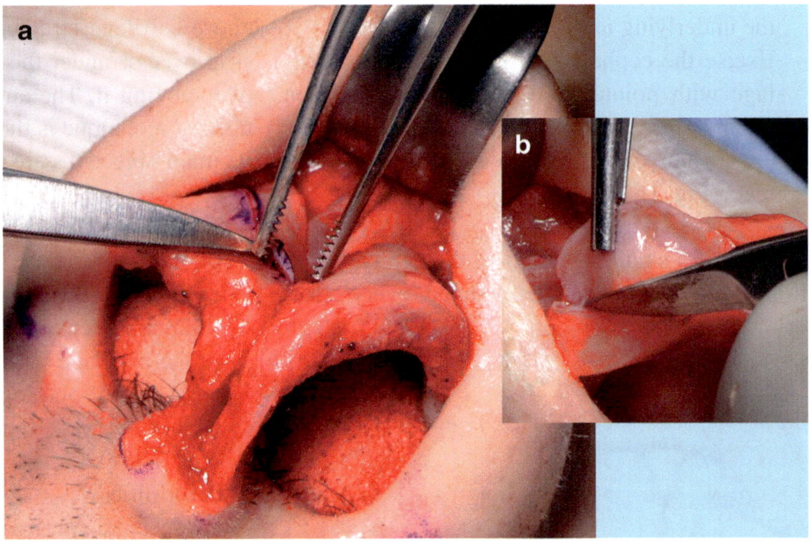

Fig. 16.85 Shaping the lateral crura. The excision of the cephalic portion of the alar cartilage is done with pointed scissors inserted between the margins of the incision and under the perichondrium taking care to avoid any mucosal tears

– Initially elevate the vestibular skin only under the dome and the medial portion of the lateral crus. To facilitate the dissection, a quantity of 0.5–0.8 cc of local anesthetic is injected under the lateral crura (Fig. 16.89a) and a small incision is performed with a 15c blade under the caudal margin close to the dome (Fig. 16.89b). With pointed scissors, a complete tunnel under the medial third of the lateral crus is created paying attention to avoid injury to the cartilage and to the underlying vestibular nasal skin. The tips of the scissors are maintained always directed towards the cartilage surface in a caudal-cephalic orientation and, with very gentle spreading movements, the avascular plane immediately over the perichondrium can be easily reached and followed (Fig. 16.90a, b). The logic of advancing from caudal to cephalic and not otherwise is due to the thinness of cephalic cartilage and

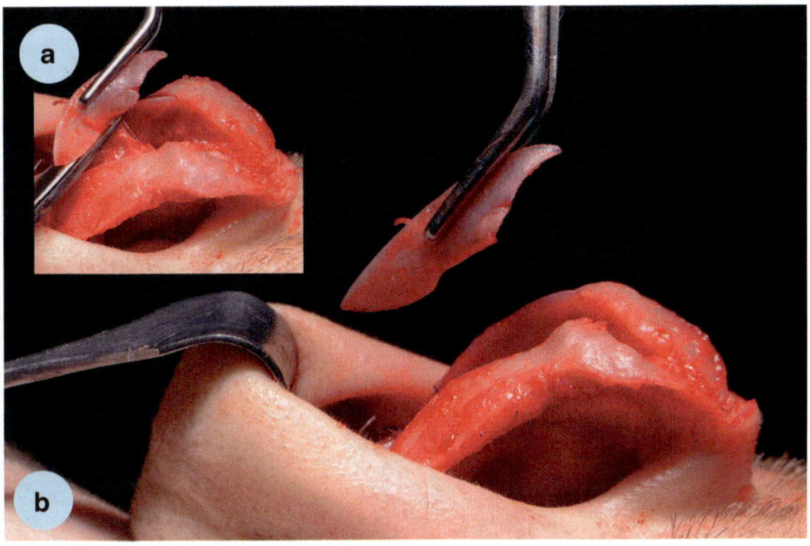

Fig. 16.86 (**a**, **b**) Shaping the lateral crura. Every effort is made to remove the cephalic portion as a single and structurally intact piece, as this can be a useful graft source for the next nasal tip reconstruction steps

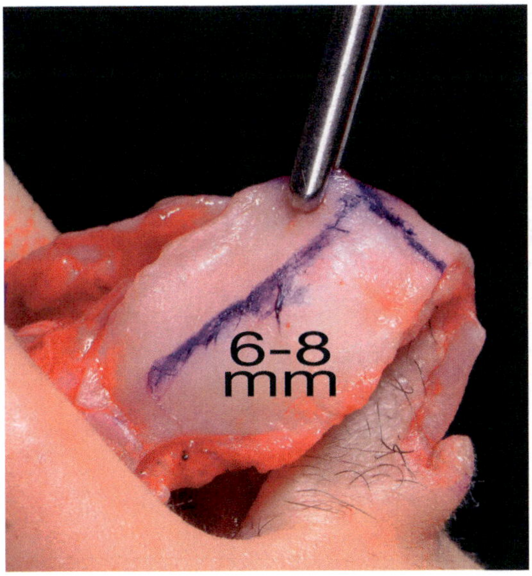

Fig. 16.87 Lateral crura turn-in flap. The cephalic excess of lateral crura that can be elevated and folded under the intact and continuous caudal strip is marked. The intact cartilage strip should maintain a width comprised between 6 and 8 mm

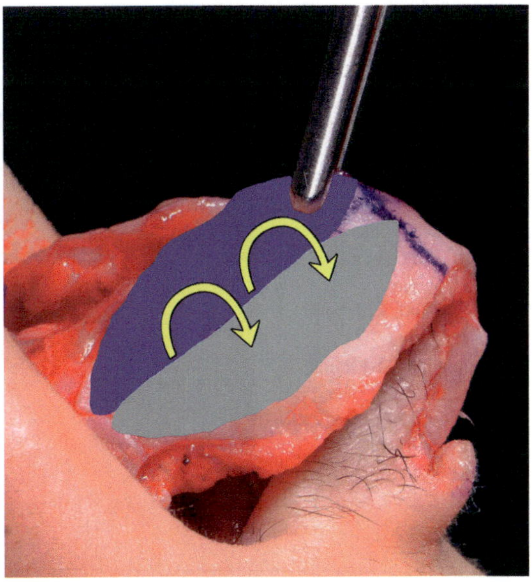

Fig. 16.88 Lateral crura turn-in flap. The area of lateral crura elevation from the underlying skin to permit a complete rotation of the cephalic flap under the caudal strip is calculated. This area is exactly double the cephalic excess area and it is specular

to the difficulty of clinically determining its irregular margin.

- Complete, with the scissors, the tunnel under the lateral crus until the expected area is elevated from the vestibular skin (Fig. 16.91). Take care not to release all the lateral crura from the skin and to maintain a small area of adherence close to the caudal margin as depicted by the dots in Fig. 16.92. Figure 16.93 shows from behind the intact vestibular skin,

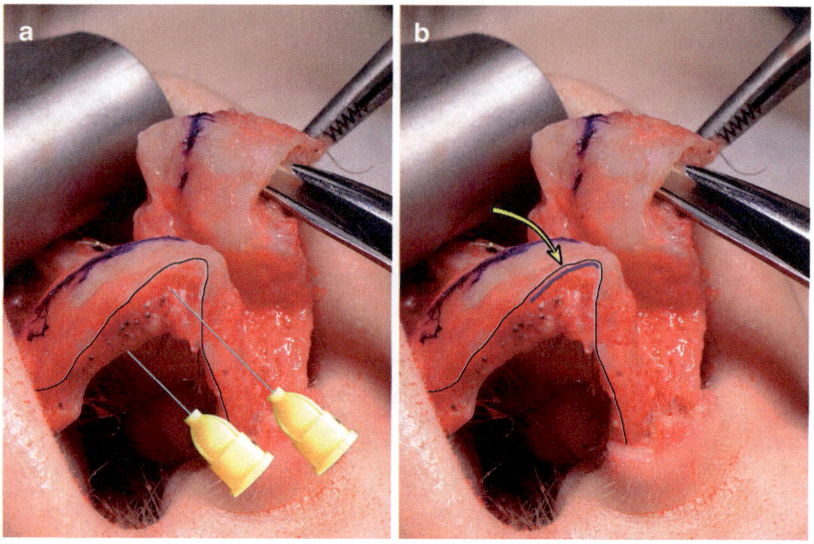

Fig. 16.89 (**a**, **b**) Lateral crura turn-in flap. To facilitate the dissection, a quantity of 0.5–0.8 cc of local anesthetic is injected under the lateral crura (**a**) and a small incision is performed with a 15c blade under the caudal margin of the lateral crura close to the dome (**b**)

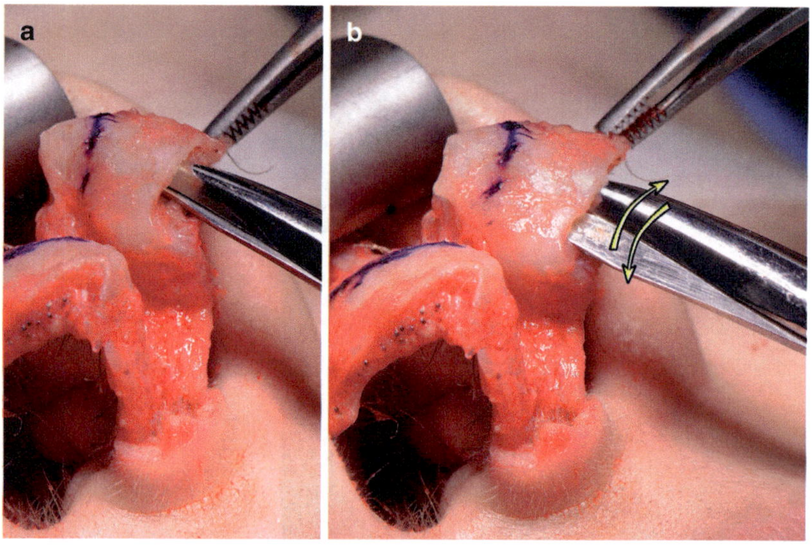

Fig. 16.90 (**a**, **b**) Lateral crura turn-in flap. With pointed scissors, a complete tunnel under the medial third of the lateral crus is created. The tips of the scissors are maintained always directed towards the cartilage surface in a caudal-cephalic orientation and, with very gentle spreading movements, the avascular plane immediately over the perichondrium can be easily reached and followed

the large area of lateral crus elevated free as well as the incomplete release of the cartilage from the skin.

- Make a partial-thickness incision, with a 15c blade, of the lateral crus along the planned line of folding (Fig. 16.94a, b).
- Turn in the cephalic excess (Fig. 16.95a, b) and stabilize it with continuous multiple 5/0 polydioxanone zigzag sutures. For convenience the first suture bite is placed closer to the dome (Fig. 16.96). The zigzag pattern (Fig. 16.97) and the rigidity of the polydioxa-

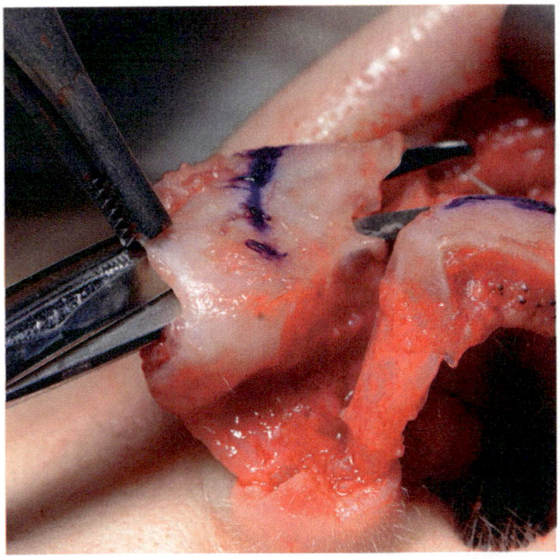

Fig. 16.91 Lateral crura turn-in flap. The tunnel under the lateral crus until the expected area is elevated from the vestibular skin is completed

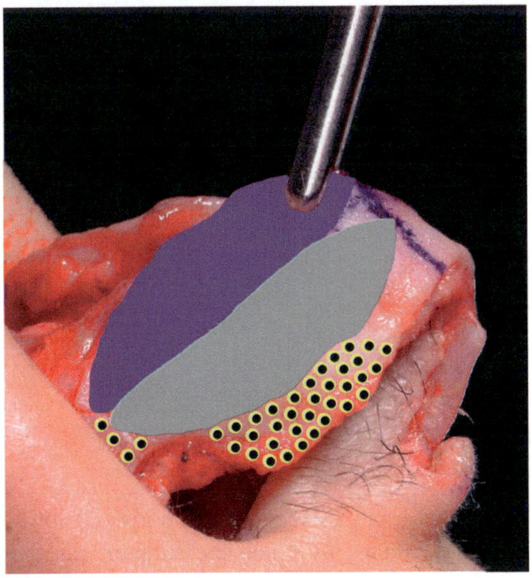

Fig. 16.92 Lateral crura turn-in flap. Take care not to release all the lateral crura from the skin and to maintain a small area of adherence close to the caudal margin (dots)

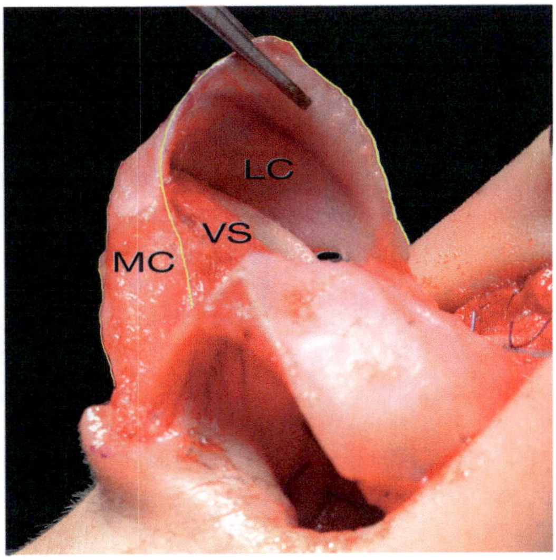

Fig. 16.93 Lateral crura turn-in flap. The intact vestibular skin after elevation from the lateral crus viewed from behind (*MC* medial crura, *LC* lateral crura, *VS* vestibular skin)

none monofilament suture improve the interface between the two cartilage strips and the straightening effects on the lateral crura realized with the turn-in flap.

- Figure 16.98a–f provides another description of the basic steps of the turn-in flap.

16.22 Creating New Surgical Domes

Ideally, each lower lateral cartilage can be divided into two small strips, one lateral and one medial, by an arbitrarily produced fold that represents the "new surgical dome." The easiest way to create a new surgical dome is with a horizontal mattress suture that determines its location and shape. Many authors propose different names and small variations for this suture such

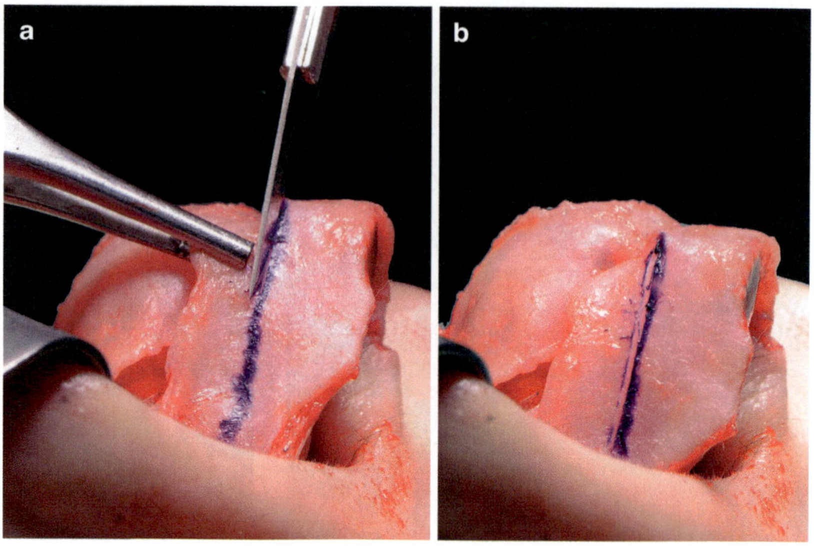

Fig. 16.94 (**a**, **b**) Lateral crura turn-in flap. With a 15c blade, a partial-thickness incision of the lateral crus is done along the planned line of folding

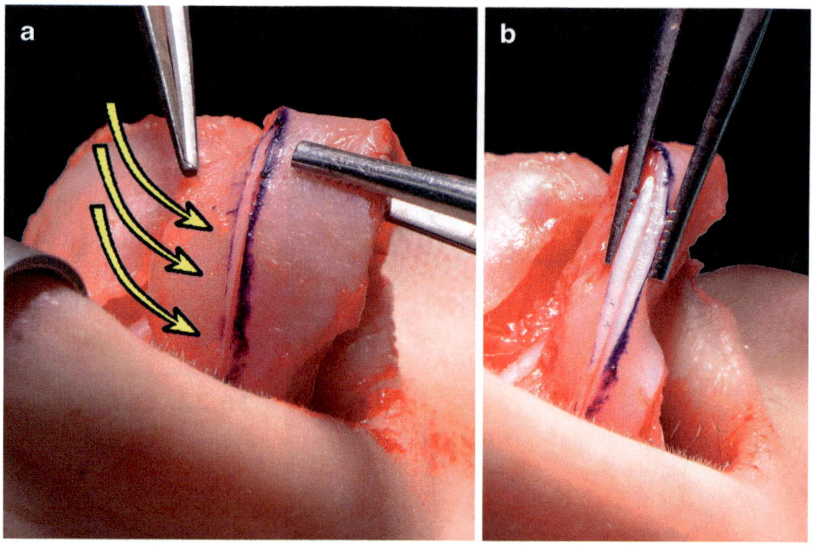

Fig. 16.95 (**a**, **b**) Lateral crura turn-in flap. The cephalic excess is then turned in and stabilized with continuous multiple 5/0 polydioxanone zigzag sutures

as intradomal suture, transdomal suture, domal modification suture, dome-spanning suture, and cranial tip suture. In consideration of the surgeon's final decision as to where to position the dome, the most logic definition of this suture is that of Rollin K Daniel: "domal creation suture."

Sometimes it is the shape of the lower lateral cartilages that "suggests" to the surgeon where the dome can be set (Fig. 16.99a, b). Other times the shape of the cartilage is so devoid of definition and folds that the surgeon will decide arbitrarily where to create the dome. Figure 16.100a, b presents a clear example of amorphous lower lateral cartilages in which the surgeon can test and finally create the best dome for the nose.

With a delicate Adson-Brown grasping forceps the cartilage can be folded slightly cranially, increasing the length of the medial segment, or caudally, increasing the length of the lateral segment, thereby changing the position of the new surgical dome. Figures 16.101 and 16.102 show the small area of the lower lateral cartilage within which the surgeon can create a surgical dome (small black dots). The three lines depict the three alternatives:

- Yellow line. In this case the new surgical dome is created inferiorly by reducing a little the length of the medial segment and elongating the lateral one. In this manner, the suture reduces the tip projection and rotates the tip downwards.
- Black line. Conversely, this line of folding creates a new surgical dome by reducing a little the length of the lateral segment and increasing the medial one. This decision increases the tip projection and rotates the tip upwards.

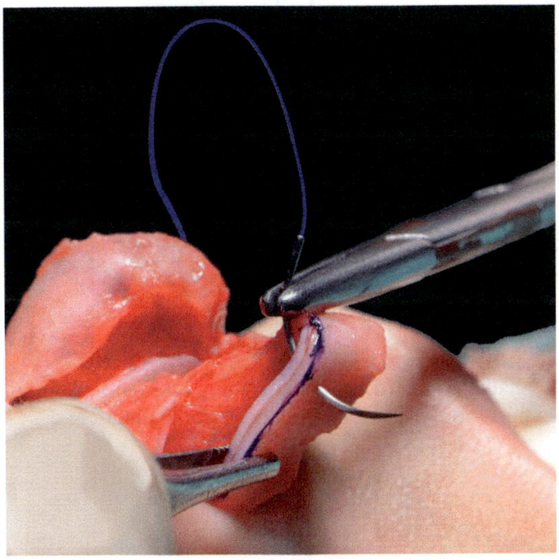

Fig. 16.96 Lateral crura turn-in flap. For convenience the first suture bite is done closer to the dome

- Yellow/black line. This intermediate line can be used as an initial test to evaluate the effect produced.

It should, however, be emphasized that variation in the setting of the new surgical dome is spatially reduced to a restricted area beyond which the suture produces unacceptable deformities to the nasal tip. Therefore the variation of projection of the nasal tip obtainable by changing the position of the domes is limited to 1–1.5 mm in terms of increase and decrease, and cannot exceed these limits. To further gain or lose projection, the surgeon should add other surgical steps described in the next chapter.

The steps to perform a domal creation suture are:

- With a 5/0 polydioxanone suture, take the first bite from middle crura to lateral crura and centered between the caudal and cranial margin of the cartilage. Care should be taken to avoid penetration of the needle into the underlying vestibular skin (Fig. 16.103).
- Take the second bite, passing from lateral crura to middle crura, close to the cephalic margin of the cartilage (Fig. 16.104).
- Progressively tighten the suture evaluating the effects that can be obtained on the cartilage (Fig. 16.105a). Overtightening this suture is a serious and frequent error. In this case, the

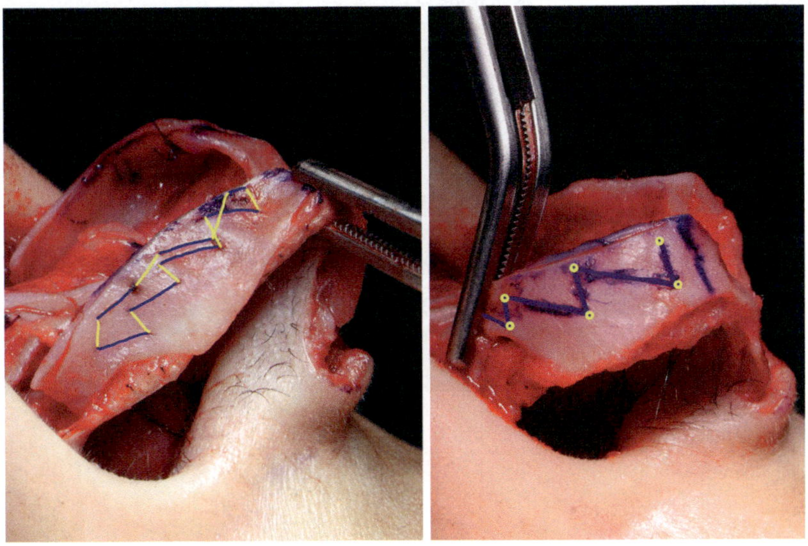

Fig. 16.97 Lateral crura turn-in flap. The zigzag pattern and the rigidity of the polydioxanone monofilament suture improve the interface between the two cartilage strips and the straightening effects on the lateral crura realized with the turn-in flap

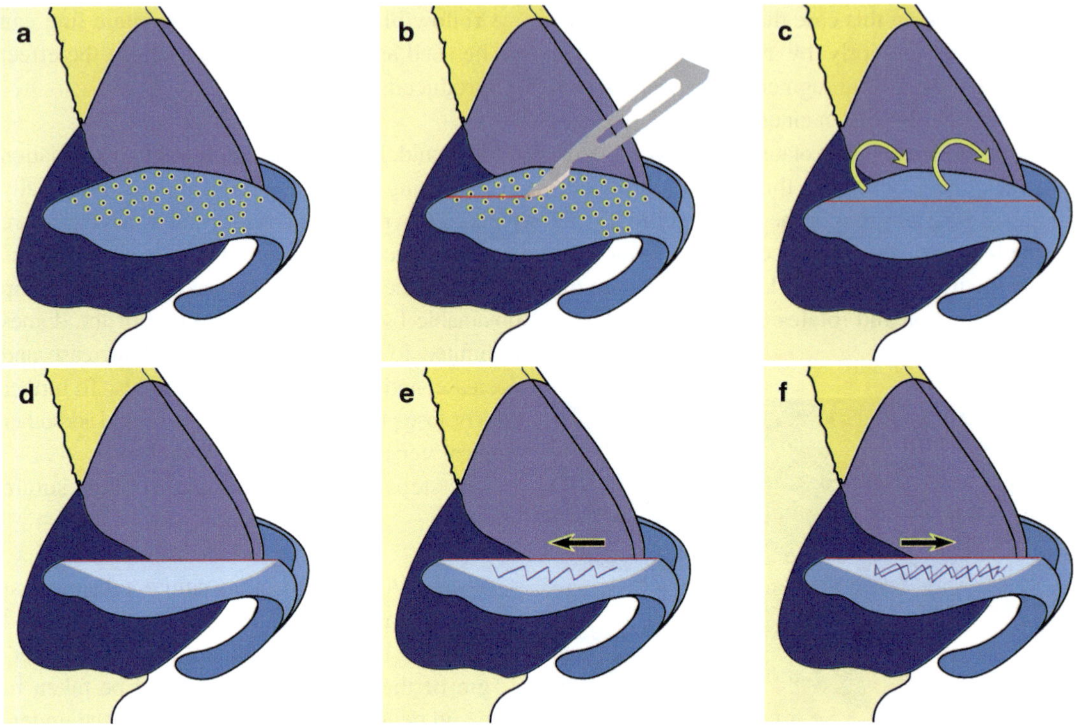

Fig. 16.98 (**a**–**f**) Basic steps of lateral crura turn-in flap. Partial undermining of the lateral crus (**a**), partial-thickness incision with 15c blade (**b**), turning in of the cephalic portion (**d**, **e**), single running suture from anterior to posterior (**f**) and then from posterior to anterior

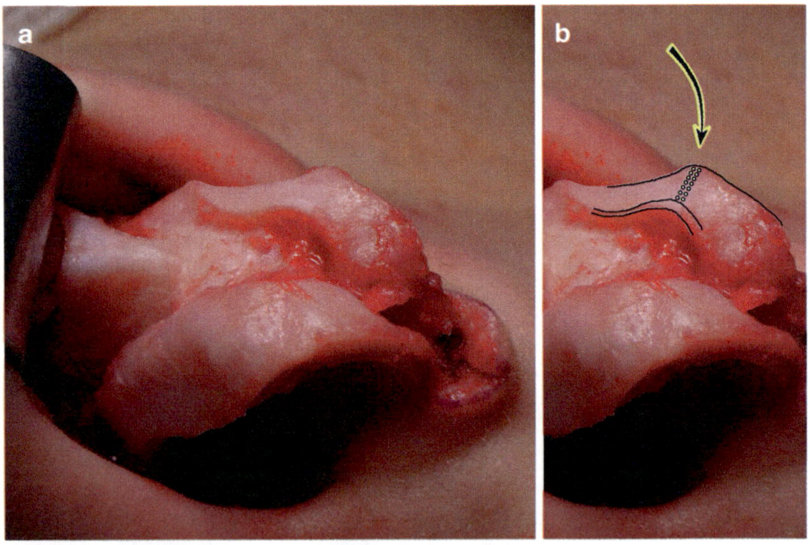

Fig. 16.99 (**a**, **b**) New surgical dome creation. Intraoperative view of a clinical case in which the shape of the lower lateral cartilages "suggests" to the surgeon where the dome can be set (arrow)

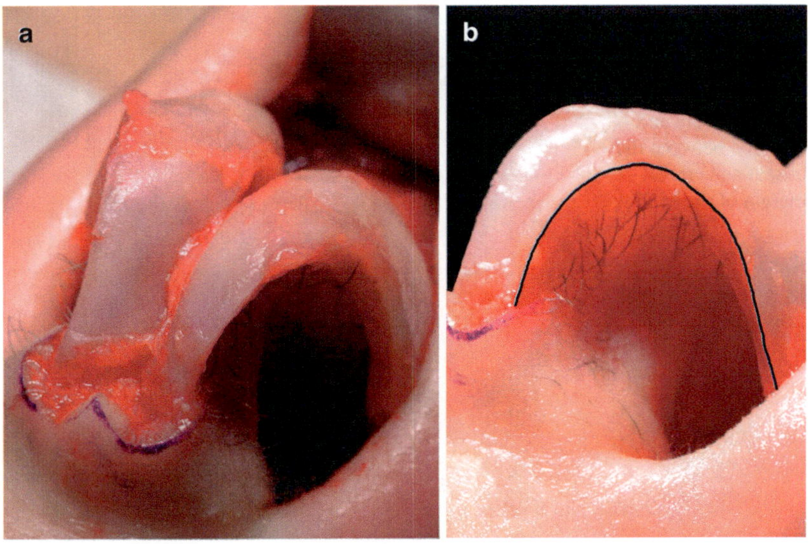

Fig. 16.100 (**a**, **b**) New surgical dome creation. Intraoperative view of a clinical case in which the lateral crus is so devoid of definition and folds that the surgeon will be obliged to decide arbitrarily where to create the dome

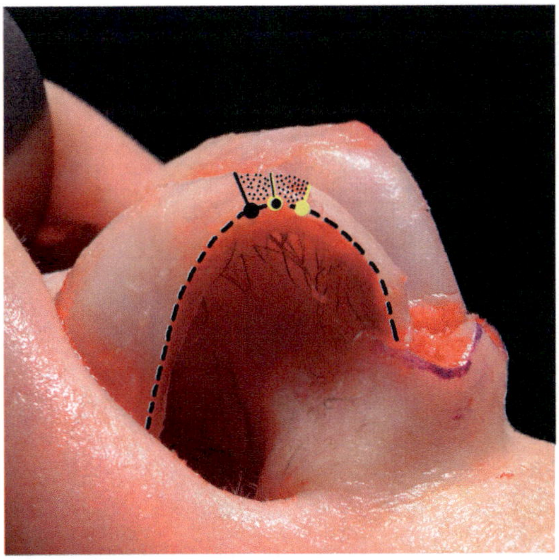

Fig. 16.101 New surgical dome creation. Intraoperative profile view. Different alternatives in setting the position of the dome (see text)

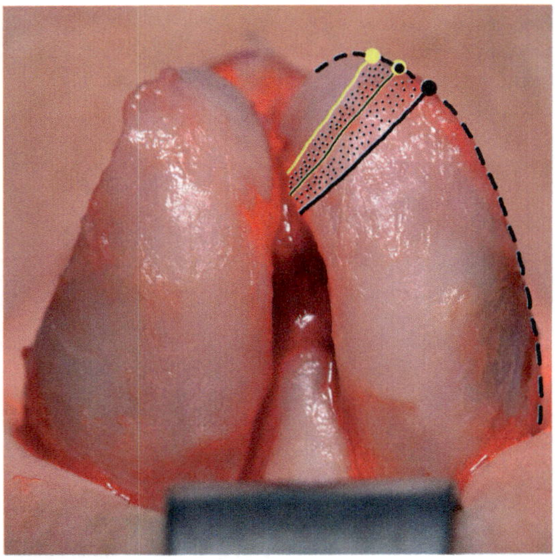

Fig. 16.102 New surgical dome creation. Intraoperative view from above. Different alternatives in setting the position of the dome (see text)

polydioxanone monofilament damages and sometimes cuts the cartilage, producing unnatural tip deformities and loss of structural stability.

Some characteristic effects of the domal creation suture are:

- Increase of nasal tip projection and structural stability in association with other tip sutures and columellar strut.
- Adjustment of domal shape and definition while maintaining a wide caudal domal margin (Fig. 16.105b).

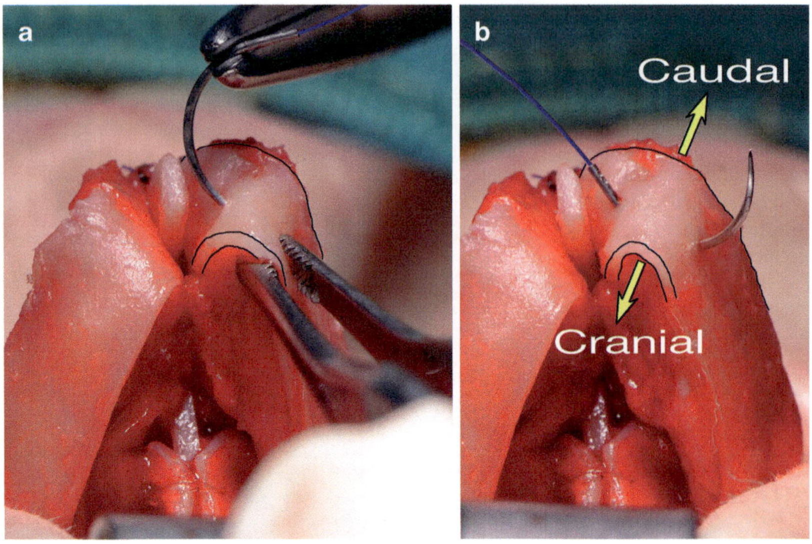

Fig. 16.103 (**a**, **b**) Steps in surgical dome creation. The first bite is done from middle crura to lateral crura and centered between the caudal and cranial margin of the cartilage

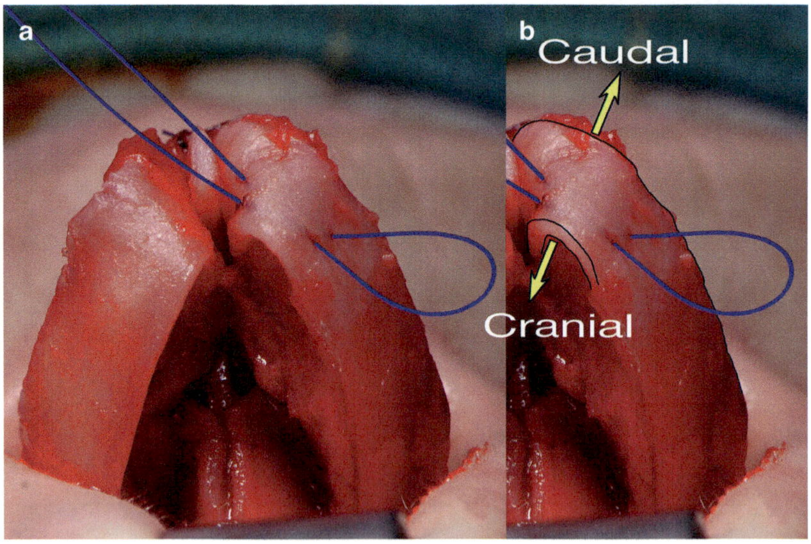

Fig. 16.104 (**a**, **b**) Steps in surgical dome creation. The second bite, passing from lateral crura to middle crura, must be done close to the cephalic margin of the cartilage

- Rotation of the lateral crura along their long axis (Fig. 16.106a, curved yellow arrow).
- Production, close to the dome, of a gentle concavity on the lateral crura that enhances tip definition (Fig. 16.106b).
- Slight straightening of the lateral crura (Fig. 16.106b).

Dealing with frequent asymmetries between the two lower lateral cartilages requires great effort and precision in suturing of the cartilages in order to obtain proportionate and symmetric domes.

The domal creation suture is a cornerstone of BOR even in the case of pre-existing well-positioned and ideally shaped domes as it stabilizes and structurally supports the cartilages during the postoperative healing process.

16.23 Domal Equalization Suture

Once set and shaped the two domes, the next step is to reduce the distance between them and stabilize the tip. The domal equalization suture, also named “interdomal suture,” is a simple

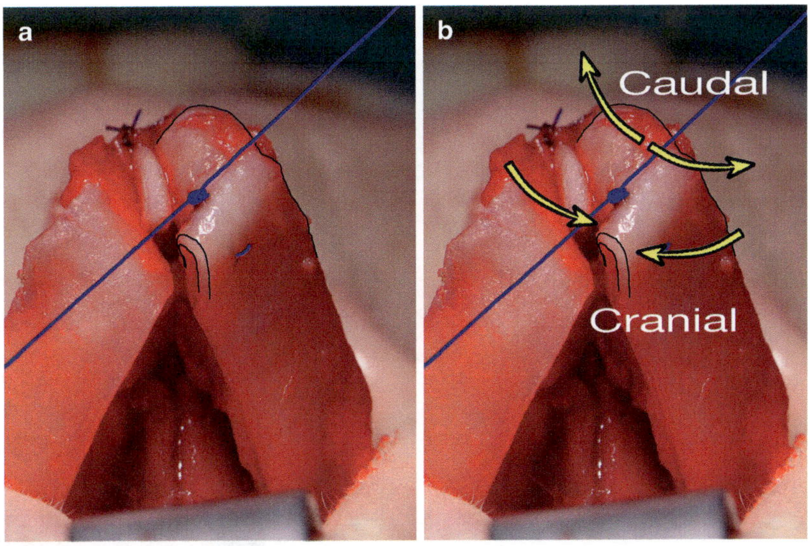

Fig. 16.105 (**a**, **b**) Steps in surgical dome creation. Progressively tightening the suture can help evaluate the effects that can be obtained on the cartilage. The cranial margin will be folded, whereas the caudal one remains extended. Overtightening this suture is a serious and frequent error. In this case, the polydioxanone monofilament damages and sometimes cuts the cartilage, producing unnatural tip deformities and loss of structural stability

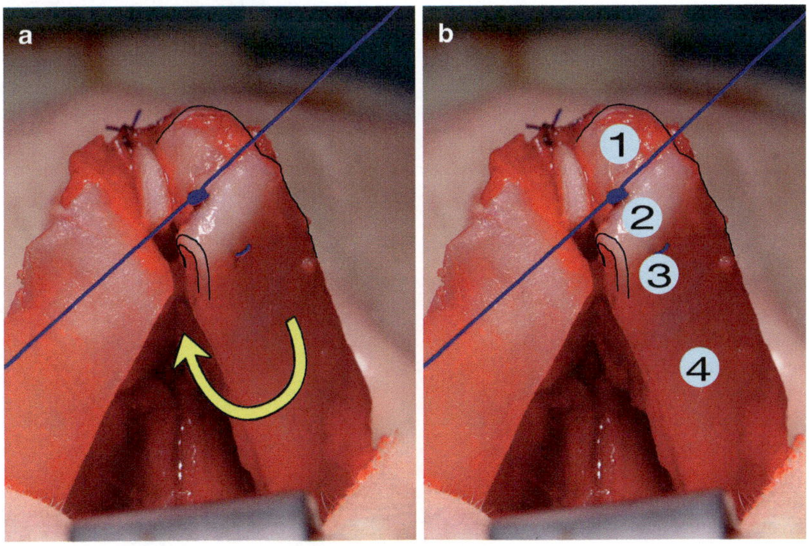

Fig. 16.106 (**a**, **b**) Effects of the domal creation suture. The lateral crura rotate along their long axis (**a**, curved yellow arrow). A wide domal caudal margin is maintained (**b1**) even if an evident fold is produced at the level of the domal cranial margin, increasing domal definition (**b2**). Immediately lateral to the dome a gentle concavity on the lateral crura is produced which enhances tip definition (**b3**). All the lateral crura appear slightly straightened (**b4**)

5/0 polydioxanone suture that brings together the two cephalic extremities of the domal fold (Fig. 16.107a). With this suture the two domes can be symmetrically placed and divergent in a caudal-anterior direction forming an angle of about 90 degrees between them (Fig. 16.107b, c).

At this stage the combination of the columellar strut with few basic dome sutures realizes a new objective: the most anterior and superior portion of the margins of the two medial crura are divergent creating a pair of "surgical middle crura." Fig. 16.108 depicts the clear angulation dividing the medial crura due to the combined effects of the anterior suture that fixes the columellar strut, the domal equalization suture, and the paired domal creation sutures. Once again, initially these anatomical details may or may not be present.

Sometimes the columellar strut profile exceeds anteriorly over the domes and should be refined with a 15c blade (Fig. 16.109). At the end of the surgery, the strut should be completely hidden and stably fixed with two or three sutures between the lower cartilages.

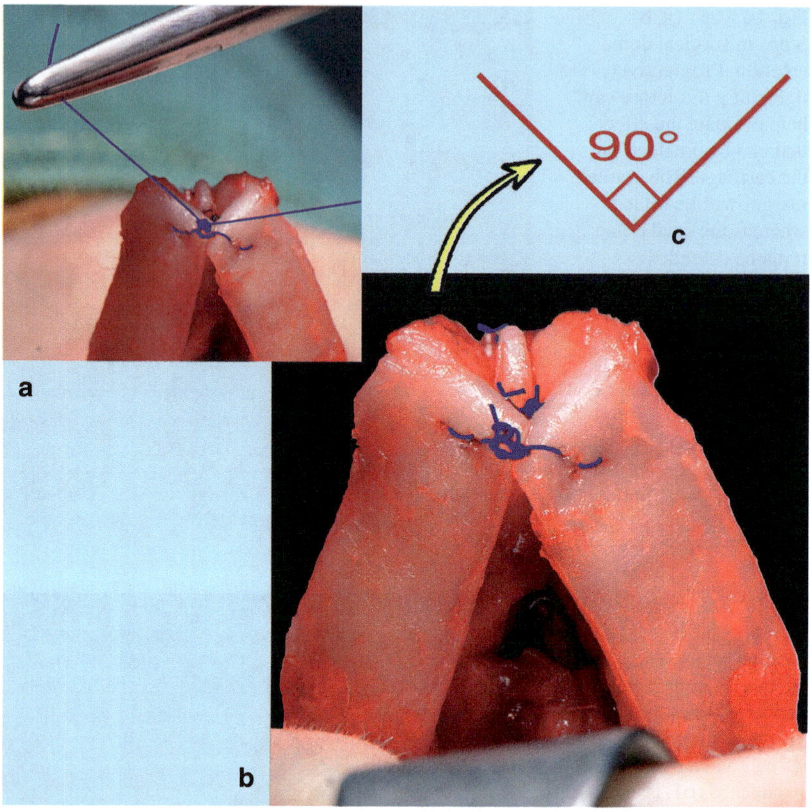

Fig. 16.107 (**a**–**c**) Domal equalization suture. This is a simple suture that brings together the two cephalic extremities of the domal fold (**a**). With this suture the two domes can be symmetrically placed and divergent in a caudal-anterior direction forming an angle of about 90 degrees between them (**b**, **c**)

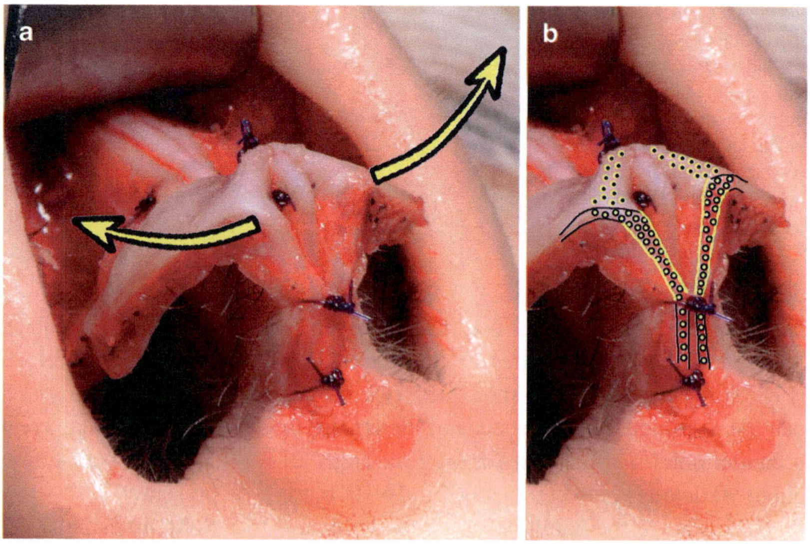

Fig. 16.108 (**a**, **b**) A clear angulation divides the medial crura due to the combined effects of the anterior suture that fixes the columellar strut, the domal equalization suture, and the paired domal creation sutures

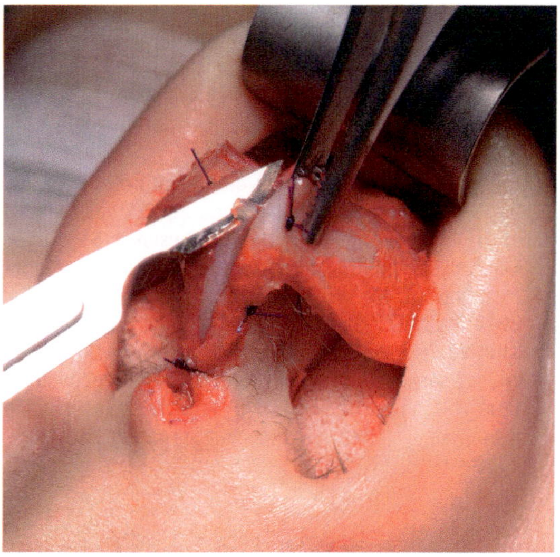

Fig. 16.109 Sometimes the columellar strut profile exceeds anteriorly over the domes and should be refined with a 15c blade

16.24 Take a Special "Surgical Time Out"

This is an important moment in the BOR sequence. It is time to check if the symmetry, strength, projection, size, and the shape of the new nasal tip harmonize with the rest of the nose. Once again, with the nasal skin flap repositioned over the nasal framework, the surgeon wears a pair of new clean gloves and wets the nose skin with sterile saline to better slide over the skin with his fingers. In 2 or 3 min, every skin subunit of the nose must be inspected visually from different points of view and palpated gently and precisely (Fig. 16.110a, b).

If the result obtained matches the ideal preoperative objectives of surgery, the next steps are quite obvious and the surgery goes rapidly towards the end. Unfortunately, this is not always

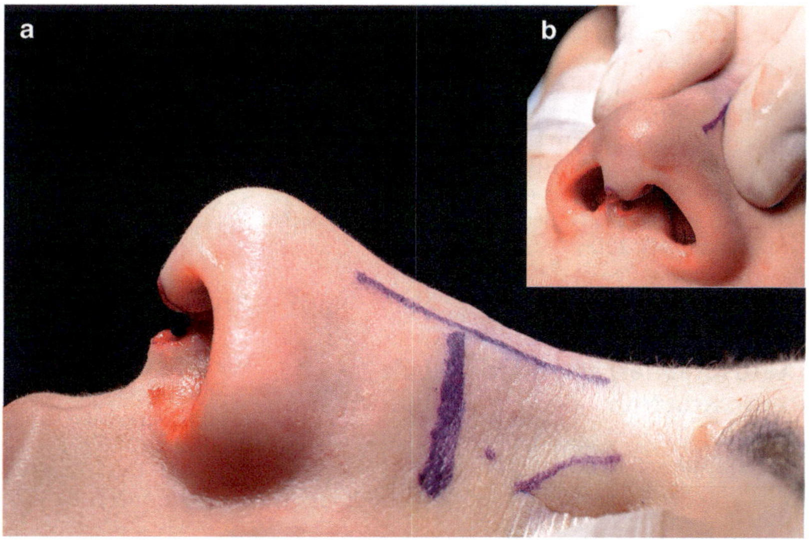

Fig. 16.110 (**a**, **b**) At this point of the surgery every skin subunit of the nose must be inspected visually from different points of view and palpated gently and precisely

the case and other steps are still necessary. With a skin marker every irregularity, asymmetry, and disproportion of the nose should be written down on sterile paper or drawn directly on the nasal skin. The next final steps are often very difficult, delicate, and challenging but the surgeon should not be forget that even a change in shape of about 1 mm in a small area of the nose could greatly change the final clinical result.

Further Reading

The description of surgical techniques can be further explored in these classic books on the open approach. They are presented here in order of publication. Even though this does not indicate the mandatory reading sequence, the historical evolution of the open approach represents an ideal way to study it. Daniel RK. Aesthetic plastic surgery: rhinoplasty. Boston: Little, Brown; 1993. p. 525–53; Jugo S. Surgical atlas of external rhinoplasty. Edinburgh: Churchill Livingstone; 1995; Tebbetts JB. Primary rhinoplasty. A new approach to the logic and the techniques. St. Louis: Mosby; 1998; Daniel RK. Rhinoplasty. An atlas of surgical techniques. Berlin, Heidelberg: Springer-Verlag; 2002; Daniel RK. Mastering rhinoplasty. A comprehensive atlas of surgical techniques. New York: Springer; 2010; Guyuron B. Rhinoplasty. Edinburgh: Elsevier Saunders; 2012; Daniel RK, Pálházi P. Rhinoplasty. Berlin: Springer International Publishing AG; 2018.

Articles on Spreader Flaps (Autospreader) and Middle Vault Reconstruction

Byrd HS, Meade R, Gonyon DL. Using the autospreader flap in primary rhinoplasty. Plastic Reconstr Surg. 2007;119(6):1897–902.

Gruber RP, Park E, Newman J, Berkowitz L, Oneal R. The spreader flap in primary rhinoplasty. Plast Reconstr Surg. 2007;119(6):1903–10.

Gruber RP, Melkun ET, Woodward JF, Perkins SW. Dorsal reduction and spreader flaps. Aesthet Surg J. 2011;31(4):456–64.

Wurm J, Kovacevic M. A new classification of spreader flap techniques. Facial Plast Surg. 2013;29:506–14.

Sabri BE, Selahattin T, Berke O, Aysenur M, Orhan O. Autospreading spring flap technique for reconstruction of the middle vault. Aesthet Plast Surg. 2014;38(2):322–8.

Avashia YJ, Marshall AP, Allori AC, Rohrich RJ, Marcus JR. Decision-making in middle vault reconstruction following dorsal hump reduction in primary rhinoplasty. Plast Reconstr Surg. 2020;145(6):1389–401.

Articles on Tip Surgery

Davis RE. Lateral crural tensioning for refinement of the wide and underprojected nasal tip: rethinking the lateral crural steal. Facial Plast Surg Clin N Am. 2015;23:23–53.

Rohrich RJ, Durand PD, Dayan E. Changing role of septal extension versus columellar grafts in modern rhinoplasty. Plast Reconstr Surg. 2020;145(5):927e–31e.

Rohrich RJ, Savetsky IL, Abigail R, Yash JA. Developing consistency in nasal tip shaping. Plast Reconstr Surg Glob Open. 2020;8(4):e2634.

Articles on Lateral Crural Turn-in Flap

Murakami CS, Barrera JE, Most SP. Preserving structural integrity of the alar cartilage in aesthetic rhinoplasty using a cephalic turn-in flap. Arch Facial Plast Surg. 2009;11(2):126–8.

Apaydin F. Lateral crural turn-in flap in functional rhinoplasty. Arch Facial Plast Surg. 2012;14(2):93–6.

Basic Open Rhinoplasty: Final Surgical Steps

17

Many sections of the previous two chapters describe indispensable or frequent surgical steps, whereas many of the next sections of this chapter are therefore dedicated to those particular situations, sometimes infrequent in daily practice, but which the nasal surgeon has to face.

The finishing surgical steps of the BOR discipline are closely related to the fine-tuning of the shape of the osseous and cartilaginous nasal framework. Rhinoplasty is a matter of fine details. The aspects to be addressed have an extreme morphological variability and there are different techniques that can be used for to achieve every single objective. In these steps, one of the surgeon's most important skills is to identify the residual intraoperative deformities deserving of improvement, prioritizing them and select the most conservative and effective corrective surgical maneuvers.

17.1 Excess of Lateral Crura Convexity

Also after the domal creation sutures, some fullness in the supratip area and a wide nasal tip may be evident. The major cause is the excess of the lower lateral crural convexity that can be viewed directly by retracting the skin flap to expose the cartilages (Fig. 17.1a–c) or palpated after repositioning the skin flap over the framework. This double check helps the surgeon to understand if the nasal tip fullness is completely created by the supporting cartilage shape and dimension or by a thick, inelastic and self-supporting skin.

The lateral crural spanning suture, a horizontal mattress suture, can shape the lower lateral cartilages by bringing them closer and improving the transition between the middle third and lower third of the nose. The absorbable 5/0 polydioxanone monofilament is passed twice in the area of the lower lateral crura responsible for convexity excess and minimally tightened, as shown in Fig. 17.2a–d. This is one of the most demanding sutures because over-tightening of the suture can narrow the nasal vestibule with airflow reduction and distortion of the nasal tip. Fortunately, also a small medial movement of the lateral crura produces an improvement of the deformity.

In the case of asymmetrical excess of lower lateral crural convexity, the lateral crural spanning suture can be done also unilaterally, one for the right side and another for the left side. In this case one or both lateral crura can be individually repositioned, anchoring the 5/0 polydioxanone monofilament suture to the dorsal margin of the septum. Figure 17.3 shows the first suture bite taken close to the upper margin of the lower lateral crura in the area of maximal convexity excess. With the second bite the suture was anchored to the dorsal margin

F. Meneghini, *Basic Open Rhinoplasty*, https://doi.org/10.1007/978-3-030-61827-8_17

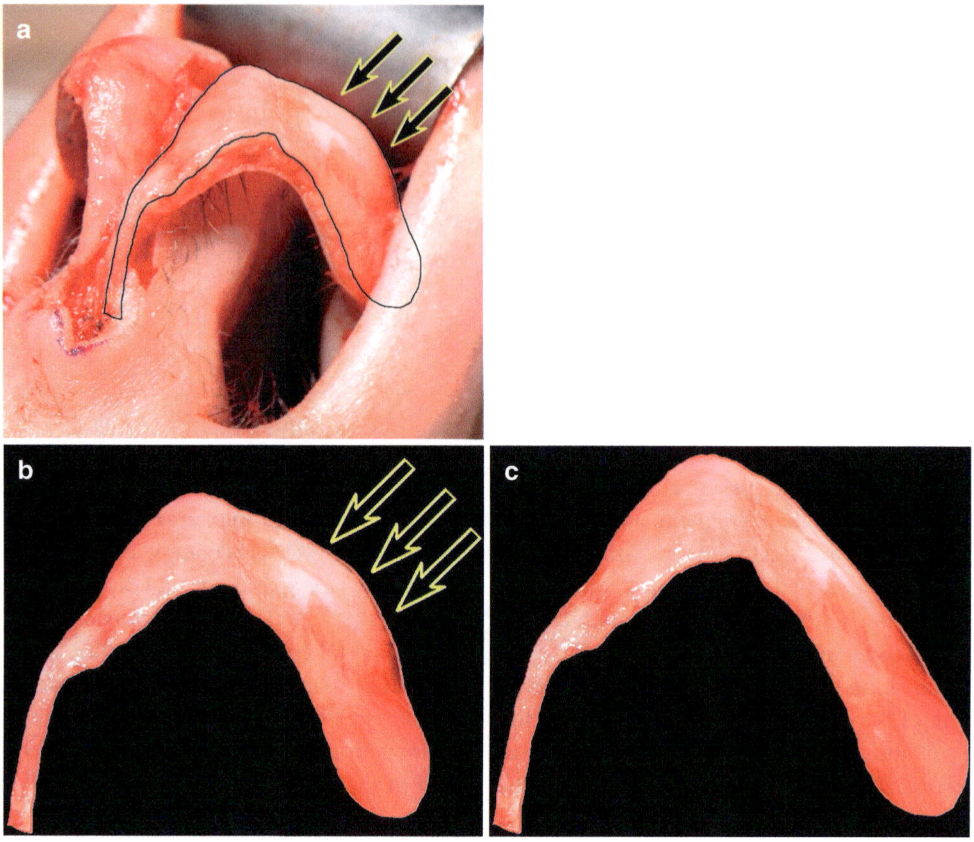

Fig. 17.1 (**a**–**c**) Intraoperative analysis of excess of lateral crural convexity indicated with multiple straight arrows (**a**, **b**). The surgeon should mentally visualize the final shape obtainable through the cephalic trim and the correction of the convexity excess (**c**)

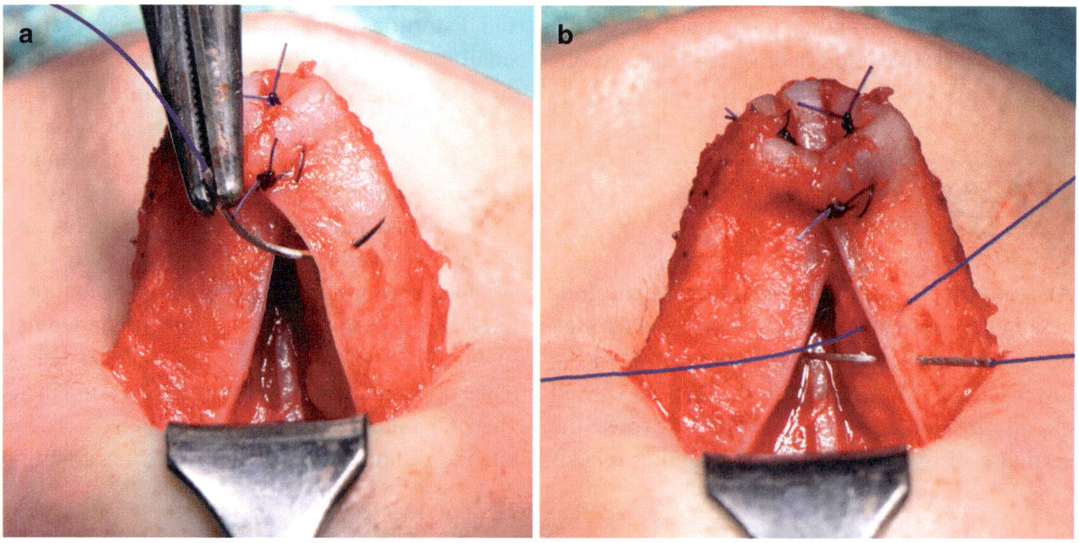

Fig. 17.2 (**a**–**d**) Lateral crural spanning suture. This is a horizontal mattress suture passed between the cephalic margins of the lateral crura at the level of maximal convexity

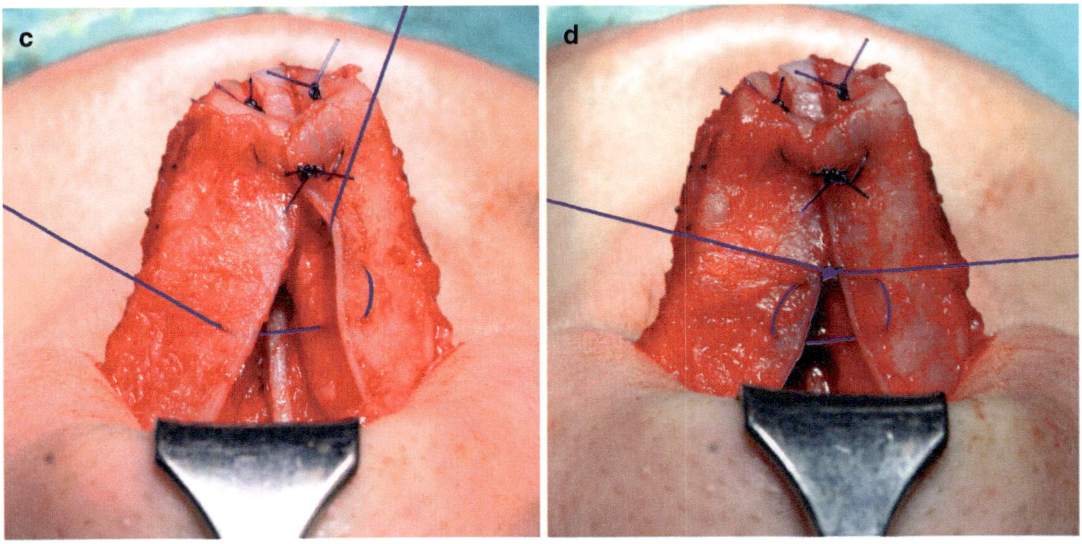

Fig. 17.2 (continued)

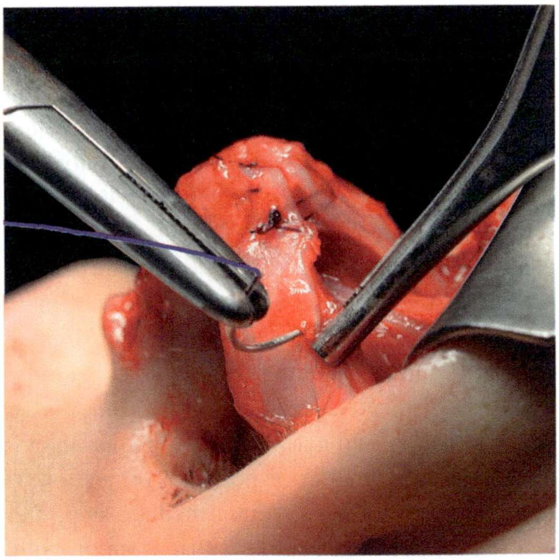

Fig. 17.3 In the case of asymmetrical excess of lower lateral crural convexity, the lateral crural spanning suture can be done also unilaterally, anchoring the suture to the dorsal margin of the septum. The first bite is taken at the level of maximal convexity of the lateral crura

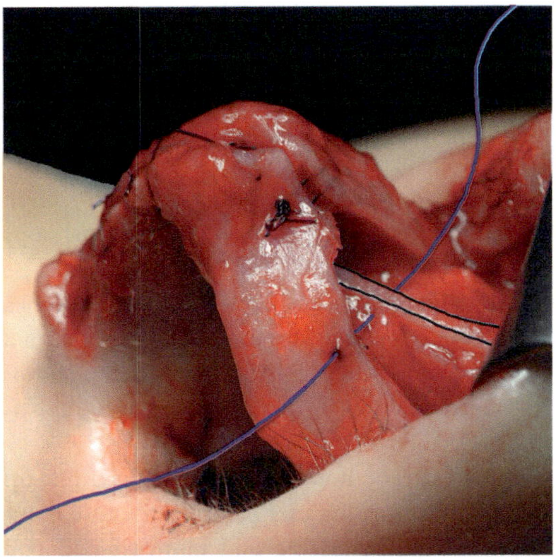

Fig. 17.4 Unilateral lateral crural spanning suture. The second bite is anchored to the dorsal margin of the septum. The third and the fourth bites pass back to the septum and then the lateral crura

of the septum (Fig. 17.4). The horizontal mattress suture was then completed with a third returning bite on the septum and the last bite done close to the first one. The suture is then tightened gently until the convexity excess is reduced and the two lower lateral cartilages appear more symmetrical (Fig. 17.5).

17.2 Over-Projected Nasal Tip

Sometimes it is quite clear from the beginning of the surgery that the insertion of the columellar strut associated with the domal sutures will produce an over-projected tip. In this case, the surgeon should resist the temptation to change

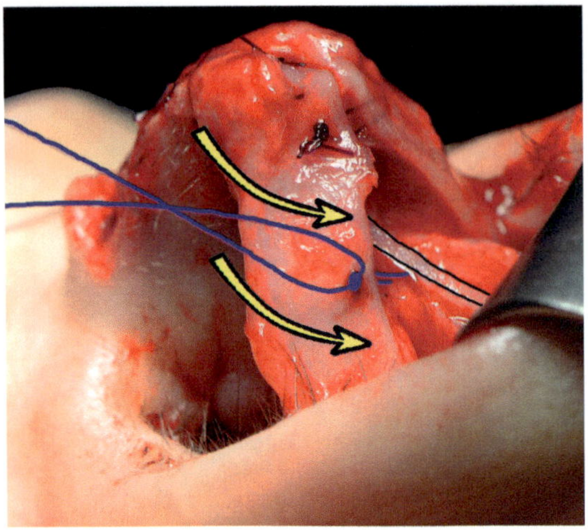

Fig. 17.5 The unilateral lateral crural spanning suture is gently tightened until symmetry with the opposite lateral crus is obtained

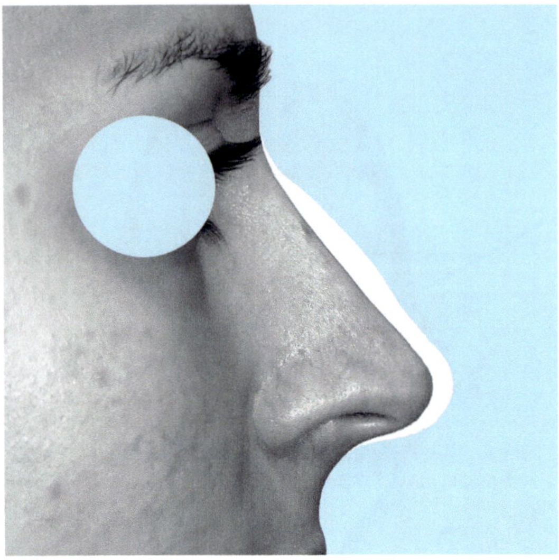

Fig. 17.6 Preoperative "Overlap" simulation in a clinical case of reductive rhinoplasty. Both dorsal and tip nasal outlines require an evident reduction of anterior-posterior projection

the basic BOR strategy and realize a reconstructed and well-shaped tip as described in the previous chapter. The reasons for doing this are more than one:

- Precisely determining the nasal tip projection before completing the standard shaping steps is a difficult task.
- Sometimes apparently over-projected domes at an intermediate surgical step can result in a perfect balance with the dorsum at the end of procedure, after the skin flap has been repositioned and sutured in place.
- Even after suturing and grafting the tip remains a floating and flexible structure compared with the stable and more rigid dorsal vault. The only physical possibility during the future healing processes is a loss of projection of the tip with respect to the dorsum and not the opposite.
- Until the nasal tip has been completely reconstituted and shaped, the true extent of the excess is not clear. Measuring in millimeters to precisely quantify the excess of tip projection is mandatory and can be considered an intermediate goal to be achieved.
- Shaping and then positioning the nasal tip is easier than positioning the tip and then shaping it.

Removal of the columellar strut in an attempt to reduce the projection of the nasal tip is a clear error. The resulting loss of projection is not predictable. Stability and symmetry of the lower third of the nose are also at risk.

The columellar strut can instead be utilized as a ruler to measure the excess. It is also a main stabilizing structure for the new repositioned domes. Figure 17.6 shows the "Overlap" simulation in a clinical case of reductive rhinoplasty. Both dorsal and tip nasal outlines require an evident reduction of anterior-posterior projection.

Figure 17.7a shows an intermediate step after resection of a 3-mm complete strip from the right medial crus. It was then sutured end-to-end and to the columellar strut to obtain a noticeable reduction of right dome projection without losing its shape or stability. As depicted in Fig. 17.7b, the temporary over-projection of the left dome and the extent of the changes obtained with the right dome can be evaluated and measured utilizing the strut as a reference.

To gain further stability and improve the contour of the nasal lobule, a long shield graft was positioned, refined and sutured in place (Fig. 17.8). Strangely, a clear reduction of the posterior-anterior projection of the nasal tip was

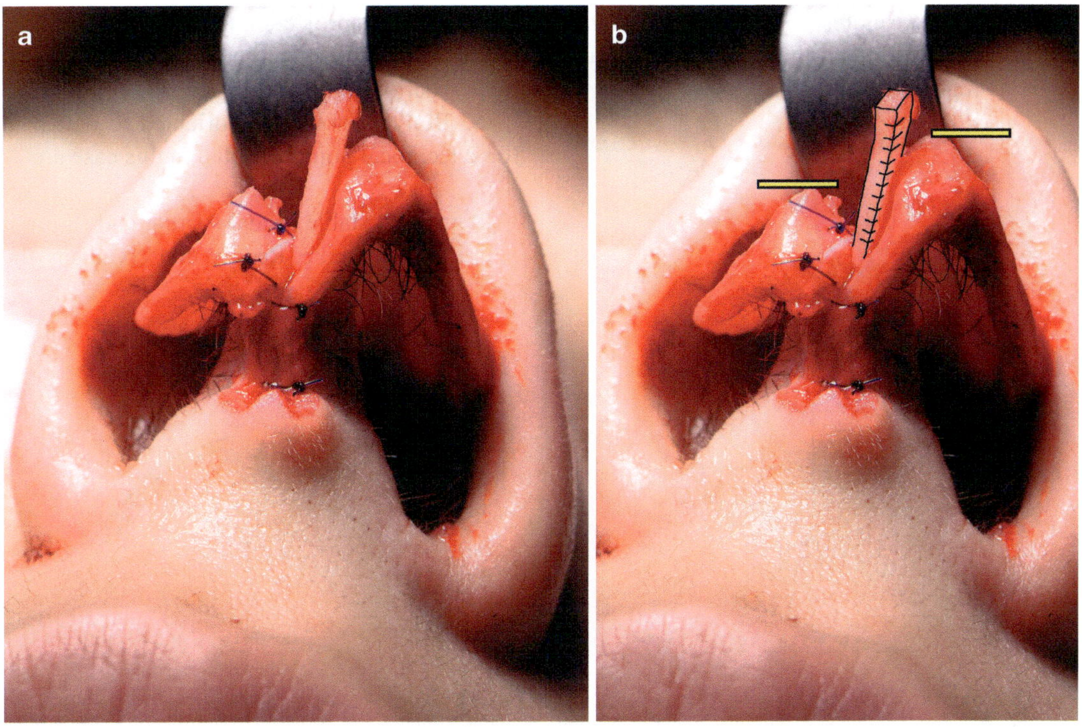

Fig. 17.7 (**a**, **b**) Over-projected nasal tip. Intermediate step after resection of a 3-mm complete strip from the right medial crus

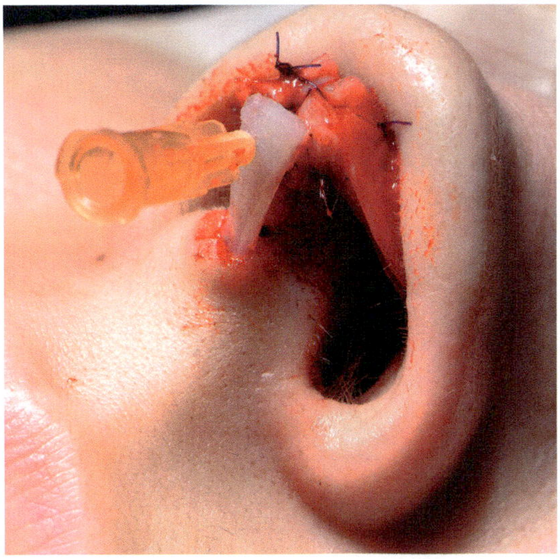

Fig. 17.8 Over-projected nasal tip. To obtain further stability and improve the contour of the nasal lobule a long shield graft was positioned, refined and sutured in place

achieved by adding two solid cartilage grafts rather than with aggressive handling and removal of the alar cartilages.

17.3 Under-Projected Nasal Tip

After the usual BOR nasal tip reconstruction steps, dealing with a slightly under-projected nasal tip is a frequent clinical situation. This intraoperative situation can also occur if a substantial confirmation of the preoperative projection of the nasal tip is expected (Fig. 17.9).

A small increase in the nasal tip projection, up to 2 mm, can be recovered with a solid graft positioned above the domes. The minimum dimensions needed for a simple tip onlay graft are 4 mm in the caudal-cephalic direction by 6 mm wide. Thus, a relatively small piece of septal cartilage may suffice (Fig. 17.10). The thickness of the piece represents the gain in tip projection. As for every solid visible graft, a minimum of three stabilizing sutures as well as a delicate work of beveling all margins in direct contact with the skin is mandatory (Figs. 17.11a, b and 17.12a, b). In this clinical case, the columellar strut is not in direct contact with the tip graft, as in the so-called “umbrella graft,” but all the 5/0 polydioxanone monofilament sutures give good three-dimensional stability to the reconstructed cartilaginous framework.

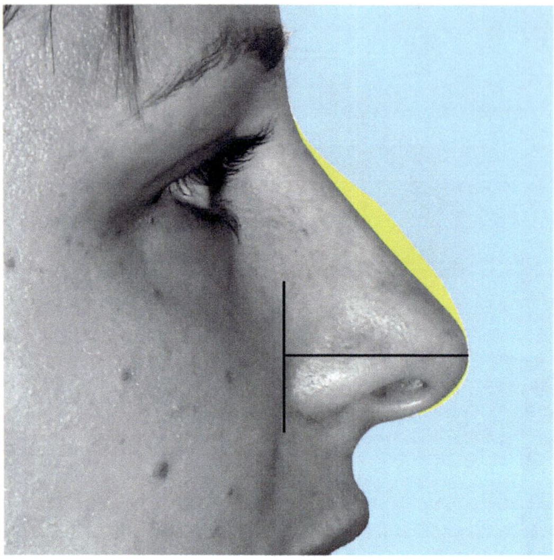

Fig. 17.9 Preoperative "Overlap" simulation in a clinical case of reductive rhinoplasty without reduction of the nasal tip projection

If greater tip projection is foreseen in the preoperative study, as in the clinical case of tip reconstruction illustrated in Fig. 17.13a–c, many of the BOR steps must be oriented to obtain it. Some technical points adopted in this case are:

– Maintain a stable caudal septum and suture it to the nasal spine. Reduce conservatively the

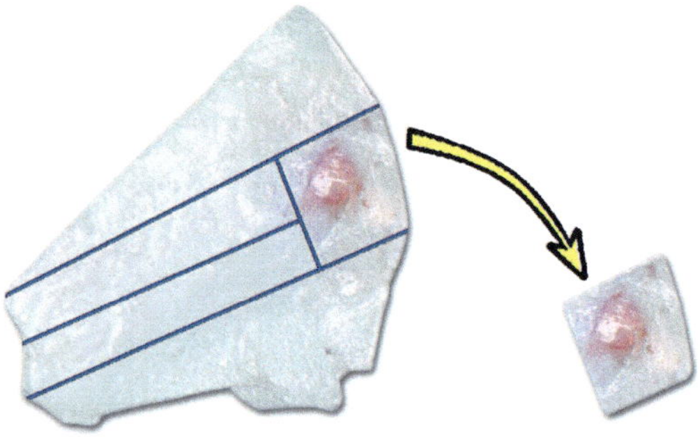

Fig. 17.10 To carve a tip graft measuring 4 mm in the caudal-cephalic direction by 6 mm wide, a relatively small piece of septal cartilage may suffice

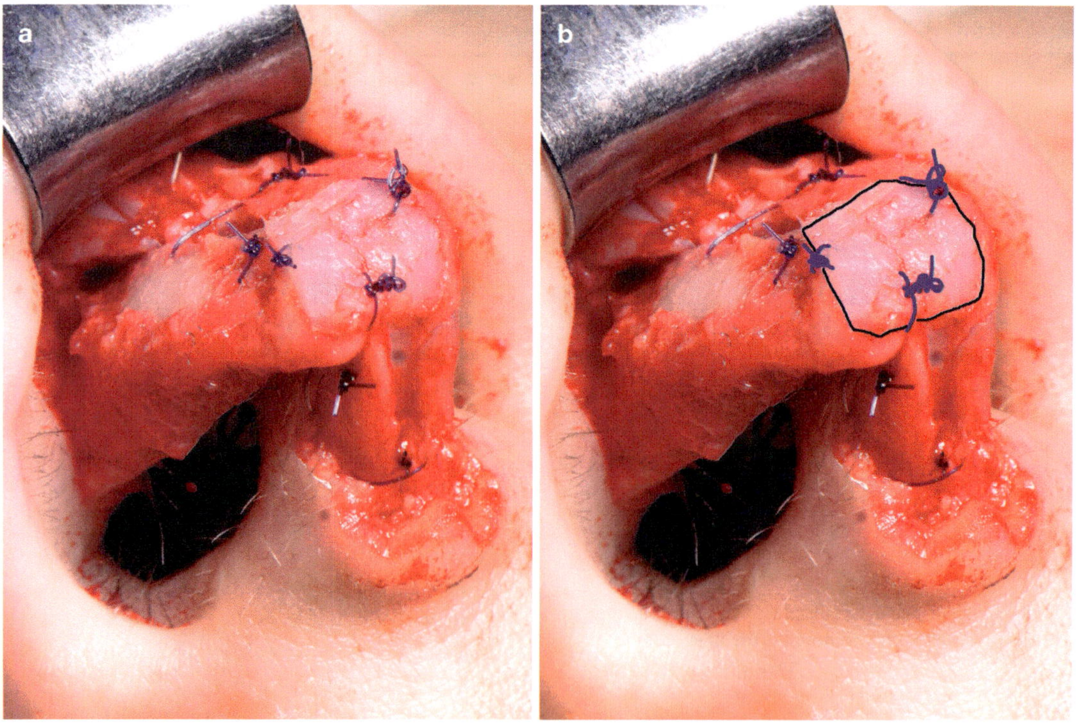

Fig. 17.11 (**a**, **b**) After the basic tip reconstruction with strut and sutures, to regain the initial tip projection a small tip onlay graft is sutured in place

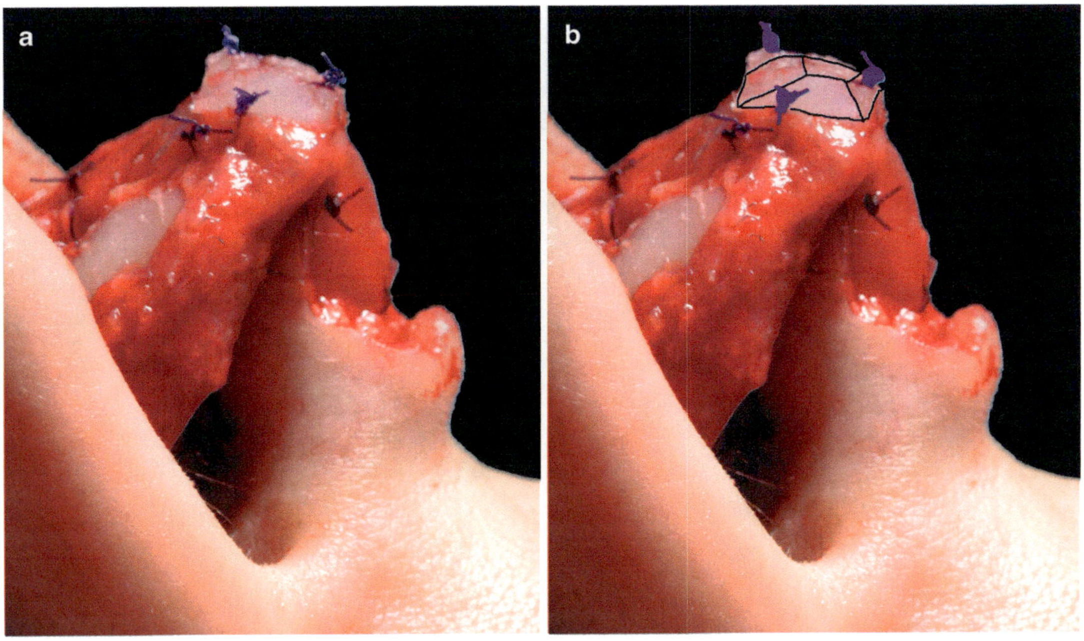

Fig. 17.12 (**a**, **b**) The lateral intraoperative view better shows the final shape of the tip framework obtained with the small onlay graft (the postoperative result of this clinical case is presented in Fig. 10.13 of Chap. 10)

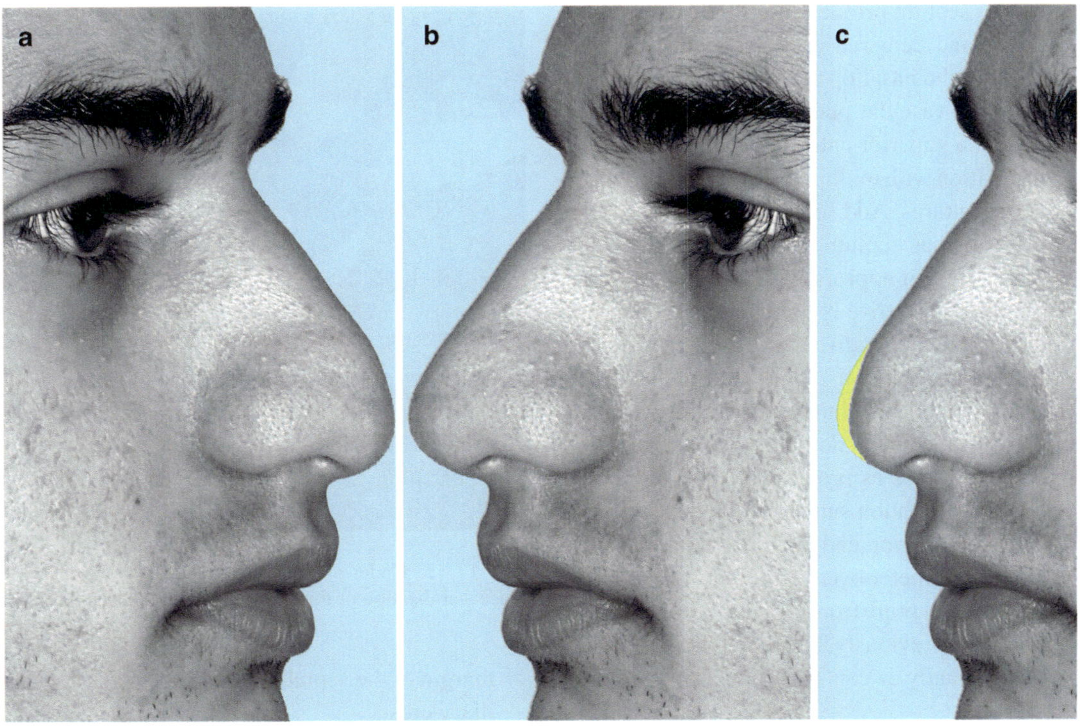

Fig. 17.13 (**a**–**c**) Under-projected nasal tip. Preoperative "Mirror" simulation. The first test with simple dorsal reduction appears inadequate and devoid of proportions (**b**). Only by associating the reduction of the dorsum with an increase in tip projection do the overall nasal proportions improve (**c**)

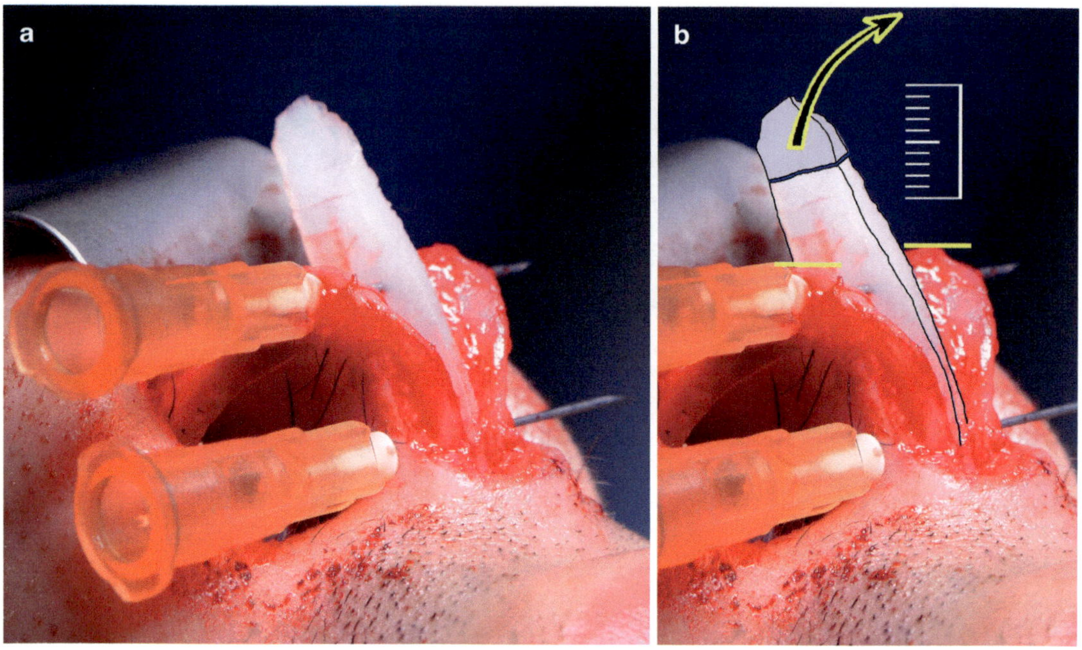

Fig. 17.14 (**a**, **b**) Under-projected nasal tip. Long columellar strut placement. The final shaping of the graft is done after the tip sutures (**b**)

caudal septum profile only if indispensable. A stable and centered caudal septum acts as a pillar in the nasal tip reconstruction steps.

- Lift with vascular pliers the membranous septum in a superior-anterior direction and fix it in position with multiple quilting 5/0 polydioxanone sutures. Add some single sutures of the membranous septum, as with the Fred[1] technique, until it appears well stabilized in position. The objective is to avoid any posteriorly directed postoperative traction to the nasal tip.
- Insert and fix a long columellar strut (Fig. 17.14a, b). Maintain it slightly protruding over the actual domal projection.
- Set the domes as projecting as possible with the dome creation suture.
- Cut the anterior end of the columellar strut half a millimeter over the domes.
- Carve a tip graft from the thickest portion of cartilage previously harvested from the septum. Usually it can be found at the inferior margin of the septal cartilage close to the maxillary crest.
- Stabilize with multiple 5/0 polydioxanone sutures the new tip complex composed by the domes and the graft (Fig. 17.15). Finally,

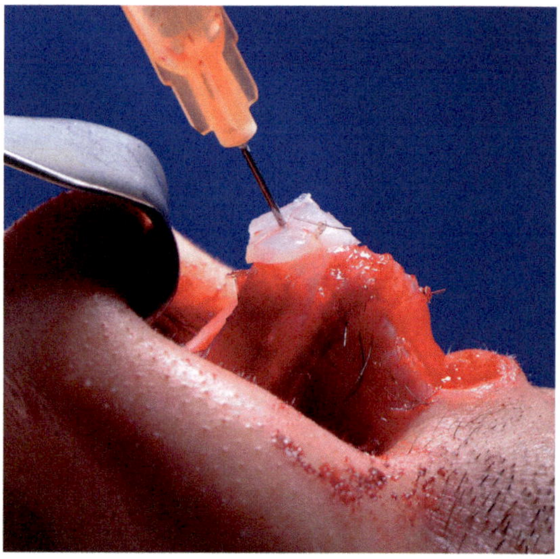

Fig. 17.15 Under-projected nasal tip. Provisional in-place stabilization of the tip graft with a fine needle

[1] Fred GB. The nasal tip in rhinoplasty: use of the invaginating technique to prevent secondary drooping. Ann Otolaryngol. 1950;59:215–23.

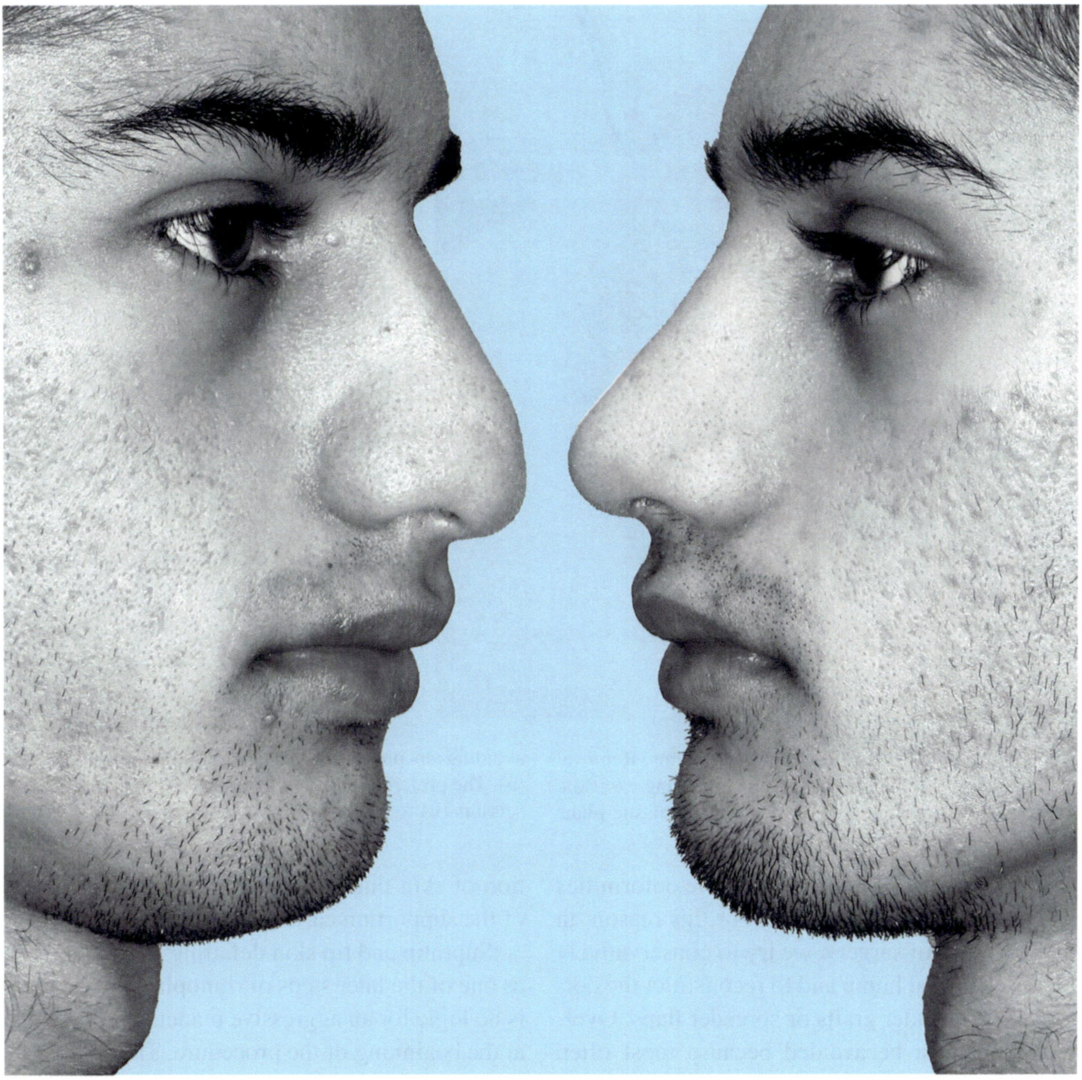

Fig. 17.16 Under-projected nasal tip. Postoperative result after minimal lowering of the dorsum and structural tip reconstruction

bevel conservatively the tip graft margins so as not to reduce its volume in search of a symmetrical result.

Figure 17.16 shows the clinical result obtained by orienting many of the BOR surgical steps towards the goal of increasing tip projection. Placement of the tip graft is only the final step of the procedure and cannot be considered the sole decisive factor of success in correcting an under-projected tip.

17.4 Nasal Thick Skin-Related Problems

Dealing with nasal thick skin requires one to respect some general principles and change the surgical techniques knowing well that probably the final results will be suboptimal. The first principle to follow consists in modifying the shape and proportion of the nose while preserving its volume. Thick and inelastic skin does not fit with a reduced new shape of the osteocartilagi-

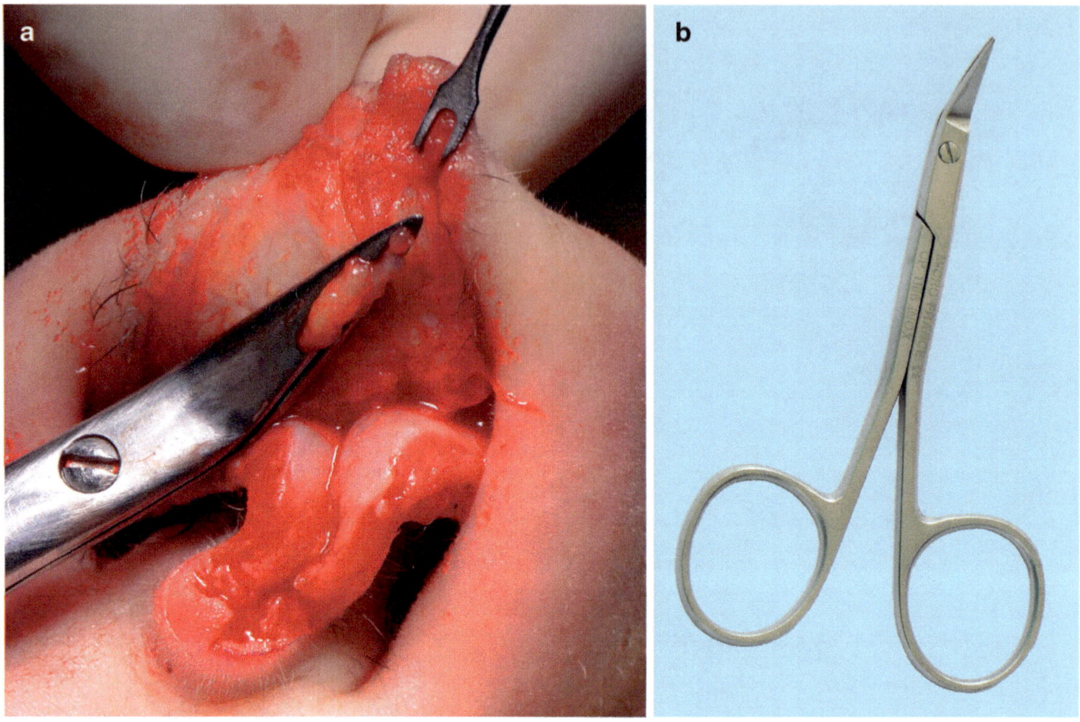

Fig. 17.17 (**a**, **b**) Thick skin-related problems. Removal of supratip and tip skin fibrofatty tissue. During excision, the scissor tips must be kept away from the tissue plane avoiding any pressure of the scissor blades against the flap (**a**). The preferred cutting instrument are angled Converse scissors (**b**)

nous skeleton, producing new visible deformities and not a pleasant correction. For this reason, in the first steps of surgery, we try to conservatively reduce the nasal hump and to reconstruct the dorsum with spreader grafts or spreader flaps. Overreduction must be avoided because most often the thick skin problems are greater at the level of the nasal tip. So, it is better not to reduce the bony and cartilaginous dorsal structures of the nose, increasing the discrepancy with the tip; rather, we should strive to equilibrate the upper, middle, and lower third projection and the width of the nose.

Also the upward nasal tip rotation should be limited to the sole correction of an acute nasolabial angle to avoid a broad amorphous short nose. As a general rule, any procedures that lead to skin excess at the end of the surgery should be avoided or at least minimized.

The management of the nasal tip and supratip region is certainly the most difficult part of this surgery. The two sides of the solution are a reduction of skin thickness and a wide reconstruction of the supporting cartilaginous skeleton.

Supratip and tip skin defatting should be done as one of the later steps of rhinoplasty since there is no logic for an aggressive maneuver on the flap at the beginning of the procedure. The safest way to reduce the subcutaneous fibrofatty tissue, as depicted in Fig. 17.17a, b, requires some basic rules:

- Evert the soft tissue envelope flap maintaining the index finger of the non-dominant hand over the supratip and tip skin surface to stabilize and control it.
- The preferred cutting instrument are the angled Converse scissors.
- During excision the scissor tips must be kept away from the tissue plane.
- Avoid applying any pressure with the blades of the Converse scissors against the flap in an attempt to remove more fibrofatty tissue.

- Only mobile and loose tissue should be removed. Most probably it is also composed of interdomal connective tissue left attached to the lower surface of the flap during its elevation.

Due to its limited effect and the risk of causing skin necrosis and scarring, defatting of supratip and tip skin should be limited to selected cases and done with extreme care.

Without doubt, in the case of thick skin, a reconstruction of the tip cartilaginous framework with solid septal cartilage grafts to ensure good support is the essential step.

Figures 17.18 and 17.19 show the intraoperative views of a nasal tip reconstruction after columellar strut placement and fixation. Also the domes were reshaped with a domal creation suture and joined together with a domal equalization suture. On careful observation an important particular cannot be missed: the great thickness of the skin flap appears completely out of scale when compared to the size of the cartilage.

A long shield graft, obtained from harvested septal cartilage (Fig. 17.20) and stabilized in place with multiple 5/0 polydioxanone monofilament sutures, can add up to 3 mm of further tip projection. The operative steps are:

- Carve the shield graft from a long triangular piece of cartilage and bevel the anterior angles and all the margins that will be in direct contact with the skin flap (Fig. 17.21a, b).

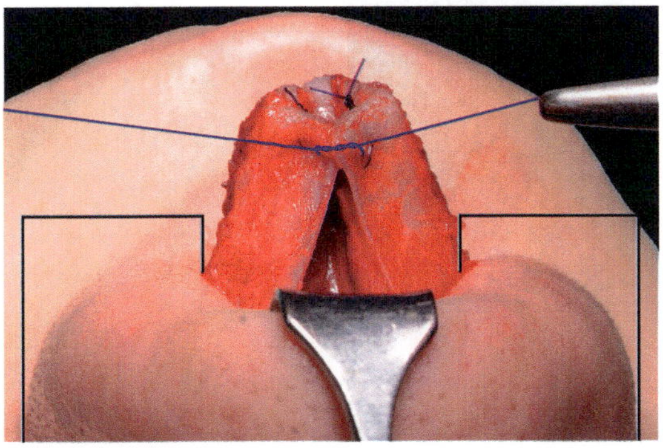

Fig. 17.18 Thick skin-related problems. Intraoperative view from above: the excessive thickness of the skin is evident in relation to the dimension of the tip framework

- Insert the long graft into the skin pocket previously created for the columellar strut at the base of columella and stabilize it temporarily with a fine needle (Fig. 17.22a, b). A short graft would not be concealed under the skin of the base of the columella with the risk of later producing an irregular notch close to the columellar scar.
- Place two sutures (absorbable 5/0 polydioxanone monofilament) in the central part of the graft anchoring it to the medial crus close to the domes. These sutures must not wrap around the margins of the graft that will probably be adapted later (Fig. 17.23a, b).

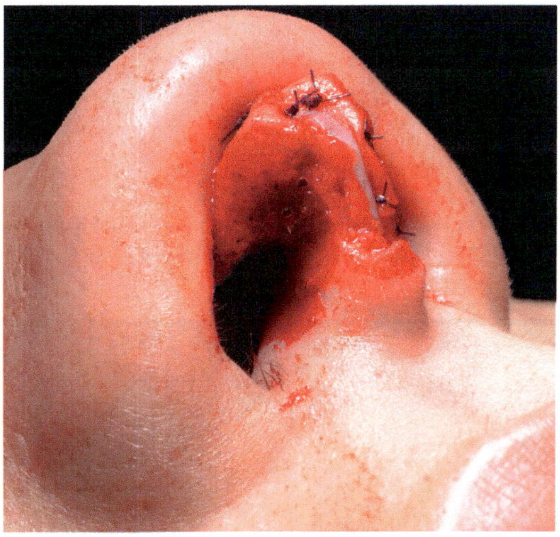

Fig. 17.19 Thick skin-related problems. Intraoperative view from below: the excessive thickness of the skin is evident in relation to the dimension of the tip framework

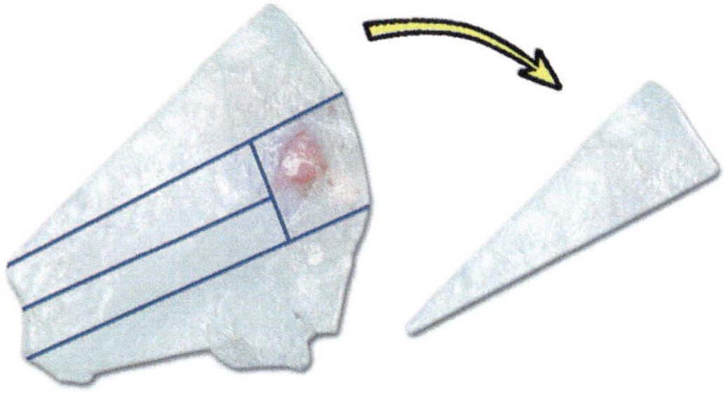

Fig. 17.20 Thick skin-related problems. To carve a long shield graft, a solid fragment of generous dimensions of septal cartilage is needed

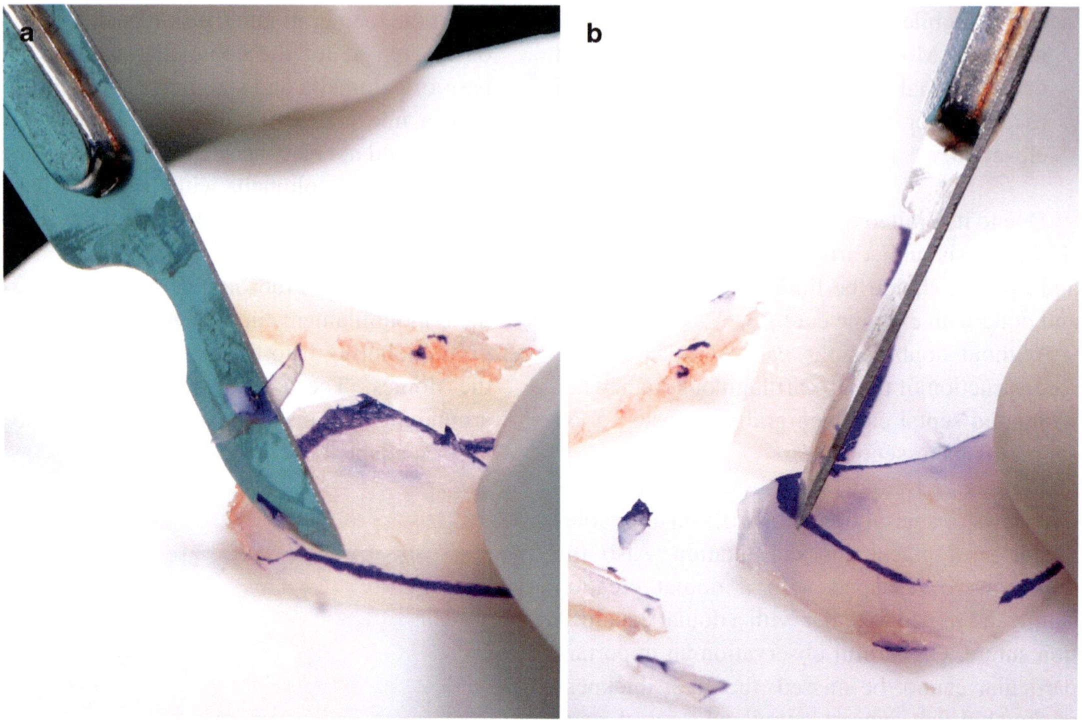

Fig. 17.21 (**a**, **b**) Thick skin-related problems. All the anterior angles as well as the margins of the long shield graft that will be in direct contact with the skin flap should be beveled

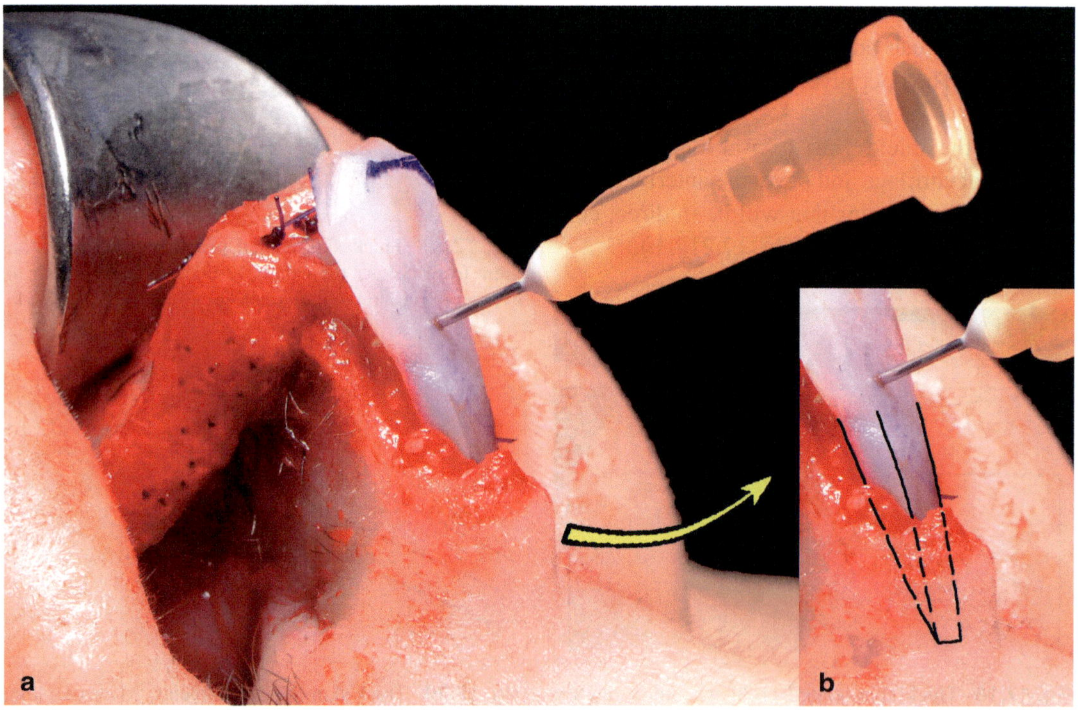

Fig. 17.22 (**a**, **b**) Thick skin-related problems. The long shield graft should be inserted into the skin pocket previously created for the columellar strut at the base of columella and stabilized temporarily with a fine needle

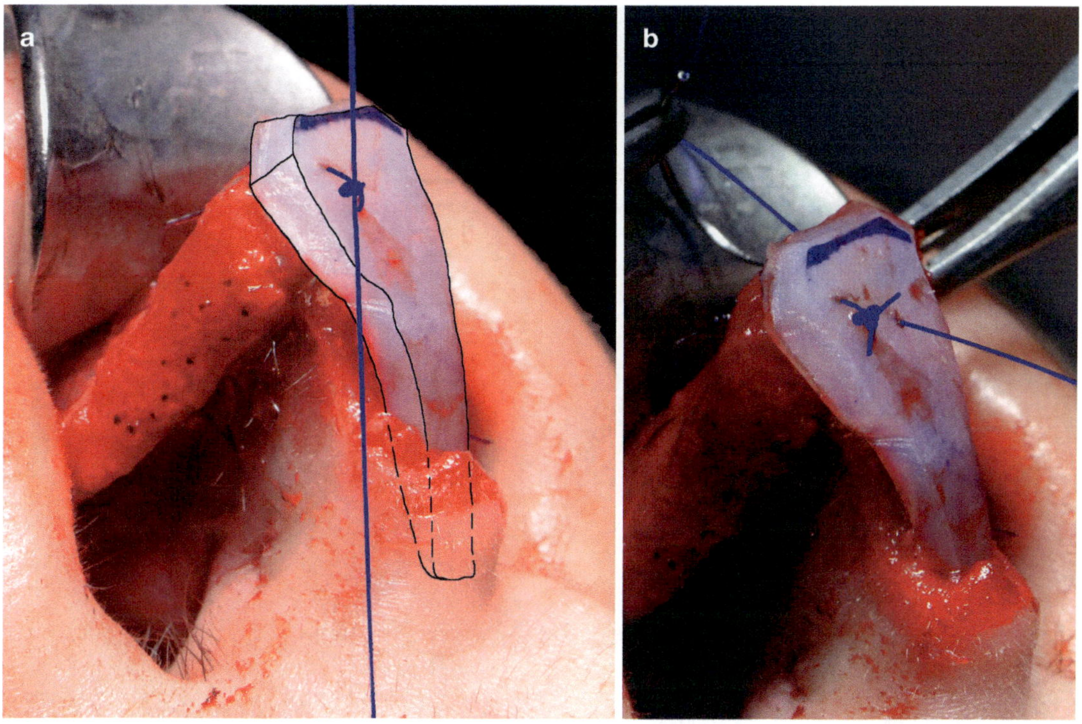

Fig. 17.23 (**a**, **b**) Thick skin-related problems. Two sutures are placed in the central part of the graft anchoring it to the medial crus close to the domes. These sutures must not wrap around the margins of the graft that will probably be adapted later

- Another stabilizing suture, wrapped to the paired medial crura, should be added close to the columellar incision to avoid any tension or protruding bulge at this level after skin closure (Fig. 17.24a). As depicted in Fig. 17.24b, with the shield graft the actual tip projection is increased by about 3.0 mm.
- The finishing of the graft is carried out after having ascertained its stability. With a 15c blade it is possible to shape the long shield graft with the aim of avoiding any excess of its margins along the edges of the future skin suture (Fig. 17.25a, b).
- To complete the nasal tip reconstruction another small graft should be carved and stabilized with one or two sutures over the two domes and in contact with the anterior margin of the shield graft (Fig. 17.26a, b).

The reconstruction of the nasal tip with multiple solid autologous onlay cartilage grafts, also named "visible grafts," must be the exception and not the rule. In thin skin patients, there is a high risk of visible deformities and asymmetries due to warping, rotation, and dislocation of the grafts as well as to skin atrophy secondary to local pressure.

17.5 Long Nose with a Narrow Nasolabial Angle

The correction of a long "aged" nose with the tip turned downward and a narrow nasolabial angle requires the application of some principles encountered in the previous sections. The main goal is to rotate the tip upward, a maneuver that requires a stable and well-reconstructed cartilage framework to retain the shape and projection of the nasal tip. So, a columellar strut and a basic tip suture technique are mandatory. The skin of the membranous septum should be lifted superiorly

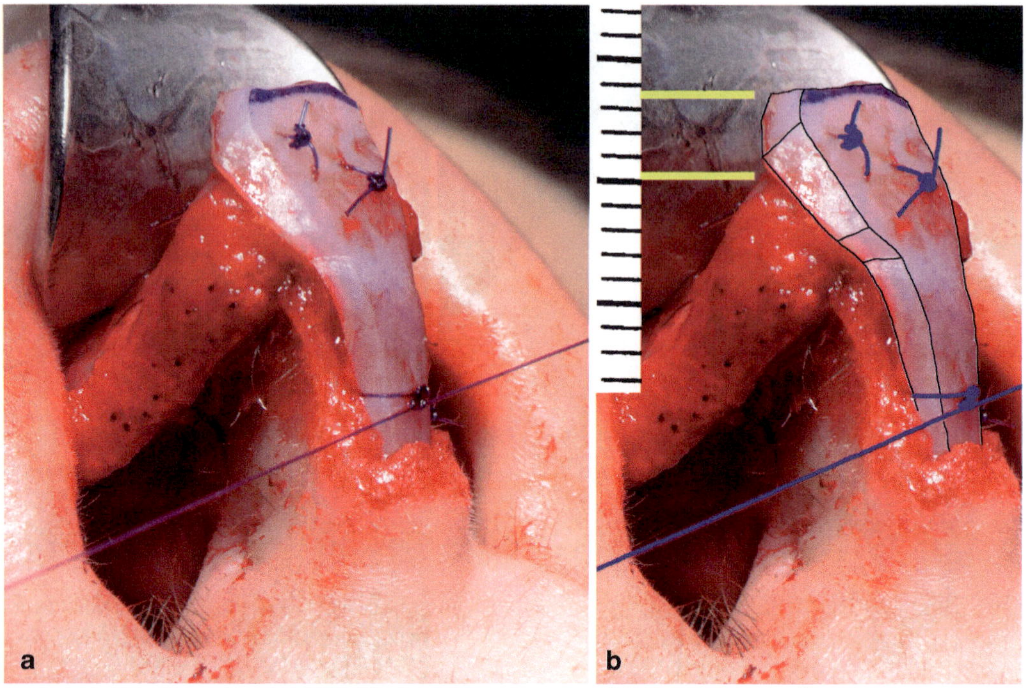

Fig. 17.24 (**a**, **b**) Thick skin-related problems. Another stabilizing suture, wrapped to the paired medial crura, should be added posteriorly close to the columellar incision to avoid any tension or protruding bulge at this level after skin closure

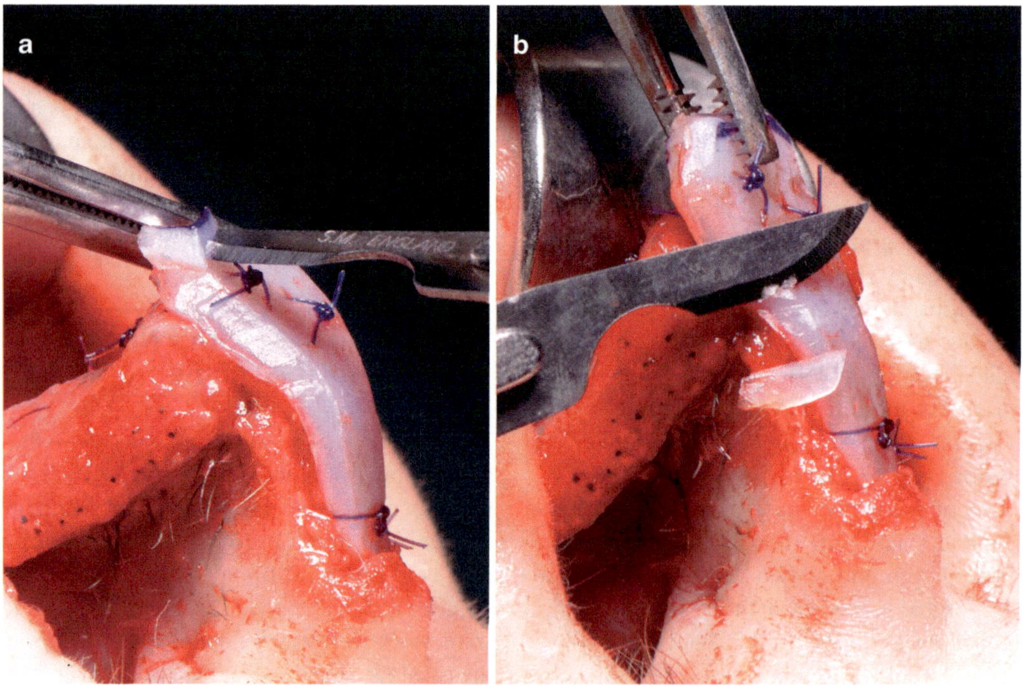

Fig. 17.25 (**a**, **b**) Thick skin-related problems. With a 15c blade it is possible to shape the long shield graft with the aim of avoiding any excess of its margins along the edges of the future skin suture

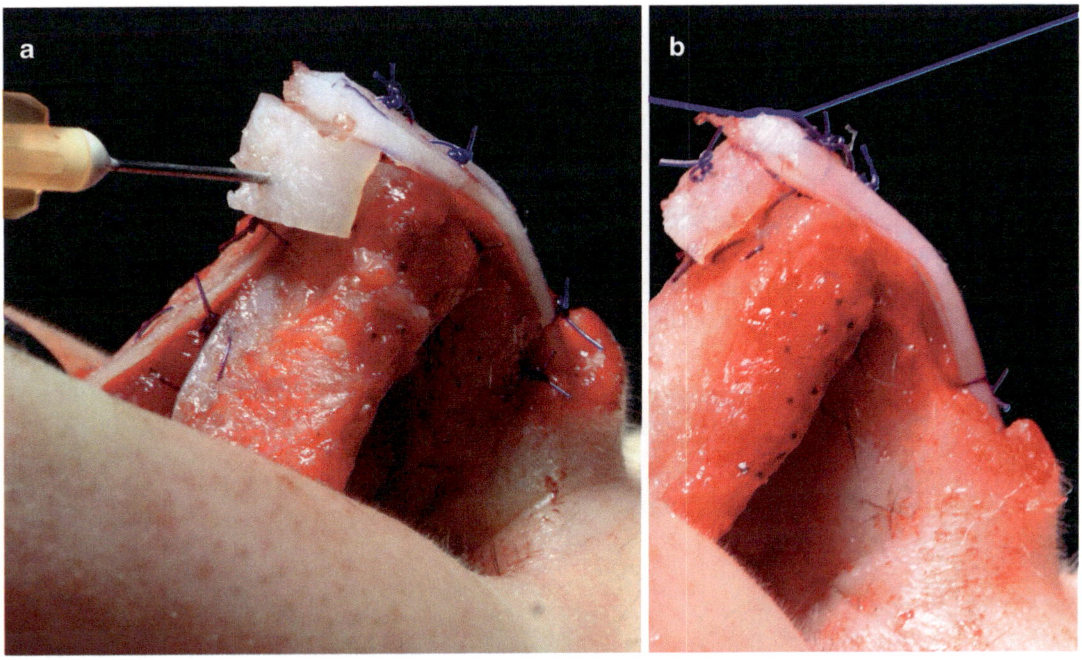

Fig. 17.26 (**a**, **b**) Thick skin-related problems. To complete the nasal tip reconstruction, another small graft should be carved and stabilized with one or two sutures over the two domes and in contact with the anterior margin of the shield graft

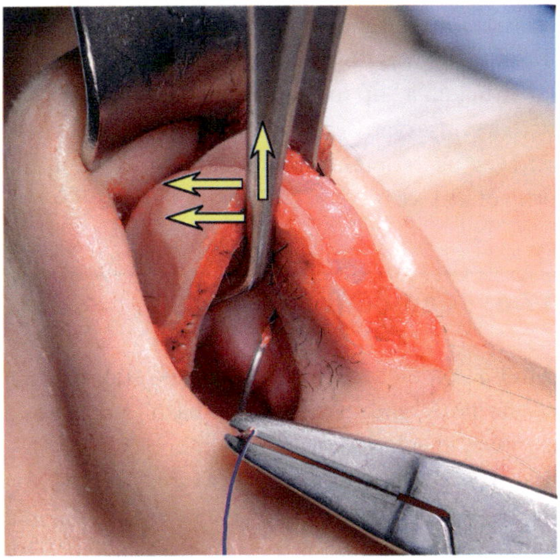

Fig. 17.27 Long "aged" nose. The skin of the membranous septum should be lifted superiorly and fixed with two or three sutures to the caudal septum to support the rotation

and fixed with two or three sutures to the caudal septum to support the rotation (Fig. 17.27); also for this reason, the excess of the caudal septum can be conservatively reduced.

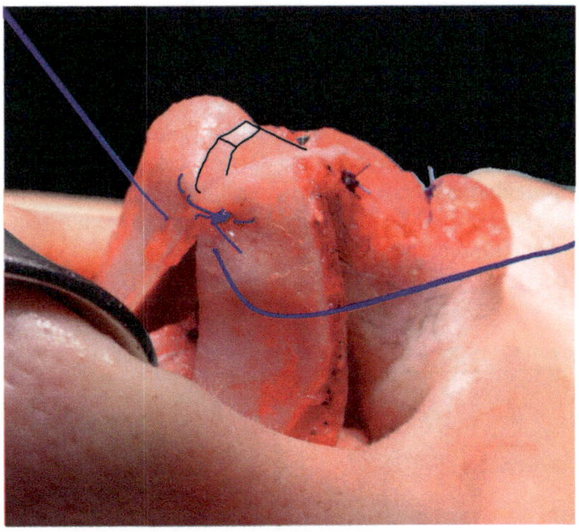

Fig. 17.28 Tip rotation long suture. This additional suture can be first passed through the medial crura, close to the superior aspect of the domes

An additional suture can be passed through the medial crura, close to the superior aspect of the domes (Fig. 17.28), and anchored to the midline of the dorsum, towards the osteocartilaginous junction, for a better rotating vector. Before applying this suture it is necessary to have shaped and stabilized the columella and the nasal tip with all the other sutures and grafts to avoid the risk of deformities or distortions. This "tip rotation long suture" must be gently tightened without overcorrecting the tip rotation (Fig. 17.29) and checked for stability with a curved DeBakey atraumatic tissue forceps (Fig. 17.30). Rather, it should be intended as a stabilizing tool applied to avoid a downward relapse that can occur progressively, sometimes months after surgery. To further obtain a long-lasting effect, it can be done with nonabsorbable 5/0 polypropylene monofilament instead of absorbable 5/0 polydioxanone monofilament.

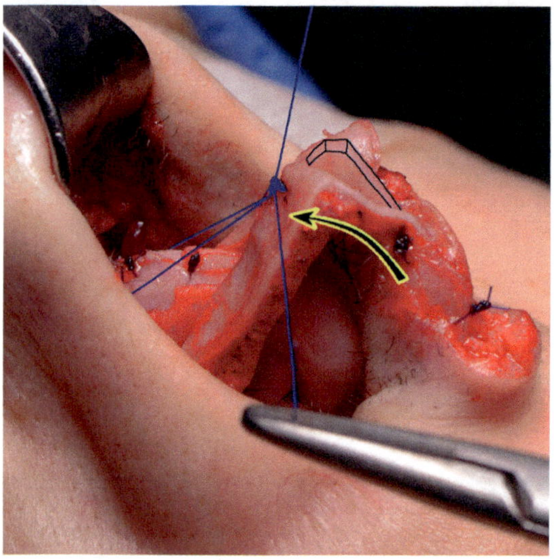

Fig. 17.29 Tip rotation long suture. The second bite is anchored to the midline of the dorsum, close to the osteocartilaginous junction for a better "long" rotating vector. The suture must be gently tightened without overcorrecting the tip rotation

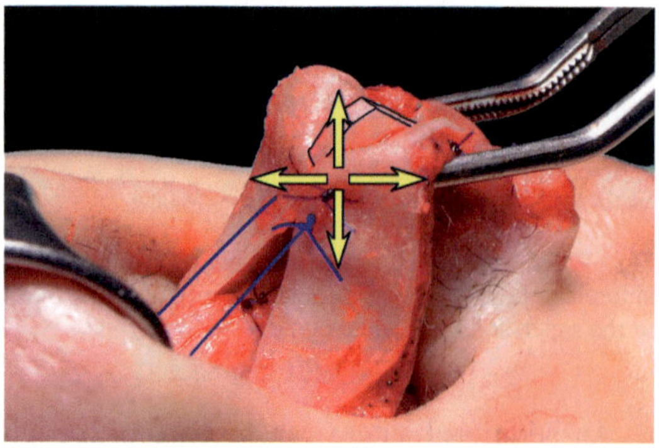

Fig. 17.30 Tip rotation long suture. The suture spatial effect on the tip is checked for its stability with a curved DeBakey atraumatic tissue forceps

However, in the case of drooping nasal tip, the most frequent cause of failure to obtain a good postoperative result probably lies in poor preoperative analysis as well as in poor communication between the patient and surgeon. Figure 17.31a shows the preoperative profile of a 60-year-old woman with an "aging nose" characterized by a small hump, long dorsum, drooping tip, and narrow nasolabial angle, whereas Fig. 17.31b illustrates the patient's desired changes in the form of an "Overlap" simulation. The requested changes are quite optimistic due to the skin excess produced by such an important reduction of the skeletal supporting structure of the nose, both in the anterior-posterior and in length dimensions. It is clear that the patient's requests do not match a realistic surgical outcome. Figure 17.32 shows a similar nasal profile of a 58-year-old patient with a less demanding esthetic request in terms of volume reduction and tip rotation. A mainly reconstructive and supporting surgery was done including a strong columellar strut and a "tip rotation long suture" combined with a conservative dorsal hump reduction which allowed us to obtain a profile similar to the initial project at 1 year (Fig. 17.33a, b).

17.6 Camouflage Grafts

After a complete reconstruction and stabilization of the bony and cartilaginous nasal structure, a rigorous check in search of small potentially visible irregularities or asymmetries should be carried out. The nose must be visually inspected and delicately palpated after perfect cleansing with sterile saline solution. The assistant and the nurse, thanks to their different points of view, can immensely help the surgeon in this fundamental analysis. In case of doubts, a further precise check can be done after suturing the columellar skin incision with two or three temporary nylon 6/0 sutures to better stabilize the skin flap over

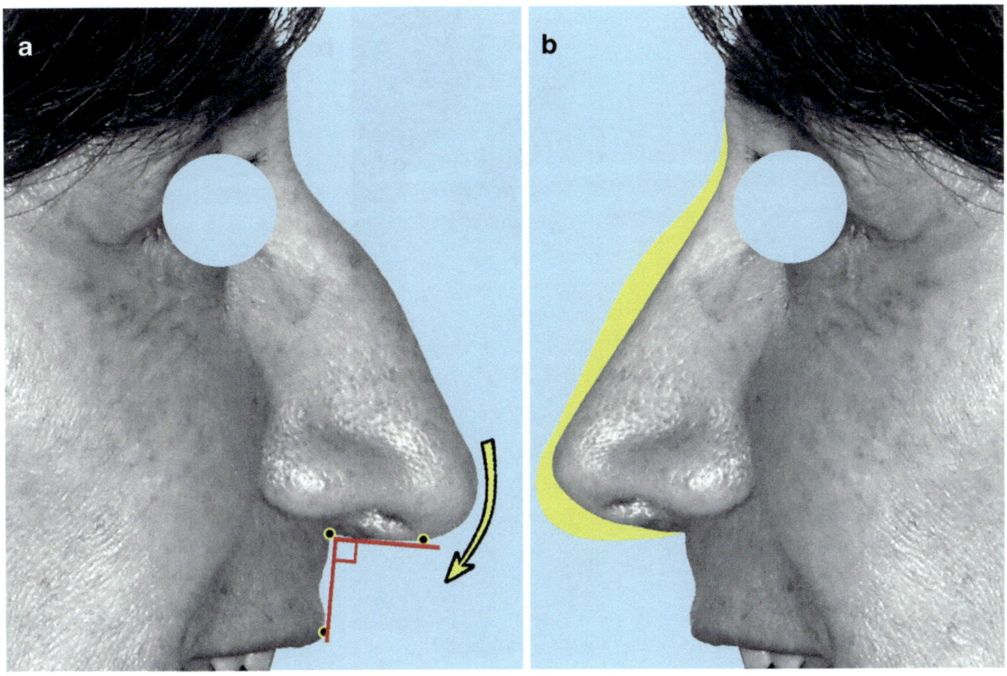

Fig. 17.31 (**a**, **b**) Long "aged" nose. Lateral right view of a clinical case characterized by a long dorsum, small hump, drooping nasal tip, and narrow nasal angle (**a**). The preoperative "Overlap" simulation based on the patient's desires is quite optimistic due to the skin excess produced by such an important reduction of the skeletal supporting structure of the nose

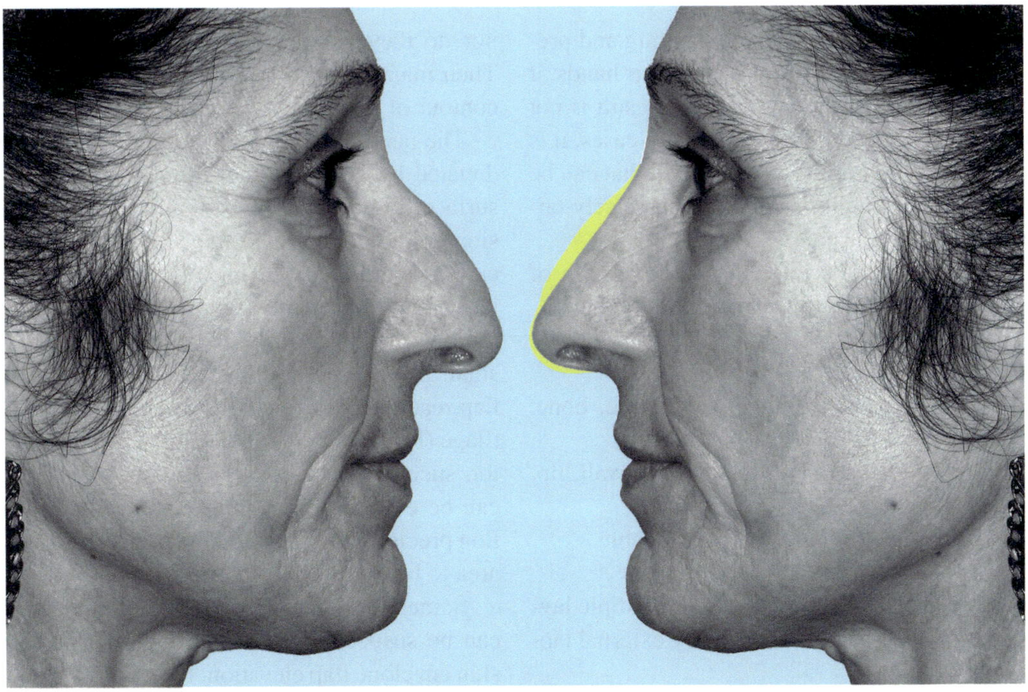

Fig. 17.32 Long "aged" nose. A similar nasal profile of a 58-year-old patient with a less demanding esthetic request in terms of volume reduction and tip rotation

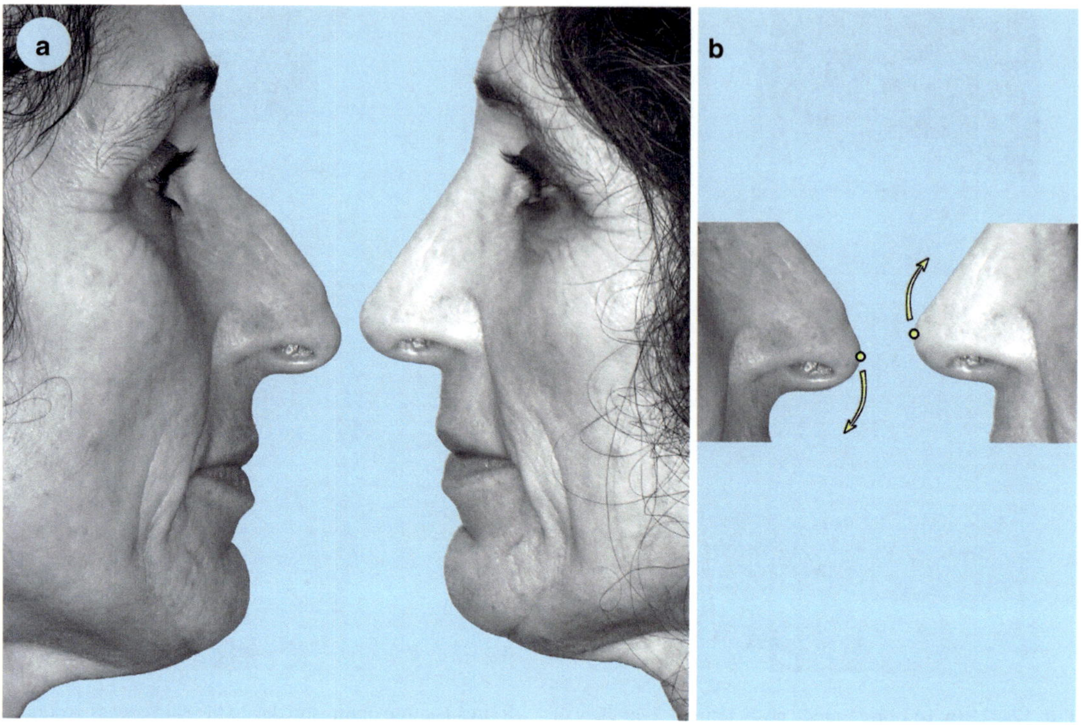

Fig. 17.33 (a, b) Long "aged" nose. The clinical result obtained in the previous patient with a mainly reconstructive and supporting surgery including a strong columellar strut, a "tip rotation long suture" and a very conservative dorsal hump reduction

the framework. Even after a demanding and precise reconstruction performed by expert hands, it often turns out that the intermediate result is not what was hoped for. In the majority of cases, it is a matter of a single and isolated detail that can be ameliorated by adding a small and precisely tailored camouflage graft.

Camouflage grafts refer to a broad group of onlay "visible" grafts that can be classified in different ways such as:

- By composition: cartilage, soft tissue, bone, and composite.
- By grafting site: radix, dorsum, sidewall, tip, ala, columella, base of columella.
- By consistency: rigid, soft, or moldable.

They can be realized in single or multiple layers and stabilized with sutures or by external taping and splinting.

In the majority of cases, camouflage grafts do not add structural support to the nasal framework nor do they have any effect on nasal function. Their main objective is to improve the shape and contour of the nose.

The need for a camouflage graft is frequently dictated by a close visual inspection of the skin surface. Figure 17.34a, b shows a small depression of the dorsum and the corresponding solid cartilage graft carved and beveled prior to its insertion. To perfectly identify the upper central margin of the depressed area to be grafted, a small needle can be transfixed through the skin flap reaching and penetrating the underlying cartilage (Fig. 17.35). With the aid of a small retractor, such as the Kasdan or similar, the skin flap can be elevated maintaining the needle in position precisely uncovering the upper margin of the area to be grafted (Fig. 17.36).

Sometimes the need for a camouflage graft can be suspected at the first look during initial skin envelope flap elevation. Figure 17.37a shows the differences and asymmetries between the lateral crura in the same subject. The left one is

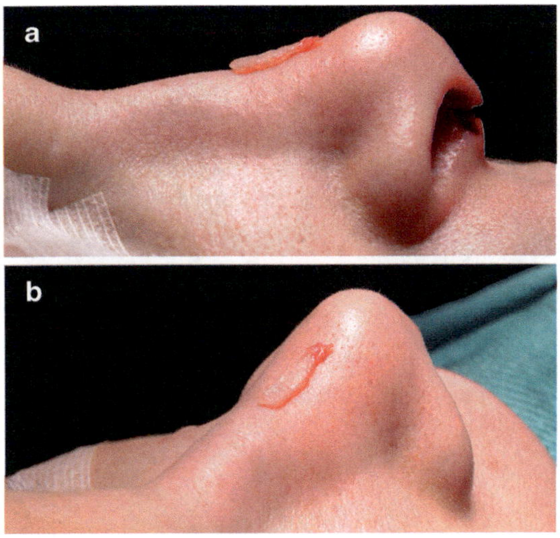

Fig. 17.34 (**a**, **b**) Camouflage grafts. Presence of a small intraoperative depression of the dorsum with the corresponding solid cartilage graft carved and beveled prior to its insertion

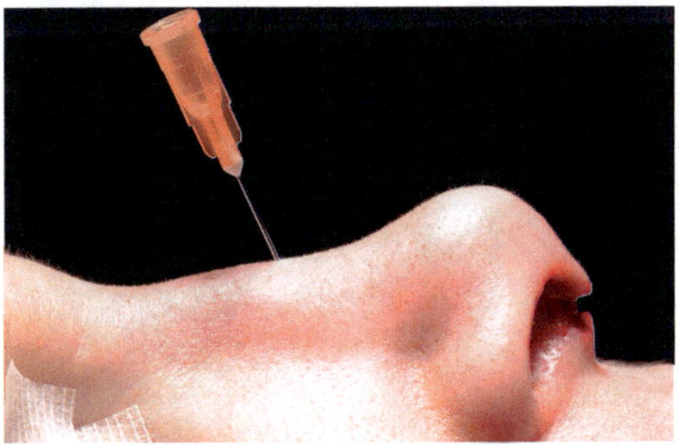

Fig. 17.35 Camouflage grafts. To perfectly identify the upper central margin of the depressed area to be grafted, a small needle can be transfixed through the skin flap reaching and penetrating the underlying cartilage

smooth and gently convex, whereas the right one is irregular and mainly concave. This initial deformity can be improved with a conservative lower lateral cephalic excision (Fig. 17.37b, c) associated with columellar strut placement and multiple sutures technique but, at the end of the procedure, some asymmetries may remain. The residual left side concavity can be refined with an onlay graft obtained from the excised convex right fragment and stabilized in place with two or

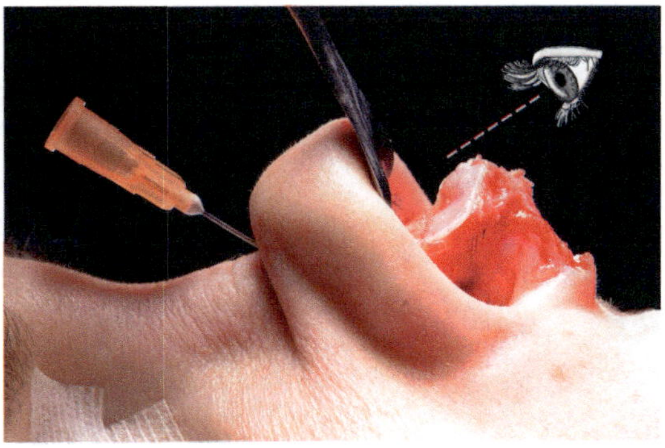

Fig. 17.36 Camouflage grafts. With the aid of a small retractor, such as the Kasdan or similar, the skin flap can be elevated maintaining the needle in position precisely uncovering the upper margin of the area to be grafted

three 6/0 polyglactin absorbable braided sutures (Fig. 17.37d). To avoid irregularities and graft visibility, the main rules are:

- The graft should not exceed both the caudal and cephalic margin of the underlying sculpted lateral crus.
- The anterior margin of the graft should lie at least 2 mm away from the domal area. A graft placed close to the dome can produce a step deformity and is at high risk of visibility in thin skin patients.
- In patients with thin skin, the anterior, cephalic and caudal margins must be thin, soft, and in direct contact with the underlying lateral crus. To release the elastic memory of the graft for a better fit, some transversal cuts can be done.

17.7 Composite Radix Graft

The preferred method to fill a deep nasal radix is with a graft of autologous temporal fascia wrapped around diced septal cartilage. Clinically, the indication to augment the nasal radix profile is rare and there are also many reasons that restrain the surgeon from grafting the nasal radix such as:

- The need to harvest temporal fascia.
- The extra surgical time required.

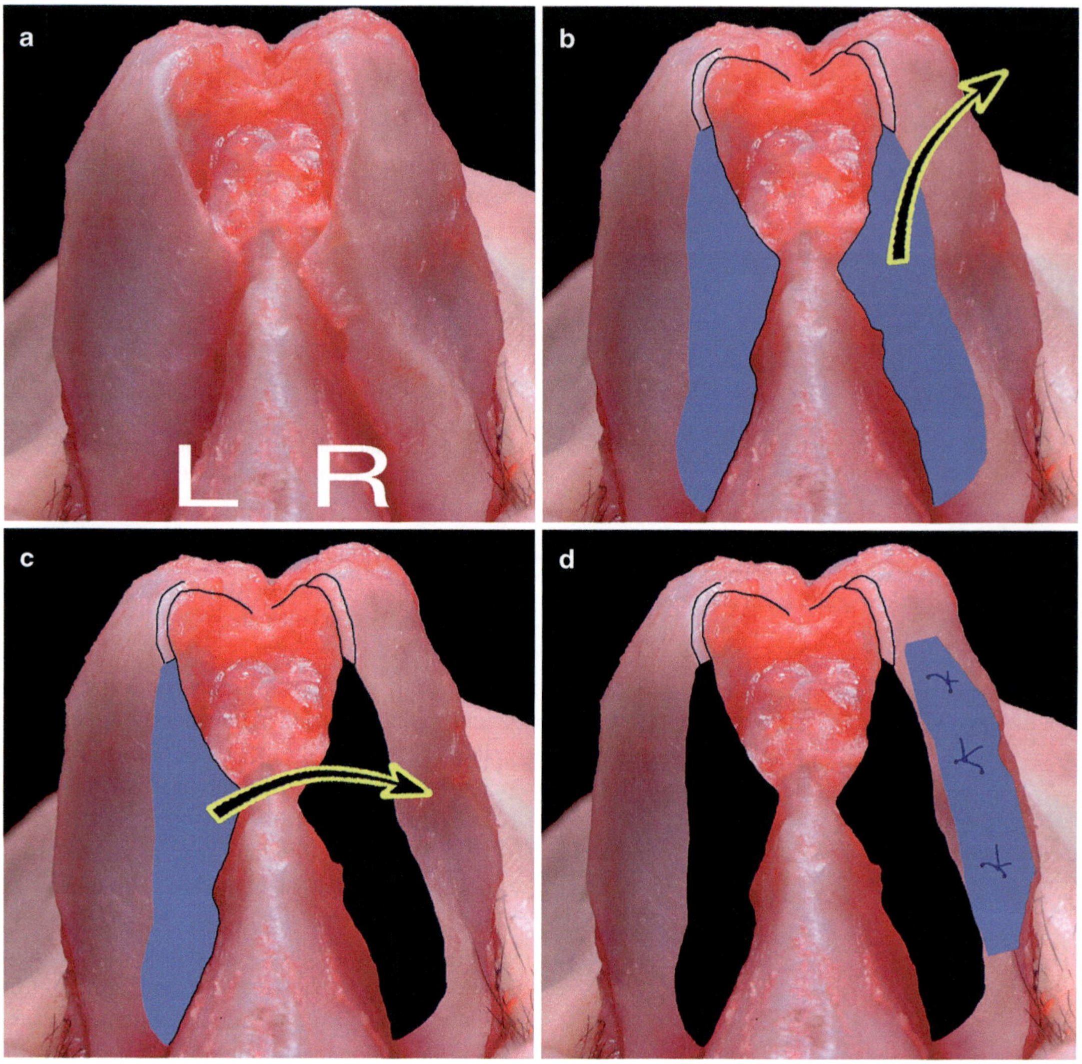

Fig. 17.37 (**a**–**d**) Camouflage grafts. Intraoperative view of an asymmetric pair of lateral crura (**a**). The left one is smooth and gently convex, whereas the right one is irregular and mainly concave. This initial deformity can be improved with a conservative lower lateral cephalic excision (**b**, **c**). The residual left side concavity can be refined with an onlay graft obtained from the excised convex right fragment (**d**)

– The limited influence of the graft in terms of the global nasal esthetic results obtainable.
– The risk of introducing profile irregularities as well as asymmetries.

The last point is probably the greatest drawback. Only a soft graft perfectly retained in the midline and precisely set in its cephalic-caudal position offers the best guarantee of a natural result. Figure 17.38 shows a clinical case of a deep nasal radix in a thick skin patient who greatly benefitted from a radix graft in order to avoid excessive hump reduction and maintain the overall nasal volume. In other words, a camouflage non-structural radix graft sometimes helps the surgeon in planning a more conservative and functionally oriented surgical treatment.

The main steps of grafting the nasal radix with the associated principles are:

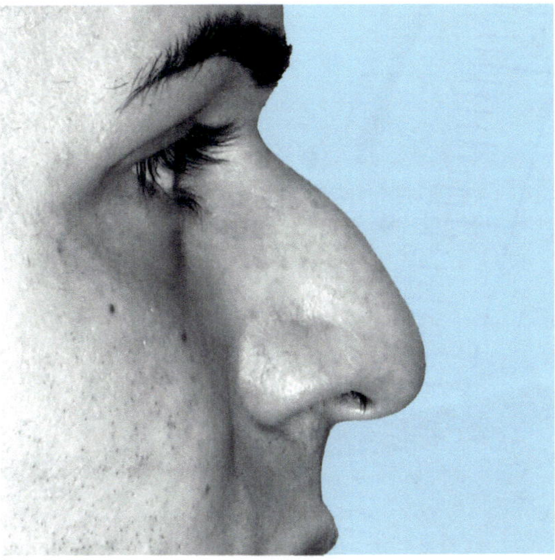

Fig. 17.38 Radix graft. Profile view of a clinical case of deep nasal radix in a thick skin patient

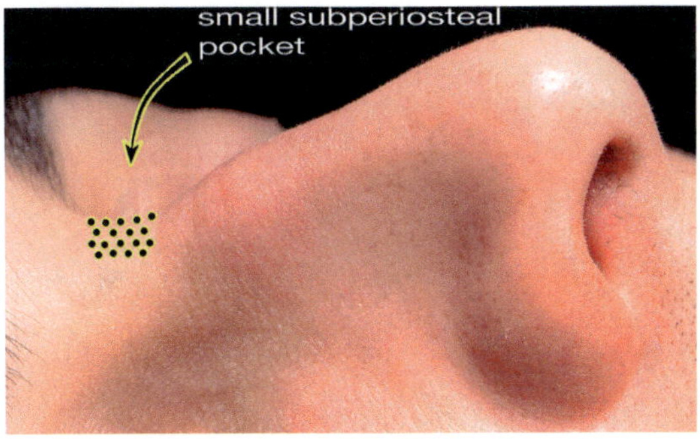

Fig. 17.39 Radix graft. At the beginning of surgery, during skin flap elevation, a small, precise and central subperiosteal pocket should be created in order to minimize the risk of lateral and upper graft displacement

- Plan the graft on the preoperative profile picture view. Usually a very small radix contour correction is needed.
- At the beginning of surgery, during skin flap elevation, a small, precise and central subperiosteal pocket, as depicted in Fig. 17.39, should be created in order to minimize the risk of lateral and upper graft displacement.
- Harvest a round piece of temporal fascia with a diameter of at least 15 mm. As an alternative to the autologous temporal fascia, a sheet of collagen membrane[2] can be used (Fig. 17.40a).
- The fascia or the collagen membrane is cut to obtain a disk of at least 15 mm in diameter and then rehydrated (Fig. 17.40b–d).
- The internal portion of the graft is obtained from small fragments of finely diced septal cartilage (Fig. 17.41).
- Suturing the collagen membrane around the cartilaginous fragments with multiple braided polyglactin 5/0 absorbable sutures provides the final assembly of the graft (Fig. 17.42a, b). The end of the suture with the needle is kept attached to the composite graft as it is necessary for the subsequent phases of positioning and stabilization (Fig. 17.43).
- The final volume of the graft greatly exceeds the need for a better nasal radix contour (Fig. 17.44). During the healing phase, the collagen membrane gradually resorbs and the diced cartilage remodels, losing part of its initial thickness.
- Utilize the polyglactin suture for positioning the graft. With the aid of a Maliniac nasal retractor, the suture needle can be passed through the skin at the level of the upper margin of the subperiosteal pocket (Fig. 17.45). A gentle suture traction, elevating at the same time the soft tissue skin envelope with the Malignac retractor, allows for easy graft positioning over the bony nasal radix under direct vision.
- Stabilize the graft with multiple Steri-Strips applied to the polyglactin suture over frontal skin. The suture should be fixed in a light upward tension (Fig. 17.46). The external polyglactin suture can be cut and removed on postoperative day 5 to 7.

Figure 17.47 shows the results 9 months after rhinoplasty with radix augmentation in a thick skin patient.

[2]Geistlich Bio-Gide porcine collagen membrane 2.5 × 2.5 cm (the author declares that he has no conflict of interest).

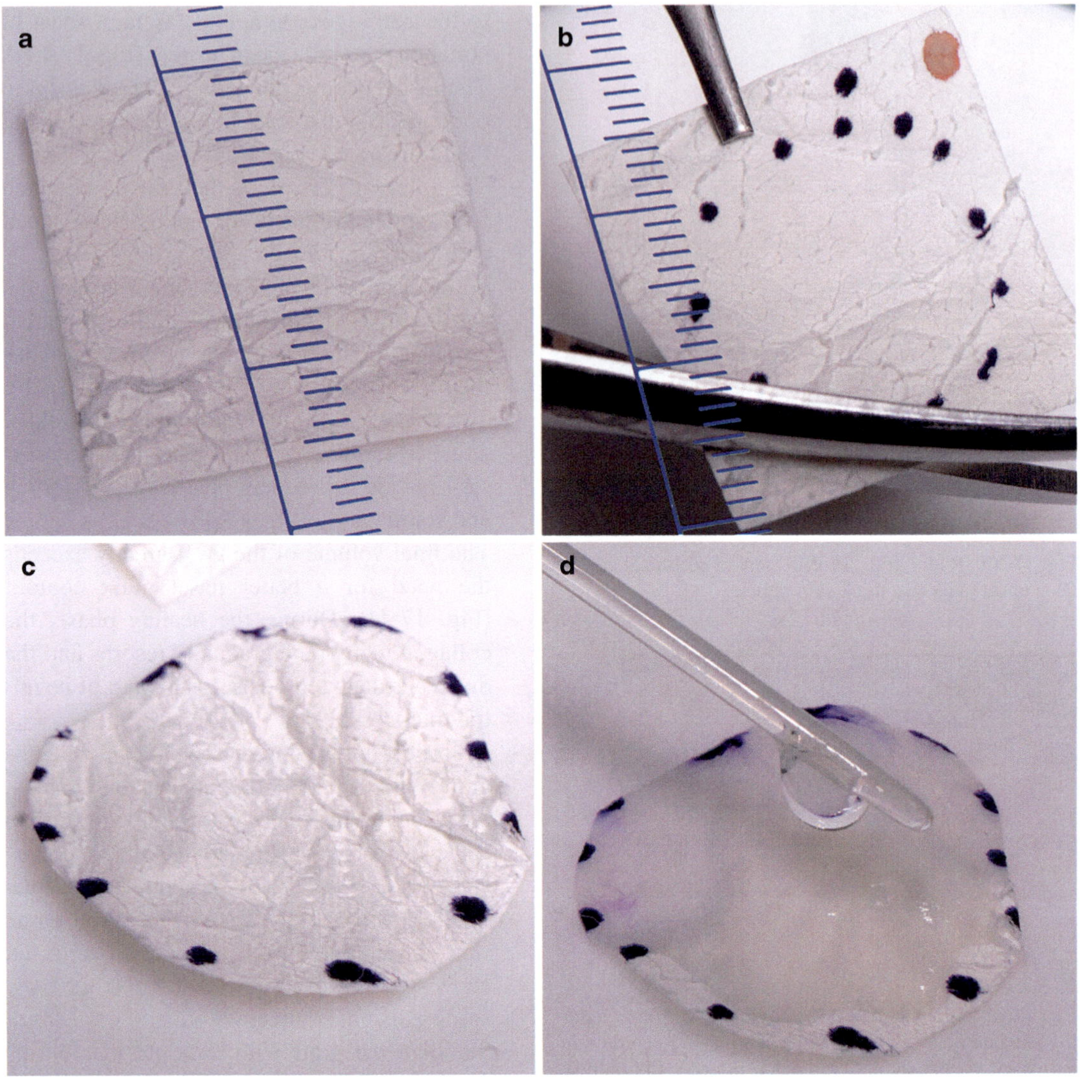

Fig. 17.40 (**a**–**d**) Radix graft. A sheet of collagen membrane can be used as an alternative to the autologous temporal fascia. It can be easily cut into the desired shape and dimension (**b**, **c**) and rehydrated with sterile saline before use (**d**)

17.8 Soft Camouflage Grafts

The natural tendency to warping of the cartilage is one of the major issues of rhinoplasty and its control increases in importance as the surgeon approaches the refinements of the nasal surface. For that reason camouflage grafts frequently require the attenuation of cartilage memory to fit perfectly the area of placement and to avoid the creation of new irregularities that may also occur months after surgery.

Reducing the thickness of the grafts may also be necessary.

Sometimes the lower lateral cephalic cartilage excision can be used as an ideal solid moldable graft without shape memory to increase thickness in any part of the nasal framework (Fig. 17.48a). The small piece can be modified and shaped as a hair comb with multiple full thickness partial cuts done with a 15c blade (Fig. 17.48b). To maintain the "hair comb graft" in a single piece, the cuts stop at a distance of 1–1.5 mm from its

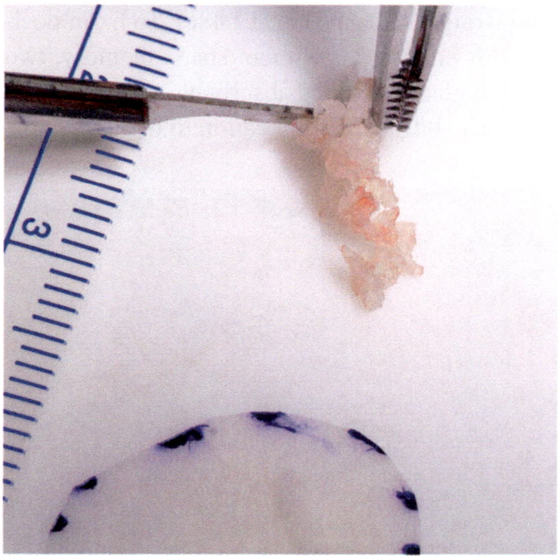

Fig. 17.41 Radix graft. Usually the internal portion of the composite graft is obtained from small fragments of finely diced septal cartilage

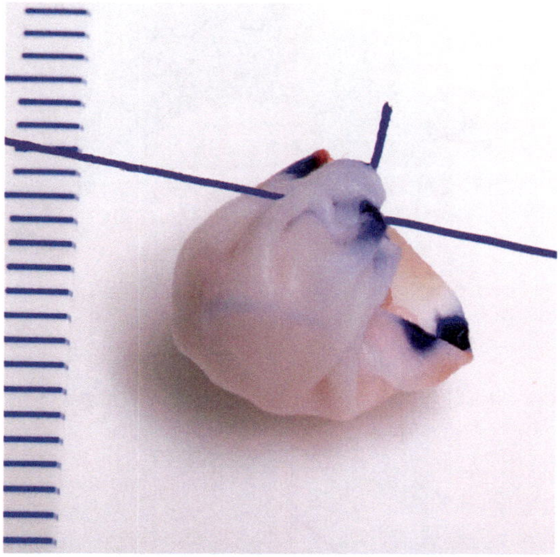

Fig. 17.43 Radix graft. The end of the suture with the needle is kept attached to the composite graft as it is necessary for the subsequent phases of positioning and stabilization

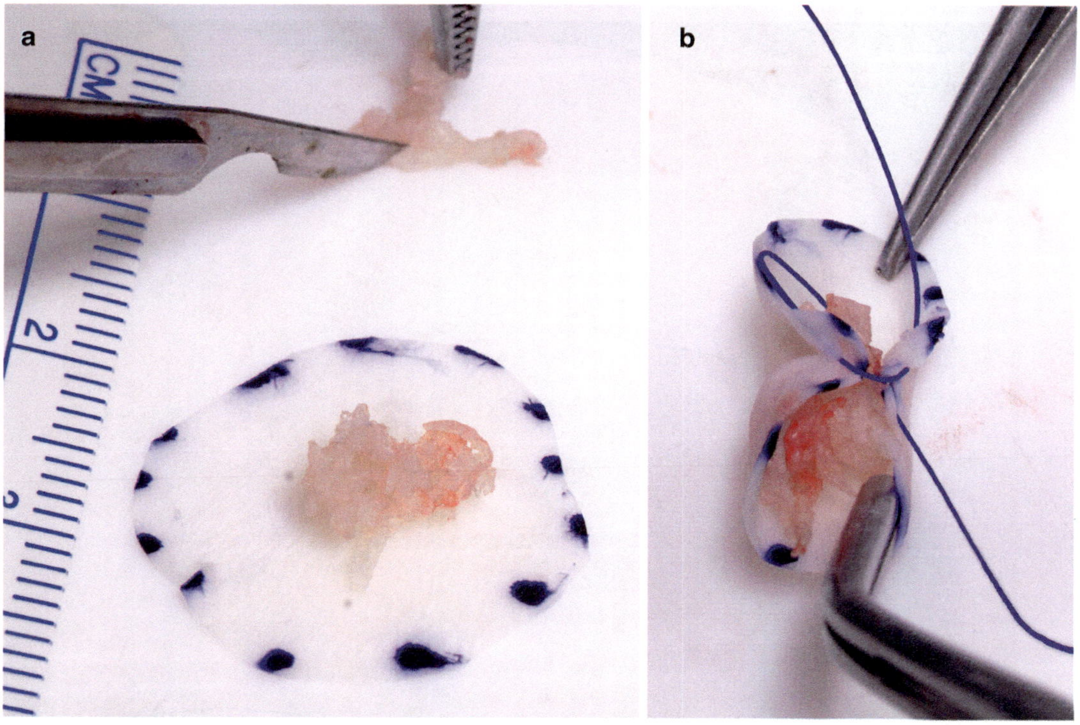

Fig. 17.42 (**a**, **b**) Radix graft. The final assembly of the graft is achieved by suturing the collagen membrane around the cartilaginous fragments with multiple braided 5/0 polyglactin absorbable filaments

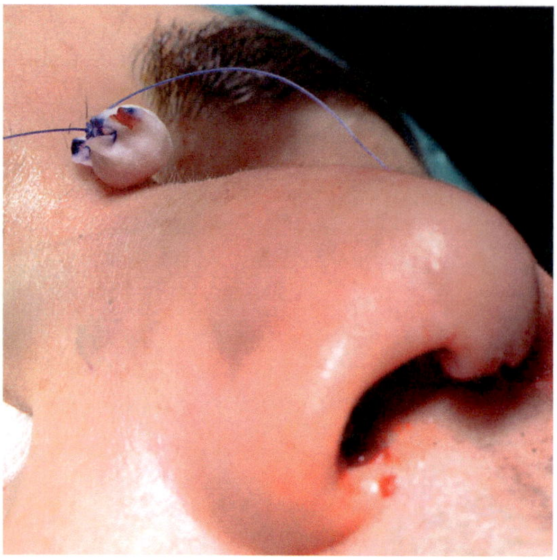

Fig. 17.44 Radix graft. The final volume of the graft greatly exceeds the need for a better nasal radix contour. During the healing phase, the collagen membrane gradually resorbs and the diced cartilage remodels, losing part of its initial thickness

long straight margin (Fig. 17.48c). To fix in position this small graft without shape memory, two 6/0 polyglactin braided absorbable sutures can be used. The only contraindication to the use of this

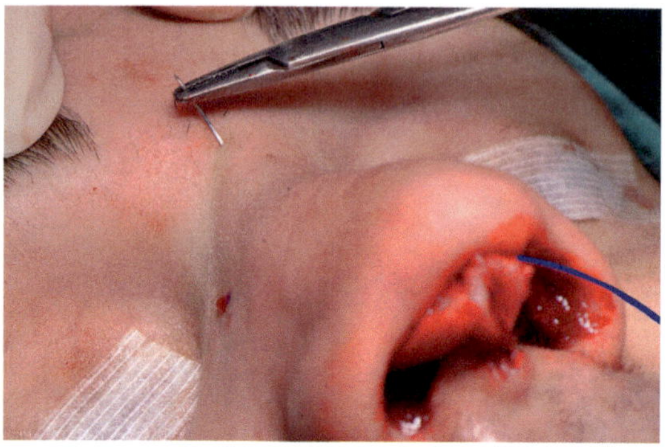

Fig. 17.45 Radix graft. Graft positioning under direct vision over the bony nasal radix. With the aid of a Maliniac nasal retractor, the suture needle can be passed through the skin at the level of the upper margin of the subperiosteal pocket. The graft is then slipped into the recipient bed

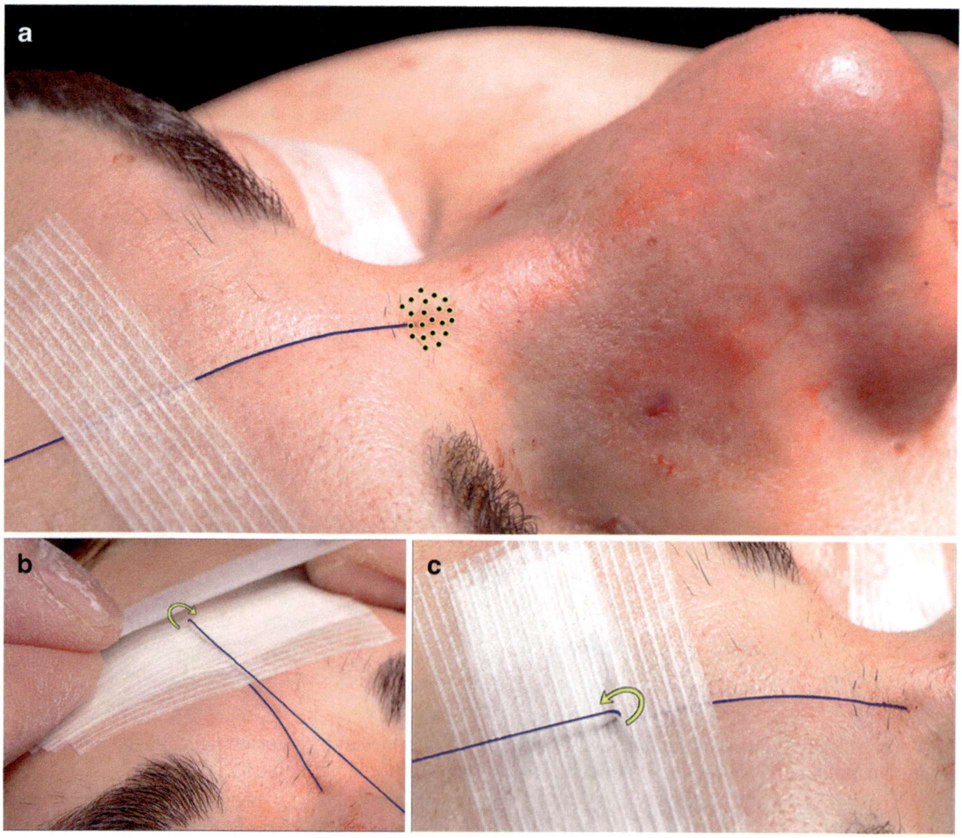

Fig. 17.46 (a–c) Radix graft. The graft is then stabilized with multiple Steri-Strips applied to the polyglactin suture on frontal skin

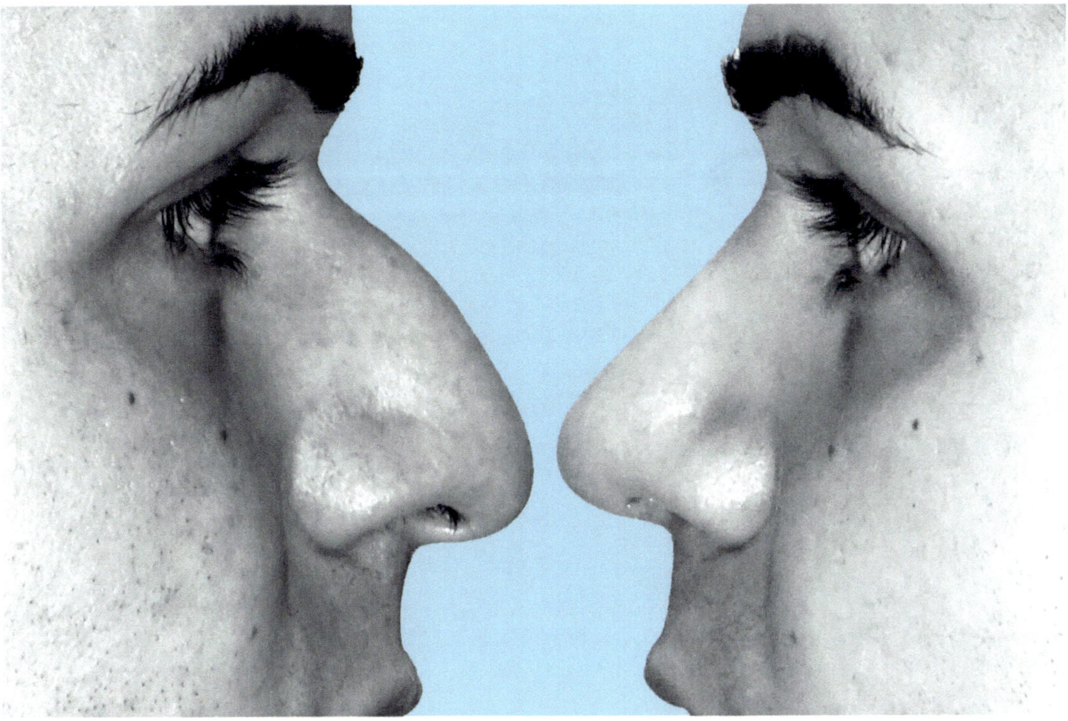

Fig. 17.47 Radix graft. Clinical results 9 months after surgery in a thick skin patient

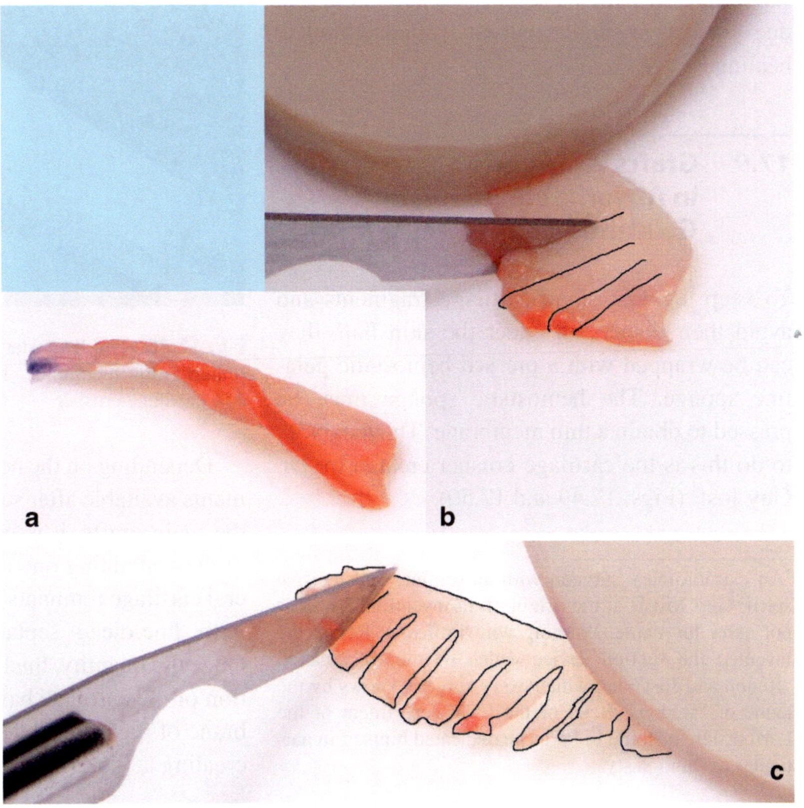

Fig. 17.48 (**a–c**) Soft camouflage grafts. The lower lateral cephalic cartilage excision can be used as an ideal solid moldable graft without shape memory to increase the thickness in any part of the nasal framework (**a**). The small piece can be modified and shaped as a hair comb with multiple full thickness partial cuts done with a 15c blade (**b**). To maintain the "hair comb graft" in a single piece, the cuts stop at a distance of 1–1.5 mm from its long straight margin (**c**)

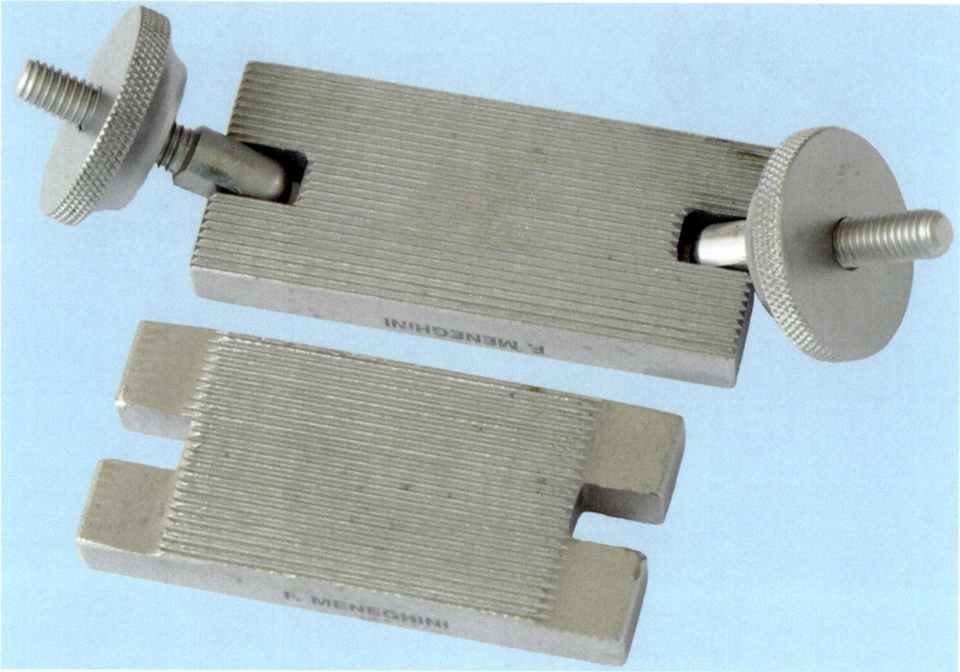

Fig. 17.49 Guy Jost cartilage crusher

graft is the increase of the central portion of dorsal profile in patients with extremely thin skin due to its potential visibility after complete healing.

17.9 Grafts Wrapped in Absorbable Hemostatic Gelatine Sponge

To keep together small cartilage fragments and avoid their dispersion under the skin flap, they can be wrapped with a pressed hemostatic gelatine sponge. The hemostatic sponge must be pressed to obtain a thin membrane. The ideal tool to do this is the cartilage crusher created by Dr. Guy Jost[3] (Figs. 17.49 and 17.50).

[3]An extraordinary surgeon with an original and incisive spirit, Guy Jost is at the origin of an invention that does not carry his name. Working with Professor Redon, he invented the suction device which he modestly called "Redon and Jost" and which every surgeon knows by the name of "Redon." Head of the ENT department of the Lariboisière hospital in Paris, he dedicated himself in particular to rhinoplasty.

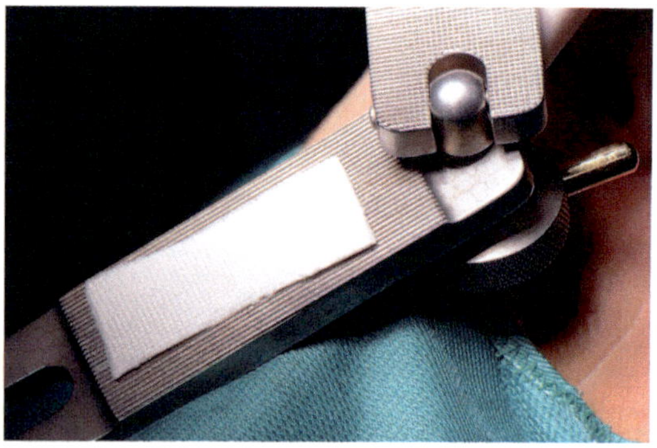

Fig. 17.50 The hemostatic sponge must be pressed to obtain a thin membrane. The ideal tool to do this is the Jost cartilage crusher

Depending on the needs and the cartilage fragments available after sculpture and positioning of the main grafts, it is possible to create wrapped grafts containing one or two layers of upper lateral cartilage remnants (Figs. 17.51 and 17.52) or with fine-diced septal cartilage (Fig. 17.53). Once the quantity, thickness, and spatial distribution of the cartilage have been set, the thin membrane of the pressed hemostatic sponge is folded creating a kind of sandwich (Fig. 17.54). For

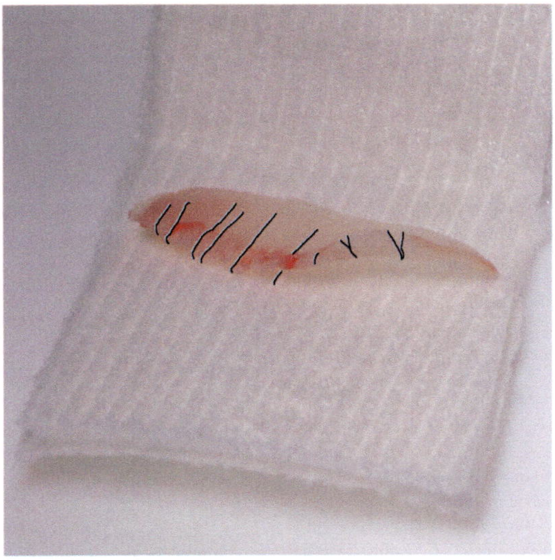

Fig. 17.51 Wrapped graft with one layer of upper lateral cartilage "hair comb graft"

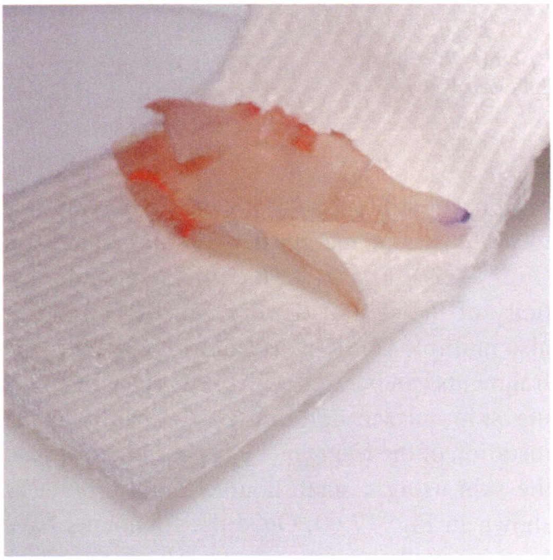

Fig. 17.52 Wrapped graft with two layers of upper lateral cartilage "hair comb graft"

better stability, when trimming the margins it is necessary to maintain a wide edge of pressed hemostatic sponge around the area containing the cartilage (Figs. 17.55a, b and 17.56). In this way, due to the extra size of the whole composite graft, the risk of displacement is limited. The position and orientation of the cartilage inside the sand-

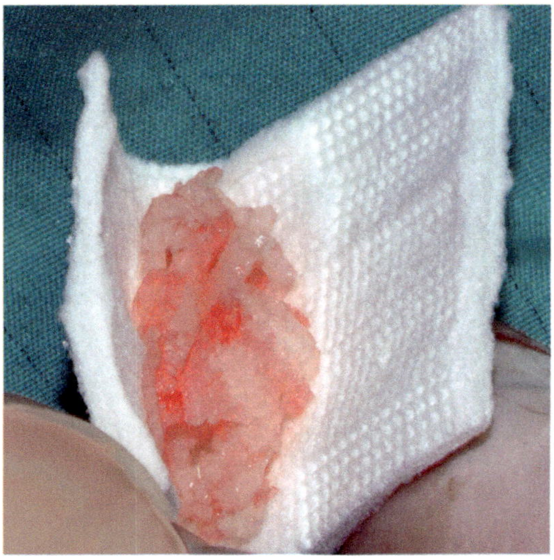

Fig. 17.53 Wrapped grafts with fine-diced septal cartilage

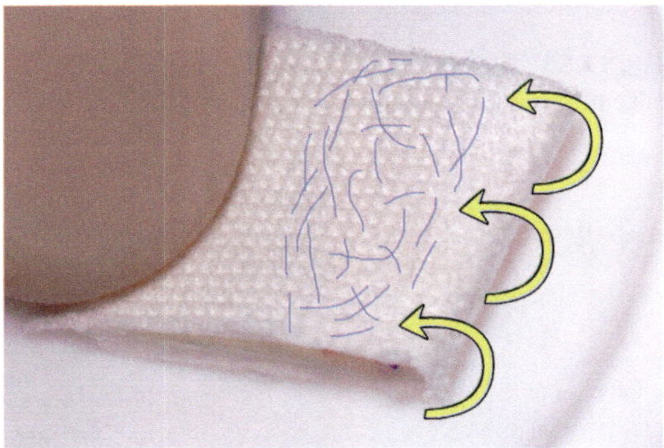

Fig. 17.54 Wrapped grafts. The thin membrane of the pressed hemostatic sponge is folded around the cartilage creating a kind of sandwich

wich should be mentally recorded by the surgeon for its subsequent precise insertion under the soft tissue skin envelope (Fig. 17.57a, b). Once the graft is positioned and the skin flap released, only very delicate pressure should be applied to promote its final adjustment (Fig. 17.58). It must be clear that after positioning this graft, the skin flap must no longer be moved or retracted. All that remains is to suture the marginal and columellar incisions and stabilize the flap with external nasal taping and casting.

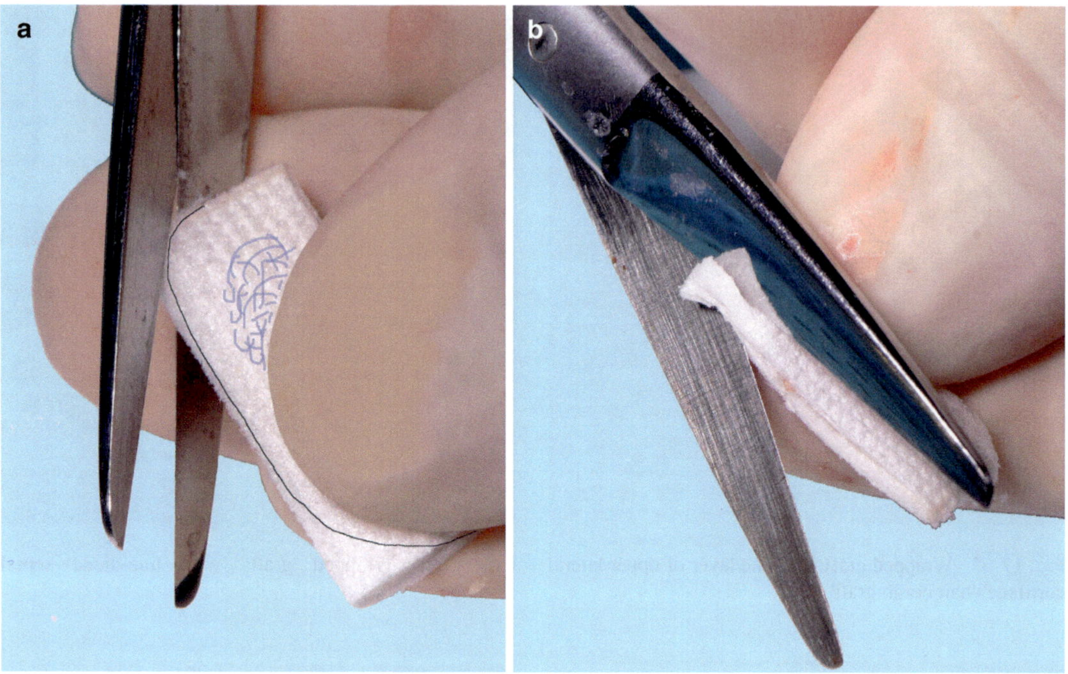

Fig. 17.55 (**a**, **b**) Wrapped grafts. For better stability, when trimming the margins it is necessary to maintain a wide edge of pressed hemostatic sponge around the area containing the cartilage

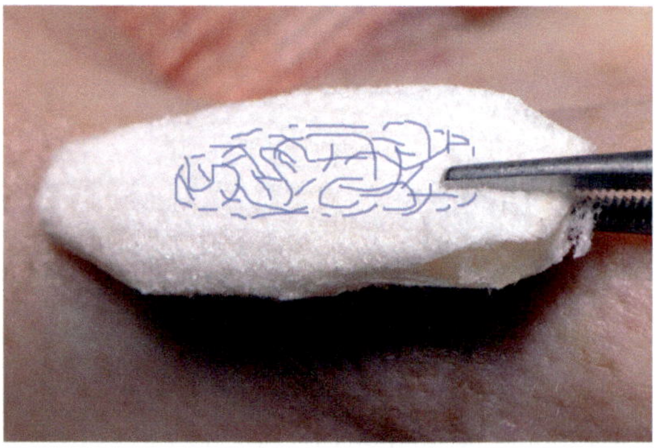

Fig. 17.56 Wrapped grafts. For better stability, when trimming of the margins is necessary to maintain a wide edge of pressed hemostatic sponge around the area containing the cartilage. In this way, due to the extra size of the whole composite graft, the risk of displacement is limited

17.10 Plumping Grafts

Plumping grafts may be used to improve an acute "masculine" nasolabial angle in female patients. They should be placed in a subcutaneous pocket at the base of the columella, inferior to the posterior margin of the columellar strut (Fig. 17.59). Thanks to the thickness and elasticity of the skin at the base of the columella, also multiple voluminous and irregular cartilage fragments can be used without any risk of creating skin surface deformities. To facilitate the insertion of the fragments it is possible to spread the skin using a small double Guthrie hook as shown in Fig. 17.60. Once the fragments have been inserted, it is important to check that there are no distortions or tensions on the posterior margin of the columellar incision, a sign of excessively anterior positioning of the plumping grafts.

17.11 Gel of Cartilage Grafts

The use of fine-diced or pressed cartilage as an injectable gel is proposed last in the surgical sequence because its use often takes place at the end of the procedure after placing the sutures of

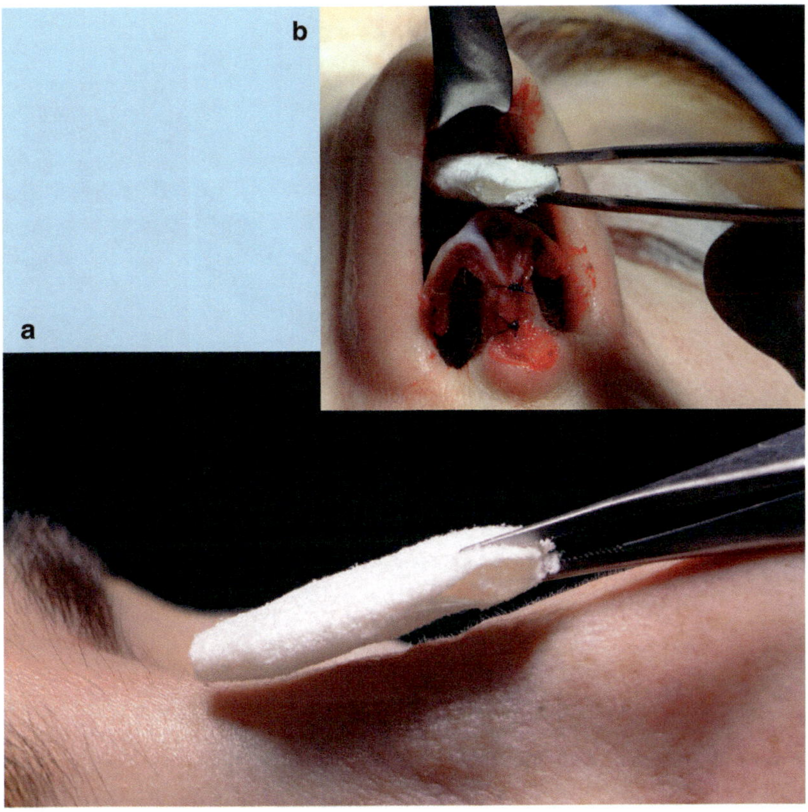

Fig. 17.57 (**a**, **b**) Wrapped grafts. The position and orientation of the cartilage inside the sandwich should be mentally recorded by the surgeon for its subsequent precise insertion under the soft tissue skin envelope

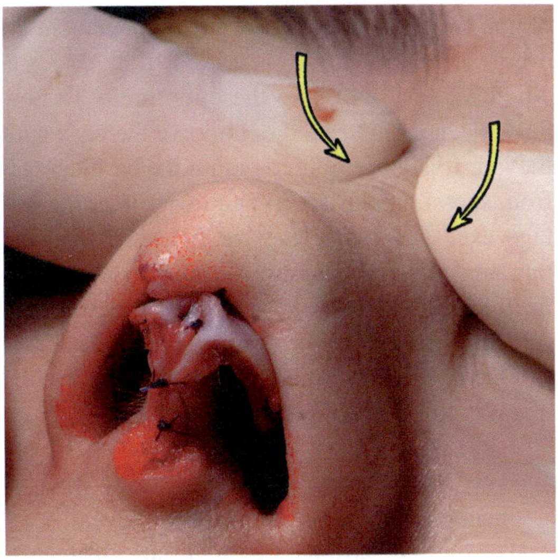

Fig. 17.58 Wrapped grafts. Once the graft is positioned and the skin flap released, only very delicate pressure should be applied to promote its final adjustment. After positioning this graft, the skin flap must no longer be moved or retracted. All that remains is to suture the marginal and columellar incisions and stabilize the flap over the graft with external nasal taping and casting

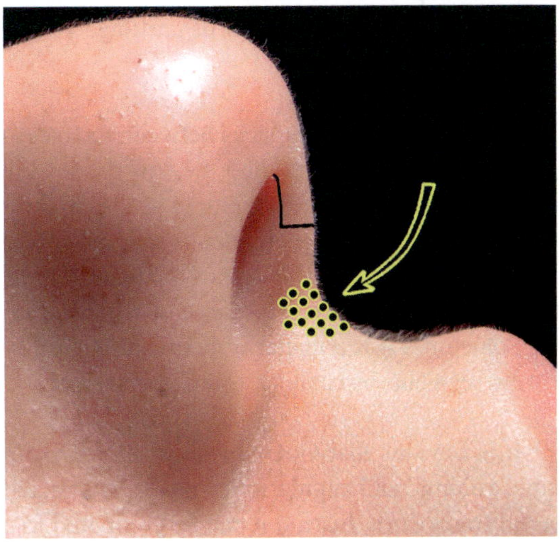

Fig. 17.59 Plumping grafts. They should be placed in a subcutaneous pocket at the base of the columella, inferior to the posterior margin of the columellar strut

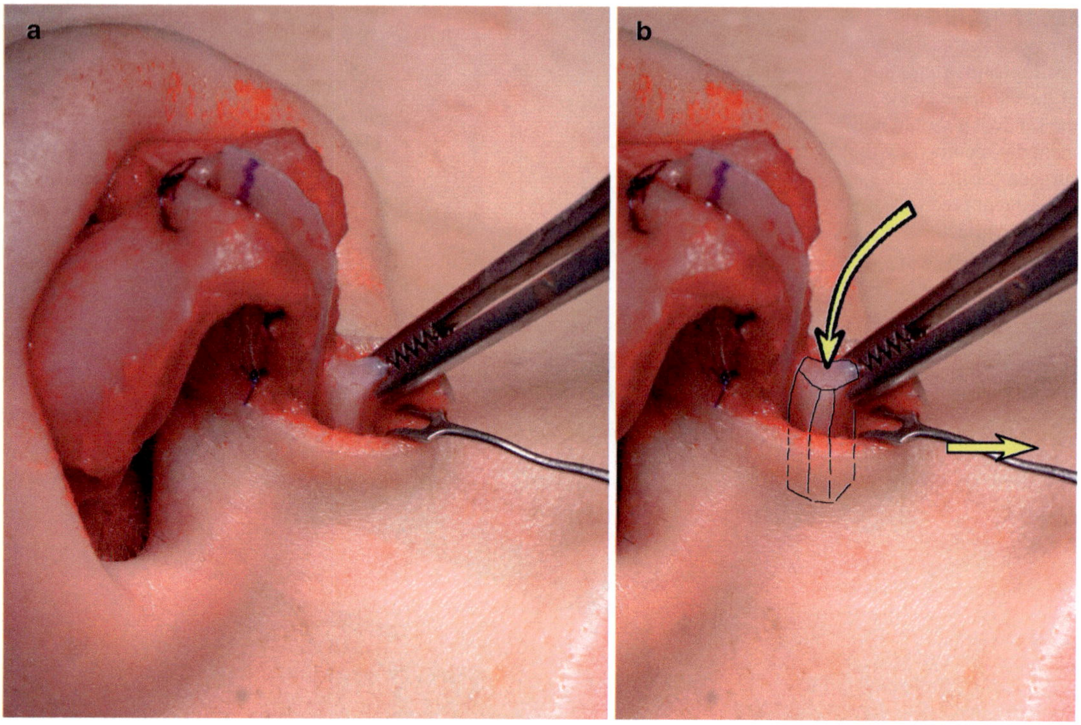

Fig. 17.60 Plumping grafts. To facilitate the insertion of the fragments, it is possible to spread the skin using a small double Guthrie hook

the skin flap at the level of columellar incision. The main indications for gel of cartilage (GoC) are two:

- Filling in the empty spaces between the osteocartilaginous skeleton and the soft tissue skin flap. The aim is to fill the empty spaces to limit the production of subcutaneous scar tissue and to fine-tune the final shape of the nose.
- Improving small irregularities and asymmetries. Sometimes it is a matter of harmonizing different segments by creating a smooth transition.

It is obvious that GoC never changes projection, volume, and angularity of the reconstructed nasal framework. Instead it can be compared to a "stucco" paste used to finish a surface or, better, to gently shape and smooth an already "good" nose. If the surgeon is not satisfied with the work done so far, it will not be the cartilage gel graft that will change the final result.

Being the last graft performed before the end of the procedure, only careful management of every piece of cartilage harvested during the whole surgery will give the opportunity to now have the amount needed to improve the nose with the gel. It is preferable to obtain the cartilage gel from septal, upper lateral and lower lateral cartilage excess. Small pieces or twisted fragments that are not otherwise usable are a good source for this purpose. Also fragments of concha or rib cartilages can be used.

One of the many methods to prepare the GoC involves the following steps:

- Both the surgeon and his assistant wear a clean pair of sterile powder-free gloves.
- The unused cartilage fragments are all cleaned with a sterile saline-soaked gauze and then placed on dry gauze. For an ideal preparation of the GoC, it is preferable that the cartilage is just moist and not dried.

- The larger-sized fragments are cut into thin strips (Fig. 17.61).
- The cartilage fragments are gently pressed one by one with a Rubin septal morselizer or alternatively with a needle holder (Fig. 17.62a, b). Care should be taken to obtain a soft uniform paste without solid pieces (Fig. 17.63). Sometimes the soft paste obtained can be composed of macroscopic fragments due to the presence of connecting fibers of perichondrium, which must be cut into smaller pieces.
- The GoC is then transferred to a 1 cc syringe after having extracted the piston from the barrel (Fig. 17.64).
- The piston is put back into the barrel (Fig. 17.65) and pressed firmly while main-

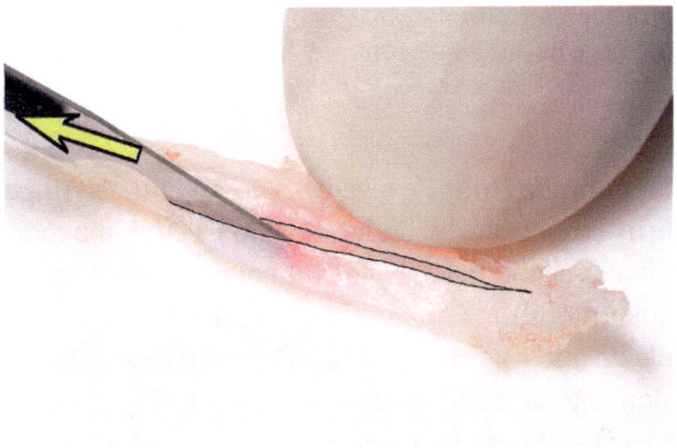

Fig. 17.61 Gel of cartilage graft preparation. The larger-sized fragments are cut into thin strips

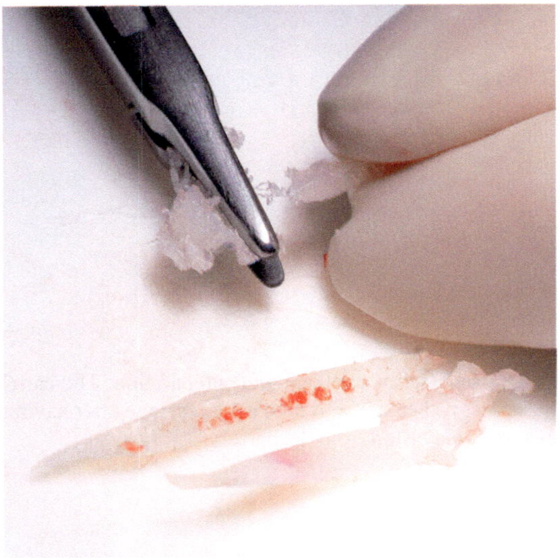

Fig. 17.63 Gel of cartilage graft preparation. Care should be taken to obtain a soft uniform paste without solid pieces

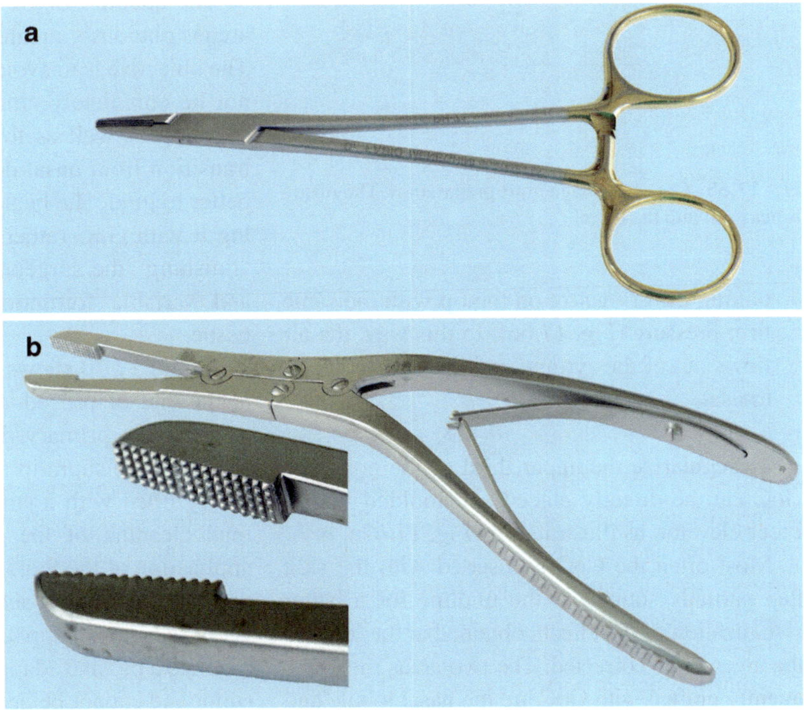

Fig. 17.62 (**a**, **b**) Gel of cartilage graft preparation. The cartilage fragments are gently pressed one by one with a Rubin septal morselizer or alternatively with a needle holder

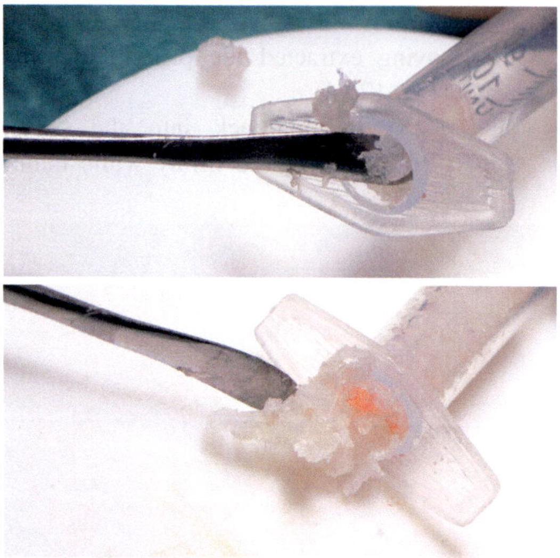

Fig. 17.64 Gel of cartilage graft preparation. The cartilage paste is then transferred to a 1 cc syringe after having extracted the piston from the barrel

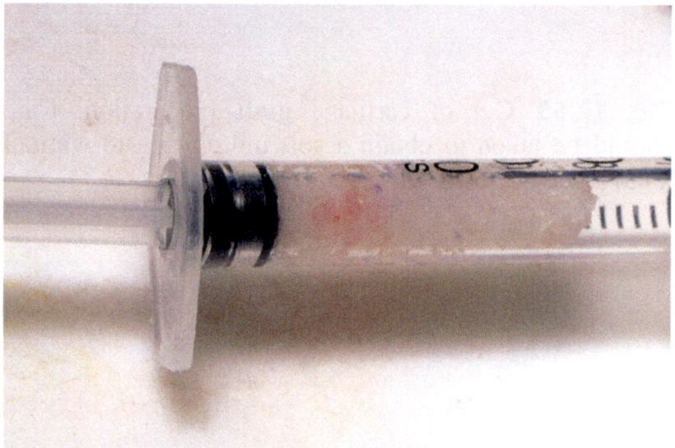

Fig. 17.65 Gel of cartilage graft preparation. The piston is put back into the barrel

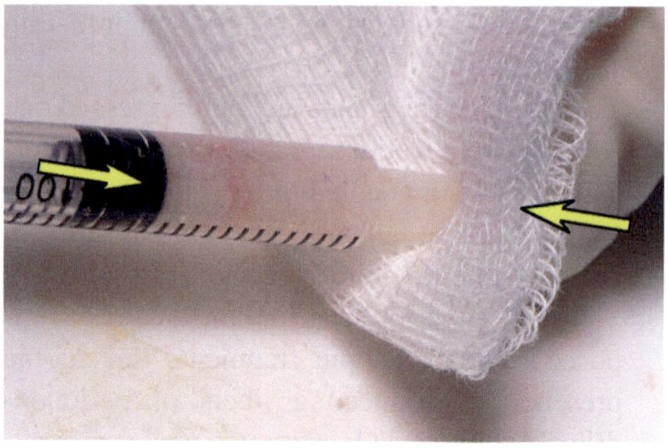

Fig. 17.66 Gel of cartilage graft preparation. The piston is then pressed firmly while maintaining the dry gauze on the tip with the same firm pressure. In this way, the air flows out of the syringe

taining the dry gauze on the tip with the same firm pressure (Fig. 17.66). In this way, the air flows out of the syringe and the GoC is ready to use.

To regularize the upper third of the nose, the GoC can be directly placed and molded with a Freer elevator, as illustrated by Fig. 17.67a, b.

Most often the GoC is inserted with the skin flap partially sutured in the midline for a better visualization of the effects obtained at the level of the areas to be corrected. The two areas most frequently grafted with GoC are the nasal lobule and the supratip (Fig. 17.68a, b). The tip of the syringe is inserted laterally under the flap through the marginal incision that has not yet been closed. A small quantity of the GoC is injected into the nasal lobule area to fill every little empty space between the skin and the cartilaginous framework (Fig. 17.69a, b). Care should be taken not to create a bump that disrupts the fine architecture of the nasal tip. Every excess of GoC must be removed with a delicate Adson Brown tissue forceps.

The quantity of GoC injected in the supratip area is obviously greater than in the nasal lobule. The objective is to avoid an empty space that cannot be completely closed later with taping and splinting as well as to create a smooth straight transition from nasal dorsum to tip. Ideally, it is better to guide the healing of the supratip by filling it with GoC rather than to leave the task of "finishing" the surgeon's work to the inevitable and variable formation of subcutaneous scar tissue.

Figure 17.70 shows the final profile obtained at the end of procedure in a male patient after conservative primary rhinoplasty. All the empty spaces in the supratip and nasal lobule areas are gently filled with a small quantity of GoC. The final cleaning of the skin and the subsequent application of the Steri-Strips must be performed with the utmost care and attention by the first surgeon. Also the application of the nasal cast requires a passive adaptation of the thermoplastic splint and cannot be delegated.

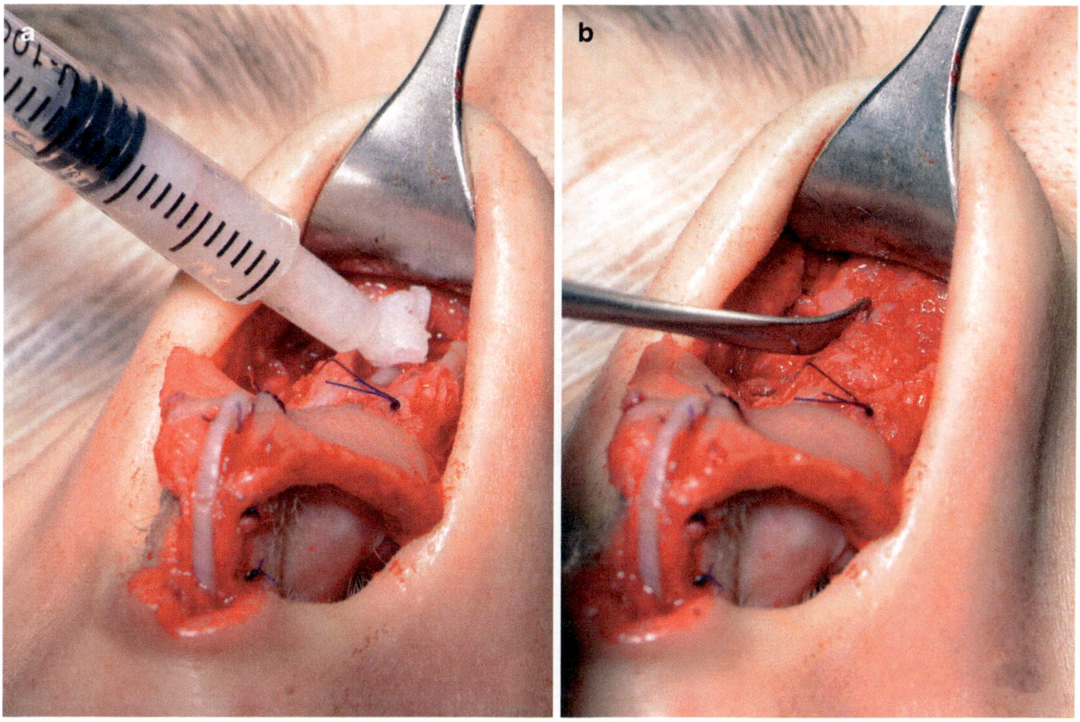

Fig. 17.67 (**a**, **b**) Gel of cartilage grafts. To regularize the upper third of the nose, the GoC can be directly placed and molded with a Freer elevator

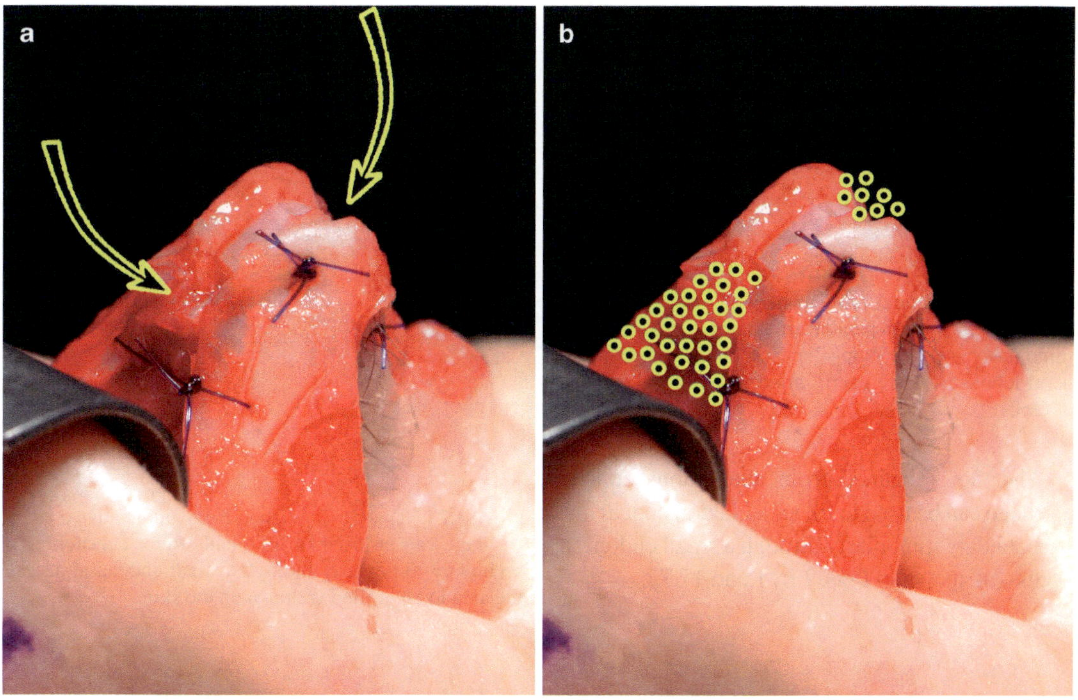

Fig. 17.68 (**a**, **b**) The two areas most frequently grafted with GoC are the nasal lobule and the supratip. The tip of the syringe is inserted laterally under the flap through the marginal incision that has not yet been closed

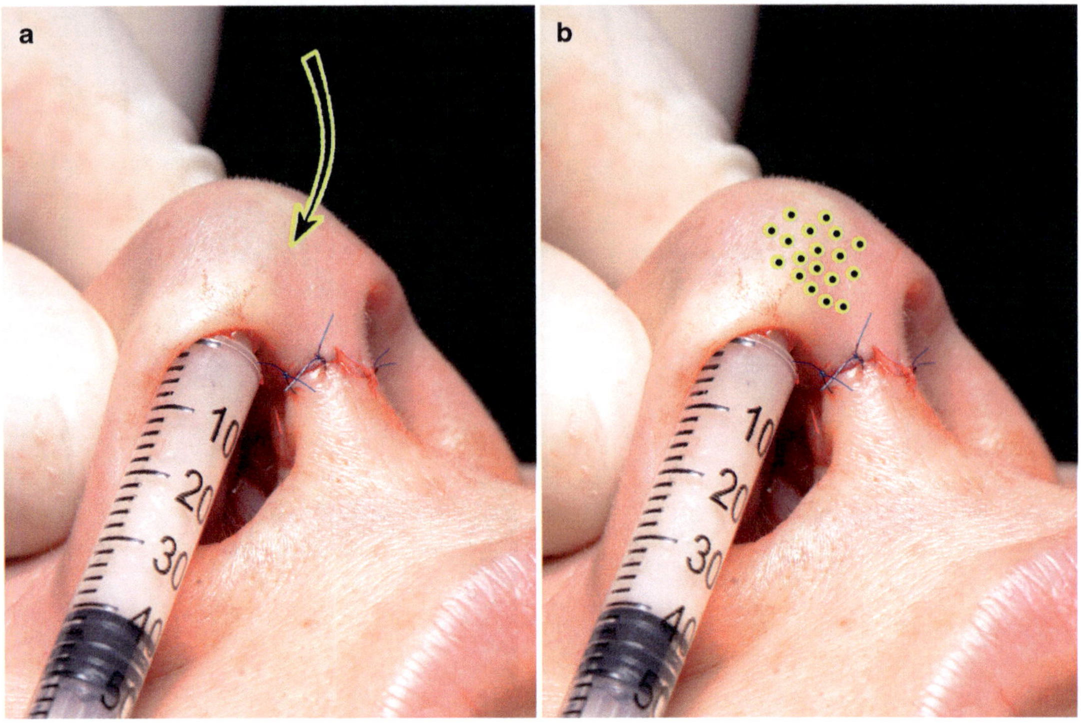

Fig. 17.69 (**a**, **b**) Nasal lobule grafting. A small quantity of GoC is injected into the nasal lobule area to fill every little empty space between the skin and the underlying cartilaginous framework

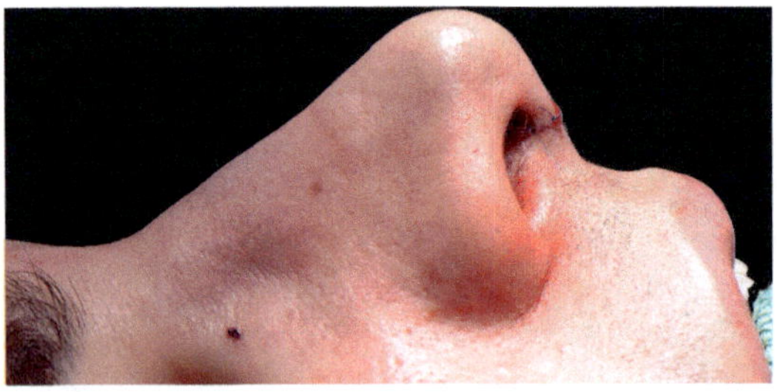

Fig. 17.70 The final profile obtained at the end of the procedure in a male patient after conservative primary rhinoplasty. All the empty spaces in the supratip and nasal lobule areas are gently filled with a small quantity of GoC

The GoC obtained from autogenous conchal cartilage can be used to fill small lateral concavities in secondary rhinoplasty through a small endonasal access, as shown in Figs. 17.71 and 17.72.

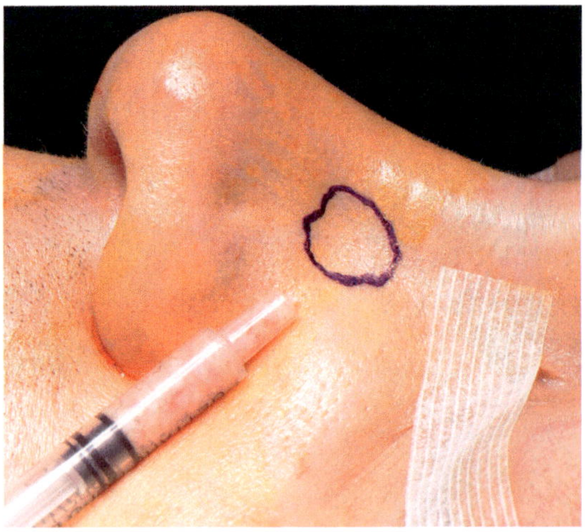

Fig. 17.71 The GoC obtained from autogenous conchal cartilage can be used to fill small lateral concavities in secondary rhinoplasty through a small endonasal access: the area to be grafted is drawn on the skin

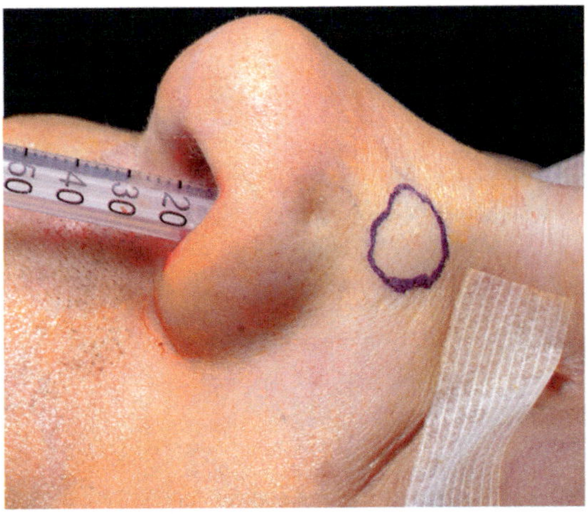

Fig. 17.72 The GoC obtained from autogenous conchal cartilage can be used to fill small lateral concavities in secondary rhinoplasty through a small endonasal access: placement of the GoC

17.12 Closure of the Marginal and Columellar Skin Incisions

The columellar incision is closed first taking care to perfectly align the angles of the skin flaps. In the past, the preferred suture material was 6-0 polypropylene non-absorbable monofilament. The suture is pigmented blue to enhance visibility. Complete removal of the monofilament is to occur within 6–8 days after surgery.

Currently the preference is for a 6-0 polyglactin absorbable braided suture with an 11 mm 3/8 circle needle. Figure 17.73a, b shows the disposition of the columellar sutures on the right side. On average, 8 to 10 single sutures are performed. Removal does not routinely require trimming and

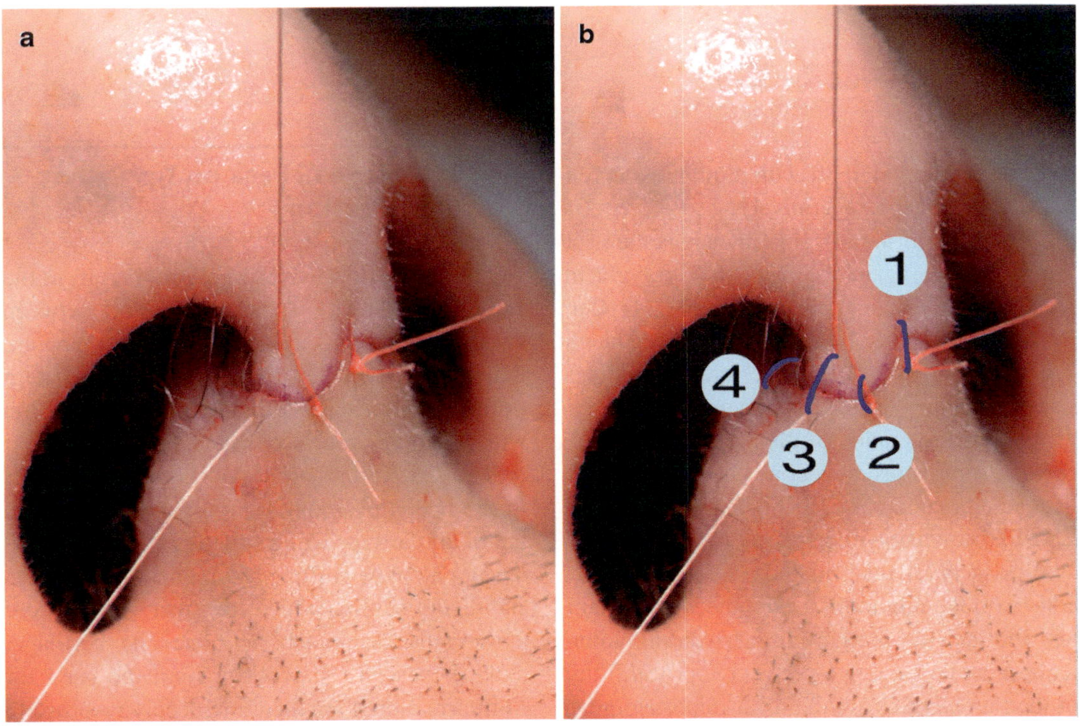

Fig. 17.73 (**a**, **b**) Columellar skin sutures

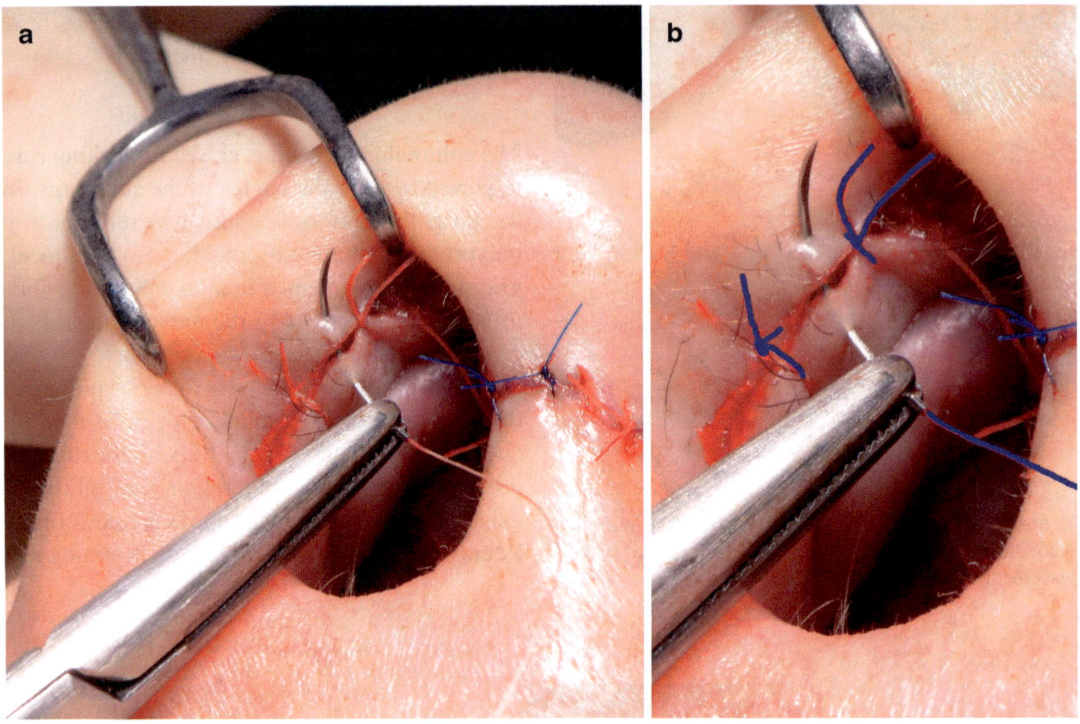

Fig. 17.74 (**a**, **b**) Marginal skin sutures

the sutures tend to fall off with minimal intervention 10–14 days postoperatively.

The suture of the marginal incisions then follows, utilizing again the same 6-0 polyglactin with 11 mm 3/8 circle needle (Fig. 17.74). Care should be taken not to include the lower lateral cartilage margin in the suture bite. Sometimes, while tightening a suture knot, a more or less evident upward retraction of the ala appears. In this case the suture must be redone changing its inclination and maintaining the bites as close as possible to the incision margins.

As a general rule, all these sutures must be done with the minimum tension needed to maintain the incision margin close. Avoiding suture tension[4] and obtaining a perfect reciprocal fitting of the flap margins are the most important goals for perfect and fast healing of the scar.

[4]Millard DR Jr. Principle number 21: Learn to Control Tension. In: Principlization of Plastic Surgery. Boston/Toronto: Little, Brown and Company; 1986. p. 345.

17.13 George C. Peck on Tip Projection

George C. Peck 30 years ago told me "If, at the end of the operation, the relationship between nasal tip and dorsal line appears perfect, you are making a mistake." He clearly advised me that tip projection is unstable and a small overcorrection with a thin tip graft is indicated.

The search for stability of the result obtained in the operating room, not only of the nasal tip but of all the supporting structures, has led to the development of grafting techniques and multiple stabilizing sutures which, together with a more conservative approach on bone and cartilage, make it possible to avoid or limit the need for overcorrection. I am therefore deeply indebted to Dr. Peck for stimulating me with his advice to include in my surgical practice all the solutions that help the stability of the result. One of the main effects on the BOR approach was to significantly increase the operating time spent in reconstructing and reinforcing the nose compared to the time spent in changing its shape.

So the decision to suture the columellar and marginal flaps should only be made if the surgeon and his assistant believe that each reconstructive step has been successfully completed, a stable result is reasonably reached, and no overcorrection is needed.

Further Reading

Daniel RK. Aesthetic plastic surgery: rhinoplasty. Boston: Little, Brown; 1993. p. 525–53.
Jugo S. Surgical atlas of external Rhinoplasty. Edinburgh: Churchill Livingstone; 1995.
Tebbetts JB. Primary Rhinoplasty. A new approach to the logic and the techniques. St. Louis: Mosby; 1998.
Daniel RK. Rhinoplasty. An atlas of surgical techniques. Berlin, Heidelberg: Springer-Verlag; 2002.
Daniel RK. Mastering Rhinoplasty. A comprehensive atlas of surgical techniques. New York: Springer; 2010.
Guyuron B. Rhinoplasty. Edinburgh: Elsevier Saunders; 2012.
Daniel RK, Pálházi P. Rhinoplasty. Berlin: Springer International Publishing AG; 2018.

Articles on Diced Cartilage Grafts

Erol OO. The Turkish delight: a pliable graft for rhinoplasty. Plast Reconstr Surg. 2000;105(6):2229–41.
Daniel RK. Diced cartilage grafts in Rhinoplasty surgery: current techniques and applications. Plast Reconstr Surg. 2008;122(6):1883–91.
Calvert J, Kwon E. Techniques for diced cartilage with deep temporalis fascia graft. Facial Plast Surg Clin North Am. 2015;23(1):73–80.
Kreutzer C, Hoehne J, Gubisch W, Rezaeian F, Haack S. Free diced cartilage: a new application of diced cartilage grafts in primary and secondary Rhinoplasty. Plast Reconstr Surg. 2017;140(3):461–70.

18 Basic Open Rhinoplasty: Alar Base Work and Final Nose Dressing

Once the suture of the columellar and marginal incisions has been completed, the nose is re-evaluated for shape and size. In case of doubts, asymmetries, or palpable irregularities, it is necessary to remove the sutures, lift the skin flap, and review every problematic detail.

If, on the other hand, the result obtained so far is fine, there may still be two points of the treatment plan to be performed:

- Approximation of excessively divergent footplates of the alar cartilages.
- Correction of a wide or asymmetric alar base.

These two optional and final steps of rhinoplasty should not be forgotten or considered less important because they can have a major influence on the esthetic and functional final result.

18.1 Approximation of the Footplates

The medial contour of the nostril aperture can be deformed and reduced in width either by a deviated caudal septum or by an excess of divergence of the footplates of the medial crura. Figure 18.1 shows a basal view of a clinical case in which both conditions are present on the right side, whereas an isolated excess of footplate divergence characterizes the left side. The ideal goal is to obtain a centered and slim base of the columella through fixing in the midline the caudal septum as well as reducing symmetrically the divergence of the footplates.

The approximation of the footplates can be better addressed later, after closure of the columellar and marginal incisions and before a possible alar base surgery.

This small adjunctive procedure can be divided into the following steps:

- Palpate the membranous septum where the footplates protrude and draw their margins with a sterile skin marker (Fig. 18.2).
- Hydrodissect the skin on each side with 0.5 cc of mepivacaine hydrochloride 2% solution with 1:100,000 epinephrine (Fig. 18.3).
- Expose the footplates with a superficial skin incision of about 2 mm (Fig. 18.4) and a gentle dissection with Converse angled scissors paying attention not to injure the underlying cartilage.
- Pass a polypropylene 5–0 nonabsorbable monofilament suture twice or four times from one footplate to the other (Figs. 18.5 and 18.6).
- Tie incrementally the knot until the desired approximation of the footplates is obtained (Fig. 18.7). As a result of the approximation of the cartilages, the nasolabial angle is filled by the protrusion of the soft tissues between the two medial crura. In the case of thin and fragile cartilages, it is preferable to double or triple the needle passages through

F. Meneghini, *Basic Open Rhinoplasty*, https://doi.org/10.1007/978-3-030-61827-8_18

Fig. 18.1 (**a**, **b**) Basal view of a clinical case characterized by deformed and reduced nostril apertures due to a deviated caudal septum towards the right side (curved arrow) and excess of divergence of the footplates of the medial crura (straight double arrow)

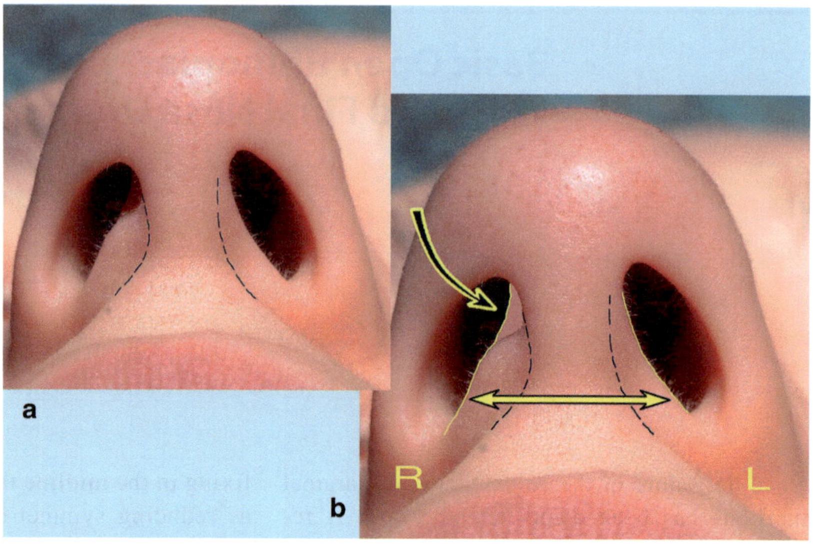

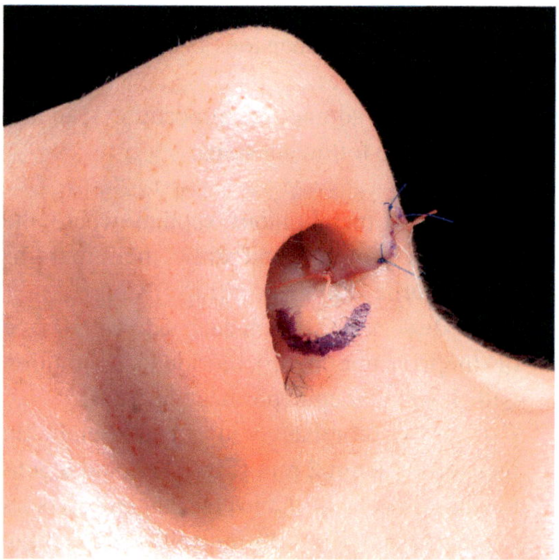

Fig. 18.2 Approximation of the footplates. The protruding posterior margins of the footplates are drawn with a sterile skin marker

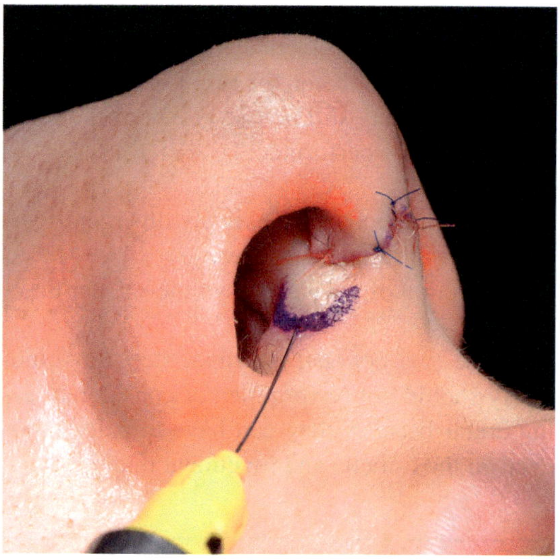

Fig. 18.3 Approximation of the footplates. With a very superficial bilateral injection of about 0.5 cc of mepivacaine hydrochloride 2% solution with 1:100,000 epinephrine the skin over the footplates is hydrodissected

the footplates to obtain the same clinical effect but reducing the overall tension of the suture and spreading the force applied over a larger area.

– If needed, suture the membranous septum skin incisions with one or two stitches of 6–0 polyglactin absorbable braided suture.

18.2 Principles and Techniques of Alar Base Surgery

A slight excess of width of the alar base is a common nasal deformity that is frequently overlooked by the patient as well as the surgeon. So,

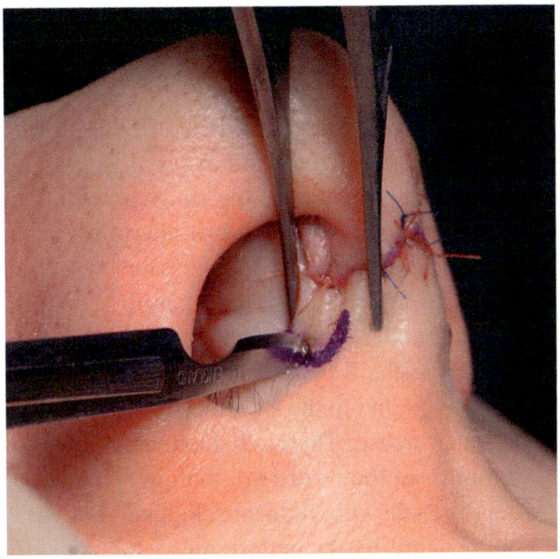

Fig. 18.4 Approximation of the footplates. Exposure of the footplates with a superficial skin incision of about 2 mm using a 15c blade and then with a gentle dissection using Converse angled scissors paying attention not to injure the underlying cartilage

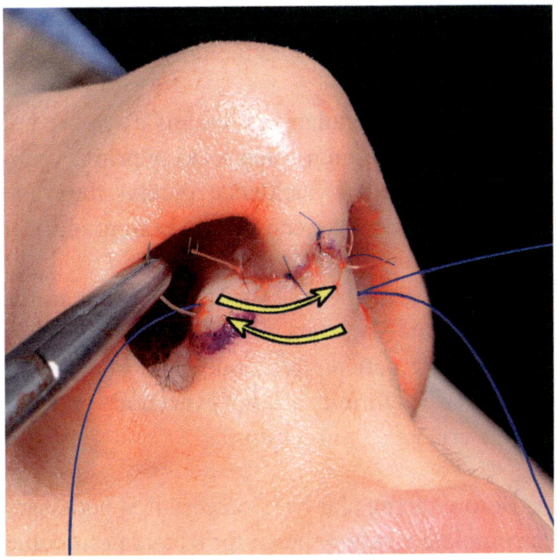

Fig. 18.6 Approximation of the footplates. From one footplate to the other, pass a polypropylene 5-0 nonabsorbable monofilament suture twice or four times through the skin incisions

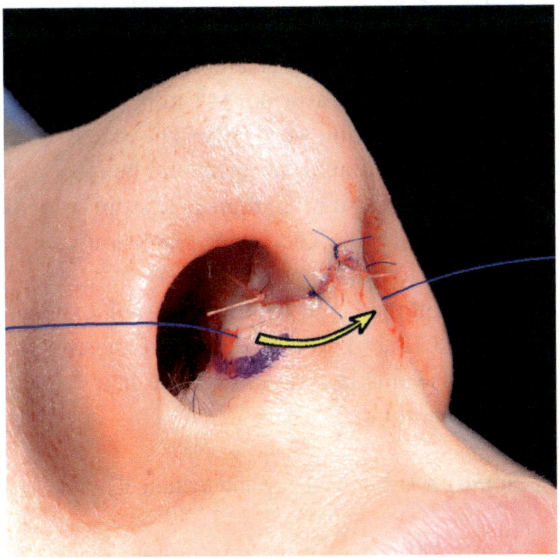

Fig. 18.5 Approximation of the footplates. From one footplate to the other, pass a polypropylene 5-0 nonabsorbable monofilament suture twice or four times through the skin incisions

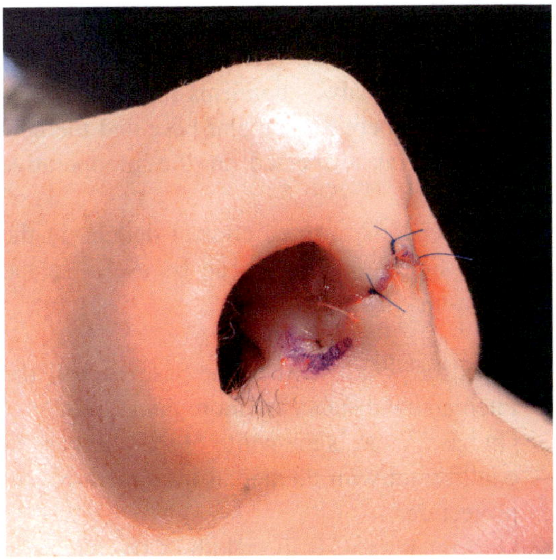

Fig. 18.7 Approximation of the footplates. The knot should be tied incrementally until the desired approximation of the footplates is obtained

changing the shape and width of the alar base is frequently indicated but rarely performed. It should always be discussed with the patient during the preoperative visits.

On review of my last 100 consecutive rhinoplasty cases, I found that some type of alar base excision was performed in only six cases. Of these six, only one patient explicitly requested a reduction of the width of the alar base at the first preoperative visit. This small percentage is probably due to several factors including:

- This patient population is mainly composed of young Caucasian women seeking primary surgery with a low incidence of alar flare and disproportion between tip projection and alar base width.
- The fear that the scars will be evident in the eyes of the observers.
- Only few patients are concerned about their alar base deformity and not everybody believes it is crucial to correct it.

Before facing alar base surgery it is necessary to completely suture the marginal and columellar incisions and the approximation of the footplates of the medial crura, if done. After cleaning the skin of the nose and the whole face with moistened gauze, it is time to review and confirm the objectives of this ancillary surgery and to measure again the extent and the design of the skin resection. The presence of previous or new asymmetries must also be reassessed. Usually this intraoperative analysis confirms the presence of an imbalance between the alar base and the new nasal shape as suspected in the preoperative analysis.

A closer look at three clinical details, in the form of simple questions, can be useful in the decision-making process:

- Does the width of the alar base exceed the intercanthal distance by more than 2 mm?
- On basal view, is the width of the alar base in equilibrium with the actual intraoperative tip projection?
- On frontal view, is the width of the alar base excessive compared to the middle third of the nose after the osteotomies?

A prerequisite for alar base surgery is that the caudal septum, the columella, and the nasal tip must be well centered in the midline both for the risk of secondary impaired nasal function and for the whole esthetic result.

In essence we can divide the most frequent alar base procedures into two subgroups with the possibility of combining them together into a third one:

- A—Alar wedge excision (Fig. 18.8a, b). The objective is to reduce the excess of alar base flare without reducing the transverse dimension of the sill of the nostril aperture. It is a 2–3 mm wide wedge skin resection (V-excision) with its lower margin set 1 mm above the alar crease. The lateral extension is limited to the 8 o'clock position for the right alar crease and to the 4 o'clock position for the left alar crease. The medial extension stops at 2 mm from the nostril sill margin. The wedge depth reaches the mid-muscle level, but without penetrating the underlying vestibular skin. These precautions are necessary to avoid retraction and deformity of the nostril aperture with functional reduction of the external nasal valve.
- B—Nostril sill excision (Fig. 18.9a, b). The objective is to reduce the "nostril show" on anterior view by a transverse reduction of the sill of the nostril aperture. The skin wedge, with a width measuring 2–4 mm, is centered in the floor quite vertically. The integrity of the nasal vestibular lining should be respected by not incising it more than 1–1.5 mm from its anterior margin. The lower extension can be set close to the wing fold.
- C—Combined alar wedge and sill excision (Fig. 18.10a, b). The objective is to narrow the alar base maximally and reduce alar flare at the same time.

Some important guiding and technical points are:

- Apply Millard's principle number 23: When in doubt, don't.[1]
- Be precise. The precision of the planned skin excision design is essential for obtaining the result (Fig. 18.11). The use of a thin-tipped skin marker is therefore recommended.

[1]Millard DR. Executional Principle number 23: When in Doubt, Don't. In: Principlization of Plastic Surgery. Boston/Toronto: Little, Brown and Company; 1986. p. 402.

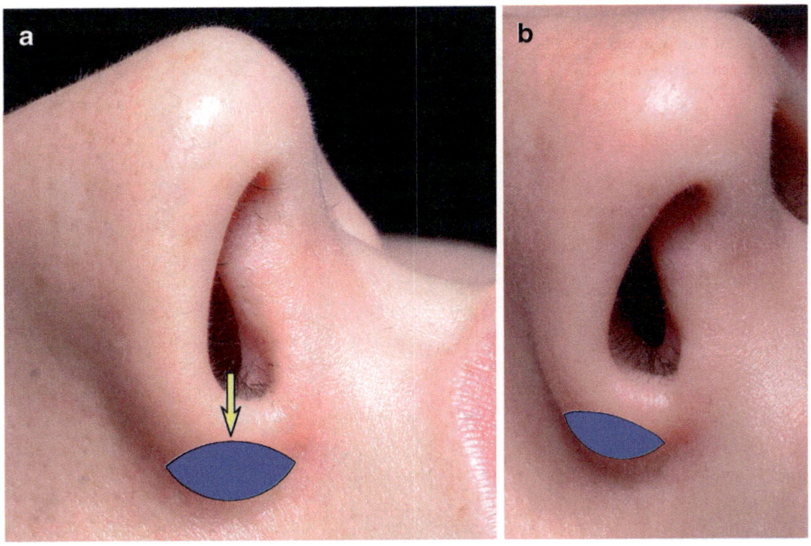

Fig. 18.8 (**a**, **b**) Alar wedge excision (see text)

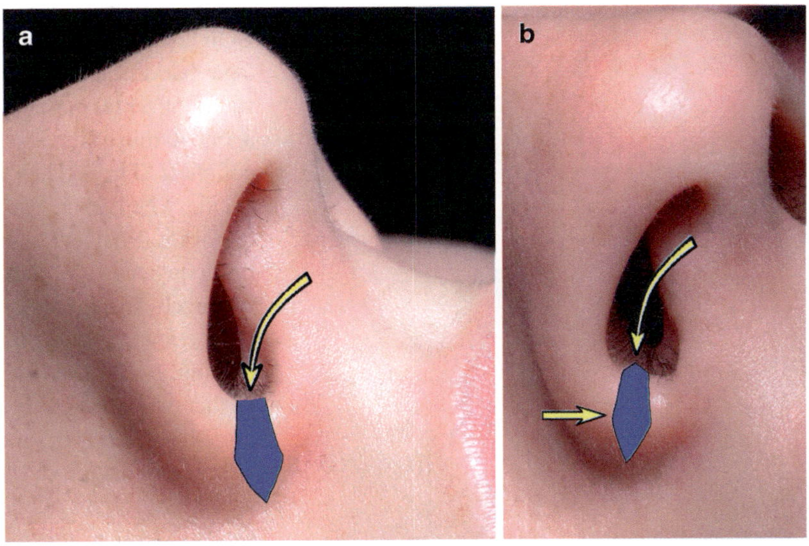

Fig. 18.9 (**a**, **b**) Nostril sill excision (see text)

- Always plan conservatively. Increasing the amount of resection if necessary is easy, whereas over-resection is exceedingly difficult to correct.
- Respect the integrity of the nasal vestibular lining by not incising it more than 1–1.5 mm from its anterior margin.
- Always use a 15c fresh blade for the skin incision and then complete the planned excision with a Colorado microdissection needle setting the electrosurgical unit at low voltage.
- Always cauterize the small bleeding vessels before suturing the flaps.
- Pass and gently tie one or two deep sutures in 5/0 polydioxanone replacing it until a perfect match of the flaps is obtained.
- Perform skin closure with 6/0 polyglactin absorbable braided multifilament or 6/0 polypropylene monofilament.

After alar base surgery, the nostril opening should be re-evaluated for shape and dimension. Frequently, the need for surgical approximation of the footplates can become evident only at this stage as depicted in Fig. 18.12.

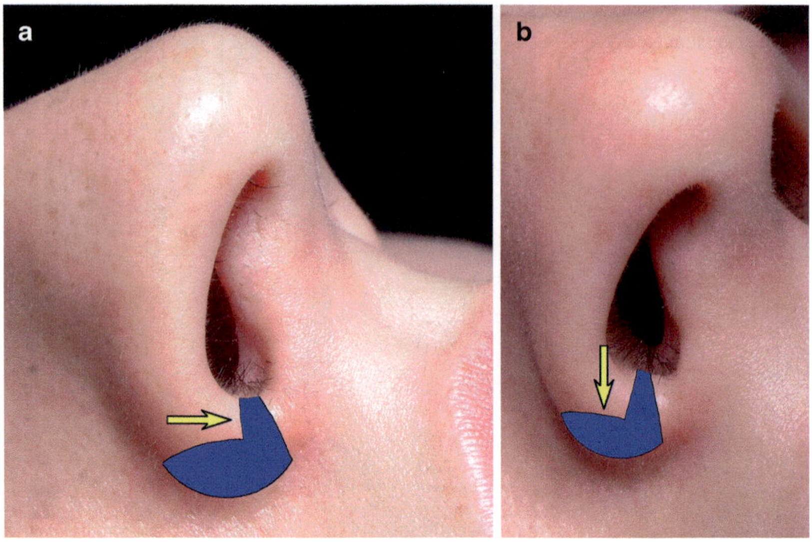

Fig. 18.10 (**a**, **b**) Combined alar wedge and sill excision (see text)

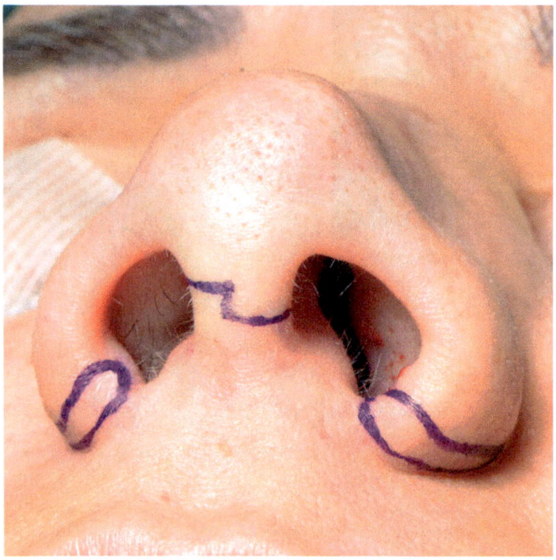

Fig. 18.11 Alar base surgery. Drawing precisely the skin incisions with a thin-tipped skin marker is mandatory

The removal of the alar base skin sutures should be done after 7–8 days, during the first postoperative visit.

18.3 Removal of Bilateral Nasal Packing

To improve hemostasis, a bilateral nasal packing with Merocel sponges soaked with tranexamic acid is done after some of the almost fixed steps of the BOR method: complete septal surgery with cartilage harvesting, turbinate surgery, and quilting suture of septal mucosa (see Chap. 16). Now, after about 40 min of more superficial work and with the complete skin incision sutures done, it is time to decide whether to keep the packing in place or remove it (Fig. 18.13). In over 50% of the patients, the sponges can be removed after analyzing retrospectively the intraoperative bleeding as well as other clinical and instrumental data related to blood clotting. In BOR leaving in place the packing for a further stabilization of the nasal framework for more than 24 h is never done. The meticulous multiple sutures of the cartilages and sometimes of the nasal bones represent the best and widely sufficient way to stabilize the recomposed nasal structures during the first postoperative period.

18.4 Taping and Splinting

After having gently cleaned and dried the nasal and facial skin, a step carried out personally by the first surgeon, the nose is taped with multiple cut-to-size pieces of R1547 Steri-Strip.[2] Figure 18.14 shows the cutting of the first strips reduced in their

[2] 3 M, R1547 Steri-Strip, 12 mm × 100 mm. The author has no conflict of interest with this or other 3 M products.

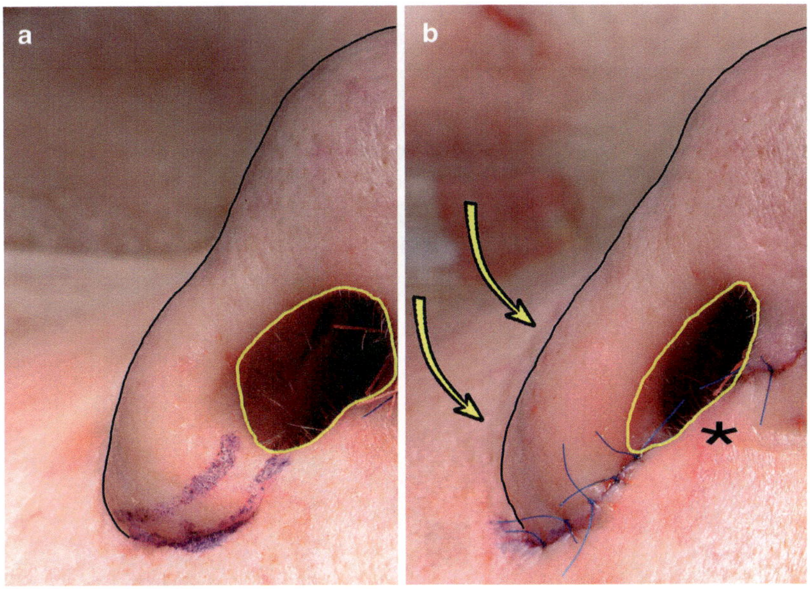

Fig. 18.12 (**a**, **b**) Alar base surgery. After alar base surgery, the nostril opening should be re-evaluated for shape and dimension. Frequently the need for surgical approximation of the footplates can be evident

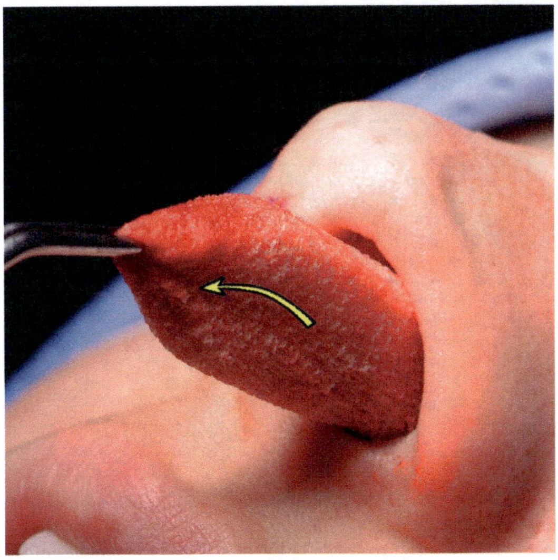

Fig. 18.13 Removal of bilateral nasal packing

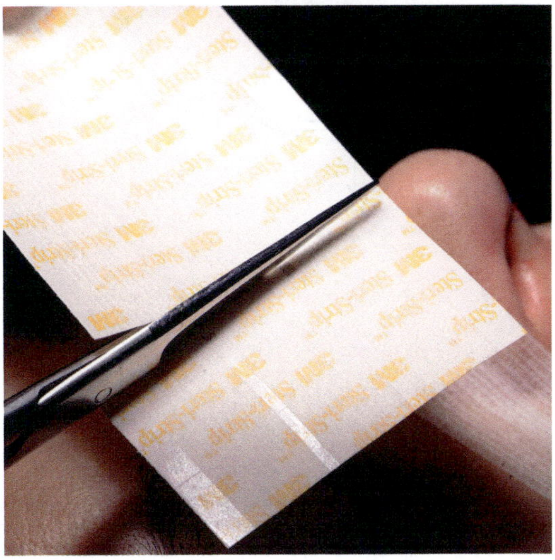

Fig. 18.14 Taping and splinting. The nose is taped with multiple cut-to-size pieces of R1547 Steri-Strip. The first strips are reduced in their length to 9 or 8 cm

length to 9 or 8 cm. The Steri-Strips are then applied to the nasal skin beginning caudally with an inferiorly and posteriorly directed gentle pressure (Fig. 18.15). Each new strip will be shorter than the previous one to which it is applied with a partial overlap (Fig. 18.16). To tape the radix area of the nose, it is essential to cut and apply small strips to leave the skin close to the palpebral commissures free.

The external dressing is then completed by applying a small and thin thermoplastic splint. A useful and inexpensive method is that of cutting out a small piece of low temperature Aquaplast from a large sheet. All pieces can be pre-cut in the shape of an isosceles trapezoid with these dimensions (Fig. 18.17):

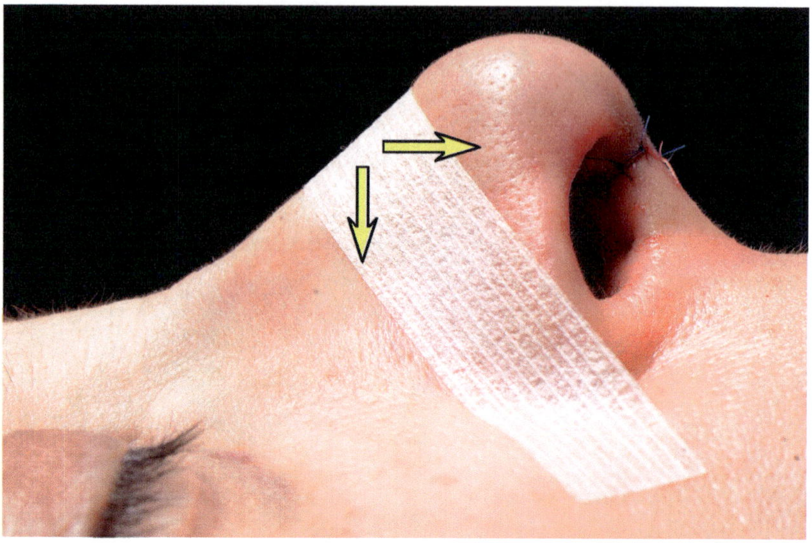

Fig. 18.15 Taping and splinting. The Steri-Strips are then applied to the nasal skin beginning caudally with an inferiorly and posteriorly directed gentle pressure

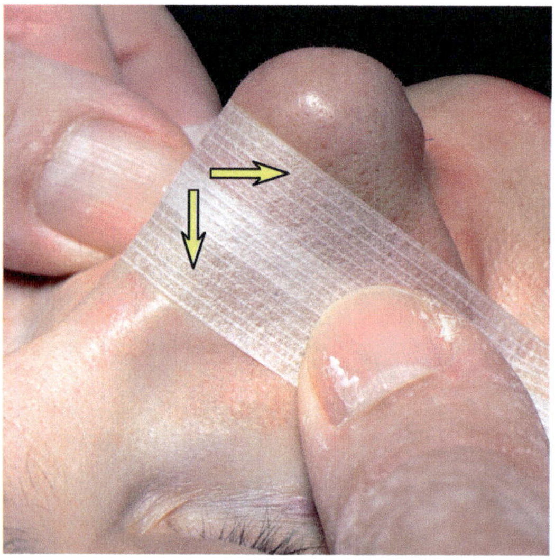

Fig. 18.16 Taping and splinting. Each new strip will be shorter than the previous one to which it is applied with a partial overlap

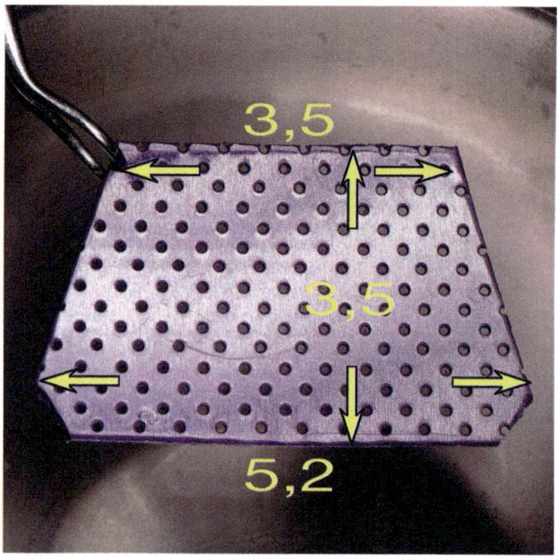

Fig. 18.17 Taping and splinting. Thermoplastic splint (Aquaplast) obtained from a large sheet and cut by the surgeon in the shape of an isosceles trapezoid

- Large lower margin: 52 mm.
- Small upper margin: 35 mm.
- Height: 35 mm.

This size is perfect for a large nose and therefore should often be reduced proportionally before being used. The nasal splint is then grasped with a small Backhaus towel clamp and held over a steel bowl while an assistant pours boiling water (Fig. 18.18). Within seconds the low temperature thermoplastic material becomes soft and it should be quickly placed and shaped over the Steri-Strip. The maneuver must be rapid but very delicate; it is not a matter of pressing vigorously to model the nasal framework but rather to create a well-adapted protective shell (Fig. 18.19). In positioning the splint, as for the Steri-Strips, it is essential to maintain an adequate distance from the skin close to the medial palpebral commissures, as indicated with the arrows in Fig. 18.20.

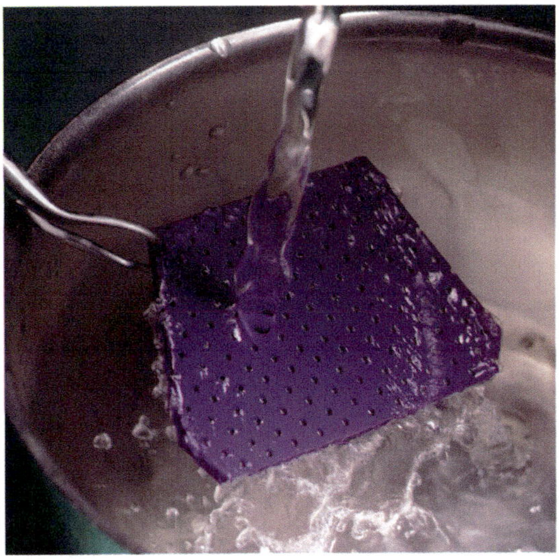

Fig. 18.18 Taping and splinting. The nasal splint, grasped with a small Backhaus towel clamp, is held over a steel bowl while an assistant pours boiling water. Within seconds the thermoplastic material becomes soft and it should be quickly placed and shaped over the Steri-Strip

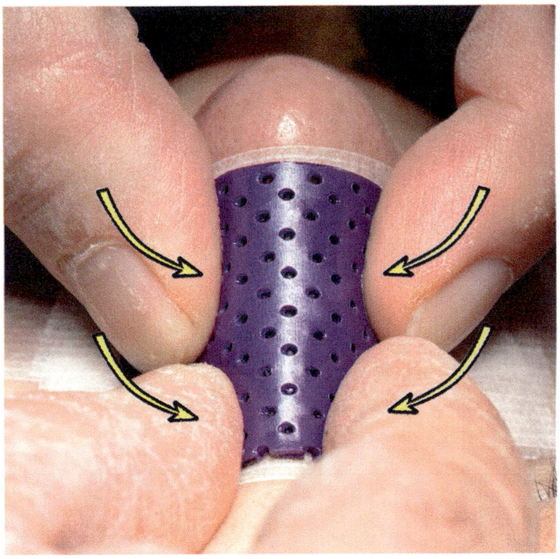

Fig. 18.19 Taping and splinting. The soft thermoplastic splint should be applied very gently, as it is not meant to shape the nasal framework but rather to create a well-adapted protective shell

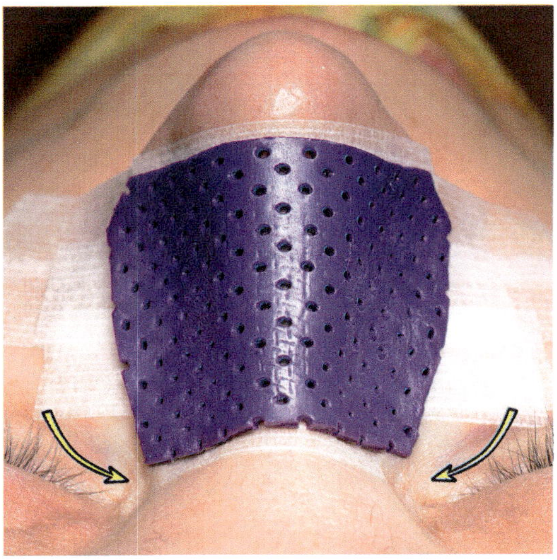

Fig. 18.20 Taping and splinting. In positioning the thermoplastic splint, as for the Steri-Strips, it is essential to maintain an adequate distance from the medial palpebral commissures

Finally, two paper plasters are applied to stabilize the nasal splint and a gauze drip pad is placed under the nose to absorb drainage.

Further Reading

Books

Guyuron B. Rhinoplasty. Edinburgh: Elsevier Saunders; 2012.

Articles on Alar Base Surgery

Guyuron B, Behmand RA. Alar base abnormalities. Classification and correction. Clin Plast Surg. 1996;23(2):263–70.

Kridel RW, Castellano RD. A simplified approach to alar base reduction: a review of 124 patients over 20 years. Arch Facial Plast Surg. 2005;7(2):81–93.

Foda HM. Nasal base narrowing: the combined alar base excision technique. Arch Facial Plast Surg. 2007;9:30–4.

19 Chin Surgery for Rhinoplasty Patients

Esthetic chin surgery is by far one of the least practiced by professionals and the most unknown among common people. In everyday practice, patients ask for an improvement in the profile of the nose often without realizing that the position and shape of the chin is somehow related to their problem. So, why does this surgery represent, from a statistical point of view, a small niche, even though it is desirable in many cases? The possible reasons are:

- Patients rarely require correction of chin deformity because they are often not fully aware of it.
- Few surgeons routinely deal with chin and nose surgery with equal competence.
- Few surgeons have had the vision and the strength to create a multidisciplinary team to deal with state-of-the-art chin, jaw, and nose surgery on an ongoing basis. Most of the time collaborations between professionals remain occasional events involving individual clinical cases.

Another negative aspect, which continues to influence chin surgery, concerns the area of origin of the specialists and the approach they prefer. Plastic surgeons and facial plastic surgeons prefer a transcutaneous submental approach with the insertion of an alloplastic implant. Maxillofacial surgeons use mainly an intraoral approach that involves one or more osteotomies, the repositioning of the chin and its stabilization, by internal rigid fixation with titanium plates and screws, in the planned position. This *modus operandi* is absurd since the decision to apply a technique in a given patient does not depend on which is more suitable but on the different basic training of the surgeons.

19.1 Clinical Analysis of the Lower Third of the Face

The study of the lower third of the face requires a preoperative photographic documentation of at least seven full-face projections: frontal, right and left oblique, right and left profile, basal and face-down (see Chap. 4). Knowledge of some points and lines described in Fig. 19.1 is also essential.

The external shape of the chin is directly related to the development of the entire mandible as well as to its grade of spatial inclination. Figure 19.2 shows the facial profile of a young female patient with a well-developed mandible in the posterior-anterior dimension as well as a gentle counterclockwise rotation of the body of the mandible. The soft tissues over the chin are well supported by the bony skeleton. The overall angles and curves from the tip of the nose to the neck outline are proportioned and esthetically pleasant. In particular, a vertical line drawn from the tip of the nose passes not too far from the

F. Meneghini, *Basic Open Rhinoplasty*, https://doi.org/10.1007/978-3-030-61827-8_19

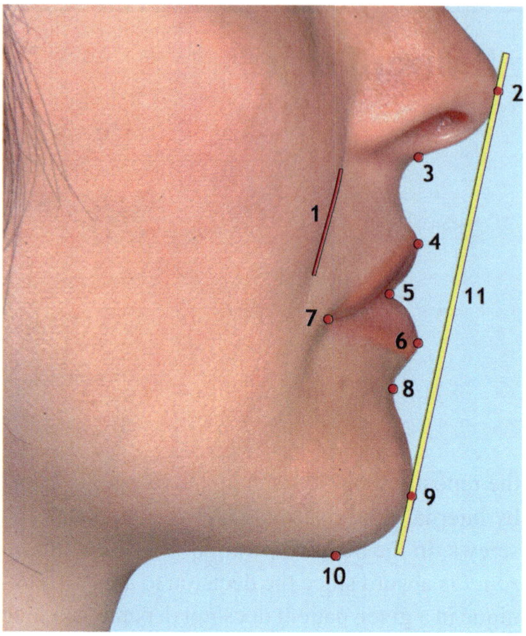

Fig. 19.1 Lower third profile. Reference points and Ricketts' lips projection reference E-line: *1* nasolabial sulcus, *2* nasal tip, *3* subnasale, *4* labrale superior, *5* stomion, *6* labrale inferior, *7* lip commissure, *8* labiomental sulcus, *9* soft tissue pogonion, *10* soft tissue menton, *11* Ricketts' E-line. The series of gentle curves from nasal tip to soft tissue menton characterize the profile of the lips

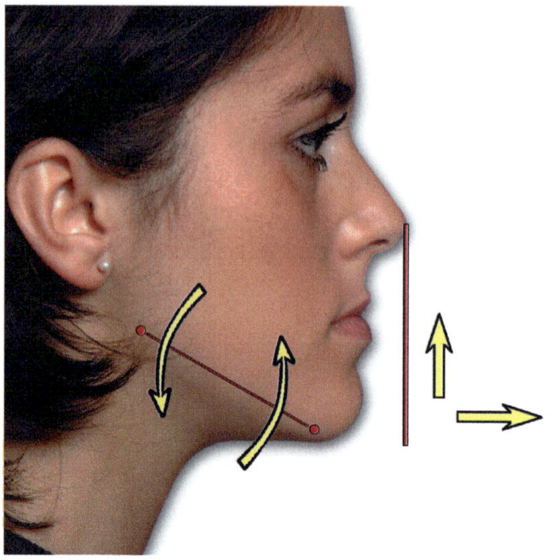

Fig. 19.2 Profile view of a young female patient with a well-developed mandible in the posterior-anterior dimension as well as a gentle counterclockwise rotation of the body of the mandible. The soft tissues over the chin are well supported by the bony skeleton. The overall angles and curves from the tip of the nose to the neck outline are proportioned and esthetically pleasant. In particular, a vertical line drawn from the tip of the nose passes not too far from the chin

chin. Figure 19.3 shows the facial profile of a young male patient with an underdeveloped mandible in the posterior-anterior dimension and a significant clockwise rotation of the body of the mandible. The soft tissues over the chin are poorly supported and several of the angles and curves from the tip of the nose to the neck outline flatten.

19.2 Cephalometric Analysis of the Lower Third of the Face

Angular and linear measurements performed on lateral cephalometric radiographs (LCR) play an essential role in orthodontic treatment and orthognathic surgery routine diagnostics. The bone morphology, the anteroposterior and vertical position of the chin, and the relationship between the skin profile and the bone profile of the chin can all be assessed from an LCR.

Many measurement methods have been hypothesized and studied statistically to define the average values for large groups of people and so to establish cephalometric norms. According to Mc Namara's cephalometric analysis,[1] in a male subject with harmonic profile the most anterior point of the bone profile of the chin (bone pogonion) should touch the line perpendicular to the Frankfurt plane drawn by the most posterior point of the bone concavity of the nose root (nasion), as depicted in Fig. 19.4.

Spradley introduced in the orthodontic literature a similar analysis for the evaluation of the most anterior point of the skin profile of the chin

[1]McNamara JA. A method of cephalometric evaluation. Am J Orthod.1984; 86: 449–469 and McNamara JA, Brudon WL. Orthodontic and orthopedic treatment in the mixed dentition. Ann Arbor: Needham Press: 1993.

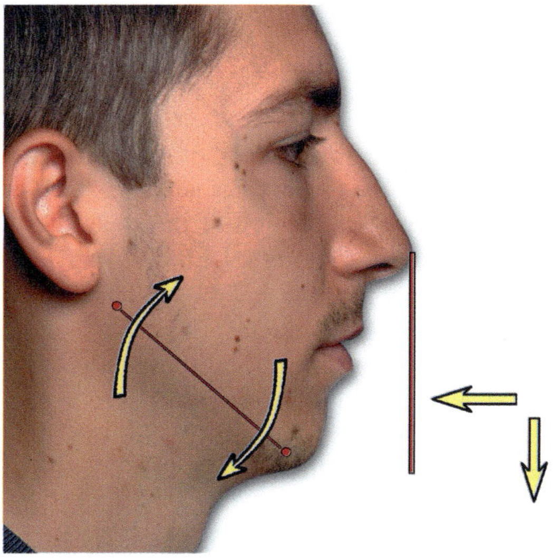

Fig. 19.3 Profile view of a young male patient with an underdeveloped mandible in the posterior-anterior dimension and a significant clockwise rotation of the body of the mandible. The soft tissues over the chin are poorly supported and several of the angles and curves from the tip of the nose to the neck outline flatten

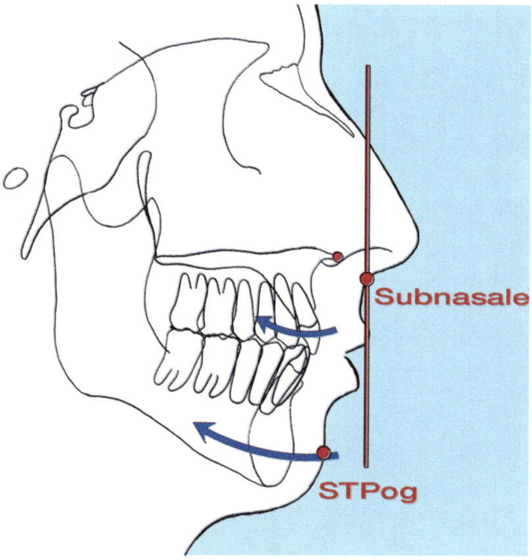

Fig. 19.5 Cephalometric analysis of a patient with a skeletal condition of clockwise rotation of both jaws secondary to the underdevelopment of the lower facial skeleton. The effect on the skin profile is an evident weak chin that is far posterior to the vertical reference line drawn passing through the subnasale

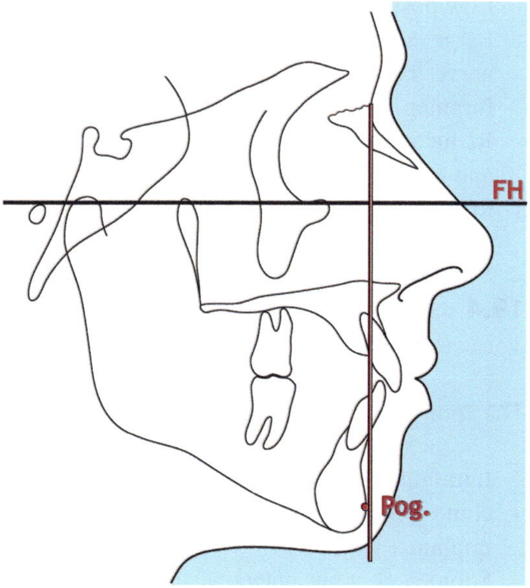

Fig. 19.4 Mc Namara's cephalometric analysis. In a male subject with harmonic profile the most anterior point of the bone profile of the chin (bone pogonion) should touch the line perpendicular to the Frankfurt plane drawn by the most posterior point of the bone concavity of the nose root (nasion)

(soft tissue pogonion).[2] Figure 19.5 illustrates a skeletal condition of clockwise rotation of both jaws secondary to the underdevelopment of the lower facial skeleton. The effect on the skin profile is an evident weak chin that is far posterior to the vertical reference line drawn passing through the subnasale. In cases like this, the surgical correction of the spatial position of the maxilla and mandible (orthognathic surgery) with movements opposite to the direction of the arrows can ameliorate the profile without performing any surgery of the chin itself. This simple chin analysis can also be done utilizing a profile view photograph, as depicted in Fig. 19.6.

Figure 19.7 demonstrates the extreme variability of the thickness of the mental soft tissues and the mismatch between the morphology of the bone and skin profile. From these two observations, derive some limitations to esthetic chin surgery

[2]Spradley FL, Jacobs JD, Crowe DP. Assessment of the anterior posterior soft-tissue contour of the lower facial third in the ideal young adult. Am J Orthod. 1981; 79: 316–325

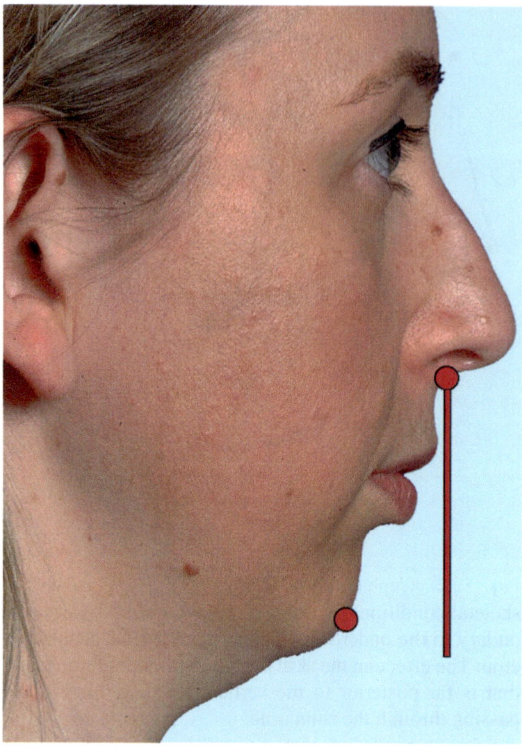

Fig. 19.6 Soft tissue profile analysis performed on a profile view photograph of a patient with extreme underdevelopment of the lower facial skeleton

such as reduced predictability and reduced effect in terms of response to bone repositioning in the case of chin osteotomy, or to increase in volume in the case of alloplastic chin implant. For example, by lengthening the chin by 4 mm the result obtained varies from subject to subject depending on the response of the soft tissues, which can sometimes be barely noticeable in the eyes of the observer. Generally, it is necessary to overcorrect the surgical movements of the bony chin to obtain the planned results at the cutaneous level.

19.3 Elements of Surgical Anatomy of the Chin

Esthetic chin surgery must safeguard the integrity of some anatomical structures:

- The inferior alveolar nerve that runs within the mandibular body and its extraosseous branch, the mental nerve (Fig. 19.8).
- The functional dental and periodontal unit of the lower frontal teeth: incisors and canines (Fig. 19.9).

For the preoperative study of the course and emergence of the mandibular nerves as well as for the study of the length of the roots of the front teeth of the jaw, the simplest and least expensive preoperative radiological investigation is the dental panoramic radiograph. Despite the inevitable distortions and limitations associated with a two-dimensional image, a panoramic radiograph is mandatory for any chin surgery. The only alternative is the CT scan of the mandible.

Figure 19.10a presents a favorable condition to chin surgery with a high course and emergence of the lower alveolar nerve and a considerable distance between the inferior mandibular border and radix of anterior teeth. By contrast, Fig. 19.10b illustrates some unfavorable conditions for chin surgery:

- Low position of the inferior alveolar nerve.
- Large terminal loop of the inferior alveolar nerve before its emergence at the mental foramen.
- Reduced vertical dimensions of the bony chin and proximity of the root of the anterior teeth to the mandibular edge.

19.4 Surgical Approaches to the Chin

The approaches are basically two:

- Intraoral, utilized both for bone surgery with chin osteotomy and for the insertion of a chin implant.
- Submental transcutaneous, utilized only for the insertion of a chin implant.

The intraoral approach starts with a horizontal incision of the anterior alveolar mucosa keeping at least 5 mm from the attached gingiva and without extending laterally beyond the projection of the root of the first premolar to maintain a safe distance from the mental foramen

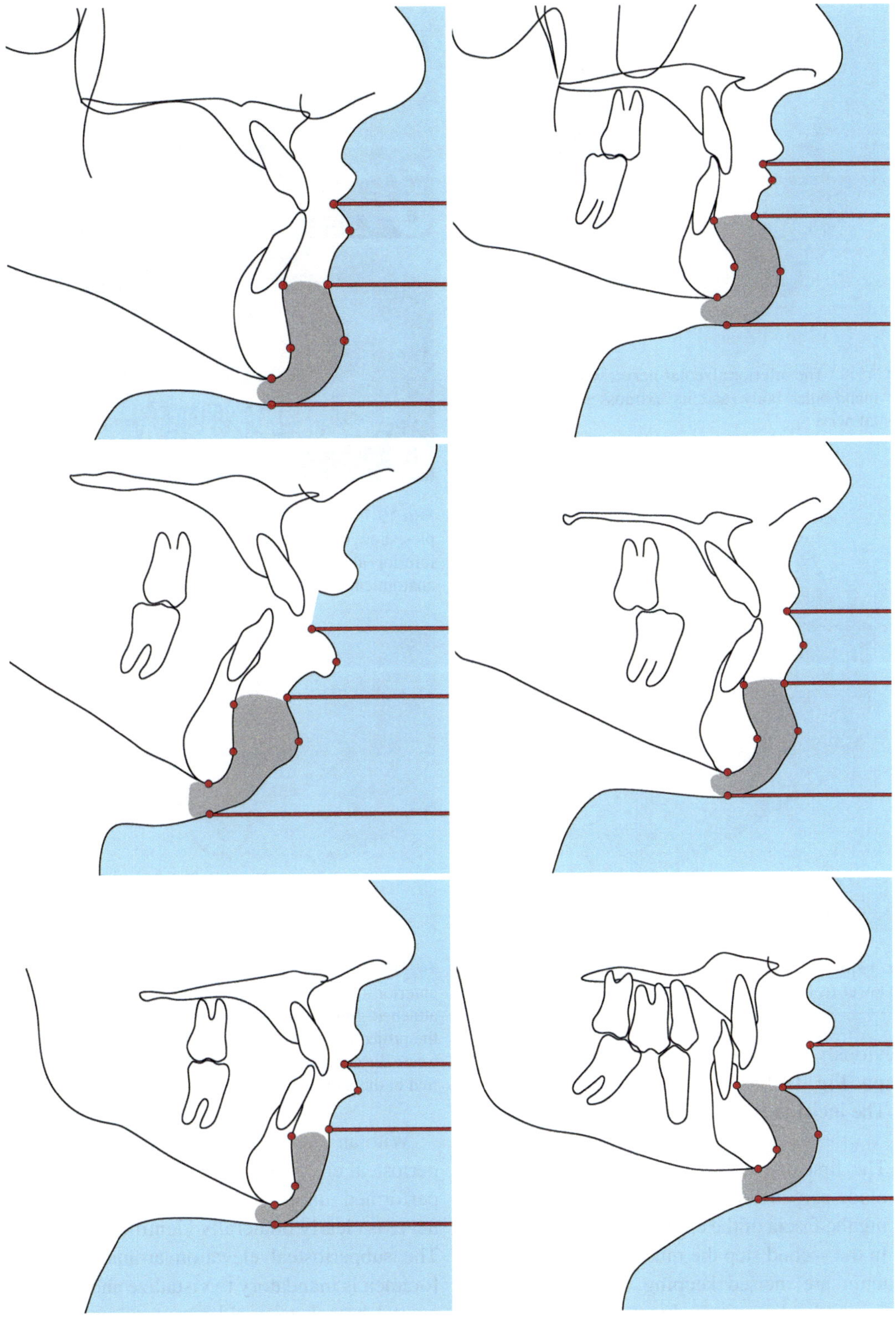

Fig. 19.7 Cephalometric tracings of the anterior mandible and soft tissue chin. Extreme variability of the thickness of the mental soft tissues and the mismatch between the morphology of the bone and skin profile

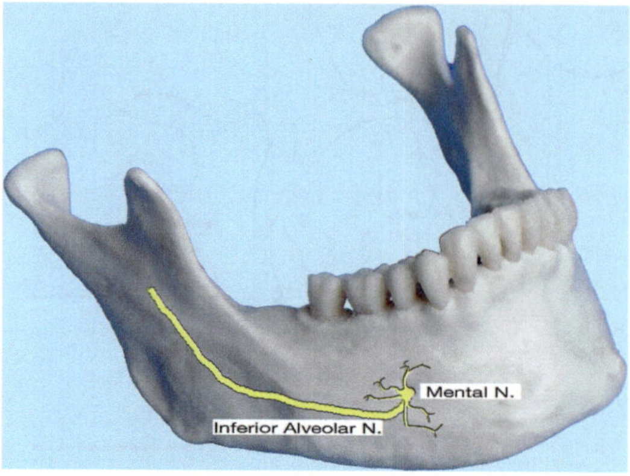

Fig. 19.8 The inferior alveolar nerve, which runs within the mandibular body, and its extraosseous branch, the mental nerve

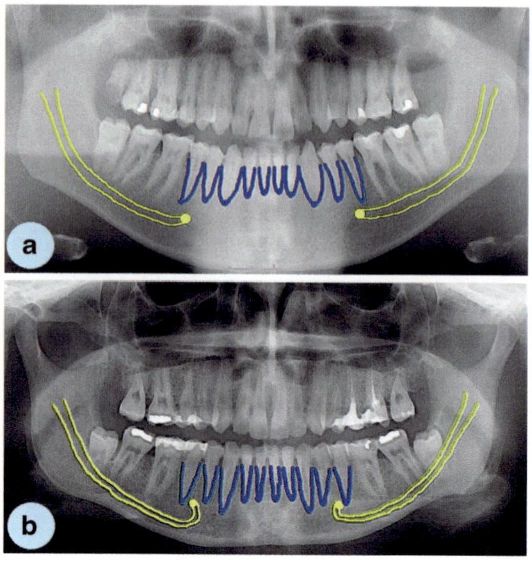

Fig. 19.10 (**a**, **b**) Panoramic radiograph. The two examples show the variables of the intraosseous course of the inferior alveolar nerve. Favorable (**a**) and unfavorable anatomical conditions (**b**) for chin surgery

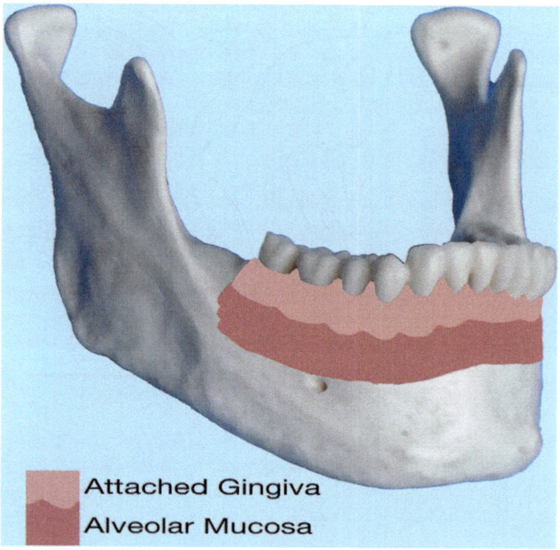

Fig. 19.9 The functional dental and periodontal unit of the lower frontal teeth: incisors and canines

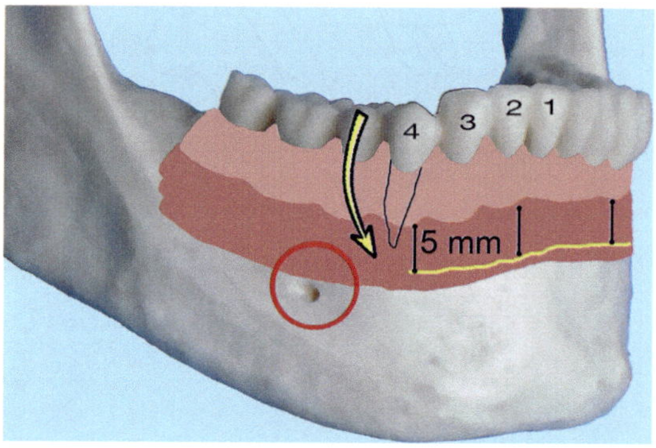

Fig. 19.11 Intraoral approach. Horizontal incision of the anterior alveolar mucosa keeping at least 5 mm from the attached gingiva and without extending laterally beyond the projection of the root of the first premolar to maintain a safe distance from the mental foramen previously identified in the panoramic radiograph

previously identified in the panoramic radiograph (Fig. 19.11).

The incision is carried out in two steps:

- The first one is carried out keeping the 15c blade perpendicular to the mucosa and reaching the fascia of the chin muscles (Fig. 19.12).
- In the second step the muscles and the periosteum are incised keeping the scalpel blade perpendicular and in direct contact with the bone surface (Fig. 19.13).

With an Obwegeser elevator, a complete subperiosteal elevation of the vestibular chin area is performed until the emergence of the mental nerve is clearly bilaterally identified (Fig. 19.14). The subperiosteal elevation around the mental foramen is mandatory to visualize and protect the mental branch to avoid any nerve injury in the subsequent surgical maneuvers (Fig. 19.15).

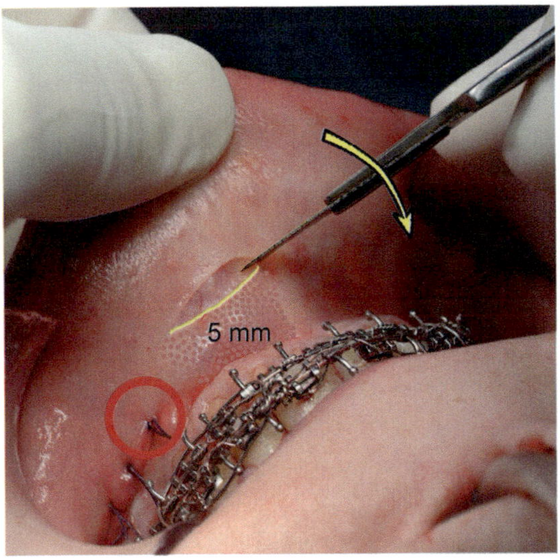

Fig. 19.12 Intraoral approach. The first pass of the mucosal incision is carried out keeping the 15c blade perpendicular to the mucosa and reaching the fascia of the chin muscles

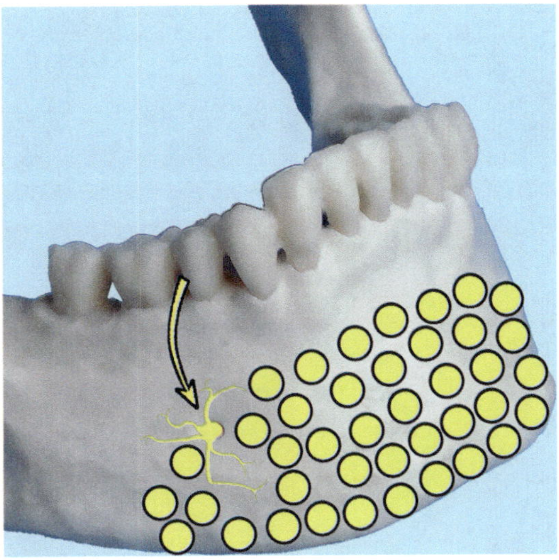

Fig. 19.14 Intraoral approach. A complete subperiosteal elevation of the vestibular chin area is performed with an Obwegeser elevator until the emergence of the mental nerve is clearly bilaterally identified

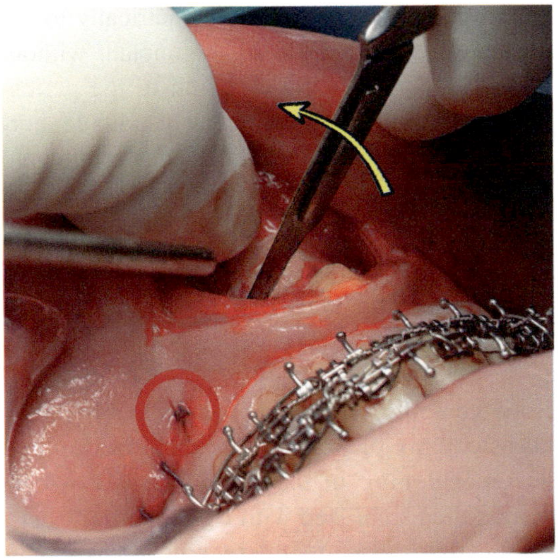

Fig. 19.13 Intraoral approach. In the second pass of the mucosal incision, the muscles and the periosteum are incised keeping the scalpel blade perpendicular and in direct contact with the bone surface

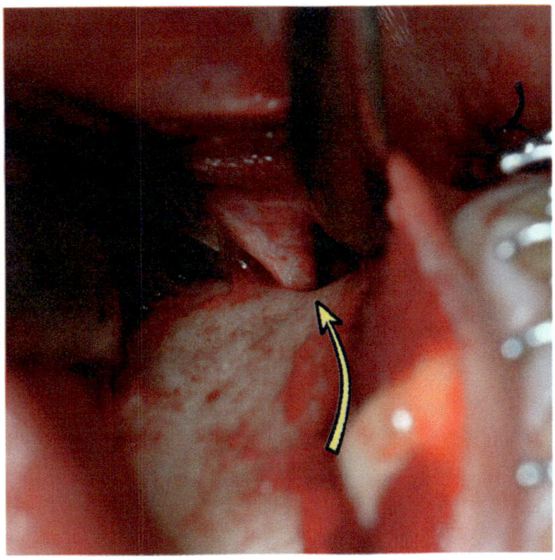

Fig. 19.15 Intraoral approach. Subperiosteal elevation around the mental foramen. It is mandatory to visualize and protect the mental branch to avoid any nerve injury in subsequent surgical maneuvers

The submental transcutaneous approach, on the other hand, requires a horizontal symmetrical submental skin incision. The lateral extension must lie within the palpable margins of the lower edge of the mandible (Fig. 19.16). If the submental sulcus is present, for a better cosmetic scar the incision is drawn 2 mm posterior to it (Fig. 19.17). The skin incision reaches the superficial subcutaneous plane utilizing a scalpel blade 15c. The fat and the platysma muscle instead are incised with a Colorado microdissection needle or similar electrocautery microneedle with the electrosurgi-

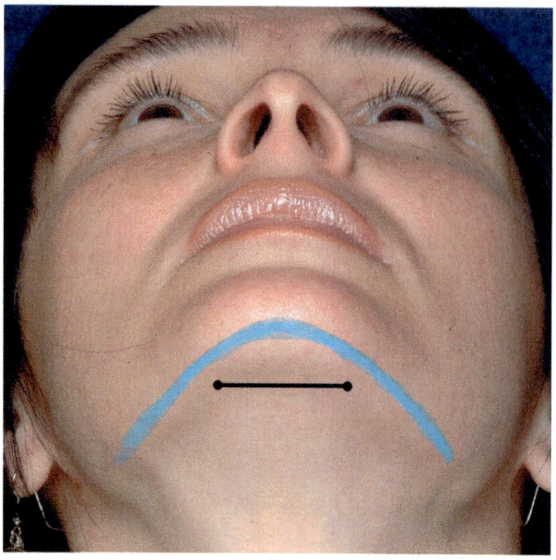

Fig. 19.16 Submental transcutaneous approach. Horizontal symmetrical submental skin incision. The lateral extension must lie within the palpable margins of the lower edge of the mandible

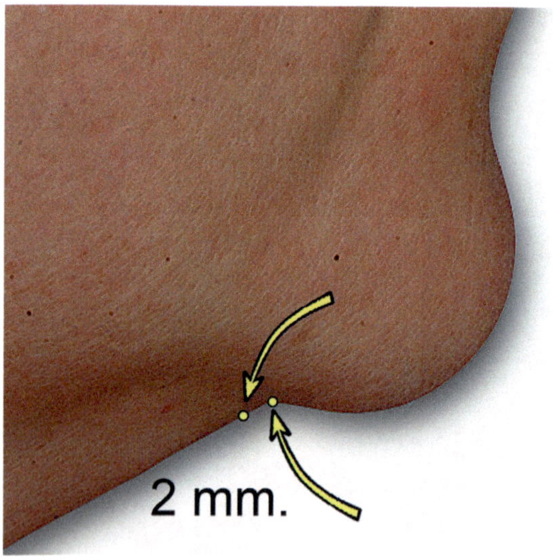

Fig. 19.17 Submental transcutaneous approach. If the submental sulcus is present, for a better cosmetic scar the skin incision is drawn 2 mm posterior to it

cal generator set at a low voltage. With the aid of a pair of double hooks or a retractor, an anterior and lateral dissection is performed under the platysma muscle until the periosteum of the inferior border of the chin is exposed. The periosteum of the mandibular edge is then incised and, with the use of an Obwegeser periosteal elevator, the chin

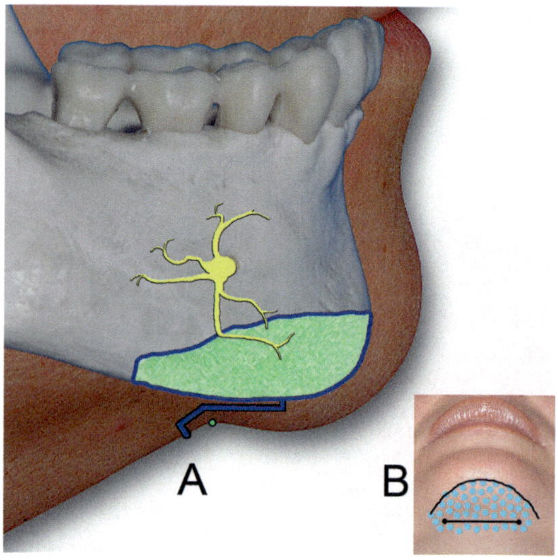

Fig. 19.18 Submental transcutaneous approach. The lateral elevation of the periosteum must be done following the mandibular border at a safe distance from the mental foramen to preserve the mental nerve

region can be skeletonized symmetrically to the extension required to insert the implant without restrictions. The lateral elevation of the periosteum must be done following the mandibular border at a safe distance from the mental foramen to preserve the mental nerve (Fig. 19.18).

19.5 Sliding Osteotomy Genioplasty

Bone genioplasty involves a complete horizontal osteotomy of the chin, its mobilization and its repositioning in the planned position. The chin is then stabilized with rigid internal osteosynthesis by means of titanium plates and screws. In the past, simple surgical steel or titanium wires were used for osteosynthesis; this method is now completely supplanted because it is not able to guarantee adequate stability during the healing phase.

The chin, once osteotomized and mobilized, can be moved forward or backward, by sliding one surface over the other, or upward, by removing an intermediate bone fragment, or also lowered, through the insertion of a bone graft (Fig. 19.19a–d). Composite movements are also

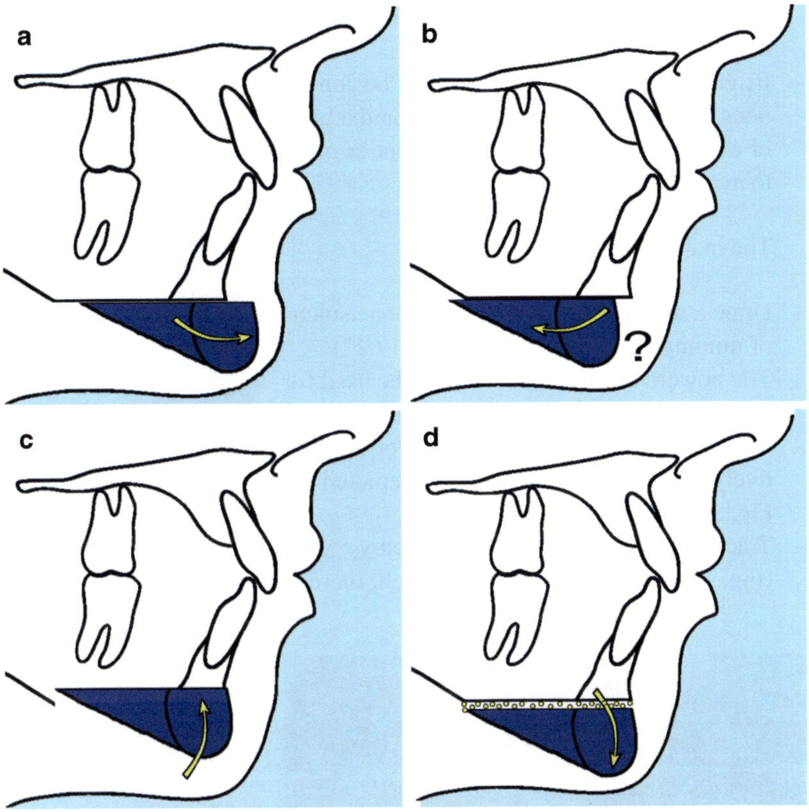

Fig. 19.19 (**a**–**d**) Sliding osteotomy genioplasty. The chin, once osteotomized and mobilized, can be moved forward (**a**) or backward (**b**), by sliding one surface over the other, or upward, by removing an intermediate bone fragment (**c**), or also lowered, through the insertion of a bone graft (**d**)

possible. The most frequent combination is the advancement of the chin associated with its vertical elongation, as depicted in Fig. 19.20. From the frontal point of view, the osteotomized segment must be repositioned symmetrically or, in the case of an asymmetrical chin, trying to center it along the median axis of the face.

Some general rules are:

- For bone genioplasty the intraoral access is mandatory.
- The chin prominence should be minimally skeletonized inferiorly to maintain the attachments of the soft tissue envelope to the osteotomized bony segment. This detail allows one to maximize the esthetic effect produced by chin repositioning.
- The planned osteotomy line cannot be marked without first having identified the emergence of the mental nerve and having reviewed the

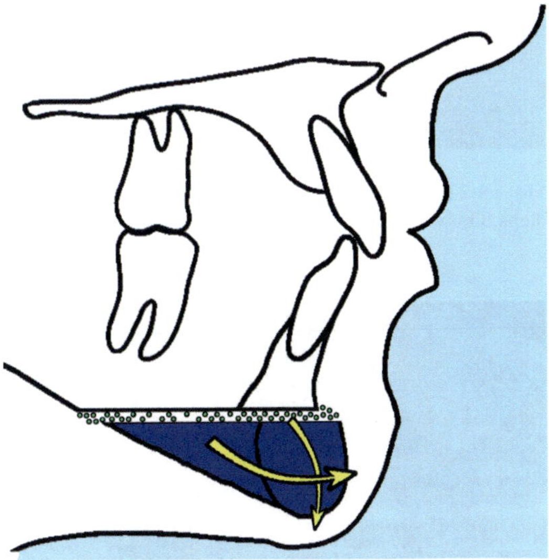

Fig. 19.20 Sliding osteotomy genioplasty. The most frequent combination is the advancement of the chin associated with its vertical elongation

course of the inferior alveolar nerve on the dental panoramic radiograph.

- Irrigation with saline solution must be continuous and abundant during the use on the bone of every kind of powered instrument in order to avoid heat damage.

The main surgical steps are:

- Draw a reference median vertical bone sulcus of minimal depth (Figs. 19.21 and 19.22).
- The powered instruments that can be used for the sulcus and subsequent osteotomies are the ultrasonic saw (Piezosurgery) or alternatively the reciprocal saw, as depicted in Fig. 19.23a, b.
- Trace the horizontal osteotomy line (Fig. 19.24a). If the level is too high, there is

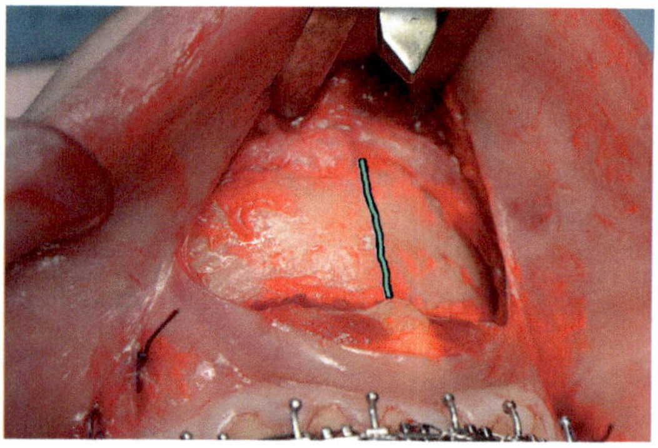

Fig. 19.21 Sliding osteotomy genioplasty: main surgical steps. Draw a median vertical reference line

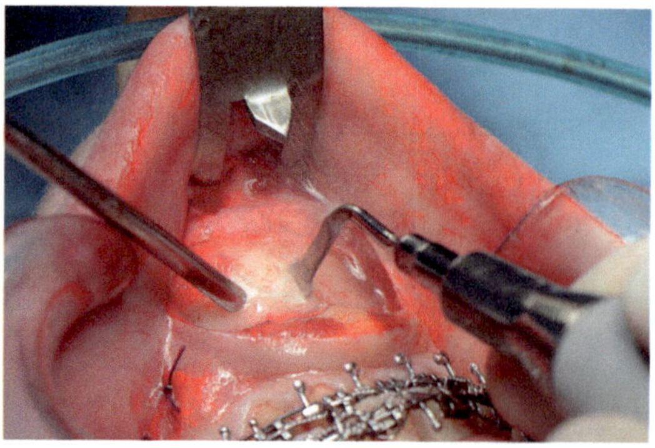

Fig. 19.22 Sliding osteotomy genioplasty: main surgical steps. Make a reference median vertical bone sulcus of minimal depth with an ultrasonic saw

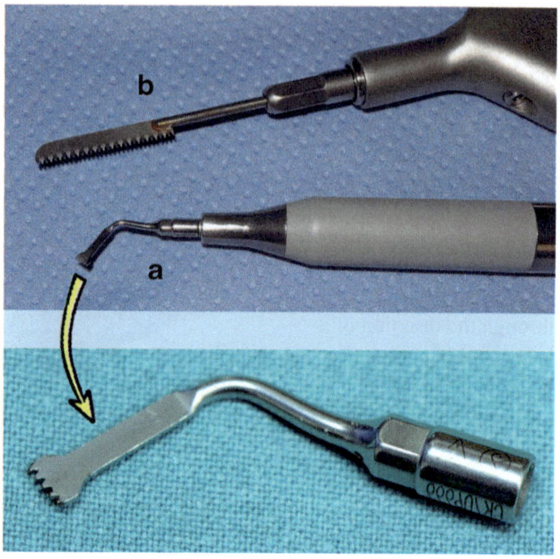

Fig. 19.23 (**a**, **b**) The preferred powered instrument that can be used for the sulcus and subsequent osteotomies is the ultrasonic saw (**a**). An alternative is the reciprocal saw (**b**)

an increased risk of injuring the mandibular nerve in its lower and anterior segment near the mental foramen and the apices of the canine teeth that have the longest roots (Fig. 19.24b). If the level is too low, the osteotomized segment is too small with the risk of producing an unnatural chin shape or a limited profile correction.

- Perform the full thickness bicortical osteotomy until the complete detachment of the mental fragment (Fig. 19.25). The last bone bridge can be fractured by gently rotating a chisel in the osteotomy sulcus (Fig. 19.26a). Before carrying out this maneuver, make sure that the lateral portion of the osteotomy is completed due to the risk of producing an iatrogenic fracture of the mandibular body or an irregular osteotomy profile.
- In the case of large chin advancement, the suprahyoid muscles should be detached from their insertion on the posterior chin utilizing the Colorado microdissection needle. A meticulous coagulation of the muscle is extremely important since, as soon as the muscle fibers are released, they retract deeply and any bleeding is no longer directly managed by the surgeon.

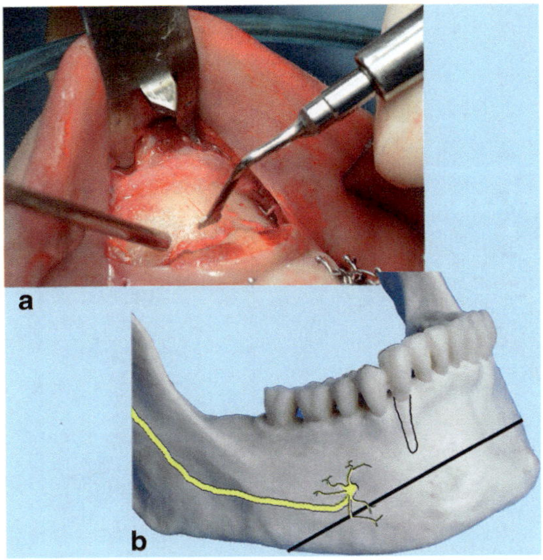

Fig. 19.24 (**a**, **b**) Sliding osteotomy genioplasty: main surgical steps. Tracing of the horizontal osteotomy line (**a**). If the level is too high, there is an increased risk of injuring the mandibular nerve in its lower and anterior segment near the mental foramen and the apices of the canine teeth that have the longest roots (**b**)

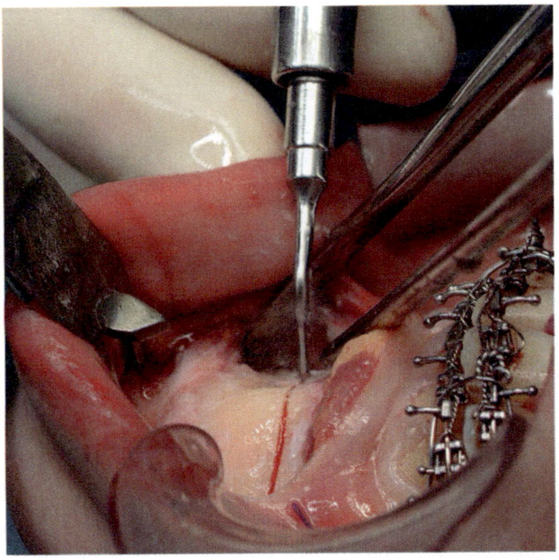

Fig. 19.25 Sliding osteotomy genioplasty: main surgical steps. Perform the full-thickness bicortical osteotomy until the complete detachment of the mental fragment

– Precise bending of osteosynthesis plates. X- or L-shaped titanium miniplates are commonly used (Fig. 19.27a–c). Alternatively, pre-bent miniplates available with various advancement distances can be used. Figure 19.28 shows the anterior repositioning and stabilization of the chin with a pre-bent titanium plate and four screws.
– If a gap is created between the two bony margins, as in the case of increase in chin height, it is necessary to fill it with an autologous bone graft or with granules of osteoconductive material such as calcium hydroxyapatite granules (Figs. 19.29 and 19.30).
– Muscle and oral mucosa suturing with 4/0 polyglactin absorbable braided simple interrupted sutures.

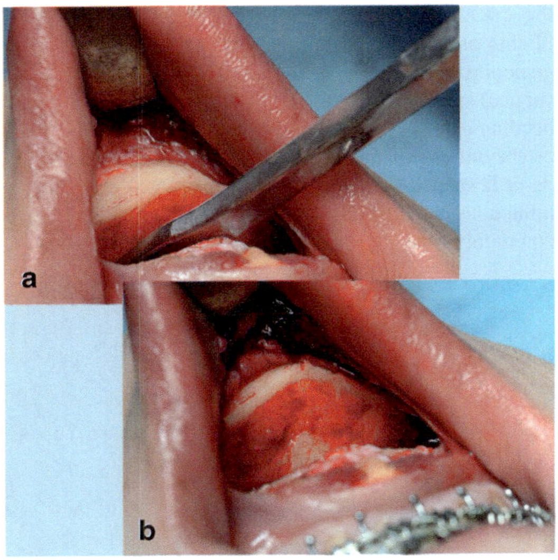

Fig. 19.26 (**a**, **b**) Sliding osteotomy genioplasty: main surgical steps. The last bone bridge can be fractured by gently rotating a chisel in the osteotomy sulcus

19.6 Alloplastic Chin Implant

Chin augmentation with solid silicone, e-PTFE or porous polyethylene implants allows the surgeon to increase the volume of the chin by acting on its posteroanterior and lateral projection. On the other hand, with this approach no real vertical increases or decreases can be obtained and it is difficult to act on a chin asymmetry. The extraoral approach is preferred owing to the increase of postoperative infections linked to the intraoral approach.

The evolution of this method has led over the years to variations in implant morphology.

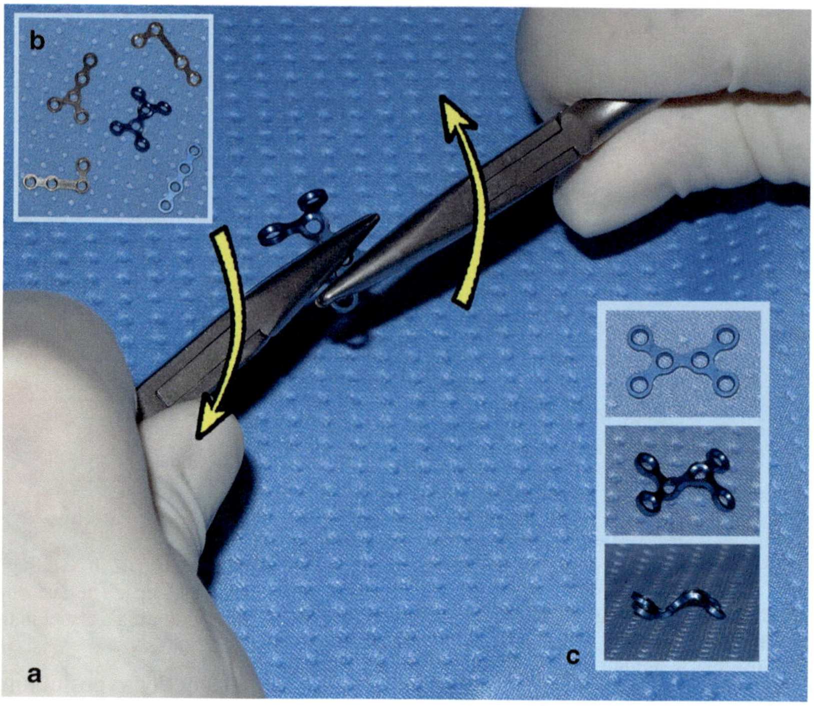

Fig. 19.27 (**a–c**) Sliding osteotomy genioplasty: main surgical steps. Precise bending of osteosynthesis plates. X- or L-shaped titanium miniplates are commonly used

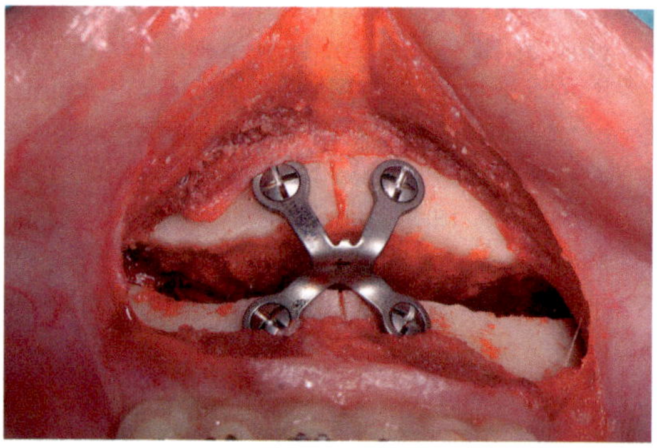

Fig. 19.28 Sliding osteotomy genioplasty: main surgical steps. Anterior reposition and stabilization of the chin utilizing a pre-bent titanium plate and four screws

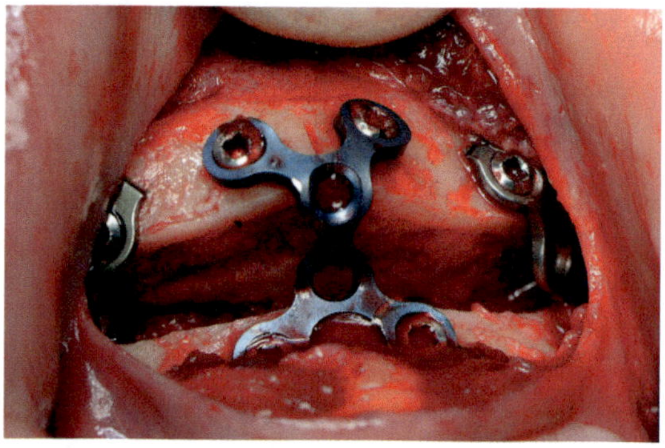

Fig. 19.29 Sliding osteotomy genioplasty: main surgical steps. A gap is created between the two bony margins in the case of a desired increase in chin height

We currently prefer wide prostheses with thin margins that can distribute the increase in volume even laterally and reduce the risk, in patients with thin skin, of visually recognizing the contours of the prosthesis. Solid silicone, e-PTFE, and porous polyethylene can be modeled with a scalpel blade or scissors allowing the surgeon to adapt a standard industrial product to the individual needs of the patient. In the case of porous polyethylene, a more rigid material, a two-piece extended implant has been studied and produced which can be inserted separately without difficulty through the surgical incision and then assembled together in the midline.

It is essential to achieve a precise and symmetrical subperiosteal soft tissue elevation slightly larger than the size of the implant.

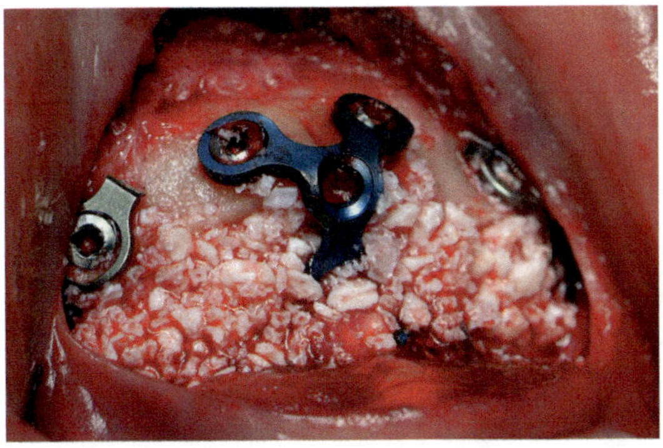

Fig. 19.30 Sliding osteotomy genioplasty: main surgical steps. If a gap is created between the two bony margins, it is necessary to fill it with an autologous bone graft or with granules of osteoconductive material such as calcium hydroxyapatite granules

Correct positioning requires that the lower edge of the implant correspond to the lower edge of the mandible. For the stabilization of the implant it is advisable to fix it in place utilizing one or two titanium monocortical screws.

19.7 Comparing Between Surgical Approaches to the Chin

Esthetic chin surgery plays a fundamental role in correcting some deformities of the young adult. Like other procedures, also this one is mostly a part of a complex and personalized treatment plan so that isolated surgery of the chin is rarely performed. The differences between the two approaches to the chin are many and the indications for their use only partially overlap.

The intraoral approach with bone osteotomy (sliding genioplasty):

- is preferable in young subjects, in corrections of asymmetries, in association with orthognathic surgery procedures.
- requires expensive and dedicated instruments (electric drill, reciprocal saw, piezoelectric saws) and specific training in maxillofacial surgery, which is rarely undertaken by professionals from other medical branches.
- exposes the patient to the risk of skin numbness and paresthesias of the lip and chin due to injury of the lower alveolar nerve for an excessively high osteotomic cut and/or unfavorable anatomical conditions. Also injury of the mental nerve during lateral skeletonization of the mandibular border can be a cause of numbness and paresthesias.
- exposes to the risk of injury to the periodontium (gingiva and alveolar bone) of the lower anterior teeth in the case of an excessively high osteotomy line and/or unfavorable anatomical conditions.
- does not allow a transverse augmentation of the chin.
- allows either an increase or a decrease in the vertical height of the lower third of the face.
- allows the improvement of an asymmetrical lower third of the face.
- is associated with a very low risk of postoperative infection and the removal of the osteosynthesis screws and plates does not cause the loss of the esthetic result obtained.

The extraoral approach with alloplastic chin implant:

- requires inexpensive surgical instruments, usually already in the surgeon's possession.
- exposes the patient to the risk of numbness and paresthesias of the lower lip and chin due to injury to the mental nerve during lateral subperiosteal elevation along the mandibular border.
- allows a transverse augmentation of the chin.
- does not allow an increase or a decrease in the vertical height of the lower third of the face.
- exposes the patient to the risk of a visible skin scar in the submental area.
- is preferable in clinical cases that require a submandibular liposuction to improve the chin neck esthetic profile.
- exposes the patient to the risk of infection and dislocation of the prosthesis from its location even after years. Early or late infection almost always requires removal of the prosthesis and the consequent loss of the esthetic result.

Each of the above points should guide the surgeon in formulating a personalized and, in many cases, unique treatment plan for each patient. Figure 19.31 shows a clinical case with

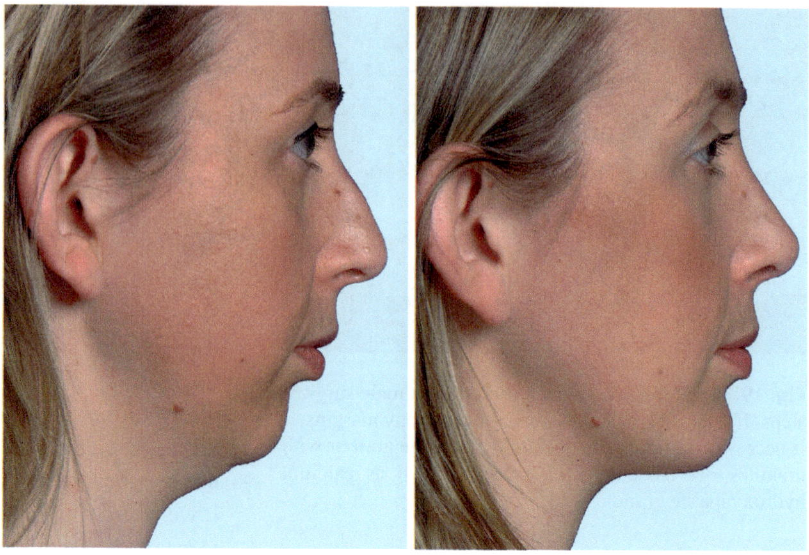

Fig. 19.31 A clinical case with nasal trauma deformity associated with mandibular deficiency. The treatment plan included a preoperative orthodontic therapy followed by surgery. The patient underwent mandibular advancement associated with chin implant, submandibular lipectomy, and open approach functional reconstructive rhinoseptoplasty in one stage

nasal trauma deformity associated with mandibular deficiency. The treatment plan included a preoperative orthodontic therapy followed by surgery. This comprised a mandibular advancement associated with chin implant, submandibular lipectomy, and open approach functional reconstructive rhinoseptoplasty in one stage.

Further Reading

Books

Guyuron B. Genioplasty. Boston: Little, Brown; 1992.
Reyneke JP. Essentials of orthognathic surgery. Chicago: Quintessence; 2019.
Steinbcher DM. Aesthetic orthognathic surgery and rhinoplasty. Hoboken: Wiley-Blackwell; 2019.

20 Cartilage and Fascia Harvesting for Rhinoplasty

The harvesting of cartilage from the nasal septum is an integral part of the BOR surgical method. Even in primary cases, the use of this source of cartilage is close to 100%.

Rarely, but even in primary patients, the septum may be considered depleted if it is mostly bony or if the cartilage is severely damaged or deformed from previous multiple traumas.

One particular skill of the nasal surgeon is to preoperatively evaluate the need for cartilage grafts, from the point of view of both quantity and quality, and to plan a sure or highly probable intraoperative time for harvesting from an extranasal donor site. In these cases, the patient must be aware of the objectives of his reconstructive surgery and of the need to harvest cartilage.

The same principles also apply to the harvesting of autologous fascia, when it is necessary to create a uniform and soft layer between the reconstructed nasal framework and the soft tissue envelope.

20.1 Conchal Cartilage Harvest

The preferred approach for conchal cartilage harvest is posterior through a linear incision placed at a distance of about 5–7 mm from the retroauricular sulcus (Fig. 20.1). The operating field should be extended to both auricles in the case that an extranasal harvesting of cartilage is planned. Before starting the skin incision the ear is prepped again with povidone-iodine solution and infiltrated anteriorly and posteriorly with two 1.8 mL dental vials containing mepivacaine hydrochloride 2% with epinephrine 1:100,000 (Figs. 20.2 and 20.3).

The length of the skin incision is about 3–3.5 cm. It is performed with the ear retracted forward and utilizing a Colorado microdissection needle with the electrosurgical unit set at a low voltage (Fig. 20.4). Special care is taken not to incise the underlying perichondrium with the Colorado tip. The supraperichondrial plane is then reached utilizing sharp scissors to expose widely the posterior concha (Fig. 20.5). The posterior auricular muscle fibers inserted to the con-

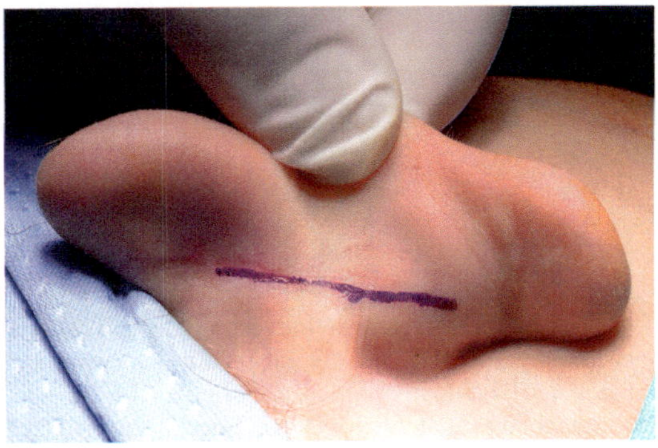

Fig. 20.1 Conchal cartilage harvesting steps. Posterior linear incision placed at a distance of about 5–7 mm from the retroauricular sulcus

F. Meneghini, *Basic Open Rhinoplasty*, https://doi.org/10.1007/978-3-030-61827-8_20

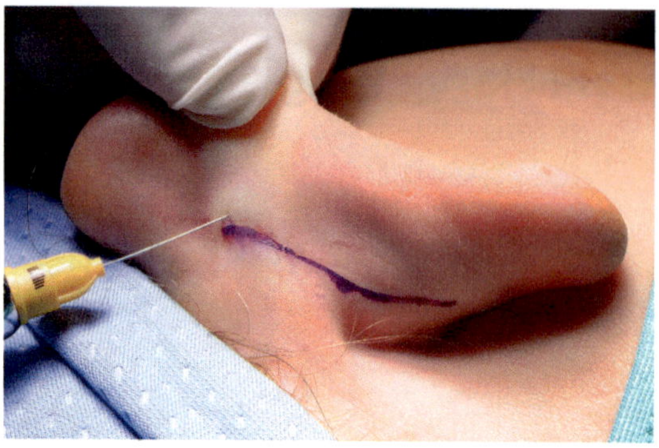

Fig. 20.2 Conchal cartilage harvesting steps. The ear is infiltrated anteriorly and posteriorly

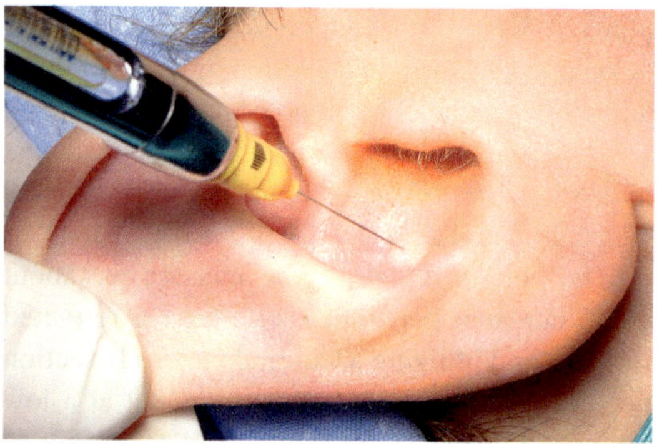

Fig. 20.3 Conchal cartilage harvesting steps. The ear is infiltrated anteriorly and posteriorly

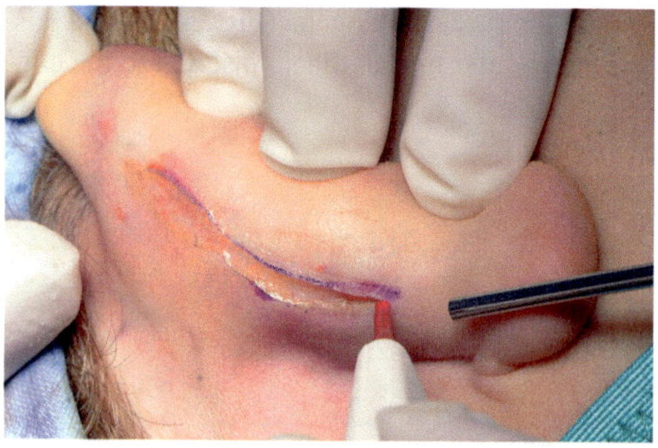

Fig. 20.4 Conchal cartilage harvesting steps. The skin incision is performed with the ear retracted forward and utilizing a Colorado microdissection needle with the electrosurgical unit set at a low voltage. Special care is taken not to incise the underlying perichondrium with the Colorado tip

cha are sectioned with the Colorado needle (Fig. 20.6).

Prior to marking and incising the conchal cartilage to be harvested, it is advisable to verify its external limit to avoid any damage to the antihelix, a highly esthetic curved prominence. The easy way is to transfix the full thickness of the auricle with two small needles positioned close to the medial margin of the antihelix, as shown in Fig. 20.7, and retract forward the ear to clearly identify the anatomical limits of the concha (Fig. 20.8).

With a fresh 15c blade, the first incision of the cartilage follows the external margin of the concha avoiding any damage to the anterior skin of the ear. An initial elevation of the soft tissue in a plane close to the cartilage is then done with a Freer or similar small periosteal elevator taking care to avoid any disruption of both the cartilage and skin (Fig. 20.9). The main objectives are twofold:

- To harvest the largest possible intact single piece of conchal cartilage (Fig. 20.10).
- To keep the anterior skin of the concha intact (Fig. 20.11).

Once the entire conchal bowl has been removed, hemostasis is completed and the surgical field cleansed with sterile saline solution. Any irregular or sharp cartilage edges are trimmed and smoothed with delicate scissors. Then the incision is closed with a running 5-0 monofilament nylon or fast-adsorbing braided polyglactin suture.

One or more cotton balls soaked with antibiotic ointment are applied posteriorly along the suture line as well as anteriorly inside the concha. At the end of rhinoplasty the ear is inspected, cleansed again with sterile saline solution and the dressing redone. A soft elastic bandage is placed around the head. Usually no drain is applied and the dressing is changed again the next day at the time of discharge from the clinic.

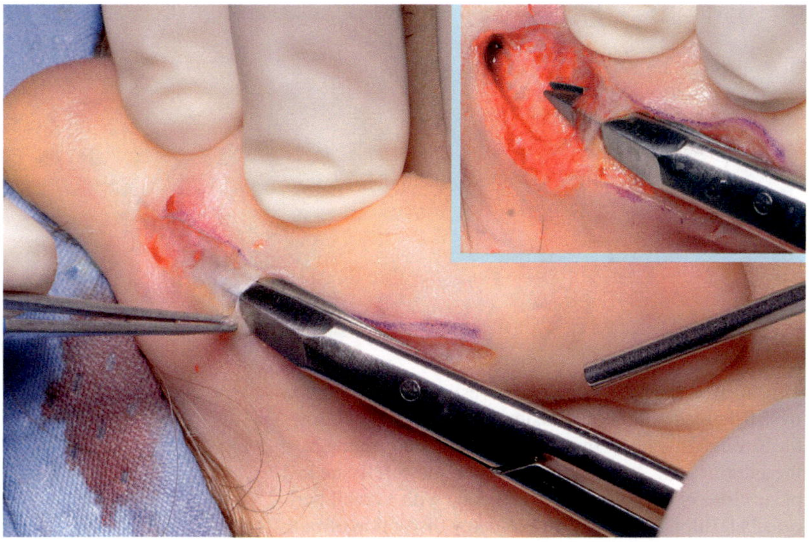

Fig. 20.5 Conchal cartilage harvesting steps. The supraperichondrial plane is then reached utilizing a sharp scissors to expose widely the posterior concha

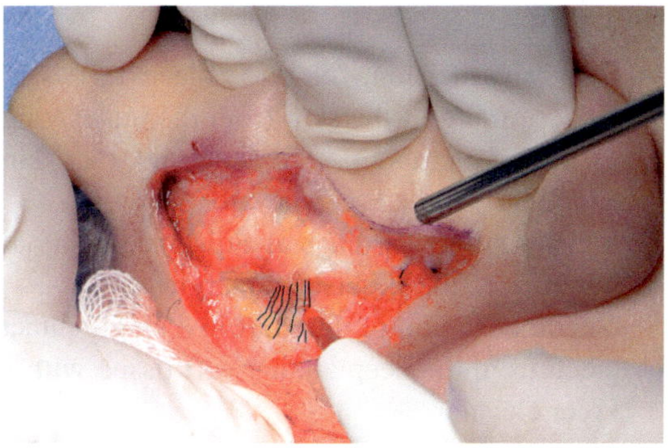

Fig. 20.6 Conchal cartilage harvesting steps. The posterior auricular muscle fibers inserted to the concha are sectioned with the Colorado needle. Once again special care is taken not to incise the underlying perichondrium

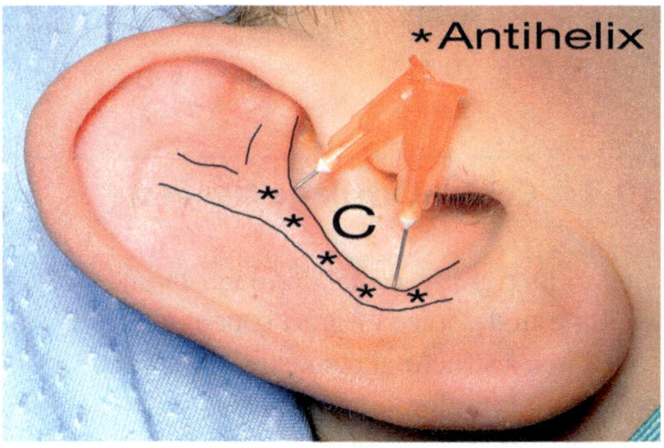

Fig. 20.7 Conchal cartilage harvesting steps. Antihelix medial limits verified using two small needles

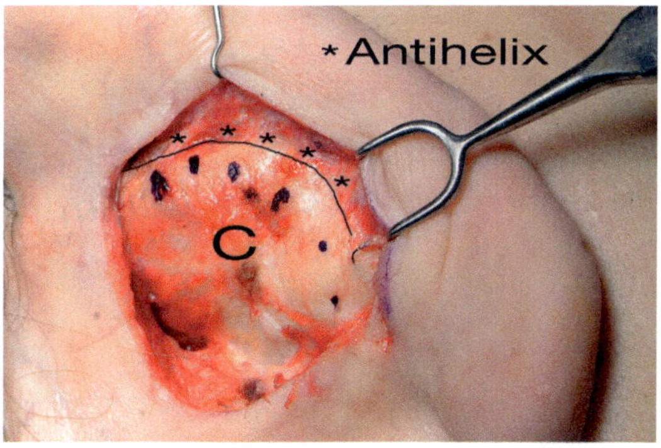

Fig. 20.8 Conchal cartilage harvesting steps. The conchal lateral margin is marked with a sterile skin marker maintaining a safe distance from the antihelix (*C* conchal cartilage)

20.2 Conchal Composite Harvest

A conchal composite graft is mainly utilized in the correction of alar rim retraction. The structure of the graft, which presents an island of skin still attached centrally over the ear cartilage, permits reconstruction of both the internal lining and the framework, with the aim of contrasting the relapse secondary to scar contraction.

The preferred approach for conchal composite grafting is anterior in the area of the cymba concha. Usually the skin island is drawn with an

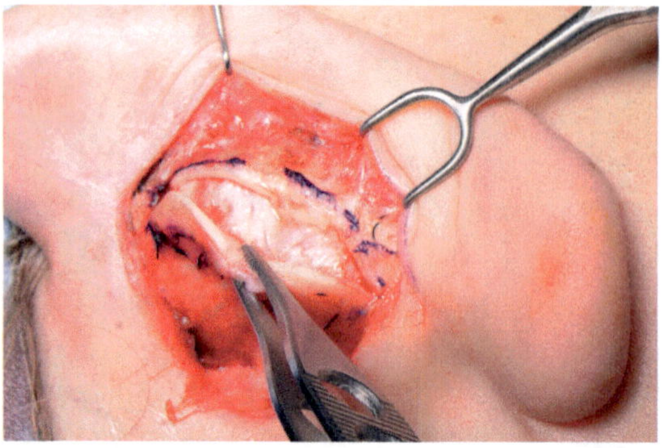

Fig. 20.9 Conchal cartilage harvesting steps. With a fresh 15c blade, the first incision of the cartilage follows the external margin of the concha avoiding any damage to the anterior skin. An initial elevation of the soft tissue in a plane close to the cartilage is then done with a small periosteal elevator taking care to avoid any disruption of both the cartilage and skin

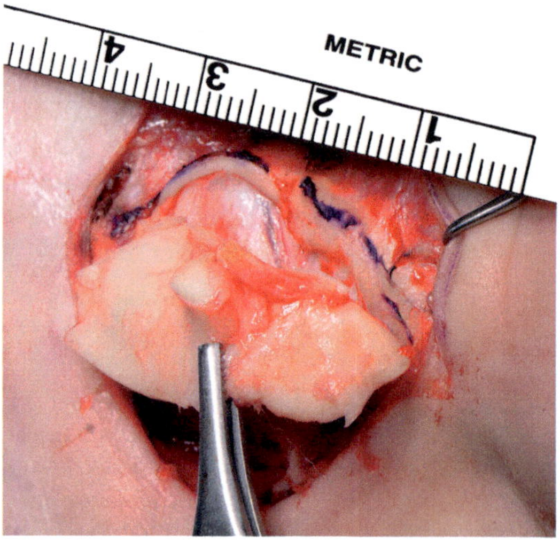

Fig. 20.10 Conchal cartilage harvesting steps. A single piece of intact cartilage is harvested

elliptical shape (Fig. 20.12). The surgeon must consider that the size of the cartilage harvested should exceed the skin margins by about 1.5–2 mm (Fig. 20.13).

The skin marked for harvesting must not be directly infiltrated with local anesthetic. Instead, multiple small infiltrations are made at a fair distance, as depicted in Fig. 20.14.

The harvesting procedure involves the following four main steps:

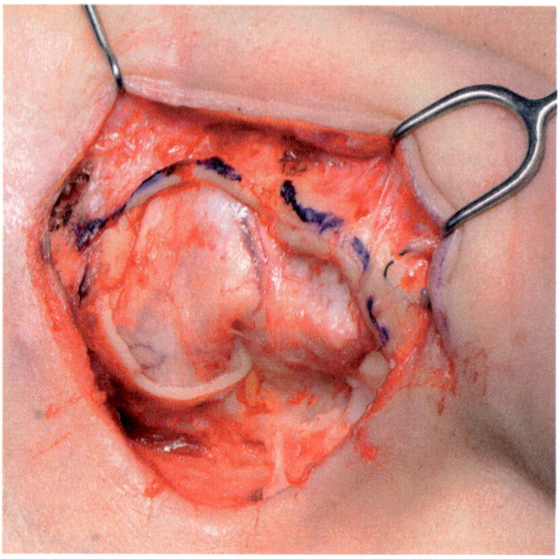

Fig. 20.11 Conchal cartilage harvesting steps. The anterior skin should be maintained intact

- Skin-only incision with a 15c blade.
- Undermining of the skin from the underlying cartilage for about 2 mm around the skin island utilizing a Freer elevator.
- Incision of the cartilage at a distance of about 2 mm from the skin island margins.
- Gentle elevation of the graft in a single intact piece from the deep areolar soft tissue with a Freer elevator.

Each maneuver must be performed without detaching the skin from the cartilage base of the graft and without utilizing electrocautery for hemostasis. Once the graft has been removed, meticulous hemostasis, wide skin undermining and closure by horizontal mattress sutures with braided fast-absorbing polyglactin can be performed (Fig. 20.15).

20.3 Costal Cartilage Harvest

Due to its rigidity, costal cartilage can be considered the first choice of graft source after the septum when a structural reconstruction is needed. In general, it is preferable to harvest a segment of the fifth or sixth rib. In female patients, the incision is set 1 cm above the medial aspect of the inframam-

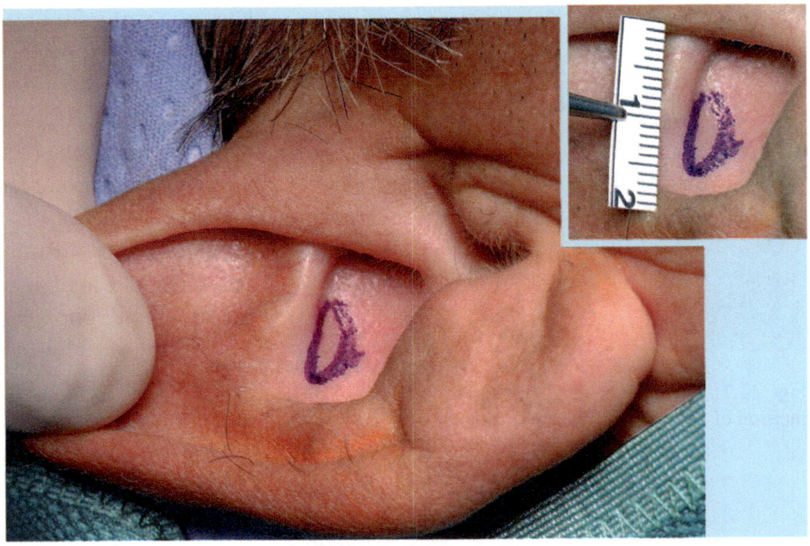

Fig. 20.12 Conchal composite graft. Anterior approach in the region of cymba concha

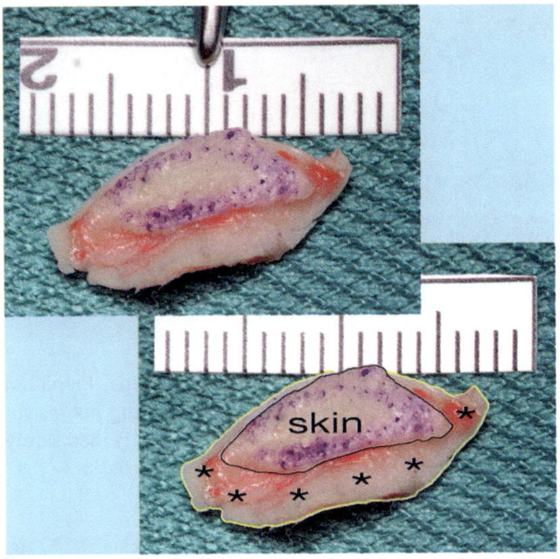

Fig. 20.13 Conchal composite graft. The size of the cartilage harvested should exceed the skin margins by about 1.5–2 mm

mary fold. Palpation helps identify the rib, and its superior and inferior margins are drawn with a sterile skin marker. A skin incision of about 3.5 cm is then drawn exactly over the rib (Fig. 20.16). The incision is made with the Colorado needle (Fig. 20.17) and the subcutaneous fat pad is dissected with Metzenbaum scissors (Fig. 20.18). Palpation continues to guide the surgeon in maintaining his instruments exactly over the rib while the assistant spreads the two skin

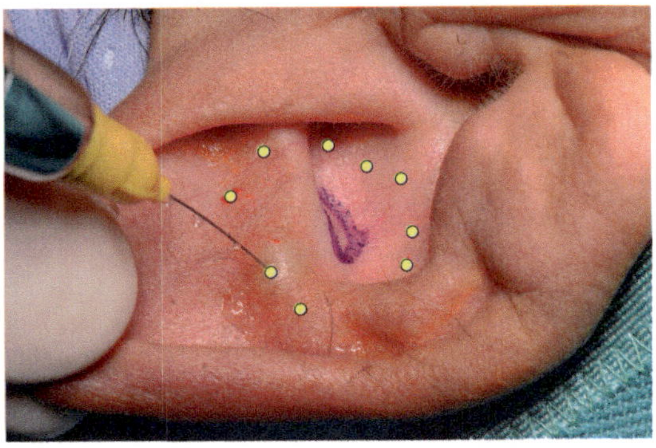

Fig. 20.14 Conchal composite graft. The skin marked for harvesting must not be directly infiltrated with local anesthetic. Instead, multiple small infiltrations are made at a fair distance from it

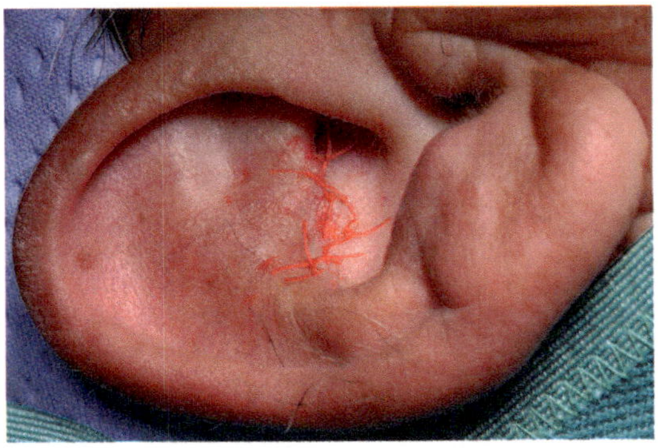

Fig. 20.15 Conchal composite graft. Skin closure by horizontal mattress suture with braided fast-absorbing polyglactin

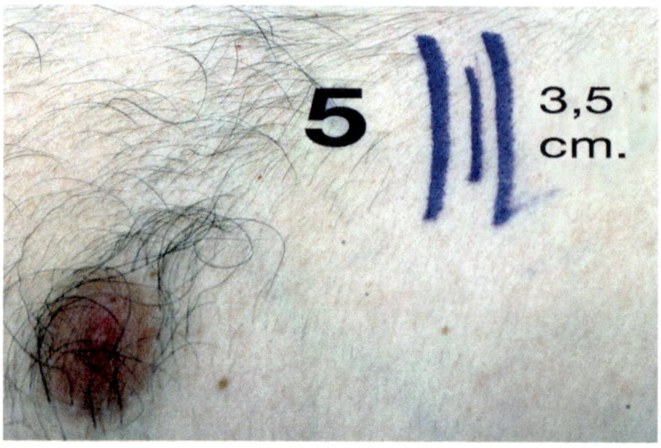

Fig. 20.16 Costal cartilage harvesting steps. The skin incision of about 3.5 cm is drawn exactly over the rib

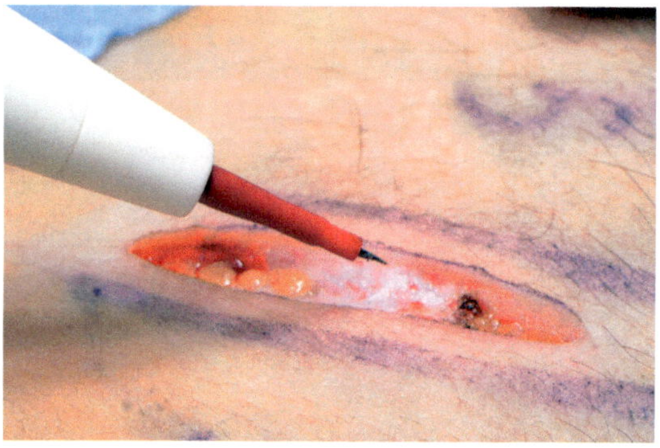

Fig. 20.17 Costal cartilage harvesting steps. Preferably the incision is made with a Colorado needle

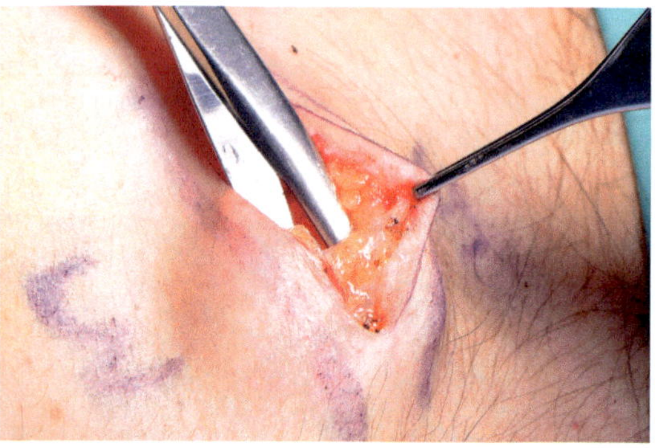

Fig. 20.18 Costal cartilage harvesting steps. The subcutaneous fat pad is dissected with Metzenbaum scissors

flaps and maintains the position. The rectus fascia is then incised with a microdissection needle (Fig. 20.19) and the dissection is deepened until the costal anterior perichondrium is reached. To obtain a strip of perichondrium that can be used later as a soft graft under the soft tissue envelope, the incision is performed inferiorly along the anterior rib and the perichondrium is gently elevated with a small Obwegeser elevator (Fig. 20.20) and removed in one piece. Figure 20.21a, b shows the anterior rib completely exposed and the overlying layers of soft tissue.

The perichondrium on either side is then carefully elevated using curved elevators and finally the perichondrium covering the posterior rib cartilage is elevated taking care to maintain its integrity. To protect the pleura for the next maneuvers a malleable ribbon retractor can be curved and inserted under the rib (Fig. 20.22). Once the surgeon is satisfied with the length of

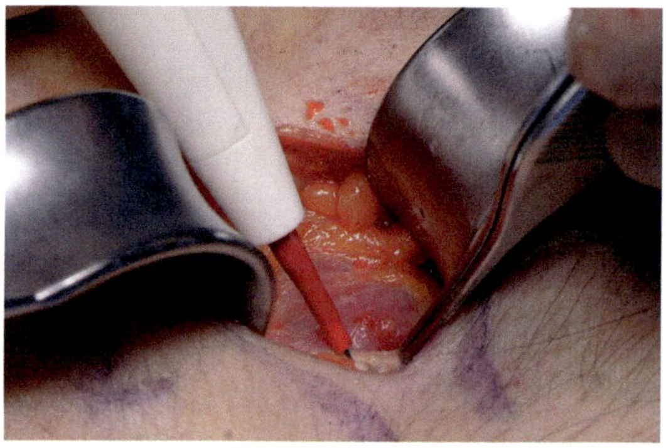

Fig. 20.19 Costal cartilage harvesting steps. Palpation continues to guide the surgeon in maintaining his instruments exactly over the rib. The rectus fascia is then safely incised with the Colorado microdissection needle

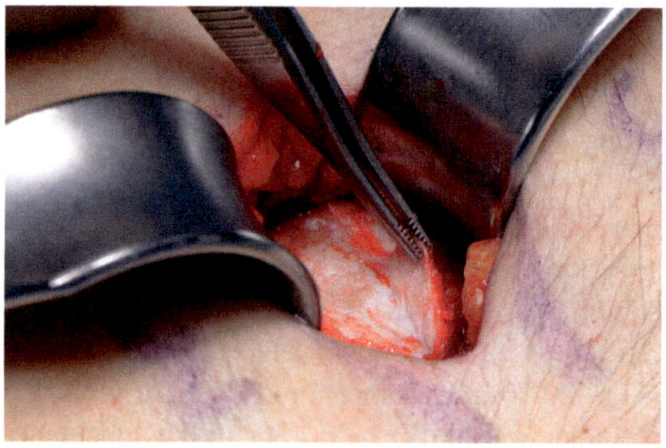

Fig. 20.20 Costal cartilage harvesting steps. A strip of costal perichondrium can be harvested before the cartilage. An incision is performed inferiorly along the anterior rib margin and the perichondrium is gently elevated with a small Obwegeser elevator

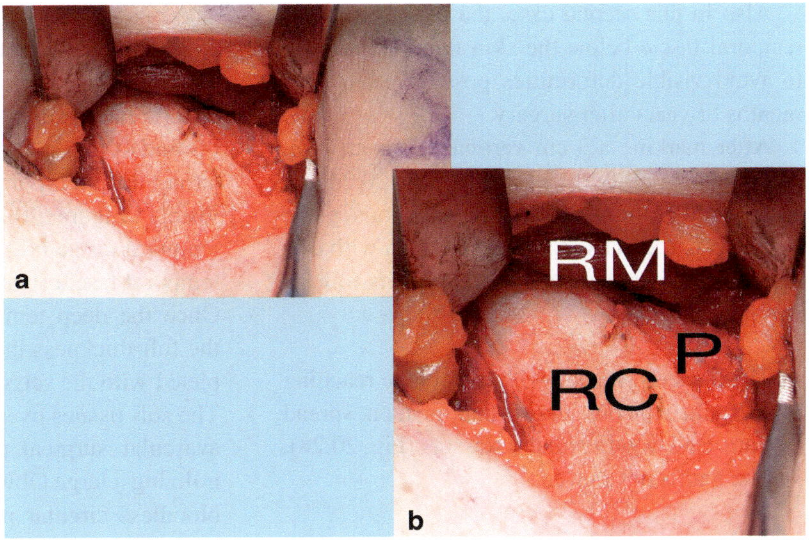

Fig. 20.21 (**a**, **b**) Costal cartilage harvesting steps. The anterior rib is completely exposed (*RC* rib cartilage, *P* elevated perichondrium, *RM* rectus muscle)

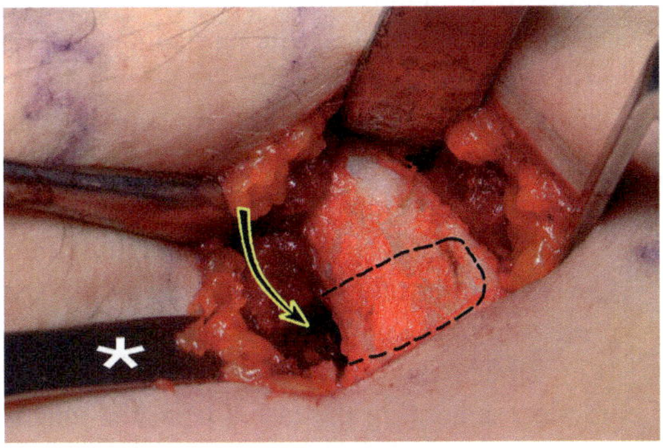

Fig. 20.22 Costal cartilage harvesting steps. The perichondrium on either side is then carefully elevated using curved elevators and finally the perichondrium covering the posterior rib cartilage is elevated taking care to maintain its integrity. To protect the pleura for the next maneuvers, a malleable ribbon retractor can be curved and inserted under the rib (asterisk)

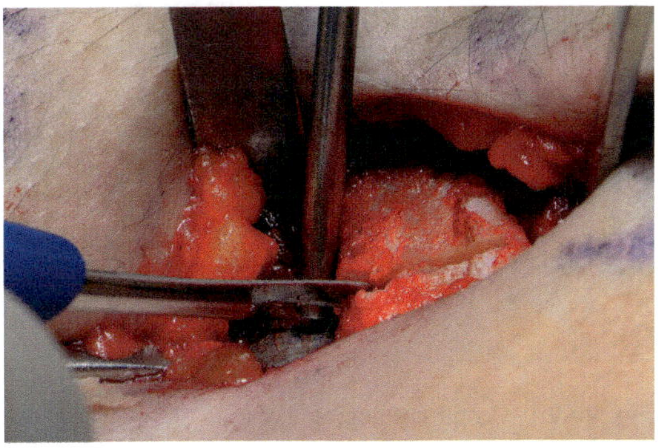

Fig. 20.23 Costal cartilage harvesting steps. The exposed cartilage is measured and divided at either end with a 10 blade, always maintaining an underlying instrument to protect the pleura

the exposed rib, the cartilage is divided at either end with a 10 blade, always maintaining an underlying instrument to protect the pleura (Fig. 20.23).

Once the cartilage graft is removed (Fig. 20.24), the deep wound integrity is checked and meticulous hemostasis is performed. The closure is multi-layered taking care to suture the muscle flap plane (Fig. 20.25a, b). Drainage is not required.

20.4 Temporal Fascia Harvest

The temporal fascia graft in rhinoplasty has essentially two uses:

- To create a uniform and soft layer between the reconstructed nasal framework and the soft tissue envelope in thin skin patients.
- To make an envelope for a diced cartilage graft to prevent spreading of the cartilage itself.

Also in this second case, the presence of the temporal fascia below the skin flap is necessary to avoid visible deformities possible even after months or years after surgery.

After marking a 3 cm vertical temporal incision line parallel to the hairline (Figs. 20.26 and 20.27) and infiltrating the subcutaneous plane with two 1.8 cc vials of local anesthesia with epinephrine, the harvesting procedure starts following these steps:

- The incision is made with a 15 blade reaching the subcutaneous tissue that is then spread transversely with pointed scissors (Fig. 20.28). The hair is not shaved.

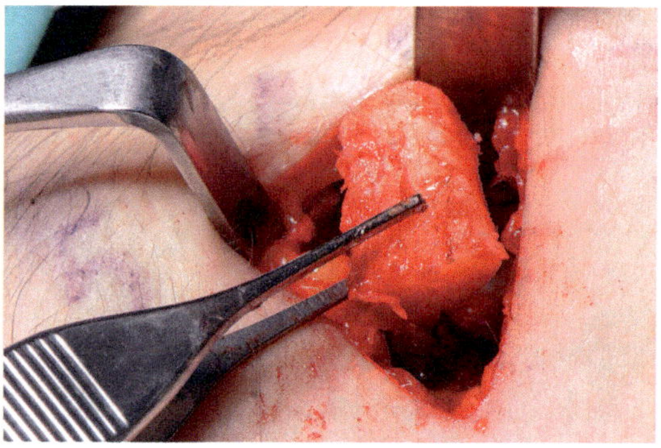

Fig. 20.24 Costal cartilage harvesting steps. The piece of harvested costal cartilage

- The tips of the scissors are maintained in a perpendicular orientation, and the spreading movements are continued until the loose superficial temporal fascia is penetrated. At the end of this step the gleaming white, intact, strong deep temporal fascia should be clearly visible. Figure 20.29 shows the superficial temporal fascia (yellow asterisk) and the deep temporal fascia (black asterisk).
- Once the deep temporal fascia is identified, the full-thickness incision can be safely completed with the scissors (Fig. 20.30).
- The soft tissues over the deep temporal fascia avascular surgical plane are easily elevated utilizing a large Obwegeser elevator creating a bloodless circular pocket having a radius of about 3 cm (Fig. 20.31).
- By pulling the skin flap upwards and downwards with small retractors or double hooks, it is now possible to draw the fascia incision line with the skin marker (Fig. 20.32). With the access obtained with a 3 cm long skin incision it is possible to draw and then harvest a single free fascia flap of about 5 × 5 cm.
- The flap is incised along its margins utilizing a Colorado microdissection needle with the electrosurgical unit set at a low voltage (Fig. 20.33) and finally easily removed under traction separating the fascia from the underlying muscular fibers (Figs. 20.34 and 20.35).

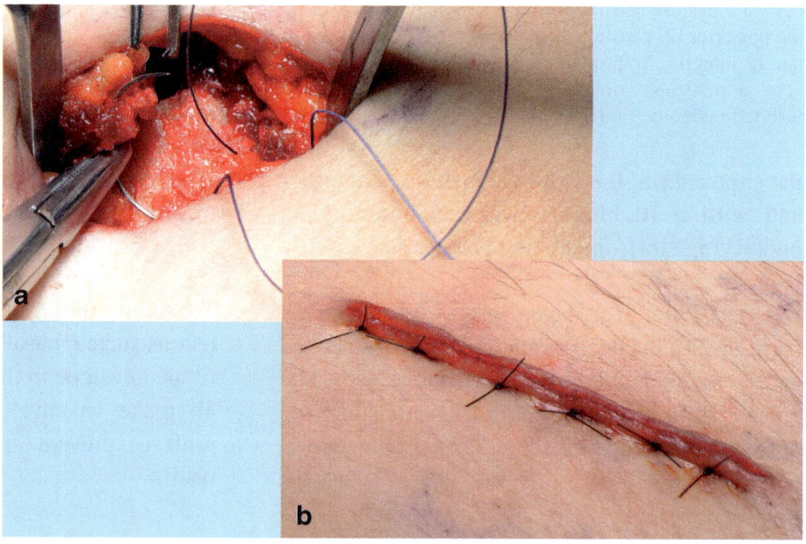

Fig. 20.25 (**a**, **b**) Costal cartilage harvesting steps. The surgical wound closure is multi-layered taking care to suture the muscle flap plane

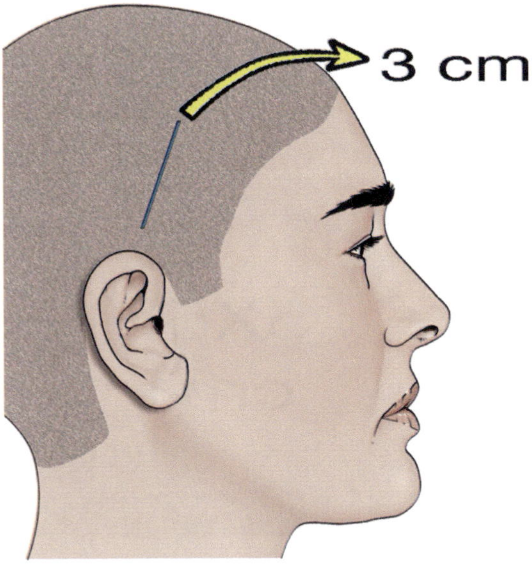

Fig. 20.26 Drawing showing the 3 cm vertical temporal incision line parallel to the hairline

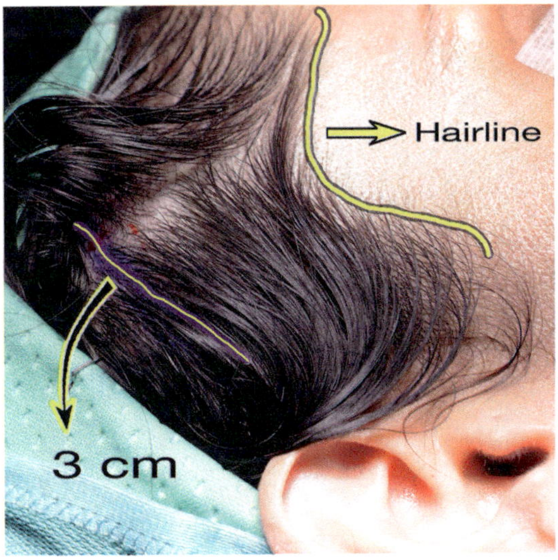

Fig. 20.27 Temporal fascia harvesting steps. The 3 cm vertical temporal incision line parallel to the hairline. The hair is not shaved

- The wound is cleaned with copious sterile saline solution and meticulous hemostasis is performed. The incision is closed with staples (Fig. 20.36). No drains or dressings are used.

Skin disinfectant and antibiotic ointment is applied three times a day for the first three post-operative days and then the patient is allowed to wash their hair with a diluted shampoo and room temperature water.

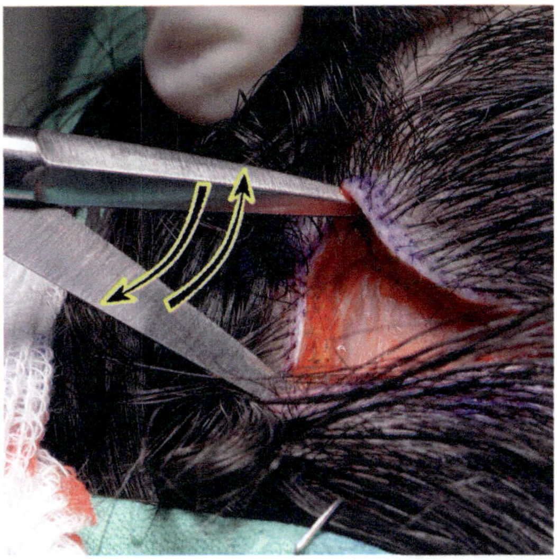

Fig. 20.28 Temporal fascia harvesting steps. The incision is done with a 15 blade reaching the subcutaneous tissue that is then spread transversely with pointed scissors

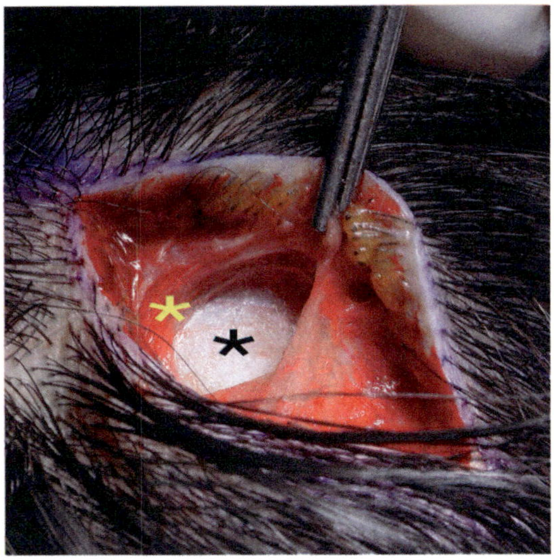

Fig. 20.29 Temporal fascia harvesting steps. The superficial temporal fascia (yellow asterisk) and the deep temporal fascia (black asterisk) are clearly visible to the surgeon

The harvested temporal fascia sheet must be temporarily stored in sterile saline solution until the final stages of the surgery, when it will be used.

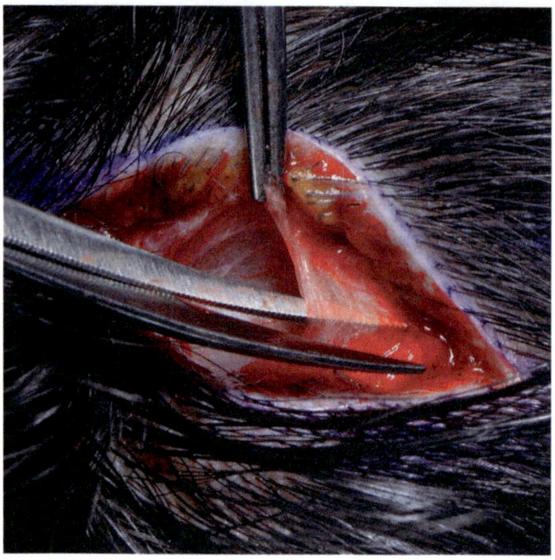

Fig. 20.30 Temporal fascia harvesting steps. Once the deep temporal fascia is identified, the full-thickness incision can be safely completed with the scissors

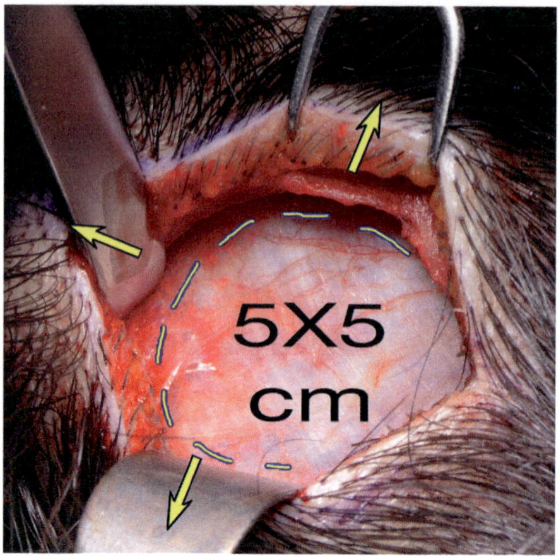

Fig. 20.32 Temporal fascia harvesting steps. By pulling the skin flap upwards and downwards with small retractors or double hooks, it is possible to draw the fascia incision line with the skin marker

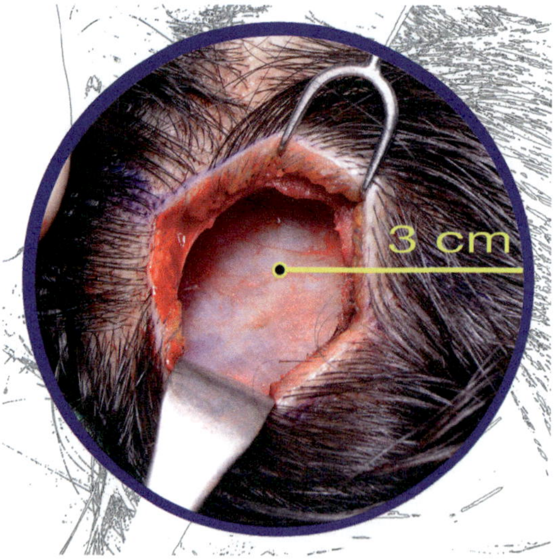

Fig. 20.31 Temporal fascia harvesting steps. The soft tissues over the deep temporal fascia avascular surgical plane are easily elevated utilizing a large Obwegeser elevator creating a bloodless circular pocket having a radius of about 3 cm

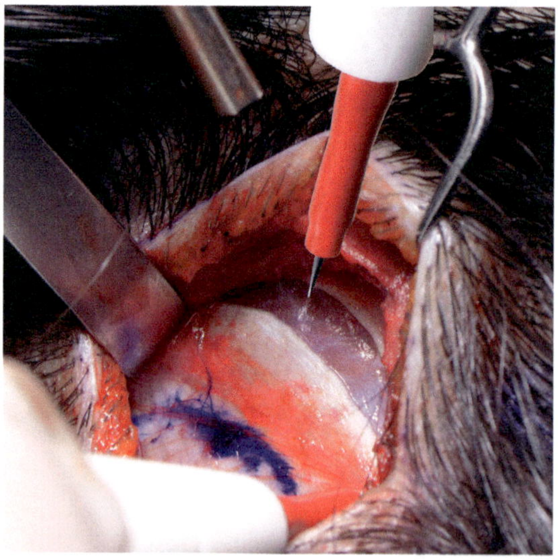

Fig. 20.33 Temporal fascia harvesting steps. The flap is incised along its margins utilizing a Colorado microdissection needle with the electrosurgical unit set at a low voltage

Only before suturing the columellar and marginal incisions is the temporal fascia uniformly and symmetrically distributed over the nasal framework and sutured in place with multiple fast-absorbing 6/0 polyglactin sutures (Fig. 20.37). To further stabilize the graft, its upper portion can be suspended with one or two frontal transcutaneous sutures, as described in Chap. 17.

Figures 20.38 and 20.39 show the clinical result obtained in a secondary case in which the

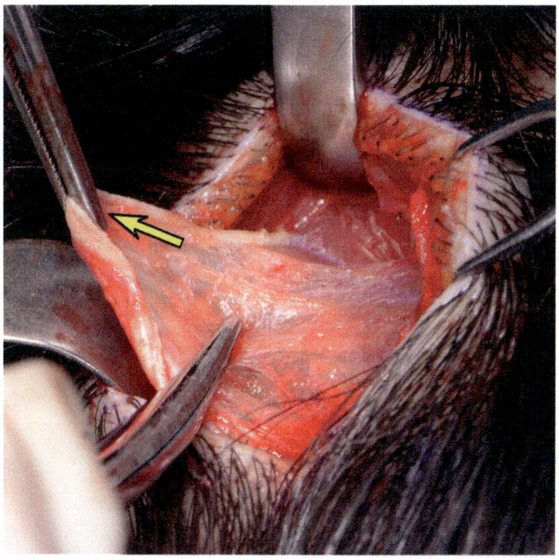

Fig. 20.34 Temporal fascia harvesting steps. Flap elevation under traction

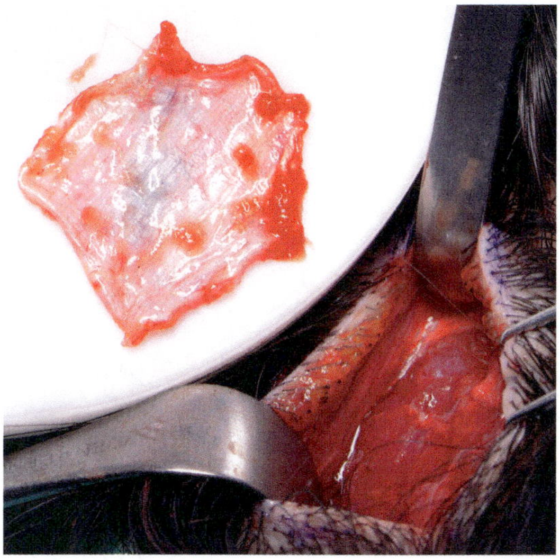

Fig. 20.35 The harvested free temporal fascia

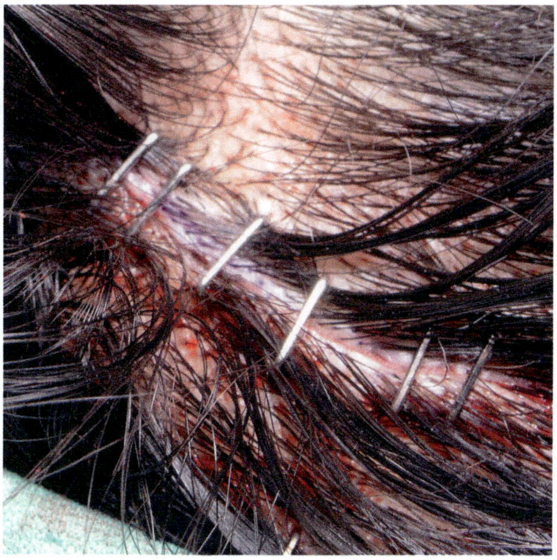

Fig. 20.36 Temporal fascia harvesting steps. The incision is closed with staples. Usually no drains or dressing are needed

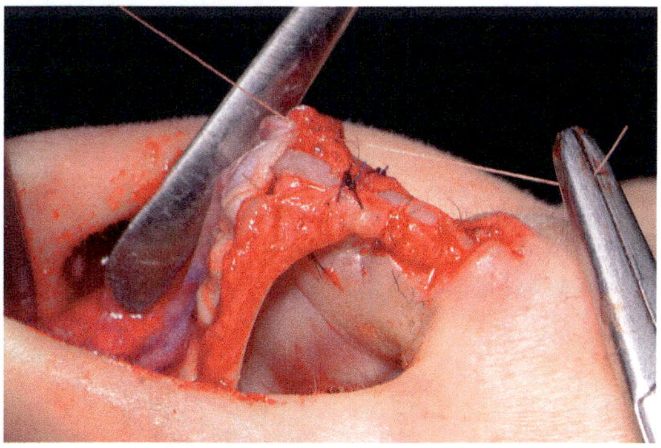

Fig. 20.37 Intraoperative view. The temporal fascia is uniformly and symmetrically distributed over the nasal framework and sutured in place with multiple fast-absorbing 6/0 polyglactin sutures

nasal dorsum deformity required not only a solid reconstruction with autologous cartilage grafts but also the insertion of a midline autologous temporal fascia graft to obtain a smooth and natural external contour. In the case of thin skin patients with secondary surgery or posttraumatic nasal deformities, the use of a temporal fascia graft can be always considered in the preoperative plan.

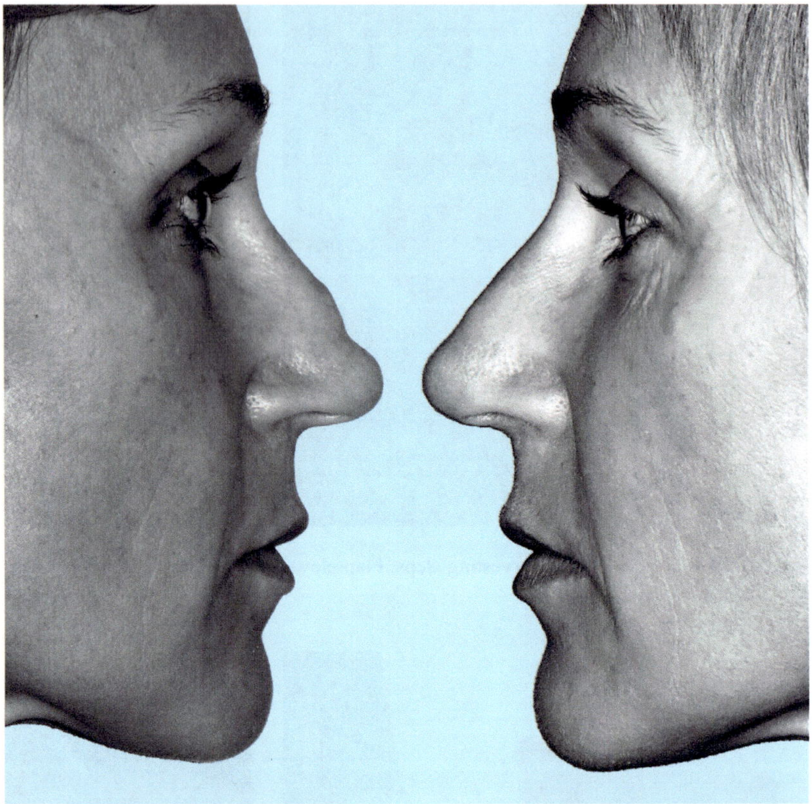

Fig. 20.38 Right profile view of the clinical result obtained in a thin skin patient after secondary reconstruction with solid cartilage grafts and temporal fascia

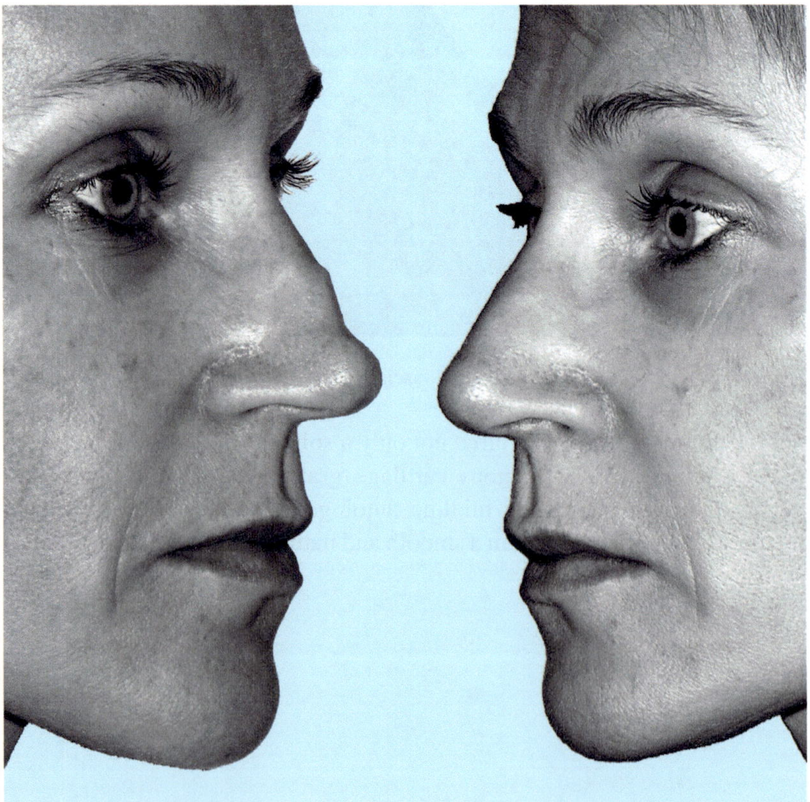

Fig. 20.39 Oblique right view of the same patient as in Fig. 20.38

Further Reading

Books

Daniel RK. Conchal harvest. In: Daniel RK, editor. Mastering rhinoplasty. A comprehensive atlas of surgical techniques. New York: Springer; 2010a. p. 234–7.

Daniel RK. Fascial harvest. In: Daniel RK, editor. Mastering rhinoplasty. A comprehensive atlas of surgical techniques. New York: Springer; 2010b. p. 238–9.

Daniel RK. Rib harvest. In: Daniel RK, editor. Mastering rhinoplasty. A comprehensive atlas of surgical techniques. New York: Springer; 2010c. p. 240–3.

Articles

Marin VP, Landecker A, Gunter JP. Harvesting rib cartilage grafts for secondary rhinoplasty. Plast Reconstr Surg. 2008;121:1442–8.

21 Postoperative Care, Complications, and Unsatisfactory Results in Rhinoplasty

Postoperative care should be well known to the patient before the day of surgery. Also the most common postoperative problems, such as nasal congestion, minor bleeding, or pain, should be mentioned and discussed during the preoperative visits. In the discipline of BOR, this information must also be given in writing. To be as thorough as possible in providing comprehensive written guidance for rhinoplasty patients, in May 2014 the author published a patient's guidebook titled "YOUR RHINOPLASTY - All you need to know about nasal surgery.[1]" Some extracts of the first English edition version of "YOUR RHINOPLASTY" will be reported here to underline the importance of clear and plainly written information in managing the patient's postoperative period as well as the occurrence of complications.

21.1 "Once the Operation is Over and You're Fully Awake,.."

Often the patient asks the surgeon what happens when he wakes up when the rhinoplasty is over. Many think it will be painful and are worried about the early postoperative period. This is the author's simple text with the information about this particular moment:

ONCE THE OPERATION IS OVER...

Once the operation is over and you're fully awake, assisted by the anaesthetist, the first thing you will need to do is concentrate on a few aspects of the immediate post-operational phase.

First of all, you will have to breathe through your mouth. So remember to breathe with your mouth open! Any pain? No, when you awake, your nose will not necessarily be painful, thanks to the personalised pain therapy designed to administer just the right level of pain relief drugs for the duration of your recovery phase.

It is possible that instead you might feel a burning sensation in your throat resembling a typical sore throat (or pharyngitis). The reason for this unpleasant sensation is due to the disinfectants and the tube that was inserted to assist your breathing during the operation. It may be useful, when you wake up, to suck on some common soothing throat pastilles.

Once in the recovery room, for the patient's comfort and safety, it helps to:

- *Use two cushions to keep the head in a slightly raised position.*
- *Grease the nostrils with balm or antibiotic ointment and replace the gauze applied by the surgeon under the nostrils every time it becomes wet with secretions or blood.*
- *Keep visits from friends and family to a minimum.*
- *Prefer soft lighting and avoid unnecessary noise.*
- *... and not take a hot shower!*

[1] Fabio Meneghini. La Tua Rinoplastica, Tutto quello che vorresti sapere sulla chirurgia del naso. First Italian edition 2014. Tempo al Libro—Faenza, Italy. English edition on fourth Italian edition: YOUR RHINOPLASTY—All you need to know about nasal surgery. 2019. Tempo al Libro—Faenza, Italy (English translation by Fabio Leopardi).

F. Meneghini, *Basic Open Rhinoplasty*, https://doi.org/10.1007/978-3-030-61827-8_21

The last sentence may seem funny but it is written for those hyperactive patients who minimize the importance of prudent behavior in the early postoperative days. The decision to insert it into the text came after more than one patient had taken a hot shower within hours of the surgery.

The acceptance of small problems and discomfort should also be mentioned and recalled immediately after:

> *PRACTICE BEING PATIENT*
>
> *It will be easier to cope with the post-operative period if you practice being patient, and are prepared to accept the minor problems that will inevitably arise, with good grace.*
>
> *To come through those days positively, it is essential that you remember to take the prescribed medication and follow the advice that you have read repeatedly in this book. Better still, learn it off by heart! You will see how being well-prepared for the operation helps you in the hours and days following surgery.*

A well-informed and highly motivated patient probably follows closely the surgeon's practical advice.

21.2 Before Discharging the Patient

Preferably the patient leaves the hospital and returns home the next morning. The surgeon meets the patient and removes nasal packing if he still has it. He carefully goes over postoperative care with the patient. The main instructions provided are as follows:

- Nasal tape and splint will remain in place for about 7 days. Your surgeon will remove them during the first postoperative visit. Keep them dry.
- During the day, internal (endonasal) nose washing using saline solution (Tonimer Normal Spray or an equivalent sterile sea water spray product) should be performed repeatedly. Nasal irrigations should be continued for the first postoperative month.
- In the evening, before going to sleep, apply a moisturizing nasal gel, such as Tonimer Nose Gel or equivalent, for the first 10 postoperative days.
- Three to four times a day for the first postoperative week, clean the nostrils with cotton-tipped applicators moistened with hydrogen peroxide. Never insert the applicator inside the nostril deeper than the length of the cotton tip. After that, with another clean cotton-tipped applicator, cover the columellar and nostril suture lines with antibiotic ointment.

The patient is instructed to begin oral antibiotics (usually amoxicillin/clavulanic acid for 5 days) and pain medication if necessary (usually ibuprofen 600 mg as needed).

To encourage the patient to respect these simple rules, the objectives of postoperative care are explained in the book as follows:

> *HOW TO RAPIDLY RETRIEVE NASAL FUNCTIONALITY*
>
> *The importance of breathing through the nose becomes clear whenever we catch a cold and we are forced to breathe through our mouths.*
>
> *During the period following the operation, the care and hygiene of your nose is essential in order to quickly recover nasal functionality. Secretions, which are produced in abundance, tend to accumulate around the openings of the nostrils and can be removed gently using 'cotton-buds' well-soaked in hydrogen peroxide. When performing this action, avoid any pulling or rubbing directly on the surgical incision (where the stitches are).*
>
> *During the day, internal (endonasal) nose washing using saline solution (Tonimer Normal Spray) should be performed repeatedly. In the evening, before going to sleep, apply a moisturising nasal gel such as Tonimer Nose Gel.*
>
> *This will prevent the formation of crusts inside the nostrils which, as well as blocking airflow, are one of the causes of pain or discomfort.*

Before saying goodbye, the surgeon reminds the patient to expect an email or a phone call from him every 2 days to discuss the postoperative evolution together. Giving direct communication channels to our patients is part of the comprehensive "Rhinoplasty" service offered.

21.3 The First Postoperative Visit

If the course is normal, the first postoperative visit is scheduled 6 to 8 days following surgery. After the patient has entered the office, this is the usual order of the steps to follow:

- Remove both the nasal cast and taping (always do this first). With a cotton swab soaked in antibiotic ointment or in skin cream, it is possible to gently lift the Steri-Strip off the nasal skin with less trauma.
- Clean the nasal skin and the nostrils.
- Remove the visible columellar sutures. The internal 6-0 polyglactin absorbable braided sutures do not routinely require trimming as they tend to fall off spontaneously the following week.
- Apply a light film of antibiotic ointment on the suture line.
- Take a complete series of facial clinical photographs.
- Write a list with the postoperative advice to be followed in the following month.

During the whole visit, it is essential to listen carefully to the patient, answer his questions, give advice on how to protect the face from the sun, explain when he can start using glasses again, how to care for and cover the ecchymosis still present and recall the light sport activities that can be practiced without the risk of traumatizing the nose.

In the case of persistent bruises under the eyes, a cream containing vitamin k oxide, such as Auriderm XO cream or equivalent, is recommended. The cream should be applied only over the ecchymosis in a thin layer twice a day, morning and evening, avoiding exposure to the sun after application.

The scheduling of the second postoperative visit depends on several factors. In the case of thick skin, persistent diffuse or localized edema, complete nasal blockage, small surface irregularities, or other problems, the appointment is fixed at 1 week. More frequently, the second visit is expected after about a month.

21.4 The Most Frequent Postoperative Complications

Postoperative complications can be divided in the following main groups:

- Hemorrhage.
- Infection.
- Persistent structural nasal obstruction.
- Septal problems.
- Visible external deformities.
- Skin and soft tissue envelope problems.

The prevention of all sorts of complications starts at the first minute of the first visit, when we investigate the patient's general state of health, and continue throughout the preoperative, intraoperative, and postoperative phases of the clinical case. The BOR discipline is strongly hinged on the prevention of complications by various means, some of which are:

- Inform the patient about the usual risks and give them some idea of their incidence and management. Provide them with an informative text containing a specific section on complications at the first preoperative visit or send it by email before scheduling the first preoperative visit. The prevention and management of complications need informed, honest, and prompt cooperation between the patient and surgeon.
- Personally follow the patient in all aspects and steps of his rhinoplasty experience.
- Always consider that there is little room for delegating to others any decisions during both surgical and non-surgical steps. Always consider the suggestions arriving from your medical team.
- Make sure you have rigorous documentation with preoperative clinical history, clinical facial photographs, and CT scan.
- Schedule at least two meetings with the patient before planning the surgery.
- Create an individual treatment plan without conflict between functional and esthetic goals.
- Avoid unnecessary nasal mucosa incisions by approaching the nose only with a columellar plus bilateral marginal skin incision.
- Perform meticulous skin and mucosal flap elevation on a proper plane (subperiosteal, subperichondrial or immediately over the perichondrium) to reduce vascular trauma.

- Minimize the removal of bone and cartilage support tissues.
- Reconstruct all nasal framework using stabilizing grafts and multiple long-term absorbable sutures.
- Meticulously suture skin incisions and any possible mucosal tears.
- Give direct communication channels to the patient and sometimes plan further postoperative visits on an individual basis.
- Offer to refer the patient with particular complications to other expert rhinoplasty surgeons.

This latter possibility is also mentioned in the informative text delivered to the patient:

A TEAM OF EXPERTS

The success of a great athlete, the performance of a new model of car, innovations in science and all that brings about improvements compared to the past, requires a team of specialists.

It may be that, for whatever reason and at any moment, the surgeon may decide to consult a colleague with a specific expertise, thus deciding to extend the team taking care of you and your nose.

Facial surgery, especially rhinoplasty, is a demanding challenge and the variables involved are many. For this reason, a patient need not worry about this decision for a consultation, as long as it is your surgeon himself contacting and introducing the colleague.

21.5 Hemorrhage

In the author's last 100 consecutive cases, two patients had early postoperative hemorrhage that required control by anterior bilateral packing with Merocel sponge. In both cases, a complex septal deviation was present preoperatively and a septoplasty was done. Nasal packing was removed the day after surgery and the patients were discharged.

In the author's experience, nasal packing is applied during surgery and maintained until the morning after surgery in less than 30% of cases. In the other cases, nasal packing is removed at the end of the surgical procedure before waking the patient up.

In the BOR discipline, the only role of nasal packing is that of promoting hemostasis since the early stabilization of the osteocartilaginous framework is totally dependent on meticulous internal sutures.

21.6 Infection

In 30 years of nasal surgery experience, 20 of which as a first operator, no acute or late infections have occurred. Although this encouraging statistical data could suggest that the nose is an organ that naturally defends itself against infections, many of the aspects codified and applied in the BOR discipline are related to controlling infections.

Some rules to minimize the risk of infection are:

- Inform the patient with all your best personal commitment and strongly request his cooperation. Patient cooperation is a prerequisite in preventing postoperative infections.
- A few minutes before the skin incision, administer 1 g of cefazolin intravenously.
- Perform skin and endonasal disinfection with half-strength (5%) povidone-iodine solution.
- Create a sterile field following the principles of draping.
- Cover the patient's entire body with sterile drapes.
- Avoid unnecessary nasal mucosa incisions by approaching the nose only with a columellar plus bilateral marginal skin incision.
- Perform meticulous skin and mucosal flap elevation on a proper plane (subperiosteal, subperichondrial or immediately over the perichondrium) to reduce vascular trauma and edema and to promote rapid postoperative healing around the skeletal framework and at the incision line.
- Gently clean all the harvested fragments of cartilage and store them in sterile saline solution inside a small capped Teflon container to avoid any contamination of the future grafts.

- Frequently irrigate the surgical field and the nose internally and externally with sterile saline throughout the surgery.
- Avoid alloplastic nasal implants.
- Avoid using nonabsorbable internal sutures, if possible.
- Perform meticulous suturing of all skin incisions and any possible mucosal tears.
- Avoid or limit nasal packing to less than 24 h. If applying packing, use only sterile Merocel sponge.
- Prescribe high frequency nose washing using sterile saline spray solution beginning early postoperatively or immediately after nasal packing removal.
- Prescribe 5 days of postoperative antibiotic therapy.
- Instruct the patient to clean the nostrils and apply a light film of antibiotic ointment on the suture line three to four times a day for the first postoperative week.
- Surround yourself with highly professional colleagues and nurse.
- Perform nasal surgery only in a hospital with excellence standards.

In the case of swelling with suspected infection, it is not recommended to rely only on the pharmacological therapy but it is absolutely necessary to incise the mucosa, drain and wash profusely with diluted antiseptic solution. Subsequent adjustment of antibiotics based on cultures is also done as well as daily office visits to inspect the nose and clean the nasal cavities.

21.7 Persistent Structural Nasal Obstruction

Postoperative nasal obstruction, after healing of the mucous membranes, can have three main types of causes more or less combined with each other:

- Pre-existing structural problems not identified or identified but not adequately treated due to inaccurate or weak preoperative studies and analysis.
- Excessive dimensional reduction of the nose with loss of volume of the nasal airway due to errors in treatment planning.
- New postoperative deformities caused by nasal surgery due to poor surgical technique. They may be visible externally or not.

The general principles of the BOR discipline to prevent postoperative structural nasal obstruction can be summarized in these points:

- Accurate nasal clinical history.
- Accurate studies of the nasal airway by CT scan.
- Accurate study of the external shape of the nose by direct inspection and standard set of photographic documentation.
- Planning every change of nasal shape conservatively and writing down the treatment plan as a comprehensive list of points. Always reconsidering the points in the plan with a view to maintaining or restoring nasal function.
- Avoiding unnecessary nasal mucosa incisions but approaching the nose only with a columellar plus bilateral marginal skin incision.
- Initial accurate intraoperative analysis of shape, thickness, structural memory, and consistency of the cartilaginous framework.
- Performing hump removal without tearing or removing the underlying nasal mucosa. The operative sequence should be bone first and then cartilage, making sure to preserve the integrity of the underlying mucosa.
- Removal of the least possible quantity of bone and cartilage tissues.
- Always reconstructing the nasal framework with long-lasting absorbable internal sutures and structural autologous cartilage grafts.
- After osteotomies, checking the bone position and stability obtained and not forgetting to suture them to the nasal septum in the case of

a tendency to unwanted displacement, hypermobility, and collapse.
- During all the stages of the surgery, constantly asking yourself if the action you are doing has a negative influence on nasal function.

It is not strange that some points to be respected to prevent infections are also suggested for the prevention of postoperative nasal obstruction.

21.8 Postoperative Septal Problems

The five main postoperative septal problems are:

- Septal hematoma.
- Synechiae between the turbinates and the septum.
- Loss of stability with more or less evident saddle nose deformity.
- Septal perforation.
- Residual septal deviation.

In the author's personal experience, none of the first four complications has ever occurred, whereas residual septal deviation is one of more common causes of revision surgery for nasal dorsal asymmetries.

Again, compliance with some general principles included in the BOR discipline is mandatory to prevent septal problems. The main ones are:

- Inform the patient about the risk of early postoperative nasal trauma on the reconstructed nasal framework and septum and strongly request his cooperation.
- Inquire preoperatively about a possible recreational use of cocaine. Rhinoplasty and septoplasty should be avoided in patients with a known history of intranasal cocaine application. In the case of surgical reconstruction of external nasal deformities, the patient must be "clean" of cocaine for at least 1 year.
- Always request a preoperative CT scan of the paranasal sinuses to study the septum as well as all the other nasal structures. Knowing in advance the degree and complexity of the septal deviation and the presence of bony spurs is helpful in determining the septal aspects of the rhinoplasty.
- Avoid any septal mucosal surgical incision.
- Respect, if feasible, the integrity of the mucosa during the procedure.
- Suture, if possible, any mucosal tears with polyglactin braided fast-absorbing suture.
- Midline caudal septal relocation is a mandatory goal of surgery. Direct suture of the cartilage to the anterior nasal spine should be considered when, after the initial steps of the septoplasty, the anteroinferior margin of the quadrangular cartilage does not lie spontaneously along the midline.
- Always stabilize the septum by suturing the dorsal margin of the quadrangular cartilage to the upper lateral cartilages and sometimes to the nasal bones utilizing 5/0 long-lasting absorbable polydioxanone monofilament. At least three horizontal mattress sutures on the cartilages and a simple one on the bone are needed.
- Consider spreader grafts or other structural grafts to reinforce and stabilize the septum.
- Avoid empty space and retain in place the two septal mucosal layers with quilting suture. The quilting suture is a fixed step of the BOR discipline and should be done after completing septoplasty and inferior turbinate surgery.

Nasal packing, especially if prolonged beyond the first 24 h, is not considered to be of any help to the healing processes nor can it be used to stabilize or keep the septum centered.

21.9 Supratip Swelling

Especially in patients with thick skin, 1 month after surgery it is not uncommon to have a still poorly defined nasal tip. Usually the most evident clinical finding is supratip swelling. Palpating the skin it must be clear that the problem is related only to the persistence of the swelling. The presence of a hard superficial deformity in the supratip area can be due to a residual excess of alar or septal cartilage as well as to a poorly fixed and displaced graft.

In the case of supratip swelling, a treatment with triamcinolone acetonide can be considered.

The major risk of treatment with triamcinolone injections is subcutaneous atrophy so it is critical that Kenalog be injected deep under the dermis in very small quantities. Because triamcinolone remains active in the tissue for 4 to 6 weeks, it should not be used more frequently than once every 2 months and should be repeated only 2 or 3 times in the event of persistent swelling. These subdermal injections should not be used in any region other than the supratip.

The simple steps and technique for the injection are:

- Shake well the vial as triamcinolone comes in a suspension rather than as a solution.
- Prefer a 1-mL tuberculin syringe with a 30-gauge needle.
- Insert the needle at 90° deep under the dermis in the upper swollen area and along the midline (Fig. 21.1).
- Aspirate to avoid injection of triamcinolone into a blood vessel.
- Inject no more than 0.1 mL of 40 mg/mL triamcinolone.

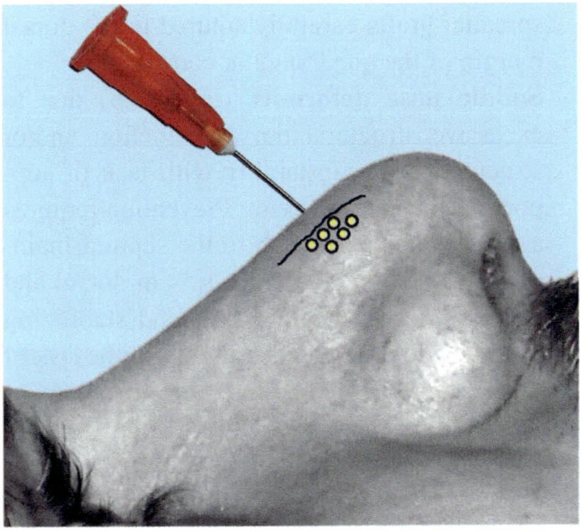

Fig. 21.1 Needle orientation used in the injection of triamcinolone in the event of supratip swelling

This prudent and limited treatment of supratip swelling has proven effective with stable results in about 80% of patients, without the appearance of secondary skin atrophy.

21.10 The Most Common Postoperative Visible Deformities

From top to bottom, the most common postoperative external deformities are:

- **Asymmetry of the bony vault** (Fig. 21.2). This can occur for multiple reasons such as: asymmetric or unstable osteotomies, unrecognized or untreated bony high (ethmoidal) septal deviation that displaces laterally the osteotomized nasal bone. Prevention requires precise intraoperative diagnosis and immediate reconstruction with unilateral spreader graft and multiple stabilizing bony and cartilaginous sutures. Sometimes also camouflage grafts at the end of the procedure are needed.
- **Rocker deformity** due to continuation of osteotomies into the frontal bone. Attempted narrowing after the osteotomies results in lateralization of the superior segment of the fractured bones, based on a fulcrum at or around the radix. In the author's experience, it is a very rare deformity suspected only in his earliest practice with the closed technique. Performing the osteotomies under direct vision with the aid of very small dedicated saws vibrating at ultrasonic frequency, the risk of unwanted osteotomy lines and rocker deformity is definitively eliminated.
- **High stairstep deformity**. A posterior and medial movement of nasal bones produced with finger pressure during osteotomy mobilization causes this deformity. It is a palpable and sometime visible stairstep close to the radix midline in thin skin patients and can be confused with the Rocker deformity. Performing the open approach, it is clearly visible with intraoperative direct visual inspection and it is easily treated with an ultrasound rasp device.

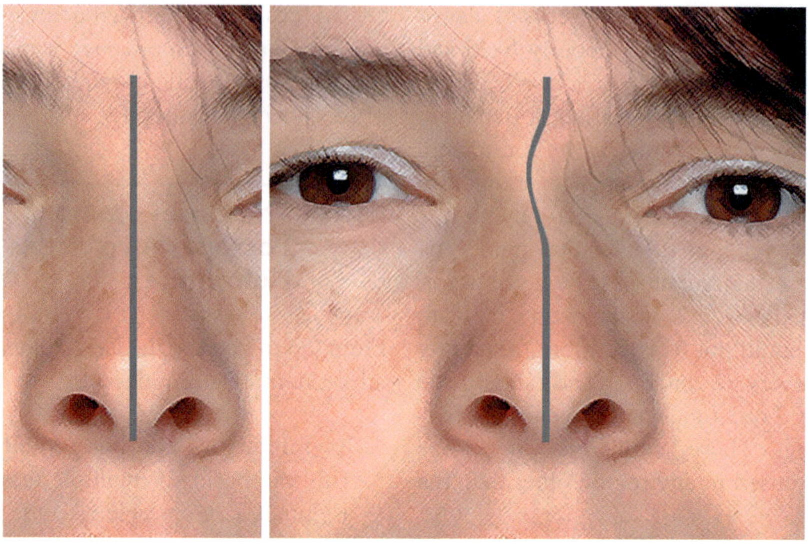

Fig. 21.2 Asymmetry of the bony vault

- **Open roof deformity**. This is a temporary deformity produced by the removal of the bone hump. The intraoperative open roof is immediately corrected with the lateral osteotomies and the medial and symmetrical movements of the lateral walls towards the dorsal profile of the nasal septum. Failure to perform lateral osteotomies and stabilize the lateral walls in close contact with the septum leaves the open roof. After the osteotomies, to fine-tune the bony dorsum width and reduce the risk of open roof deformity, a stabilizing suture of the two nasal bones to the septum is recommended.
- **Asymmetry of the middle vault** (Fig. 21.3). More frequently this can be due to septal deviation. Prevention requires precise intraoperative diagnosis and dorsal septal straightening with spreader grafts and multiple stabilizing bony and upper lateral cartilage sutures to the dorsal margin of the septum. Sometimes refinements with camouflage grafts are needed.
- **Inverted-V deformity**. This refers to an upside-down V-shaped indentation between the free margin of the nasal bones and the upper lateral cartilages. The main cause of the inverted-V is a rotation of the upper lateral cartilages in an inferior and posterior direction following hump removal and osteotomies (Fig. 21.4). Since an upper lateral cartilage collapse against the septum reduces the nasal airway, a more or less severe functional impairment is associated with the external deformity. Prevention requires a conservative treatment plan that limits the dorsal reduction or contemplates a mandatory reconstruction of the nasal dorsum with spreader flaps or spreader grafts carefully sutured to the dorsal margin of the quadrangular cartilage.
- **Saddle nose deformity** (Fig. 21.5) due to excessive structural dorsal reduction and/or structural septal instability with lack of support for the nasal dorsum. Prevention requires a conservative approach to the septum maintaining a stable and strong 1.5-cm dorsal and caudal strut. Structural grafts and stabilizing sutures are recommended to reduce the risk of this severe esthetic and functional problem.
- **Lateral stairstep deformity** (simply called stairstep deformity). This is due to improper placement of the lateral osteotomy line at a

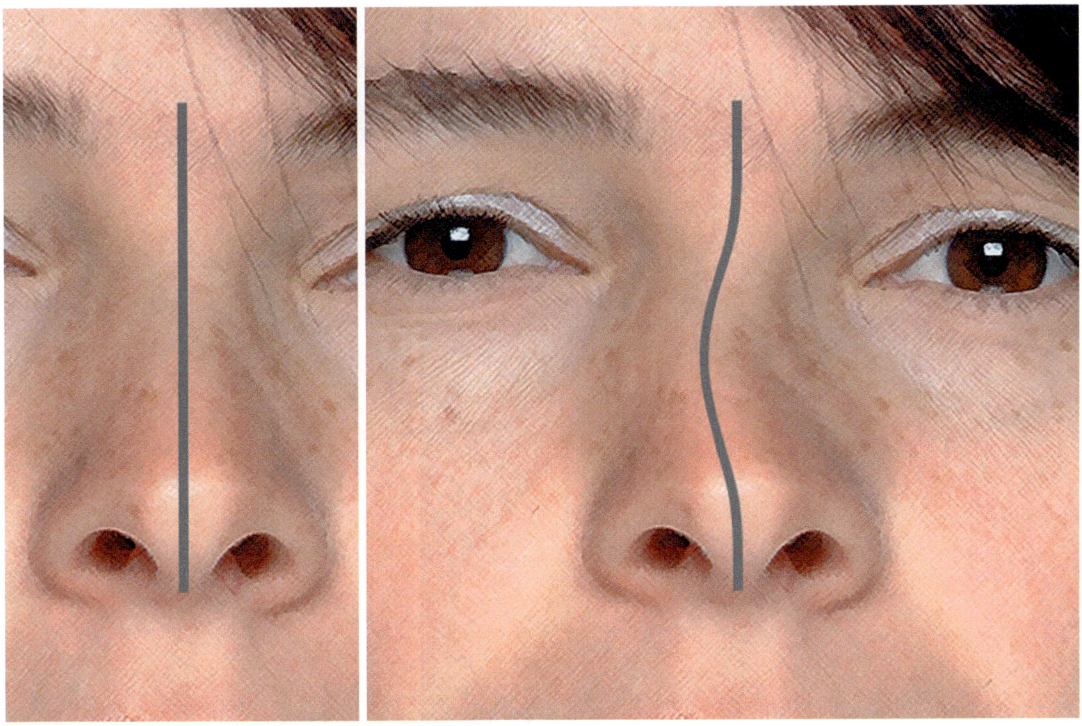

Fig. 21.3 Asymmetry of the middle vault

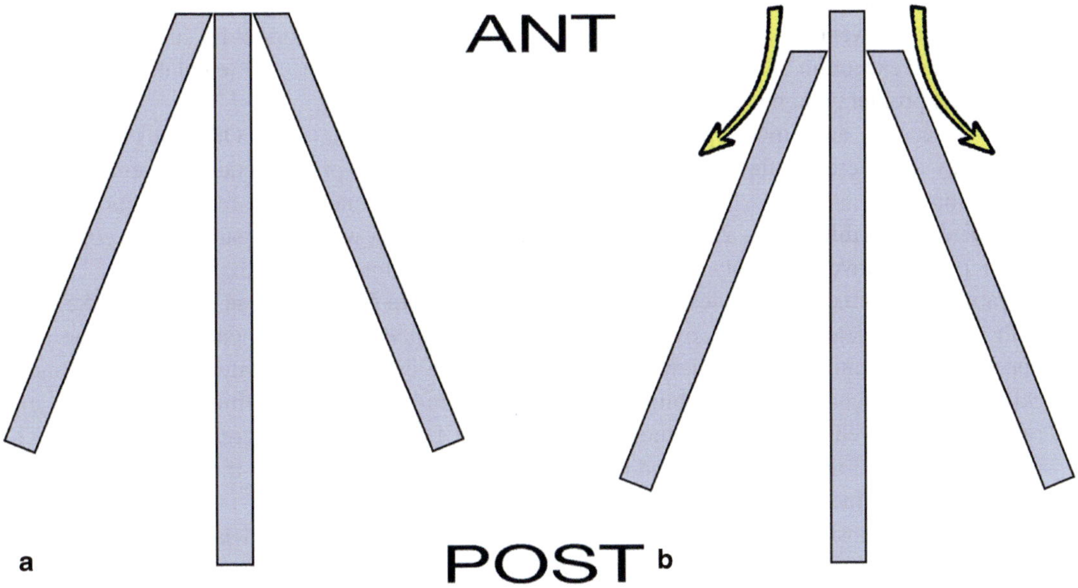

Fig. 21.4 (**a**, **b**) Cause of inverted-V deformity. Posterior slippage of the upper lateral cartilages following osteotomies and hump removal

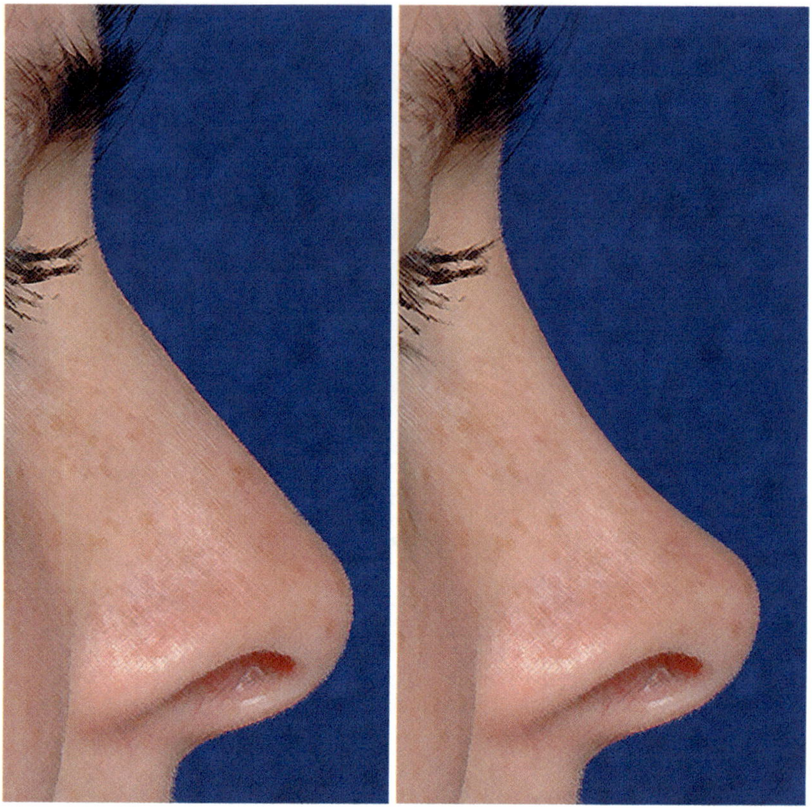

Fig. 21.5 Saddle nose deformity

level too anterior on the ascending process of the maxilla. Prevention requires meticulous planning and execution of the nasal osteotomy lines. This problem can be partially improved with a second and more posterior new osteotomy and therefore the best course is its prevention.

- **Pollybeak deformity** (Fig. 21.6). This is a stable postoperative deformity in which the supratip fullness is more or less associated with a down-rotated tip and over-resected upper nasal dorsum: in profile view, the typical dorsal nasal convexity resembling a parrot's beak. Prevention requires meticulous planning of dorsal reduction, balanced in both bony and cartilaginous components, as well as precise spatial positioning of the nasal tip. Pollybeak deformity should not be mistaken for the more frequent postoperative soft supratip swelling.
- **Tip asymmetry** (Figs. 21.7 and 21.8). This deformity can have many causes combined with each other such as residual caudal septum deviation, incorrect tip sutures, and interference between the caudal septum and columellar strut.
- **Tip ptosis** (Fig. 21.9). Often this represents a more or less pronounced recurrence secondary to an inadequate reconstruction of the framework without a supporting columellar strut and internal stabilizing sutures.
- **Nasal tip bossae**. These are "knoblike" protuberances of the alar cartilages at the level of the domes or just lateral to them. Bossae are more evident in thin skin patients and can be caused by aggressive surgical techniques, which weaken the rim strips near the domes.
- **Pinched tip** (Fig. 21.10a, b). This can be a sign of over-resected lateral crura and excessive tightening of nasal tip sutures. In the past it was a stigma of interrupted rim strip techniques. In the case of thin and structurally weak alar cartilages, the prevention of second-

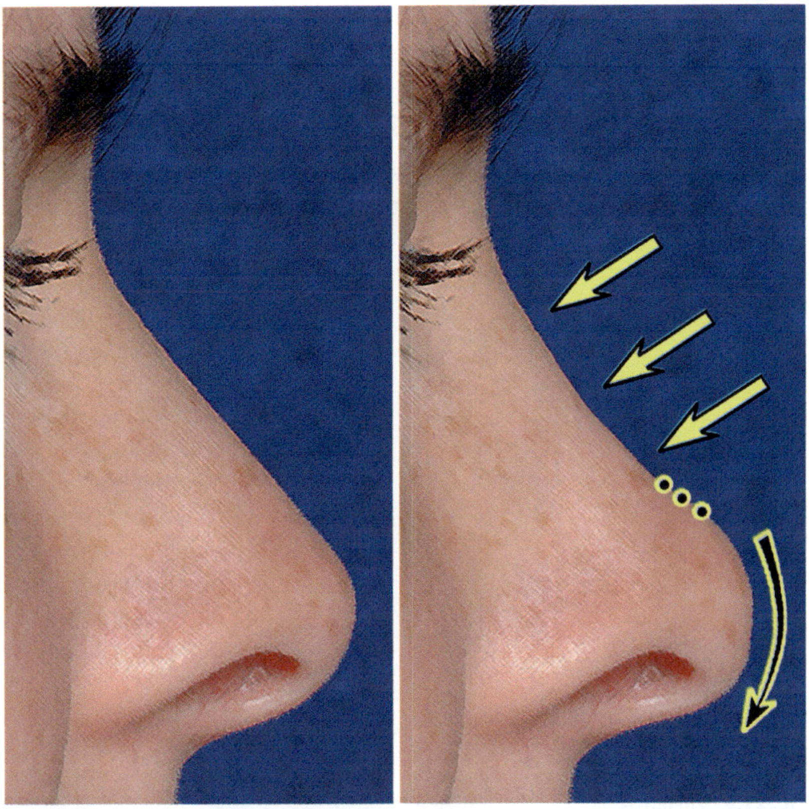

Fig. 21.6 Pollybeak deformity. This is a stable postoperative deformity in which the supratip fullness (dots) is more or less associated with a down-rotated tip (curved arrow) and an over-resected upper nasal dorsum (three straight arrows)

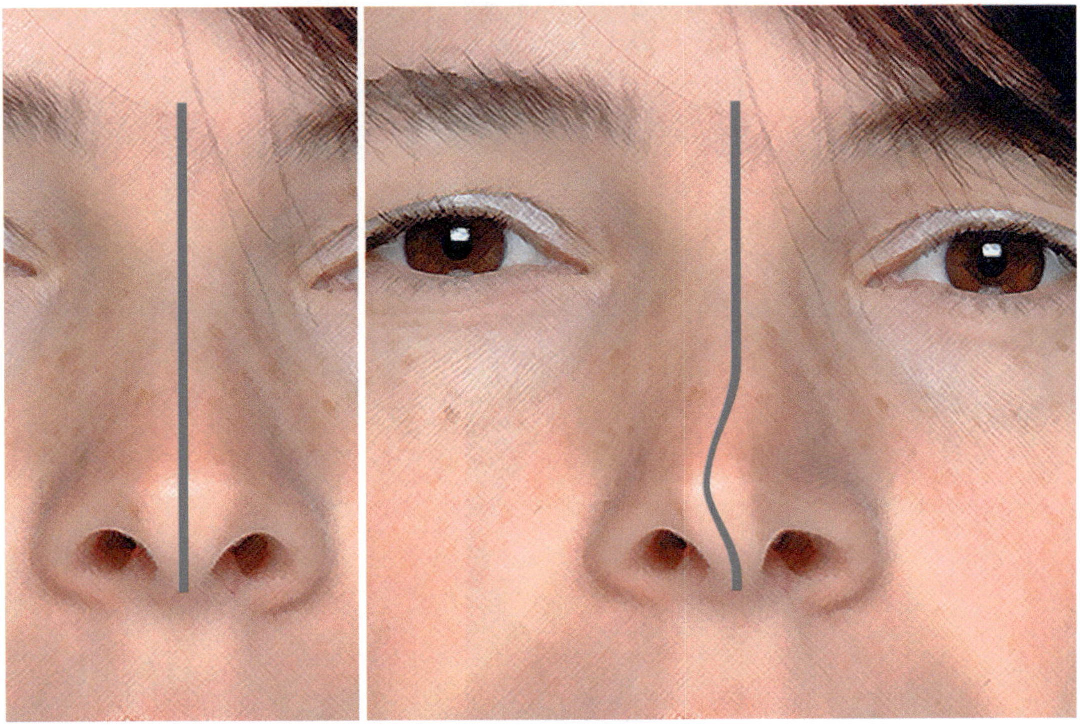

Fig. 21.7 Tip asymmetry (frontal view)

ary tip deformity can require reinforcement of the lateral crura with a turn-in flap and structural grafts.

- **Poorly defined tip**. This deformity is more frequent in thick skin noses mostly when a loss of tip projection occurs. Over-resection and lack of structural reconstruction should be avoided.
- **Nostril asymmetry** (Fig. 21.11). The possible causes are residual caudal septal deviation, errors in handling and suturing together the lower lateral cartilages and spatial interference with contact between caudal septum and columellar strut that displace the columella.
- **Visible grafts**. Causes are the poor carving of the graft or its displacement due to insufficient stabilization with multiple sutures. A precise written description of the grafts used during surgery is necessary to diagnose this deformity that often becomes evident months later.

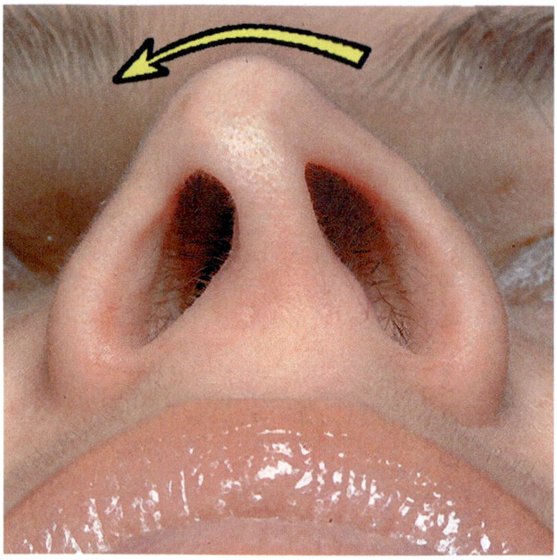

Fig. 21.8 Tip asymmetry (basal view)

Fig. 21.9 Tip ptosis

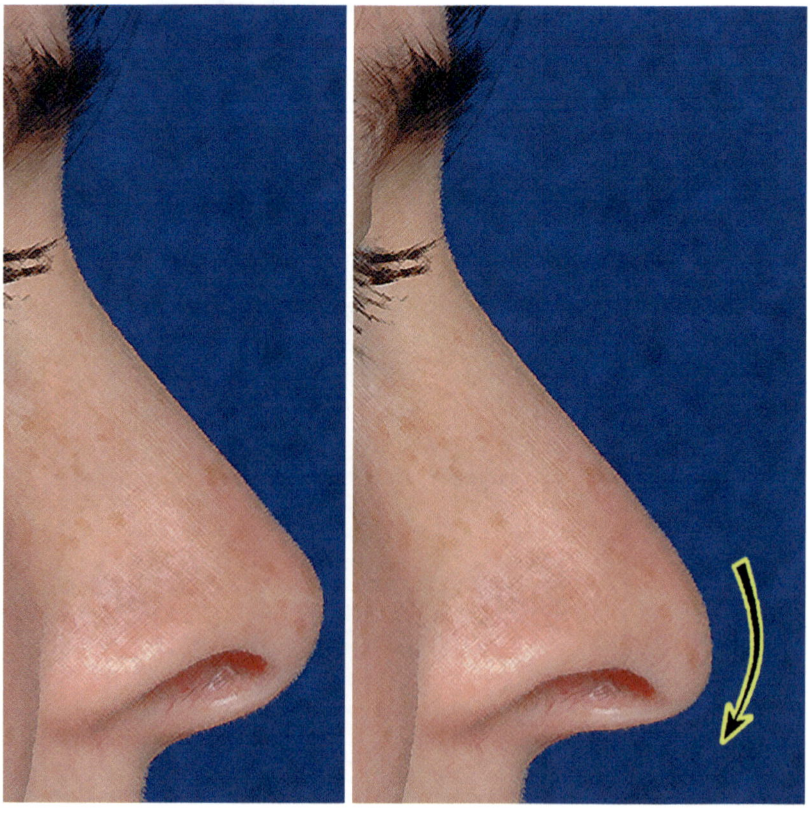

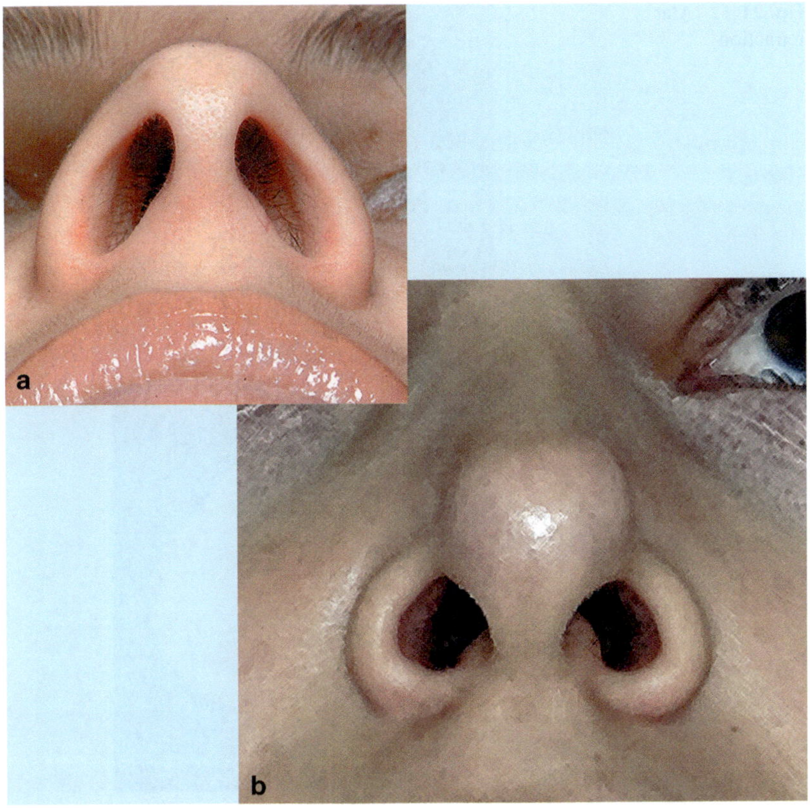

Fig. 21.10 (**a**, **b**) Normal not operated (**a**) and pinched nasal tip secondary to aggressive endonasal tip surgery (**b**)

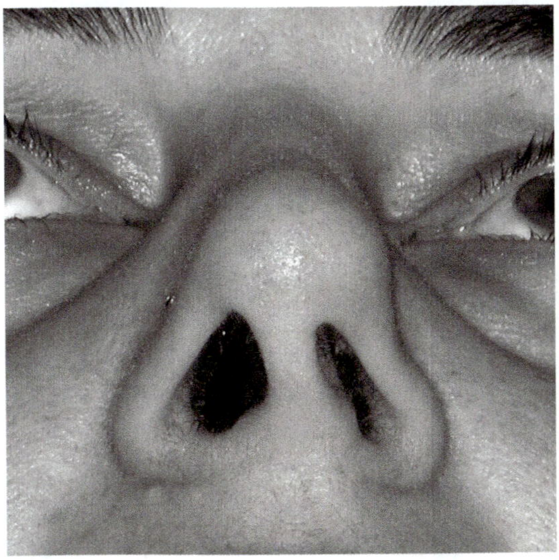

Fig. 21.11 Nostril asymmetry

- **Alar retraction** (Fig. 21.12). This has several surgical causes such as over-resected lateral crura, upward orientation of the lateral crura by errors in nasal tip suturing technique, overly tight closure of the marginal incision.
- **Columellar retraction** (Fig. 21.13). This can be secondary to over-resected caudal septum, excessive upward traction of the columella with quilting septal sutures, poorly executed "tongue-in-groove" sutures for tip stabilization, or failure to correct a short nose with a septal extension graft.

21.11 "THE MOST FREQUENT COMPLICATIONS" Explained to the Patient

Several times in the written information given to the patient it is necessary to mention the possible postoperative complications and the way to deal with them. These are some of the texts used for this purpose by the author in his patient book "YOUR RHINOPLASTY":

Fig. 21.12 Alar retraction

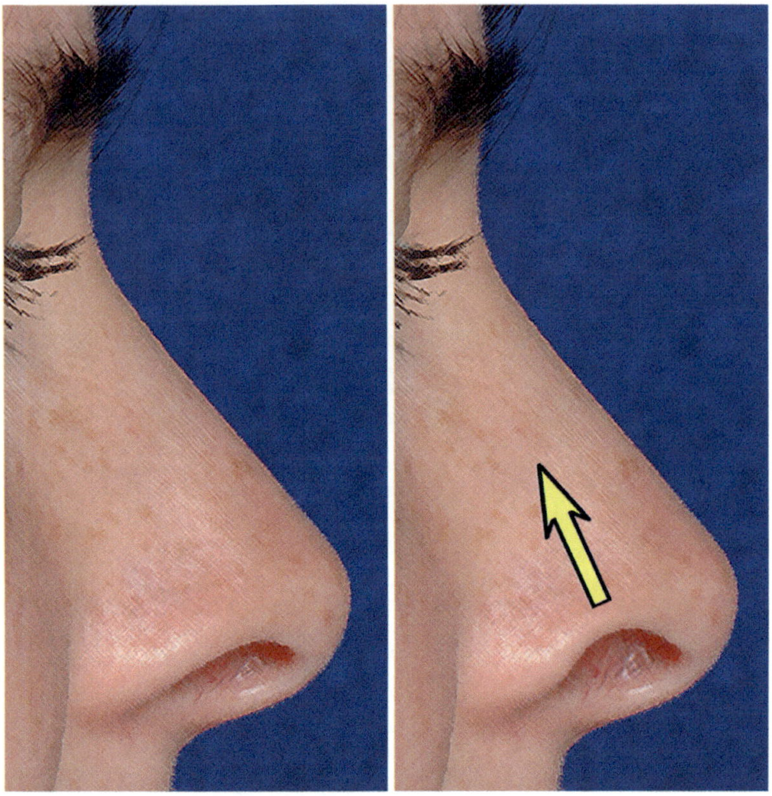

Fig. 21.13 Columellar retraction

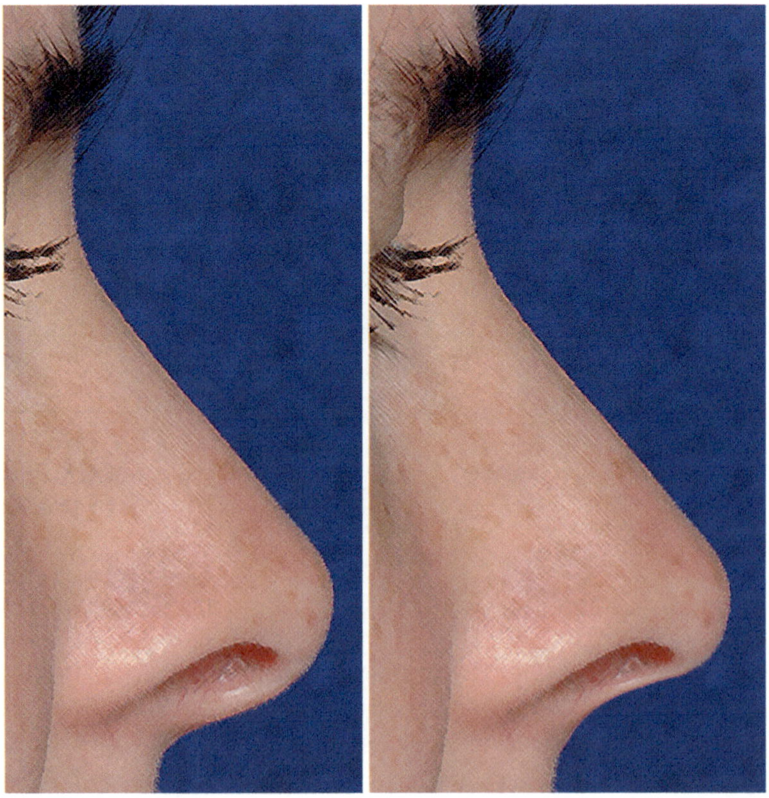

THE MOST FREQUENT COMPLICATIONS

Major complications are extremely rare when rhinoplasty is performed by expert hands on a well-informed and collaborative patient.

Inconveniences as a result of the operation are usually minimal. The main drawback derives from the fact that (nasal) breathing is hindered due to increased secretions, and it is simply a case of putting up with it for a few days.

Following septoplasty or turbinoplasty, the increased flow of air through the nose can unsettle a patient, but again, it is just a matter of getting used to this new sensation.

The mucous membrane that covers the nose internally needs time to heal, and the swelling and irritation will resolve themselves in the first six to seven weeks. My advice is to avoid aggressive decongestant medications in sprays or drops and to wait for spontaneous healing of these internal mucous membranes.

Excessive bleeding is rare in rhinoplasty (an incidence of probably less than five percent). However, should this occur the recommendation is to pack the nose once again or to cauterize the small blood vessel that is still bleeding.

After rhinoplasty surgery, small irregularities may appear which, in some cases, require subsequent corrections. I consider it preferable to accept the possibility of an eventual 'touch-up' to the nose as the alternative to a more aggressive initial operation. Many repeat procedures are of a minor nature and of short duration.

Infection is a possible complication of any kind of surgical procedure, but happily it is extremely rare in the nose, where serious infection could damage nasal tissues.

A sudden sneeze, a small trauma or inadvertent manipulation can displace the nasal structures resulting, at worst, in loss of the form or symmetry of the nose obtained by the operation. If these incidents are readily acknowledged, they can often be corrected without subjecting the patient to another operation.

The septal cartilage behaves like a spring and if moved, tends to return to its position of rest. To correct a septal deviation it is therefore necessary to weaken the 'spring'. The septum also represents an important brace for the nose. For this reason it is vital to find a compromise between straightening the septum and its support function, and to advise the patient that incomplete correction and/or asymmetrical nasal deformity may be residual conditions.

Some aspects of the healing processes are beyond control. If some areas do not heal properly or there is excessive production of scar tissue, internal or external (visible) deformities may appear. Rarely, septal perforation may occur but this can be improved or corrected by a subsequent procedure.

In rare cases, a change in the sense of smell has been reported. While in my personal clinical experience I have not found residual problems concerning the sense of smell, these are theoretically possible.

All the complications of rhinoplasty mentioned are unusual but, despite the use of all the appropriate surgical measures, they cannot be totally excluded. They have been listed, not to alarm the patient, but rather to offer the most complete information possible.

UNSATISFACTORY OUTCOMES

As I have said before, this type of surgery is not magic. When both the aesthetic and the functional results are not satisfactory, we have to accept this eventuality and look for the underlying causes of failure. To make this assessment we can:

- *Verify all the previous steps (planning and execution of the operation, treatments and post-operative behaviour).*
- *Acquire new documentation of the condition with further consultations and tests.*
- *Request an eventual consultation from an expert colleague.*

However, in time most patients report being satisfied with the results achieved with nasal surgery.

Also limiting factors are an aspect of surgery that must be clearly explained to patient:

ACCEPT WHAT YOU CANNOT CHANGE

In all fields there are circumstances we have to face up to. There are things we can change, things over which we can exercise control. But there are also things we cannot do anything about.

Even in the best hands, rhinoplasty has its limits and boundaries, and it is important that these are addressed, clarified and above all accepted.

A long nose can be shortened, a long face, not.

A large nose can be shrunk, but it can never be made small.

A wide tip can be improved, but it can never be made tiny.

When the nose is not centred in respect to the face (other terms to define this condition are deviation or asymmetrical nose), our expectations for the operation have to be for a partial centring, because perfect alignment would be difficult to achieve.

Discuss these limiting factors with your surgeon beforehand, apply them to your specific case and remember to accept what you cannot change!

Further Reading

Books

Tebbetts JB. Primary Rhinoplasty. St. Louis: Mosby; 1998.

Guyuron B. Rhinoplasty. Edinburgh: Elsevier Saunders; 2012.

Daniel RK, Pálházi P. Rhinoplasty. Heidelberg: Springer; 2018.

Articles

Surowitz JB, Most SP. Complications of rhinoplasty. Facial Plast Surg Clin N Am. 2013;21:639–51.

22 A Clinical Practice Focused on Rhinoplasty

How to build a clinical practice focused on rhinoplasty? Like many human activities, it is a matter of an infinite series of rules and of four main boundaries. Knowing, improving, and applying these rules while remaining within the boundaries is mandatory, so it is advisable to start studying them and repeating them almost every day of our clinical practice. The most important word of the last sentence—you found it for sure—is "**improving.**" The undoubted fact that every surgeon is called to **improve** the rules and vary his boundaries makes rhinoplasty a tricky and fascinating practice for our lifelong journey.

This chapter, more than of the rest of this book, is dedicated to every young surgeon who still does not know if rhinoplasty will be their working passion. The aim is to offer the basis for an identikit of the rhinoplasty professional. It starts with the boundaries, continues with a long series of rules, suggestions, and personal considerations and finally ends with a little story about something that happened to the author many years ago during a rhinoplasty course held in Philadelphia.

22.1 Boundaries

In an abstract form, the field of rhinoplasty can be viewed as a box with four sides. Each side of the box represents a group of boundaries for the surgeon. This is only a simplification but every day he must act respecting these boundaries:

- **Moral Boundaries**. These concern the surgeon's ethical behavior towards his patient and all those involved in the professional activity.
- **Technical Boundaries**. In this broad category we find the manual skills, the basic medical knowledge, the specific knowledge of the surgeon in the field of rhinoplasty, the professionalism of the medical team, the medical facility, the instruments and the electromedical devices used, and much more.
- **Legal Boundaries**. These refer to all the rules conforming to or permitted by the law as well as the established medical rules.
- **Physical Boundaries**. These are subject to the laws of nature. The biological aspects, including the patient's physical and mental health conditions, fall into this category.

Boundaries must not be perceived as obstacles or impediments; instead, they circumscribe an area so large as to make rhinoplasty a very interesting and rich field of study and work.

Figure 22.1a–c divides the way of conceiving rhinoplasty boundaries into three main situations:

- A large area perfectly delimited by borders in which a surgeon can find his way into the profession. For a few of these surgeons, remaining in this area offers a unique, ever-changing and fulfilling activity (**a**).
- A small area where the surgeon struggles to find a good level of professionalism and is

F. Meneghini, *Basic Open Rhinoplasty*, https://doi.org/10.1007/978-3-030-61827-8_22

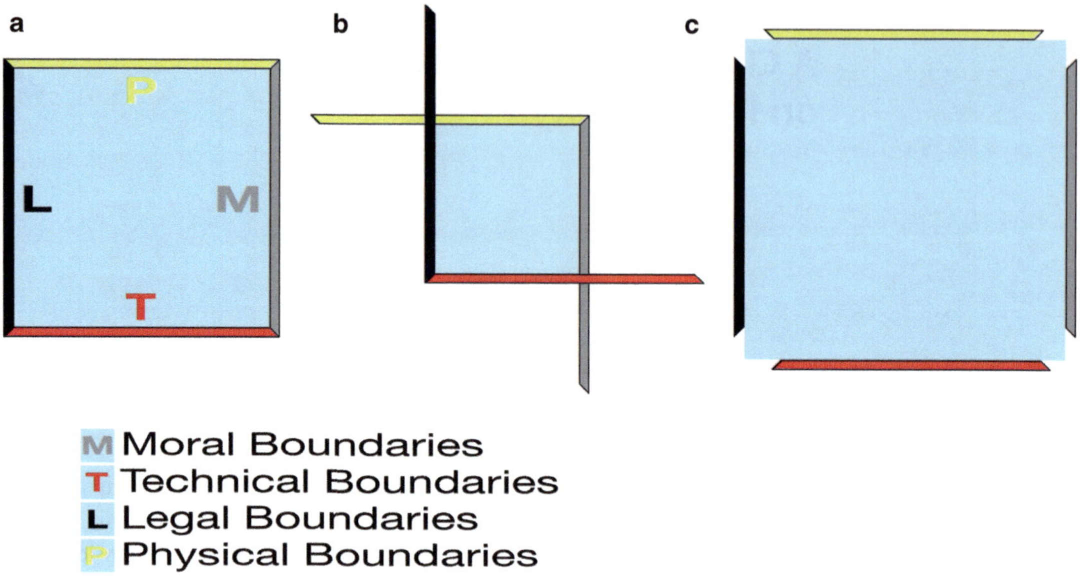

Fig. 22.1 (**a**–**c**) Boundaries (see text)

unable to offer his patients a high level of performance in human, medical, and surgical terms (**b**). These surgeons usually continue to repeat the same mistakes blaming external factors and avoiding a personal commitment to improve their performance.

- An area not perfectly delimited from which it is easy to escape simply by failing to respect the rules, leading to a high risk of causing damage to patients and to yourself (**c**). Outside the borders, there is no room for integrity and professional growth.

22.2 Prepare a Path of Self-Selection for New Patients

Out of a hundred patients who contact a surgeon for esthetic nasal problems:

- Many of them are not yet ready to start a course with the surgeon.
- Others will never be ready.
- There are some "timewasters" who request a visit for rhinoplasty knowing well in their hearts that they will never undergo rhinoplasty in their life.
- Some book a first visit but then fail to show up and we will never know anything about them.
- Still others ask for something that the surgeon cannot give them. *"I have already had a rhinoplasty to make my nose smaller but I would like it even smaller."*
- Some young males are unaware of the normal proportions of the nose. *"I don't know exactly what I want... but you are the expert.... you know very well which nose is right for me!"*
- It may happen that someone has an acceptable request but uses a bizarre way to explain it. *"I want Brad Pitt's nose!"*
- For strange reasons very few persons want an imperfect or even a deformed nose and help you in imagining it with a precise example. *"I want Silvester Stallone's nose!"*

The list goes on and on and every surgeon should have a preoperative path and rules that allow for a guided and logical Patient Self-Selection (PS-S).

The next four sections illustrate some PS-S rules for a professional practice focused on rhinoplasty.

22.3 Orient Your Professional Communication to Patient Self-Selection

The first and most important point concerns the contents of your professional website. My current home page opens with four slides for the visitors:

- You've never liked your nose? Maybe it's too big?
- Having trouble breathing through one or both nostrils?
- Did your nose suffer a trauma that may have made it look crooked?
- Have you already had surgery, but aren't satisfied with the outcome?

Just below we find:

- Fabio Meneghini, M.D.
- RHINOPLASTY.

There is no doubt about the audience to whom the site is addressed. All website contents, such as texts, images, drawings, and links, clearly refer to nose surgery. The topic of chin surgery is also inserted as an additional procedure to the main one: rhinoplasty. All visitors to the website will therefore fall into one of these two distinct categories: those interested in nose surgery, who will find every corner of the site dedicated to them, and all the others, who will exit immediately.

For consistency, in any other form of communication, such as articles, interviews, public speaking, meetings, webinars, and on the social media, I introduce myself as: Dr. Fabio Meneghini, Rhinoplasty Expert.

22.4 Orient Your First Direct Contact with a New Patient to PS-S

Before the first office visit, there are two possibilities for a new patient to communicate directly with me: by sending a message or with a telephone call. In either case, it is a perfect opportunity to continue the process of patient self-selection (PS-S).

In addition to answering questions and requests from the patient, always looking for the clearest and simplest language, I have a perfect opportunity to give them some information:

- My job as a surgeon is dedicated only to nasal surgery.
- The cost of the first consultation and what it includes.
- The closest location to make the first consultation.

Attached to the written message or immediately after the phone call, I send them my book titled "YOUR RHINOPLASTY" in PDF format to provide further written basic and structured information on nasal surgery (see also the Sect. 22.28 in this chapter).

22.5 "WHY ISN'T THE FIRST CONSULTATION FREE?" and PS-S

I am strongly opposed to the policy of offering a first surgical consultation for free. This way, I keep away the "timewasters" and probably some of those "not yet ready to start."

If a patient asks me why I do not offer a free first consultation, just for clarity and professionalism, I have a small text, shared with other colleagues, which I send as answer:

> WHY THE FIRST CONSULTATION IS NOT FREE, UNLIKE THOSE OFFERED EVER MORE FREQUENTLY BY MANY ESTHETIC SURGEONS?
>
> Because the specialist, when he carries out a first consultation with a view to operating, needs time to listen to the patient and to observe and examine them. He needs time to think and reflect.
>
> Having sufficient time allows the doctor to provide a professional consultation of high quality, including:

- gathering a complete case history (anamnesis),
- performing an in-depth examination of the patient,
- determining the appropriate plan for the treatment,
- providing a thorough explanation of the proposed operation and any possible alternatives, convalescence, outcomes, and possible complications,
- photographic illustration of the methodology and outcomes,
- prescriptions for preoperative exams and medication,
- compilation of consent forms and documentation.

Having the necessary time available allows the patient to ask useful questions in order to further their understanding and receive any clarifications they may want.

A specialist who is not constrained to earning exclusively by operating is free to provide a truly neutral and objective opinion. On the other hand, a doctor who provides the initial consultation for free and only earns if a patient decides to undergo surgery could be tempted to try and persuade the patient to have surgery without having thoroughly explained any limits and possible complications.

Medical examination requires a constant commitment to professional updating (congresses, courses, publications, etc.) which are both expensive and essential in order to offer patients the best and most up-to-date treatment.

Because the cleanliness, hygiene, and organization of a medical practice demand commitments (and related expenses) to guarantee the necessary standards of health and safety for patients.

A serious and reputable professional does not need to attract patients with free consultations.

22.6 Meet the Patient at Least Twice Before Surgery

The time spent talking to the patient is never wasted. A golden rule for PS-S is to plan at least two preoperative visits of at least 40 min each. Ideally, at least a week and no more than a month should pass between the first and second visit. If the patient sets the date of the surgery more than 3 months after the second visit, it is necessary to add a short meeting a few days before the surgery to review the treatment plan together once again.

During the consultation, I openly say to every patient:

- There is a double choice behind this surgery: the patient has the right to choose his surgeon but the surgeon must also choose his patients.
- I am always in favor of the patient contacting another colleague for a second opinion as long as he is an expert in rhinoplasty.
- The date of the surgery will be set only on the explicit request of the patient who must feel free to make an unhurried decision.
- We can only go to the operating room with a detailed, explained, shared and written treatment plan built on the preoperative CT scan and clinical facial photography. Vagueness of the treatment plan is dangerous!

After the second visit, a small percentage of patients, who are uncertain about what to do, reserve the right to decide whether or not to continue towards surgery, but we never hear from them again. I personally don't recommend calling these patients unlike other colleagues who pay a secretary for a "recall strategy." The objective of the preoperative pathway, from the new patient's first glance at the website to the end of his second visit, is to offer a precise and personalized information service and let a spontaneous PS-S process take place.

22.7 Ask Your Patient About Three Important Points

Parallel to the process of PS-S, a completely different task is that of the surgeon who must personally decide which patients are to be operated on and which are not.

Many patients answer the surgeon's doubts without any need to ask them questions. Their spontaneous narrative is clear, logical and contains all the surgeon needs to know. Sometimes this is not the case and we have to ask some direct and precise questions. Here are the three most important:

1. Is he requesting surgery driven by a personal desire or by external pressure? When two sisters or two friends ask to have a consultation together, it is very likely that one is being "dragged" into this new adventure by the other and that the surgeon must decide which of the two deserves surgery and which does not.
2. Has the patient's desire been stable and present for a long time? If the answer is no, it is advisable to postpone the surgery and fix a new consultation a few months later.

3. Has he read and understood the information in the book that I sent before or personally gave him during the first visit? Reading and understanding the information is a fundamental sign of collaboration and commitment on the patient's part that encourages the surgeon regarding the patient's personal motivation and commitment to do his best throughout the process.

22.8 Ask Yourself Three Questions

Rollin Daniel, in his books on rhinoplasty, always recalls that he spent a lot of time preoperatively deciding whether to operate or not because he has learned the hard way that "the preop course is finite, but the postop course is infinite."

The surgeon must necessarily develop a sensitivity to listening to his inner voice mostly when it advises him not to operate on that patient.

Another suggestion is to ask yourself three simple questions:

- Will a rhinoplasty make a significant improvement to this patient's nose?
- Do I think I am able to do something important to help this patient?
- Do I want this person in my practice?

If the answer is "no" to any one of these questions, it is better not to operate.

22.9 How to Maintain a Continuous Professional Relationship with Your Patient

Even after years, whatever the outcome of the surgery, every patient is ideally still your patient. As there are no other possibilities, this rule must be accepted and managed in the best possible way. To maintain your reputation at good levels over time there is nothing better than to "work" on your own patient population and:

- Continue to inform patients all about your services through newsletters, brochures, social media messages, and your website. Do not delegate the content of your communication to other people. Get help but, if you have any doubts, read three times for three consecutive days everything that will become public for a long time.
- Take care of your old patients (but also of friends and colleagues) who refer new patients repeatedly. Thank them as often as you have the opportunity. They are a valuable part of your ethical internal marketing strategies.
- Reply to every message, even to a simple Merry Christmas message.
- If a patient has asked to speak to you on the phone, call him when you can take at least a few minutes for an undisturbed, quiet talk. If you don't remember him perfectly, prepare for the telephone conversation by opening his pictures on the laptop to be sure to personalize each phrase on the person. By looking at his face your memory can recover small details, a particular situation, or an anecdote that happened even 10 years earlier. You should be in the best condition to make a new positive first impression again.
- If a patient sends you a complex message with several questions or with unusual incomprehensible requests, offer to speak on the phone or invite him to reserve a postoperative visit. The risk of misunderstanding is always just around the corner.
- As always, when talking to a patient avoid cold abrupt answers like "yes," "no," "maybe" followed by a long silence. Answer in simple words and give some examples. My communication has improved since I started comparing the nose to a house with its roof, walls, doors, and spaces.
- Never antagonize the patient. Rather, give him as much support as possible and let him know that you are by his side.

And, if the reason for contact is a postoperative problem or an unwanted outcome, always offer a free follow-up appointment.

To manage this activity dedicated to our previous patients, it is necessary to have a folder for each of them in the memory of our computer where to collect not only the material of strict medical value but also the email messages and anything else that concerns them.

22.10 Everything You Must Delegate

In many human activities, delegating some tasks is essential and often leads to wealth, widespread improvement of products or services, and reduction of work stress. Delegating some tasks to others also has the aim of increasing the time available to us to dedicate ourselves to what we do best, which either requires our own personal expertise or which the other team members are not able to carry out as well.

For those who want to engage in a clinical practice focused on rhinoplasty, one of the first objectives to be achieved is to delegate all those medical and surgical activities without a direct relation to nasal surgery.

Early in my clinical practice, I was part of a multidisciplinary surgical team of nine surgeons who were in charge of cleft lip and palate, craniofacial and dentofacial deformities, head and neck cancer, and facial trauma. We all collaborated every day with neurosurgeons, oral surgeons, ENT surgeons, ophthalmologists, orthodontists, dermatologists, physiatrists, and speech therapists. Our motto was: "Total Facial Rehabilitation." In this department, nasal surgery, almost all performed in cleft lip and palate patients, accounted for less than 5% of all procedures.

Thirty-five years later I am still fascinated by that formative and human experience but I have renounced or delegated many of these activities to other colleagues.

Choosing a path in professional life is essential and today my practice consists of about 90% rhinoplasty and 10% orthognathic surgery. It is a small professional niche that I have chosen with the aim of offering my patients a high level of human, medical, and surgical performance.

But, beyond this general logic, working in this particular professional niche I've had to create a long list of non-delegable tasks and the number of points seems to be growing continuously. You can find it in the next section.

22.11 Everything You Can't Delegate: A List

For a clinical practice focused on rhinoplasty I advise you not to delegate:

- The safety of your patient.
- The safety of your team.
- The preparation and control of the contents of your communication such as text, images, and videos.
- Collecting your patients' questions in a notebook to have a personal source of topics for creating new contents for your future communication activity.
- Answering the questions that potential new patients send by email.
- Offering a short direct telephone interview to any new patients that require it. This service can be provided on an optional basis but, if your decision is to activate a preliminary direct contact with patients, it cannot be delegated to personnel or assistants.
- Conducting the first preoperative visit.
- The shooting of a complete set of preoperative clinical facial photographs.
- Preparing the photographic material and the profile simulations for the second preoperative visit.
- Conducting the second preoperative visit.
- Personally conducting all the surgical steps.
- Writing the description of the surgical operation. It should be done as soon as possible so as not to forget any steps of the procedure.
- Conducting all the postoperative visits. Each time, don't forget to shoot a complete set of clinical facial photographs.
- Asking the patient for authorization to use his pre- and postoperative photos for scientific reasons and for communication, including on electronic media.
- Any disputes of the result obtained by patients.
- Creating and maintaining your personal surgical instruments set.
- The final evaluation of the results obtained through the study of pre- and postoperative

photographs. Do not forget that this is one of the most important steps for your professional growth.

22.12 Time and Commitment: Related Numbers

The development of a clinical practice focused on rhinoplasty also depends on some numbers.

To acquire a new surgical competence you need a lot of time (numbers) that can be divided across attending the operating room of experienced nasal surgeons (numbers), reading books (numbers), watching the surgery on recorded videos (numbers), attending live surgery at meetings and courses (numbers), exploring the anatomy and trying out surgical techniques in cadaver-lab sessions (numbers), and of course, operating on your own patients (numbers).

The last group of numbers, your rhinoplasty clinical cases per year, should be monitored during your entire professional life for quantity. If, after years of activity, less than 50 rhinoplasties are done per year, you must face the problem of lack of continuity and reduced mental and manual training. And the clinical practice cannot be focused on rhinoplasty due to its low productivity in terms of revenue.

From 50–100 clinical cases per year all the previous issues improve on condition of having rigorous patient selection rules and a schematic surgical approach, such as the BOR method, to maintain a high level of proficiency.

With over 100 clinical cases per year, the goal of having a clinical practice focused on rhinoplasty is finally achieved also from the point of view of economic sustainability, while exceeding 200 cases per year puts your professional practice at risk from the point of view of maintenance of standards and time that you personally dedicate to each individual patient.

Obtaining consistency and reliability of clinical results needs numbers!

22.13 Self-Discipline Matters

Some definitions of self-discipline are: the ability to control one's feelings and overcome one's weaknesses; the ability to pursue what one thinks is right despite temptations to abandon it. Another one is the ability to control yourself and to make yourself work hard or behave in a particular way without needing anyone else to tell you what to do.

Self-discipline concepts applied to rhinoplasty practice are wide and full of implications. It is clear that much of the clinical outcome depends on a single person, the surgeon, and that a self-discipline-oriented behavior is just what he needs.

22.14 The Rule of Changing Rules

Some rules are universal and, instead of changing them, a better idea is to defend them. But sometimes it happens that experience and research give rise to new rules or change some of the old ones.

A problem that plagues many experienced surgeons in their professional middle age is that they reject new ideas and rules. Their favorite inner phrases contain often the three "MY-MY-MY." Here's an example: "In MY hands MY technique works well in almost all of MY patients."

Fortunately, in rhinoplasty there are and there will be new ideas and new rules worthy of being known and practiced.

22.15 Read the Classics Again from Time to Time

I am not referring to Kafka, Joyce, and Tolstoy but in rhinoplasty, as in literature, we find some authors who have given the best articles and books ever.

I don't think I have to recommend a list of my favorites, certainly questionable, or a long series of names in alphabetical or temporal order. But I cannot avoid recommending to every young surgeon a very inspired and committed author, Dr. Rod Rohrich of Dallas. For years I have read and sometimes reread everything he has written on the topic of rhinoplasty. But his horizons have always been wide and everything regarding the medical, technological, economic, organizational, ethical, and moral practice that a nose surgeon must face every day has been dealt with by Dr. Rohrich in his many articles.

I recently reread a short article from 2001 where, at the end of the text, he gave 20 tips on how to do marketing while remaining a doctor in the eyes of his patients, his staff, and colleagues. Here they are:

- Create a focused mission statement for your practice.
- Become a patient in your own office. Make your practice user-friendly.
- Empower your office staff as your representatives. There should be no weak link in your chain of excellent patient care.
- Do not underestimate the word-of-mouth power of your patients.
- Let patients know all about your services through newsletters, brochures, and your website.
- Become involved locally and speak to community, hospital, and auxiliary service organizations.
- Take care of your practice champions (patients who refer patients repeatedly). Make them a part of your internal marketing strategies.
- Exceed patients' expectations and experiences with their initial consult and preoperative and postoperative care.
- High tech still means high touch. Establish a useful and helpful personal website with links to your local, state, regional, and national societies Internet addresses.
- Greet your patients with a handshake, and sit down during your patient consultation.
- Survey your patients periodically about your practice.
- Develop effective communication skills to improve your ability to listen to your patients.
- Provide your patients with visual and educational materials before their initial visit.
- Manage your schedule so that you are on time. Avoid delays, and entertain patients while they wait. If you are late, notify your patients so that they can make an informed decision to wait or to reschedule.
- Use your own or your societies' brochures or newsletters to communicate your areas of expertise.
- Become a cost-effective practice in a managed-care environment.
- Pick one objective that allows you to measure and track your results.
- Work cooperatively with a motivated and talented staff. Reward them for their merit and loyalty to you, your patients, and your practice.
- Develop and maintain a positive image of your practice regionally and nationally.
- Enjoy yourself, and instill humor in your practice. Like your life, your practice is not a dress rehearsal.

22.16 Essential Equipment: Part I

For those who start their practice as a rhinoplasty surgeon, purchases are very important and it is right to first choose the essential tools, also thinking about saving. For simplicity, we can divide the equipment into two main categories:

- Tools for patient documentation and data storage.
- Surgical instruments indispensable for nasal surgery (see next sections).

If you do not have a dedicated fixed office or if you work in different locations, one of the first needs is to have an ultralight and portable system. For convenience it must be transportable within a small backpack. Today the total weight of a high-end camera with zoom lenses and small built-in flash, ultimate technology slim laptop with a 13.3″ display, and a 3 terabyte portable hard-disk is less than 1.650 kg. The quality of the photographic documentation obtainable is good and comparable with that obtained from fixed professional systems as it depends more on the experience and ability of the professional than on the weight and cost of the instruments.

Another technological advancement is the possibility to connect a smartphone to a short and thin endoscope with a built-in LED light source. With this portable and light system it is possible to capture and store preoperative and postoperative endonasal still images and video. The total weight is 450 grams including the smartphone.

What does this all mean? I think that a rigorous, standardized and high-quality patient documentation is within everyone's reach. The availability of instruments is wide and affordable and the results depend only on the surgeon's self-discipline.

Some final technical advice on this topic is:

- The computer screen must not be less than 13 inches to allow at least two people, usually the surgeon and the patient, to see every detail of the portraits, profile simulations, and CT scan images.
- The system must run Adobe Photoshop or a similar software application for image editing and photo retouching and DICOM Viewer software to load, view, and store CT scan images.
- The camera must have an adjustable zoom on a medium telephoto lens that allows framing of the patients' faces while maintaining a distance of at least 1.20 m from the subject.
- Even years after the first visit and surgical treatment, it must always be possible to recover quickly all the patient's documents.

22.17 Essential Equipment: Part II

I firmly believe that it is not right to buy the complete surgical kit proposed by Dr. T. or by Dr. G. with the risk of spending a large amount of money and only to utilize part of it. Surgical instruments are like fingerprints: everyone has their own.

Some instruments, specifically dedicated to rhinoplasty and designed by the fathers of this discipline, have been surpassed by others designed for other fields of surgery. Joseph's nasal dorsum elevator is outdated, aggressive, and should be discarded from any catalog and its use discouraged. Instead, the elevator proposed by Obwegeser for maxillofacial surgery, thanks to its thin and curved drop-shaped end without edges, is a perfect instrument to elevate the periosteum from the nasal bones, the radix, and the frontal process of the maxilla. Unfortunately, it rarely if ever appears in the sections "Instruments for Nasal Surgery."

Another example: for handling cartilages during rhinoplasty the most utilized instrument is the Adson-Brown forceps. Each end has two rows of seven teeth that fit exactly to the corresponding rows of the other end when tightening the forceps (Fig. 22.2a). Many authors suggest morselizing the cartilage with the Adson-Brown ends to obtain a softer and more pliable tissue by breaking its inner structure. But obtaining this effect is rarely necessary. Again, the Adson-Brown forceps are small and straight and difficult to handle when working in-depth and in confined surgical fields (Fig. 22.2b). It can happen that the operator's or assistant's hands obscure the view using the Adson-Brown. For all these reasons, I have included a couple of curved DeBakey dissecting forceps into my nasal surgical set. They permit gentle handling of the cartilage with almost no risk of damaging it and they maintain the hands further away from the surgical field. The rounded margin of the forceps ends as well as the less aggressive surfaces that come into contact with the tissues, designed for more fragile tissues such as blood vessels, are definitely elements of improvement when compared with the Adson-Brown forceps. A curved DeBakey dissecting forceps is also invaluable to work in the depth of the surgical field and inside the nasal septum or nasal cavities. Once again, an indispensable tool for me was found looking beyond the products designed and produced for nasal surgery.

Today, after years of experience, I would not feel comfortable without my set of surgical instruments because I would not be sure of the sharpening of the chisels. Without my surgical instruments in certain moments of surgery I would have to stop and think about how to move

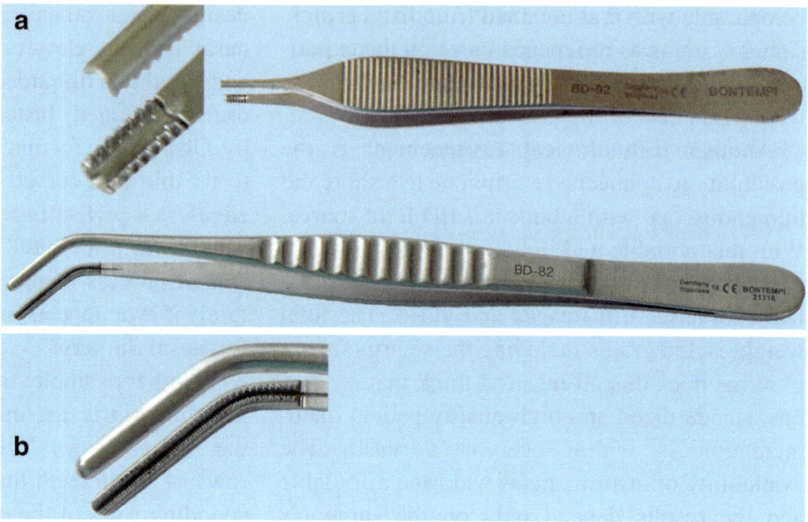

Fig. 22.2 (**a**, **b**) Adson-Brown forceps (**a**) and curved DeBakey dissecting forceps (**b**)

my hands, I would probably be slower than usual and, in the end, more tired.

Professional growth is also linked in some way to continuous improvement and knowledge of working tools.

22.18 Essential Equipment: Part III

If a surgical instrument has some defects, for example it is too expensive or too fragile, too aggressive with the tissues, or simply weighs too much, you can try to find an alternative in the market.

Sometimes, however, it is better to design and test a whole new one.

In my personal set, I have four different instruments that I have conceived myself for rhinoplasty. It took years of attempts, creating prototypes, rough at first and then increasingly precise and refined, and so more suitable for the purpose.

Early in my practice as a surgeon I had the great privilege of meeting an elderly craftsman, Mr. Bruno Galiazzo. I fondly remember his invaluable help and the hours spent in his mechanical laboratory for the creation of new instrument prototypes. Subsequently, after his death, I still continue to collaborate with his successor, Mr. Gabriele.

Now the four definitive instruments are also available for my colleagues. Of course, I have not asked the manufacturer for any royalties to keep the final price of the instruments as low as possible.

22.19 Become Passionate about Portrait Photography

A suggestion more than a rule: in the early years of your nasal surgery practice, never miss an exhibition of portrait photography and fill your library with Man Ray's and other portrait books. The faces fixed in the photos of the great photographers are a very rich source for studying every detail, the proportions and the smallest deformities of the face and in particular of the nose as well as the most pleasant way to devote ourselves to our work during our free time.

22.20 The Most Conservative Option Is Often the Best Choice

The BOR procedure makes the conservation of bone and cartilage structures a major goal. The surgeon who convinced me more than anyone else of the importance of this principle, as it applies to rhinoplasty, is John B. Tebbetts. Another principle directly connected to the previous one envisages that every surgical action is performed with small increments and that it is preferably reversible during the operation. Only when the removal of a tissue fragment is considered inevitable to obtain the desired result, is it carried out.

22.21 The More Conservative Option Should Not Be Confused with the Simpler One

There is no room for simplification in rhinoplasty surgery. Here's an example. The suture of the upper lateral cartilages to the septum is more stable if at least three stitches are placed. Sometimes during surgery, after performing osteotomies, it appears that the upper lateral cartilage rests perfectly along the dorsal margin of the septal cartilage. What a perfect opportunity not to suture the cartilages to each other! Unfortunately, simplification—in this case the reduction of the surgical time by two maybe 3 min by omitting the sutures—poses a serious, increased risk of late dorsal deformities such as asymmetries or inverted-V deformity and can lead to nasal valve collapse.

22.22 A Reconstructive Approach

The nasal framework must be completely stabilized with sutures at the end of rhinoplasty. Also the nasal bones, after osteotomies and mobilization, can be safely sutured to the dorsal septal margin. To make small holes on the nasal bones for sutures we have at least three safe and simple possibilities, ultrasonic, electric drill and manual drill perforation … and no excuse for not using them.

22.23 Two Honesty Tips

Honesty tips are infinite.

A precious one is to take care to avoid raising false expectations in your patient, which means avoiding failures, which means avoiding litigation.

Another tip is never to deny the evidence. If complications or visible deformities appear in the postoperative period, do not negate the evidence or underestimate the problem with your patient.

22.24 Be Less Responsive and More Understanding with Your Patients

In the relationship with your patients but also with your collaborators, a reactive attitude is full of stress. We feel pressurized and put pressure on those around us. One of the main problems of this behavior is that of making hasty decisions concerning patients, collaborators as well as ourselves.

A sympathetic reaction instead means a relaxed mood. We have clear ideas. Sometimes it's just a matter of waiting a minute for a better idea to come. We are at our best and we help others to be.

This behavioral rule applies both to talking with the patient, from whom you need all the collaboration he can give, but also to the operating room during the surgery, when you need all the collaboration of your colleagues and staff.

22.25 Mentorship

As a young surgeon you can do many things except reflecting on your past experiences as a key to understanding. The solution exists and must be addressed as soon as possible: find a mentor. My advice is not to limit your request for mentorship over time, in an educational institution, in a geographical area, or based on a mentor's age.

Personally, I have had many mentors who have helped me enormously in many fields of surgery. Even today I know that I can count on many of them. Mentor and apprentices are not two rigid and regulated categories. The relationship between them is free and changeable. Many times it materializes when drinking coffee around a table, or sending a message with a few questions, or with a phone call when both have some free time. Each mentor has his own way and time to make himself available to the young person. If you're in the operating room with him, I've found that a perfect time to talk to the mentor is at the end of his surgery, when he is taking off his gloves and protective mask.

The advantages of mentorship for a young surgeon are obvious: trust, solidarity, ideas, guiding principles, tips, and advice. A map to follow faithfully.

For the mentor there is the joy of helping, of feeling esteemed and necessary. There is the pleasure of teaching, the privilege of reviewing with others his work experiences, and the idea of passing the baton.

Remember that the mentor is someone who likes to share their ideas and experiences with others. It is not necessary to formalize one's situation and define an agreement. Mentoring almost always includes some characteristics typical of friendship and interpersonal esteem.

Often the best rewards for your mentor is to promise him that when you are able to, you will also do the same for someone else.

22.26 How to Join a Private Practice Facility

A surgeon who focuses his practice on nasal surgery is uncommon in the field of medical and surgical centers dedicated to esthetics. For such a surgeon, the opportunities are not lacking. So to start a private practice, I advise you to look for a multidisciplinary team of colleagues where nobody deals with nasal surgery. In this way you will enrich the team and avoid conflicts of interest.

22.27 Add Highly Professional Specialists to Your Extended Team

A strategy closely related to decreasing concerns and increasing success is certainly this: hire professionals above you, more qualified, somehow better than you. This is essential to your success.

22.28 The Power of a Gift

As you already know, since May 2014 I've given a personal gift, a small book, to each new patient.

Even a small gift like this has its functions. I use it to let people know what the surgeon thinks about rhinoplasty. Explain what are the achievable goals and the difficulties to overcome. And writing it in a book is better than saying it.

Only you can make known how much passion and commitment you dedicate to rhinoplasty. And writing it is better than saying it.

In a book you can also describe the characteristics of a good patient, who can have important advantages from nasal surgery. And writing it in a book is better than saying it.

But above all, a gift is a gift, a kind way to start, to welcome a person.

Don't underestimate the power of a gift.

22.29 Collect Your Patients' Questions and Write Your Unique Book

How did I write the book "Your Rhinoplasty?" And how can you accomplish something like that?

To begin with, you must always have a notebook with you where you can write and collect the questions that every patient asks you, even the strange ones. In a few years, you will have the perfect material to write a 100 small chapters, each of which contains a thoughtful and correct answer to the 100 most frequently asked questions.

With this method, when you write for your patients, you will be guided not only by what you can learn from more experienced colleagues but also by your unique and unrepeatable experiences. When you write you can't forget how interesting and rich your professional life is.

The 100 chapters will then be divided into groups. A good idea is to start with "YOUR NOSE AND HOW IT WORKS" and finish with "WHAT TO DO AFTER YOUR OPERATION."

The next step is to collaborate with a writing expert who knows nothing about rhinoplasty or noses. Your goal is to produce a simple text for ordinary people and not for professionals.

And finally you have to find a publisher who believes in your project.

But remember, it all starts with a notebook.

22.30 Become Aware of the Passion Factor

As you approach rhinoplasty, the key question that, sooner or later, you must answer is "*Do I want to dedicate myself to this activity because I really love it?*". If you have read this book only once, it is not yet time to ask yourself this question. First you still have to enter the operating room 10, or better 50, times to see a nasal surgeon at work and read again this and other books.

If you have already graduated in medicine there are miles of different employment possibilities, all equally beautiful, difficult, and interesting as rhinoplasty. It is difficult to find another field among human activities as vast as medicine.

22.31 One Day in Philadelphia

Dear colleague, you still have a few lines to read. I thought long and hard about how a book on rhinoplasty should end and finally decided to tell a little story.

***

If I remember correctly it was November 2000. I was at "The Penn Rhinoplasty Course," a very important international rhinoplasty course, organized in Philadelphia for a small group of young surgeons. It was afternoon and the cadaver-lab was one of the most important practical lessons of the entire course.

One of the exercises I had to do in front of the instructors was to perform lateral osteotomies of the nasal bones with a guarded two-millimeter osteotome. The first step was a small stab incision on the left vestibular nasal mucosa just over the piriform aperture margin, followed by a limited subperiosteal elevation over the frontal process of the maxilla. The next and most demanding step was producing a regular low-to-high osteotomy line. Holding firmly the nose of the specimen's head with the index and thumb fingers of my non-dominant hand, I then precisely positioned the guarded osteotome against the left margin of the piriform aperture.

The angulation of the instrument was checked and approved by the two instructors: the course director and a famous professor from Chicago. Their eyes quietly confirmed to me that the osteotomy could begin. Even though I had done nasal osteotomies many times, I was enthused by the idea that, for once, I could do it guided by two such important and recognized colleagues.

I said "taptap" and the Philadelphia professor gave two hammer strokes on the osteotome. The osteotome, as usual, was then rotated in a more parallel direction to the nasofacial junction and I said "taptap" several times and the instructor gave several series of paired hammer strokes until the osteotomy was done. At the end of the procedure, the two professors and I were absolutely satisfied of the result obtained. "Very well," said one of them.

Finally, we made an inspection that can only be performed in the cadaver-lab. After having incised the skin of the nasal back at full thickness, we elevated the flap to directly check the lateral osteotomy. The disappointment we all felt was great: the nasal wall that we thought was intact was fragmented into three small pieces of bone!

This little story has a lot to do with the practice of rhinoplasty, a surgery that is not totally under the surgeon's control and that often reserves unexpected events even when it is done in the best conditions. The only defense against the thousand variables, we said in Philadelphia, is to work with passion, perseverance, light and precise hands, using the right instruments, applying sound surgical principles, and maintaining humility. A difficult task.

Further Reading

Books

Meneghini F. Your rhinoplasty—all you need to know about nasal surgery. Faenza: Tempo al Libro; 2019.

McCollough EG. The elite facial surgery practice. New York: Thieme; 2018.

Williams E. The white coat entrepreneur. Charleston: Advantage; 2020.

Williams E. Rhinoplasty. North Charlestone: CreateSpace Independent Publishing Platform; 2013.

Articles

Rohrich RJ. Streamlining cosmetic surgery patient selection—just say no! Plast Reconstr Surg. 1999;104(1):220–1.

Rohrich RJ. The market of plastic surgery: cosmetic surgery for sale—at what price? Plast Reconstr Surg. 2001;107(7):1845–7.

Rohrich RJ. Mentors in medicine. Plast Reconstr Surg. 2003;112(4):1087–8.

GPSR Compliance

The European Union's (EU) General Product Safety Regulation (GPSR) is a set of rules that requires consumer products to be safe and our obligations to ensure this.

If you have any concerns about our products, you can contact us on ProductSafety@springernature.com

In case Publisher is established outside the EU, the EU authorized representative is:

Springer Nature Customer Service Center GmbH
Europaplatz 3
69115 Heidelberg, Germany

Batch number: 10731407

Printed by Printforce, the Netherlands